EDITORS
Sergio Candiotto Pietro Ruggieri

MINIMALLY INVASIVE HIP ARTHROPLASTY

Surgical approaches and procedures

MINIMALLY INVASIVE HIP ARTHROPLASTY
Surgical approaches and procedures

ISBN 978-88-97162-99-5

Publishing coordination: Giuseppe Roccucci
English translation: Giulio Edoardo Vigni
Editing: Rachele Villa
Design and layout: Massimo D'Onofrio
Illustrations: Massimiliano Crespi - info@max-medicalillustrator.com

Printing: Starprint srl
First edition: May 2023

PUBLISHER
Griffin srl unipersonale
Via Don Luigi Meroni 58 - 22060 Figino Serenza (Como) - Italy
Tel. + 39 031.789085
customerservice@griffineditore.it
www.griffineditore.it

Preface

The profound cultural changes, the favourable results obtained with minimally invasive techniques in other surgical branches and the promising contributions from new technologies also force orthopaedic surgery to adapt. It therefore leads to the implementation of those technical and procedural changes capable of making the surgery more tissue-friendly and the clinical outcome more favourable and stable over time.

Reduced surgical aggressiveness, shorter surgical times, less tissue damage, less blood loss, less post-operative pain (with an easier pharmacological control), shorter hospital stays, earlier functional recovery and quicker acquisition of the final result represent the fundamental aspects of minimally invasive surgical techniques.

However, there are also aspects more pertinent to surgical pathophysiology in the use of minimally invasive techniques with reduced tissue damage. These include reduced endocrine imbalances (cortisol, catecholamines, etc.) and reduced release of pro-inflammatory chemotactic substances (interleukins, prostaglandins, etc.), muscle cytolytic enzymes and thromboplastin-like factors. It is now well established that reducing this unfavourable 'immunohistochemical network' can only benefit the post-operative metabolic balance and functional recovery, especially considering the lower risks and greater patient satisfaction.

In our discipline, there are now numerous areas of application of minimally invasive techniques. For example, arthroscopic procedures are becoming more and more widespread and versatile, as are the innovative solutions introduced in traumatology, such as the MIPO techniques in certain complex tibial fractures.

Prosthetic hip surgery is a field that is showing remarkable clinical results with the minimally invasive technique, as it can also rely on other promising aspects such as the possibility of adapting this innovative method to special conditions (elderly people, compromised clinical conditions) that make it preferable to traditional techniques.

Moving increasingly towards minimally invasive surgery has been a great effort given the increased complexity and difficulty of these surgical acts. The learning curve can be long and difficult, representing for many an obstacle in daily practice. Sometimes there have also been disappointments, due to some inevitable failures in the learning and development phases of these techniques.

However, the difficulties, problems, complications and mistakes that are possible with these innovative techniques have always constituted for us reasons for deep critical examination, confidence and the will to improve. Our casuistry is now extensive and well-established. In our practice, good results clearly prevail and at the same time there are fewer complications and tissue damage compared to traditional techniques, which are still widely performed.

Minimally invasive surgery, in our as in other surgical branches, is a 'philosophy', an irreversible and now indispensable choice. This is something we deeply believe in because of its credibility and reliability, which is destined to be refined and spread to many other surgical fields.

Sergio Candiotto **Pietro Ruggieri**

Authors

Editors

Sergio Candiotto
Hip and Shoulder Surgery Unit, Abano Terme General Hospital, Padua, Italy

Pietro Ruggieri
Department of Orthopaedics and Orthopaedic Oncology, University of Padova, Italy

Stefano Basso
Orthopaedics and Traumatology Unit, San Candido Hospital, Bolzano, Italy

Alessandro Berni
Department of Orthopaedics and Traumatology, Modena University Hospital, University of Modena and Reggio-Emilia, Italy

Enrico Bertugli
Department of Orthopaedics and Traumatology, Modena University Hospital, University of Modena and Reggio-Emilia, Italy

Luca Bianchi
Department of Orthopaedics and Traumatology, Modena University Hospital, University of Modena and Reggio-Emilia, Italy

Antonio Camporese
Hip and Shoulder Surgery Unit, Abano Terme General Hospital, Padua, Italy

Serafino Carta
Department of Orthopaedics and Traumatology, Siena University Hospital, Italy

Fabio Catani
Department of Orthopaedics and Traumatology, Modena University Hospital, University of Modena and Reggio-Emilia, Italy

Matteo Cengarle
Hip and Shoulder Surgery Unit, Abano Terme General Hospital, Padua, Italy

Maria Chiara Cerchiaro
Department of Orthopaedics and Orthopaedic Oncology, University of Padova, Italy

Stefano Concheri
Department of Orthopaedics and Traumatology, S. Antonio Hospital, Padua, Italy

Lucia Coppola
Rehabilitation and Functional Recovery Department, S. Antonio Hospital, Padua, Italy

Daniele Coraci
Department of Neuroscience, Section of Rehabilitation, University of Padova, Italy

Vittore Costa
Hip and Prosthetic Surgery Unit, Humanitas Gavazzeni Hospital, Bergamo, Italy

Elia Creta
Scientific Institute Auxologico Capitanio Hospital, Milan, Italy

Raffaele De Caro
Institute of Normal Anatomy, University of Padova, Italy

Agostino De Felice
Scientific Institute Auxologico Capitanio Hospital, Milan, Italy

Florian Fischer
Scientific Institute Auxologico Capitanio Hospital, Milan, Italy

Mattia Fortina
Department of Orthopaedics and Traumatology, Siena University Hospital, Italy

Andrea Fossali
Scientific Institute Auxologico Capitanio Hospital, Milan, Italy

Alessandro Geraci
Department of Orthopaedics and Traumatology, San Valentino of Montebelluna Hospital, Treviso, ULSS 2 Marca Trevigiana/Veneto, Italy

Alessandro Giovannini
Rehabilitation and Functional Recovery Department, S. Antonio Hospital, Padua, Italy

Giovanni Francesco Grano
Department of Orthopaedics and Traumatology, Bassano del Grappa Hospital, Vicenza, ULSS 7 Pedemontana/Veneto, Italy

Guido Grappiolo
Hip Diseases and Replacement Surgery Unit, Humanitas Clinical and Research Center - IRCCS, Rozzano, Milan, Italy; Livio Sciutto Foundation Biomedical Research in Orthopaedics Onlus, Campus Savona, Italy

Salvatore Gravinese
Hip and Shoulder Surgery Unit, Abano Terme General Hospital, Padua, Italy

Francesco La Camera
Hip Diseases and Replacement Surgery Unit, Humanitas Clinical and Research Center - IRCCS, Rozzano, Milan, Italy; Livio Sciutto Foundation Biomedical Research in Orthopaedics Onlus, Campus Savona, Italy

Frédéric Laude
Clinique du Sport, Paris, France

Andrea Marcovigi
Department of Orthopaedics and Traumatology, Modena University Hospital, University of Modena and Reggio-Emilia, Italy

Stefano Masiero
Department of Neuroscience, Section of Rehabilitation, University of Padova, Italy

Francesco Melan
Operative Unit of Orthopaedics and Traumatology, Hospital of Adria, Rovigo, ULSS 5 Polesana/Veneto, Italy

Giuseppe Necci
Rehabilitation and Functional Recovery Department, S. Antonio Hospital, Padua, Italy

Nelson Ojeda
Hip and Shoulder Surgery Unit, Abano Terme General Hospital, Padua, Italy

Elisa Pala
Department of Orthopaedics and Orthopaedic Oncology, University of Padova, Italy

Maria Pavlidou
Department of Orthopaedics and Traumatology, Bassano del Grappa Hospital, Vicenza, ULSS 7 Pedemontana/Veneto, Italy

Vanni Benito Petrachi
Scientific Institute Auxologico Capitanio Hospital, Milan, Italy

Silvia Pierantoni
Hip and Shoulder Surgery Unit, Abano Terme General Hospital, Padua, Italy

Dario Pizzuti
Rehabilitation and Functional Recovery Department, Movement analysis laboratory, Abano Terme General Hospital, Padua, Italy

Alberto Procura
Hip and Shoulder Surgery Unit, Abano Terme General Hospital, Padua, Italy

Alberto Ricciardi
Department of Orthopaedics and Traumatology, Venice Hospital, ULSS 3 Serenissima/Veneto, Italy

Beatrice Ricciardi
Department of Orthopaedics and Traumatology, Venice Hospital, ULSS 3 Serenissima/Veneto, Italy

Alberto Rigato
Rehabilitation and Functional Recovery Department, Movement analysis laboratory, Abano Terme General Hospital, Padua, Italy

Alberto Rigon
Rehabilitation and Functional Recovery Department, Movement analysis laboratory, Abano Terme General Hospital, Padua, Italy

Riccardo Ruggeri
Hip Diseases and Replacement Surgery Unit, Humanitas Clinical and Research Center - IRCCS, Rozzano, Milan, Italy; Livio Sciutto Foundation Biomedical Research in Orthopaedics Onlus, Campus Savona, Italy

Filippo Selleri
Department of Orthopaedics and Traumatology, Modena University Hospital, University of Modena and Reggio-Emilia, Italy

Carla Stecco
Institute of Normal Anatomy, University of Padova, Italy

Jacopo Tagliapietra
Hip and Shoulder Surgery Unit, Abano Terme General Hospital, Padua, Italy

Lucrezia Tognolo
Department of Neuroscience, Section of Rehabilitation, University of Padova, Italy

Giulio Edoardo Vigni
Department of Orthopaedics and Traumatology, University of Palermo, Italy

Renato Villaminar
Rehabilitation and Functional Recovery Department, Movement analysis laboratory, Abano Terme General Hospital, Padua, Italy

Marco Zamperetti
Hip and Shoulder Surgery Unit, Abano Terme General Hospital, Padua, Italy

Contents

General considerations on minimally invasive surgery. 'The stress response to surgery'

Sergio Candiotto*, Vittore Costa**, Antonio Camporese*, Stefano Concheri***, Salvatore Gravinese*, Giulio Edoardo Vigni****, Alberto Procura*

*Hip and Shoulder Surgery Unit, Abano Terme General Hospital, Padua, Italy
**Hip and Prosthetic Surgery Unit, Humanitas Gavazzeni Hospital, Bergamo, Italy
***Department of Orthopaedics and Traumatology, S. Antonio Hospital, Padua, Italy
****Department of Orthopaedics and Traumatology, University of Palermo, Italy

Introduction

The aim of minimally invasive surgery is above all to reduce Surgery Stress and to favourably influence the Stress Response to Surgery, a constant and ambivalent reactive phenomenon in its clinical effects.
In general surgery and in the various specialist branches into which it has been divided over time, there has always been a strong interest in reducing aggressiveness and tissue damage for the best clinical results and the fewest possible complications.
Initially, in minimally invasive techniques, the length of the surgical incision, the extent of muscle damage and the duration of the procedure were of exclusive importance. Later, however, scientific studies also emphasised other favourable aspects of a general nature (histochemical, immunological, endocrinological, neurological, cardio-respiratory, etc.).
The limitations, which nevertheless presented themselves, derived from the objective steepness of the learning curve of minimally invasive techniques, with associated problems and complications. These steps required a strong cultural change, the availability of complex technologies and sometimes the use of artificial intelligence (PCs and robots).
In abdominal surgery, where the push for mini-invasiveness has prevailed until now, access to the peritoneal cavity has become possible even through natural orifices (oral, rectal, vaginal or bladder - 'NOTES surgery' / natural orifice translumenal endoscopy surgery), or by using the umbilical scar ('NOTUS surgery' / natural orifice translumenal umbelical surgery) to perform certain procedures, such as cholecystectomy, nephrectomy, appendectomy, etc. [50].
The 'scarless surgery', which represents the reasoned extreme of this minimally invasive trend, has always fascinated surgeons because of the possibility of performing the procedure without visible skin scars and reducing tissue damage.
The development of tissue sparing surgery (TSS) has laid the foundations and technical principles that are indispensable in modern surgical branches. Orthopaedic surgery has been no exception to this. Numerous surgeons have in fact progressively modified procedures using minimally invasive techniques in the various areas of modern orthopaedic and trauma surgery (arthroscopy, MIPO in certain fractures, nailing in long bones, hip prostheses, etc.).
In hip surgery in particular, 'reduced' variants of traditional approaches (anterior, anterolateral, lateral and posterior) have been developed. Numerous acronyms have been introduced: MIS Minimally Invasive Surgery,

MAS Muscle Sparing Approach, LIS Less Invasive Surgery, MIS Mini-Incision Surgery, RIS Reduced Invasive Surgery and RTTS Reduced Tissue Trauma surgery.

We prefer the latter definition (RTTS), proposed by C.S. Ranawat [53], because it identifies the essentiality of minimally invasive surgery. This is that of limiting damage to the tissues involved, particularly the muscular tissue. However, it is important to define the real advantages of minimally invasive surgery, which are far from being theoretical, as shown by clinical experience and scientific research. We must mainly remember the clinical-organisational criteria, the properly clinical criteria and, finally, those inherent to surgical pathophysiology. It is above all the latter that have made the greatest contribution to the minimally invasive choice, because they thoroughly explain the body's behaviour in response to the surgical act ('stress response to surgery').

Clinical-organisational criteria. Prosthetic hip surgery with the minimally invasive technique includes a shorter operation time, shorter hospital stay, faster rehabilitation phase, reduction of the 'convalescence' phase as a faster functional recovery and an earlier return to the patient's own functional standard. It is also possible to treat more 'complex' patients (age, comorbidities, etc.), who would have clinical conditions that would preclude their suitability for surgery with traditional surgical techniques.

These parameters also play an important role in defining care costs. This is an issue that also has obvious repercussions on health policies, which must be reconciled with the increasingly difficult balances of economic policy.

Clinical criteria. Minimally invasive hip replacement surgery is characterised by the following: a shorter surgical skin incision, less blood loss, reduced need for blood transfusions, less muscle damage, less intensity and easier post-operative pain control, less need for analgesic drugs, fewer complications (instability, infections, heterotopic ossifications, fractures), a rarer and milder impairment of cognitive status in the elderly, a lower incidence of gastro-intestinal problems and a faster transition to the post-surgical phase. Such advantageous conditions are of particular interest to the patient, who 'suffers less and recovers faster', and to the in-patient ward for easier care management.

Great importance is attributed to 'post-operative recovery', defined as 'the process of regaining control over physical, psychological, social and habitual functions and returning to pre-operative levels of independence and psychological state' [3].

The criteria for defining recovery are now centred on the patient (absence of symptoms, ability to carry out regular activities, recovery of work and quality of life) and no longer on purely managerial criteria (length of hospital stay, material costs, etc.) [46].

The reasons for a 'difficult and delayed recovery' are fatigue, residual pain and functional impairment. These are closely related to the extent and duration of surgical stress [10,29]. Fatigue is a core element of the disease, described as 'an indefinable weakness throughout the body that requires sitting or lying down after minor tasks' [24,28,58,78].

Improving the patient's pre-surgical phase, by defining a preparatory pathway that integrates with advantages of the minimally invasive surgical technique, favours a faster and simplified recovery, with a lower incidence of 'fatigue syndrome' symptoms.

Henrick Kehlet's multimodal approach to surgery, which is fundamental in this field, implies knowledge of the 'patient-specific factors' capable of influencing functional recovery, qualifying the surgical risk, obtaining the 'predicted recovery profile' and studying the pathophysiological processes underlying the surgical act and the body's reaction [40,41,42,60,61,76].

Surgical pathophysiology. It is essential to know the clinical features of surgical stress ('stress trauma surgery') and the body's response to surgical trauma ('stress response to surgery') [22,23]. Every surgical trauma produces significant cellular and tissue damage, particularly to muscle, skin and blood. Damage can occur by direct mechanism, through surgical approach, incision, dissection and tissue excision, tension produced by retractors, ligation of vessels and mobilisation of anatomical structures. Indirectly, on the other hand, surgical trauma acts through blood loss, haematoma formation, altered tissue perfusion, changes in microcirculation and through the indirect effects of anaesthetic procedures [26,61,68].

The muscle prevails, particularly in hip surgery, as the vulnerable tissue in terms of quantity. It acts mainly as a 'biological' substrate, for the local and general immune-endocrine-metabolic changes that its injury may induce (fig. 3).

The rich presence of nociceptors in the dermis and hypodermis also makes the skin an important algogenic target of surgical aggression, both due to direct damage to the nociceptors themselves (incision, dissection, excision, tension produced by retractors, ischaemia, haematoma, etc.), and due to the prolonged stimulation of them by chemical mediators in the post-operative inflammatory phase.

Reducing intra-operative bleeding, due to the shorter surgical time and the shorter extension of the incision/tissue dissection, and limiting haematoma formation in the surgical 'dead spaces', are also fundamental aspects to counteract the harmful effects of blood dispersion and its degradation factors.

Therefore, it is obvious that any surgical procedure must seek to reduce stress trauma surgery and favourably influence the stress response to surgery, reducing or counteracting its potentially negative effects.

The stress response to surgery has many points in common with the trauma response to traumatic injuries in general. The surgical act (surgery trauma stress), which is at its basis, in fact repeats all the steps of the general traumatic event (trauma stress) and induces a response to the surgical trauma through a series of endocrinological, immunological, histochemical and haematological changes (tab. 1) [6,14,16,26,34,37,43,48,52,75].

The current concept of trauma response basically follows the original scheme of DP Cuthbertson (1932) [22,23], who identified the general response of the organism to trauma in the metabolic ebb and flow phases. This is characterised by a brief initial decrease and a subsequent protracted increase of the metabolic activity.

Any modification of cellular activity and tissue response to trauma exploits the mechanism of 'intercellular signalling'. In fact, all substances included in the trauma response to surgery (hormones, immune response, cytokines, prostaglandins, complement fractions, glutamine, metal ions, proteins, lipids, carbohydrates) act as 'communicators' of cellular or tissue activation or depression. These have local and general effects depending on the extent of the surgical trauma and the quantitative changes in these cellular mediators [6,28,69].

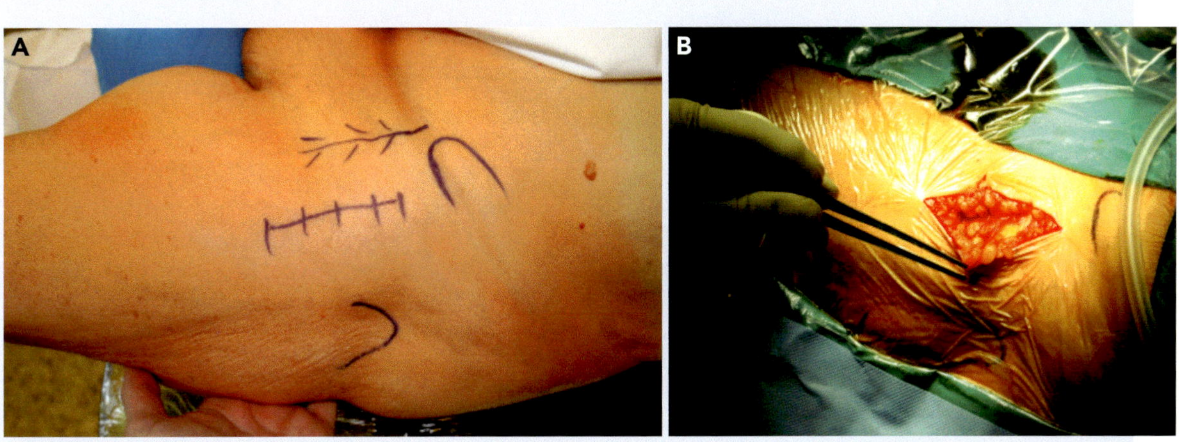

Figure 1 The anterior minimally invasive technique. A) The site and the reduced extent of the skin incision. B) The exposure of the fascial plane

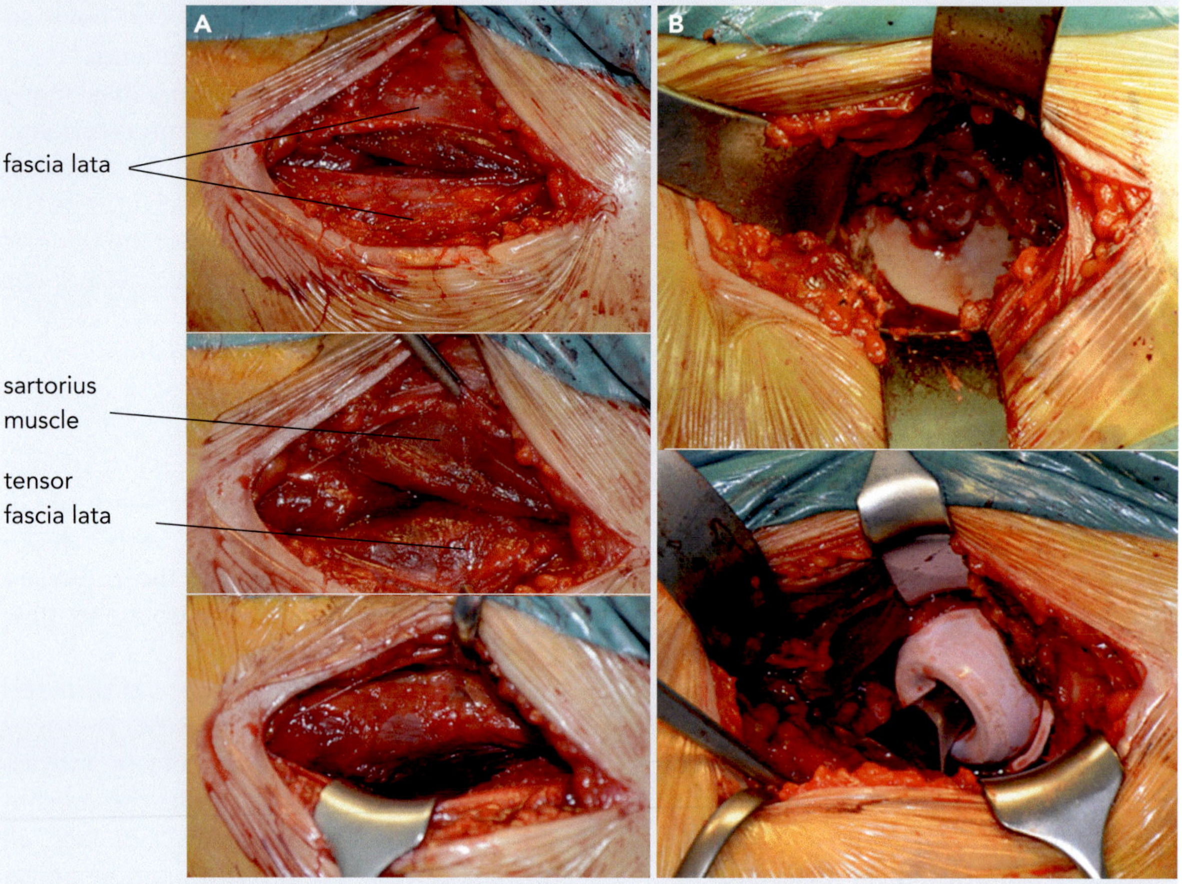

Figure 2 Intraoperative photos of the anterior minimally invasive surgical approach. A) The intermuscular deepening after the fascial incision. B) The exposure of the acetabulum and the prosthetic implant. Using this technique the respect of the soft tissues, in particular the muscular tissue, is extreme

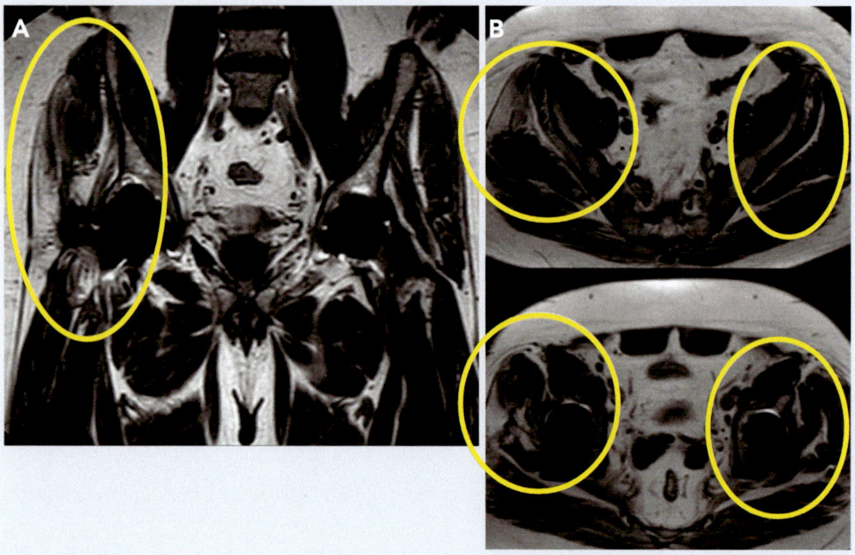

Figure 3 MRI evaluation. The changes in muscle tissue produced by two different surgical approaches can be compared: standard lateral approach (on the right) and anterior minimally invasive access (on the left). Note the marked involvement of the gluteus medius and gluteus minimus muscles on the right. Partial fibro-adipose degeneration of the damaged muscle tissue is present. Alterations are evident both in the coronal (A) and in the transverse planes (B)

Table 1 Changes induced by surgical trauma

Sympathetic nervous system activation
Endocrine 'stress response' (primary pituitary secretion, insulin resistance)
Immunological and haematological changes (cytokine production, citokines, acute phase reaction, neutrophil lucocytosis, lymphocyte proliferation)

Neuro-endocrinological aspects

Surgical stress activates the sympathetic nervous system and the hypothalamic-pituitary-adrenal axis, with an increase in the corresponding hormone secretion [14,16,22,23,34,74] (tab. 2). The effect is to increase catabolism, with mobilisation of substrates and an increase in cellular energy sources, and to promote hydrosaline retention, to maintain fluid volume and cardiovascular homeostasis.
The surgical act is in fact a powerful activator of pituitary ACTH and adrenal cortisol secretion, with increases detectable as early as a few minutes after the start of the surgical act. Growth factor (GH), prolactin (PLTH) and pituitary endorphin (without metabolic effects the latter) also increase.
Cortisol plays a role in glucose, protein and lipid metabolism. It increases blood glucose, promotes lipolysis and stimulates gluconeogenesis. It also has anti-inflammatory activity, inhibiting the accumulation of macrophages and neutrophils in the area of tissue inflammation. It also counteracts the synthesis and release of inflammation mediators, in particular cytokines and prostaglandins.
The increase in vasopressin (posterior pituitary), linked to the extent of the trauma and the presence of any complications, promotes fluid retention by acting on renal function and lasts for 3 to 5 days. Adrenal aldosterone, due to pituitary activation, and the renin-angiotensin system, due to sympathetic nerve stimulation, also increase with surgical stress [22,23].
Hypothalamic activation by the sympathetic autonomic nervous system also produces an increase in catecholamines (Noradrenaline and Adrenaline) from the adrenal medulla and the release of Noraepinephrine from the pre-synaptic nerve endings. The effect will be predominantly cardiovascular, with an increase in heart rate and blood pressure, and to a lesser extent on the visceral organs (liver, pancreas and kidneys) with activating effects on metabolism, especially glycaemic metabolism.

Table 2 Hormonal changes induced by surgical stress

Anterior pituitary	ACTH	Increase
	GH	Increase
	TSH	May increase or decrease
	FSH/LH	May increase or decrease
	PLTH	Increase
Posterior pituitary	AVP (vasopressin)	Increase
Surrene	Cortisol	Increase
	Aldosterone	Increase
	Catecolamine	Increase
Pancreas	Insulin	Often decrease
	Glucagone	Increase
Thyroid	Thyroxine	Decrease

Other endocrinological aspects

Insulin, a key anabolic hormone, decreases after induction of anaesthesia and during the surgical act, with indirect catabolic effects and hyperglycaemic response. Glucagon, on the other hand, increases transiently after the surgical act, although it does not appear to particularly affect the 'impaired glucose tolerance' phenomenon.

Surgical stress increases the secretion of glucostatic hormones (glucagon, cortisol and catecholamines) and induces the production of pro-inflammatory factors (cytokines and PGE). These substances are capable of promoting insulin resistance and glycaemic imbalance [34,59,60,71,72], especially if this is a pre-existing condition prior to surgery [33,73].

TSH and T3 levels decrease with the surgical procedure for reasons that are unclear and possibly related to circulating levels of catecholamines and cortisol [22,23]. The levels of gonadotropins (FSH and LH) are variable, with values rising or falling after surgery, while testosterone and oestradiol tend to decrease. The endocrine response to surgery ultimately consists of a secretory increase in catabolic hormones with activation of metabolism (glucose, protein, lipid) and correction of the hydro-electrolyte balance, basically to provide additional energy sources to the body and to support cardiovascular homeostasis.

The endocrine response is largely activated by neuronal afferents. These, from peripheral sensory endings stimulated by surgical trauma, reach the hypothalamus, the structure at the base of the neuroendocrine response, via ascending nerve pathways (vertebral sensory roots and posterior spinal cords).

Histochemical background

Cytokines are a group of low molecular weight molecules, including interleukins and interferon. They are produced by leukocytes, fibroblasts and endothelial cells as an early response to tissue trauma and play an important role in inflammation and immune response [62].

They act on the surface receptors of numerous target cell types and interfere in their protein synthesis. They govern the so-called **'acute phase response'** [39,62,67], which comprises a wide range of local and systemic reactions. They play a predominant role in the inflammatory response to surgical trauma, with general inflammatory effects ('systemic inflammatory state') and local effects at the site of tissue trauma. After trauma, mainly interleukin-1 (IL-1), interleukin-6 (IL-6), interleukin-8 (IL-8), interleukin-10 (IL-10) and tumour necrosis factor-alpha (TNF-alpha) are released, forming the **'cytokine network'**.

Cytokine concentration is low and unidentifiable under basal conditions. Their production, on the other hand, undergoes a marked increase as a result of surgical trauma, which expresses the degree of tissue damage. The released factors, in particular the predominant IL-6, activate macrophages and monocytes in the damaged tissue.

The local and systemic damaging effects produced by the cytokine network decrease in low-trauma procedures, while they increase in more aggressive procedures (arthroplasty, colorectal surgery, vascular surgery, etc.).

Cytokines are an indicator of tissue damage and a predisposing condition for complications. In particular they are so for the infectious risk, as they interfere with the immune, metabolic and haemocoagulative response [28,43,56].

The **acute phase response**, mainly managed by cytokines (tab. 3), is characterised by fever and certain tissue and metabolic changes, in particular through the production in the liver of acute phase proteins **(APP, Acute Phase Proteins)**. Consequently, PCR, fibrinogen, alpha1 globulin and alpha2 (APP positive) increase and albumin, transferrin, alpha1 lipoprotein and beta-lipoprotein (APP negative) decrease. In particular, hepatic PCR synthesis follows the increase in IL-6 linearly [22,23].

The acute phase results in the release of pro-inflammatory mediators at the traumatised site, which have the following tasks: to circumscribe the inflammatory focus through microvascular thrombosis and fibrin deposition in the interstitium, to modulate blood

Table 3 APR - Acute Phase Response

Fever
Granulocytosis
Production of acute phase proteins in livery
CRP
Fibrinogen
Alfa2-macroglobulina
Changes in serum concentration of transport proteins
Increased ceruloplasmina
Decrease in transferrin, albumin and alfa2-macroglobulina
Changes in serum concentrations of divalent cations (copper increase, zinc and iron decrease)

flow and vessel wall permeability, to attract and activate circulating leucocytes, to facilitate proteolysis, phagocytosis and to trigger tissue repair (scavenger action).

Particular types of cytokines, referred to as **'alarmins'** (DAMP Danger Associatet Molecular Pattern, which include HMGB1 (High Mobility Group B1) and HISP (Heat Shock Proteins), strongly activate monocytes (especially the CD14+ subpopulation). The changes in intercellular communication induced in monocyte subgroups within 24 hours after surgery are able to favourably characterise the speed of recovery from fatigue, pain and functional impairment of the patient [6,11,15,28,69].

Surgical trauma also activates the metabolism of arachidonic acid (from membrane phospholipids) in numerous cell groups, with a marked increase in its derivatives (prostagladines, prostacyclins, thromboxanes and leukotrienes).

These substances contribute to multiple actions (tissue inflammation, platelet aggregation, nociceptor stimulation, smooth muscle contraction, vasodilation, vascular permeability, local oedema, pain threshold and body temperature). The increase in cytokines in particular is associated with that of prostaglandins, especially PGE2, either by direct stimulation ('induced event') or by sharing the generating mechanism [56].

Certain complement factors (C3bc, TCC/C9b-e) also increase for a short phase after surgical trauma (2 days) and can form **MAC** (cell membrane attachment complex) with a cytolytic effect. They cooperate with the pro-inflammatory and vasomotor action of cytokines and prostaglandins [9,56].

All these substances concur, during the peak phase (4-5 days), in supporting the local and systemic inflammatory response to surgical trauma and in reducing the immune response. The concentration and duration of action of cytokines, prostaglandins and complement have a direct relationship with the extent of surgical trauma and cell and tissue damage. At the same time, however, they prove capable to some extent of activating granulocytes, T cells, monocytes and phagocytosis.

Cytokines are also able to stimulate the secretion of catecholamines from the adrenal [56] and pituitary ACTH. Cortisol secretion also increases reflexively, but with a negative feedback mechanism, as the increase in cortisol tends to inhibit that of the cytokines themselves [39].

The traumatic event also activates the haemocoagulative cascade. Pro-inflammatory cytokines and prostaglandins interfere with coagulation in a prothrombotic direction. They act with a direct action on factors XII, VII and X, either by enhancing coagulation abnormalities or by promoting thromboplastin activation (basic or through the release of thromboplastin-like factors from damaged muscle tissue). Platelet activation secondary to tissue trauma (vessel laceration, endothelial injury, collagen exposure, contamination, etc.) may also contribute to the pro-coagula-

tive tendency [4,19,31,49].
Certain metal cations may change blood concentration (zinc and iron decrease, capper increase), as a response to surgical stress, in relation to a decrease in plasma transport proteins [67].

Metabolic background

The surgical act increases the secretion of glucostatic hormones (glucagon, cortisol and catecholamines) and induces the production of pro-inflammatory factors (cytokines, PGE, complement fractions, ROS). These substances are capable of altering glycaemic metabolism leading to an increase in glycaemia and promoting insulin resistance [34,60,71,72].
The possible presence of a pre-surgical glycaemic imbalance may aggravate post-surgical metabolic dysfunction [33] and promote its complications, particularly infection [73].
Surgical stress and the endocrine-metabolic response also have a significant effect on protein metabolism. Healthy patients undergoing elective major abdominal surgery can lose up to 40-80 g of nitrogen, which corresponds to approximately 2 kg of skeletal muscle [44]. Protein hypercatabolism, which sets in after surgery, is accentuated in patients with hyperglycaemia and in poor health [60]. Protein deficit predisposes to delays in patient mobilisation, poor respiratory function and immune deficit, with increased infectious risks and prolonged hospitalisation [60]. In contrast, patients with a favourable nutritional status show less protein loss and insulin resistance [17,77].
Post-operative metabolic control is fundamental, including early resumption of the oral diet (if possible for the type of surgery) and nutritional supplementation, to counteract the catabolic phenomena induced by the stress response [5,12].
Lipolytic activity (on triglycerides) during surgical stress as a result of hormones (GH, ACTH, cortisol, catecholamines; insulin deficiency) leads to an increase in glycerol and fatty acids. Glycerol acts as a substrate for hepatic gluconeogenesis, contributing to the increase in blood glucose and insulin resistance [22,23].
ROS (Reactive Oxygen Species) are the product of mitochondrial cellular activity as a result of oxidative stress, secondary to a variety of conditions and in particular the inflammatory state. These oxidising agents play a predominant role in intercellular communication (signalling pathways) and act on the nervous, cardiovascular and immune systems. They control cell apoptosis in pathological tissues. In excess, however, they can play a cytotoxic role [63,64,66,79]. Increased ROS are also capable of damaging lipids, proteins, DNA and vascular permeability [16,34].

Fluid balance

Surgical stress results in increased levels of catecholamines, inflammatory cytokines, prostaglandins, vasopressin, renin/angiotensin, aldosterone and other substances that induce renal hydro-saline retention and promote blood hypercoagulability [61].
It is important to maintain adequate intravascular volume and good tissue perfusion. These conditions are jeopardised by the procedures themselves (surgical and anaesthesia), especially by the condition of intraoperative vasoplegia, without overloading the patient with fluids and salts. In the postoperative period, restoration of normovolaemia is important [13].

Gastro-intestinal function

The intestine, which has an intricate nervous system, mucous membranes with a high rate of cell turnover and tissues specialised in the absorption and secretion of substances, is very sensitive to inflammatory changes induced by surgical stress.
The effects of sympathetic nerve stimulation and systemic inflammation, supported by elevated ROS (Reactive Oxigen Species) values and other histochemical mediators (cytokines, PGE2, complement fractions), alter intestinal function. Motility is reduced (up to ileus) and

permeability with parietal oedema, causing prolonged hospitalisation and the need for additional treatment [8,16].

In this field, better results are known to be achieved with laparoscopic surgery compared to open procedures [51], especially when combined with spinal anaesthesia techniques and less use of opioids [35,38].

Effects of the anaesthesiological procedure

The anaesthesiological procedure is able to condition the stress response to surgery. Peripheral anaesthesia and its short duration of use appear to provide the best conditions for an advantageous immuno-metabolic/endocrinological control with a less demanding stress response [36].

Heavy opioids (Fentanyl) and propofol reduce glucose imbalance compared to inhaled general anaesthesia techniques. These drugs, through predominantly hypothalamic inhibition, tend in fact to reduce pituitary secretion, particularly of ACTH, GH, cortisol and catecholamines [22,23,32].

Some drugs used in the past (Etomidate and dl Thiopental) had revealed a reversible inhibition of adrenal production of cortisol and aldosterone [2,45]. Benzodiazepines (Midazolan) inhibit the cortisol response by acting at the hypothalamic-pituitary level [2,45,22,23].

Clonidine, a central antihypertensive with sympatholytic alpha-2 agonist action, also inhibits the stress response mediated by the sympathetic nervous system. In fact, this limits the vasoconstriction produced by alpha-1 receptors [1].

Neuroaxial anaesthesia inhibits the ascending and descending nociceptive stress response pathways. Thus, in pelvic and lower limb surgery, spinal anaesthesia attenuates the endocrine and metabolic response. This is because somatic and sympathetic nerve stimulations from traumatised tissue have a lower afferency to the central nervous system and the hypothalamic-pituitary axis.

This phenomenon improves insulin sensitivity, decreases protein catabolism and reduces energy demands to maintain a neutral or positive nitrogen balance with less protein loss [59,60]. Blocking efferences to the adrenal medulla and liver also counteracts the hyperglycaemic response [22,23,25].

Inhibition of the stress response is however a common feature of anaesthesia procedures (general or spinal). The lower risks involved in peripheral blocks, however (thromboembolic complications, pulmonary function, cardiac complications and gastrointestinal function) make them preferable to general procedures [7,40,41,42,47].

Tissue hypoperfusion

In hip surgery, the tissue most anatomically involved and most vulnerable to surgical gestures is the muscle tissue. The surgical incision of the muscle and its tendons alone would be sufficient not to define the surgical act as minimally invasive.

Minimally invasive accesses should strictly adhere to the technical principle of **'muscular sparing and not detachment'**. The fundamental aspects of tissue damage are: surgical incision of the muscles, tissue hypoperfusion, intensity and duration of the pressure exerted by the retractors on the muscles.

Tissue hypoperfusion, especially due to impaired microcirculation, is a condition of great importance and closely related to surgical aggression. It may be regional and contiguous to the affected area, or general. It may result from blood loss, decreased ventilation, prolonged maintenance of low blood pressure, the presence of ischaemic devices, patient position with possible 'intravascular fluid shift', excessive prolongation of the procedure, and exposure to low temperatures in the operating theatre.

Intra- and post-operative bleeding and residual post-surgical haematoma are the fundamental aspects underlying cellular damage, due to the resulting tissue hypoperfusion, increased local pressure and the action of blood-degrading factors.

Tissue hypoperfusion also contributes to the development of the **'systemic inflamma-**

tory response syndrome', with a cascade of events leading to cellular dysfunction, mainly due to depression of mitochondrial activity, resulting in reduced ATP production [16].

The 'muscle damage reaction' includes the phenomena triggered by the release of substances contained in the myocell, such as glutamine, myoglobin and calcium and sodium salts, potassium, magnesium, phosphate and enzymes such as CPK, CKM and LDH. Although essential for cellular function, these substances are harmful if released rapidly and in large quantities.

Attempts to quantify muscle damage by post-operative measurement of CPK, CK-MM and myoglobin in the minimally invasive and standard technique have not shown conclusive or unequivocal results. However, it confirmed the lower muscle tissue damage caused by the reduced-aggression procedures [27,70].

Glutamine is the most abundant free amino acid in the human body and plays a key regulatory role in several cellular processes, including: metabolism (oxidative fuel, gluconeogenic and lipogenic precursor), cell integrity (promotes proliferation, especially at the enteric level, and counteracts apoptosis), protein synthesis, antioxidant activity, reduction of insulin resistance, increase in insulin synthesis and extracellular matrix (ECM). It also regulates the expression of many genes related to metabolism, signal transduction, cell defence and repair, and intercellular signalling function [18,20].

In response to surgical trauma and increased cortisol, glutamine is released from muscles and taken up by splanchnic organs and the immune system. The function of immune cells is largely dependent on the availability of glutamine. During hypercatabolic circumstances, the demand for glutamine increases considerably, which can lead to glutamine deprivation and a consequent impairment of cellular function and the cellular and humoral immune response [68].

In addition to cytokines, the tissue damage produced (muscle in particular) by surgery results in the release of numerous substances such as calcium, sodium, potassium, prostanoids, bradykinin, NGF (nerve grow factor), substance P and CPK. These substances prove capable of increasing the sensitivity of peripheral nociceptors in the area of surgical trauma. Substance P, however, can extensively sensitise tissue nociceptors (contiguous or distant), even if not directly affected by the surgical trauma [26].

Stimulation of nociceptors by this group of substances may continue at a distance from the surgical stress. They may also lead to sensitisation of the central nervous system via NMDA receptors located in the posterior horn of the spinal cord and promote the development of hyperalgesia, allodynia and chronic post-surgical pain [52].

Skin damage, due to the surgical incision, prolonged and forced tension of retractors and inadequate management of the surgical wound, may involve nociceptors in the dermis and hypodermis, which are usually richly represented.

Algogenic 'stimulation' of nociceptors can be protracted over time and be the basis of chronic post-surgical pain. Noteworthy is **'PISC' (Peri-Incisional Sensorial Changes)**, which is characterised by alterations in sensitivity and nociception of a more or less extensive skin area around the surgical incision. This can be found in any part of the body and for any type of surgery. However, this seems at least partly related to the extent and duration of the cutaneous surgical trauma [30].

Cognitive status

Effects on cognitive status may occur in the post-operative period (POD post-operative delirium; POCD post-operative cognitive decline). These conditions are sometimes unexpected and not preceded by particular patient states, such as advanced age, poor education, attention disorder and the presence of metabolic syndromes [26]. The high intensity of surgical stress and its response may contribute to neurological sequelae with cognitive impairment [21].

Decreasing the intensity and duration of surgical stress, modulating the stress response, attenuating the phase of systemic phlogosis, reducing the release of cytokines and other mediators of phlogosis, reducing the post-operative use of drugs (particularly long-acting benzodiazepines), careful infusion therapy and multimodal analgesic strategies, have proved to be the ways of counteracting the onset and progression of cognitive disorders [54,55].

Conclusions

The surgical act inevitably causes stress to the organism, of varying magnitude. This will be in relation to the anatomical structure involved, the type of tissue, the extent and duration of the surgical stress and the post-operative management. The resulting tissue damage (surgery trauma stress) results in a multi-sectoral involvement of variable magnitude (immunological, endocrinological, neuroendocrine and histochemical), which partly mimics the phases of general trauma stress.
The stress response to surgery is a constant effect of an ambivalent nature. To a certain extent, it has a protective and compensatory role in local or general imbalances caused by the surgical act, which can contribute to immuno-endocrinological homeostasis.
Beyond this, the extent and duration of the response, adrenal activation, the increase in the cytokine network and the immune imbalance, can instead determine regional and general tissue damage of varying magnitude, also capable of evolving subsequently by self-aggravation.
Hence the need to reduce surgical stress by respecting all the conditions capable of mitigating harmful intra- and post-operative situations (extent, intensity and duration of stress, tissue damage caused, blood loss and intra-operative gestures).
In our activity, for a long time and with a large case history, the adoption of techniques with reduced surgical aggressiveness has allowed us to appreciate the numerous advantages of mini-invasiveness.
After completion of the steepness learning curve, we have noted a considerable increase in favourable clinical results and, conversely, a considerable reduction in the problems and complications associated with traditional prosthetic surgery.
Even in our experience, however, the learning curve proved to be long and not easy, initially marked by a transient increase in intra- and post-operative complications, which were then greatly reduced with the acquisition of a well-established surgical standard.
Therefore, the two fundamental points that deserve great attention are the recognition of the technical difficulties in minimally invasive surgery and overcoming the challenging learning curve that this modern surgical concept imposes.
It must be admitted, however, that most of the scientific knowledge concerning stress trauma surgery and stress response in minimally invasive surgery comes mainly from experiences and studies in other surgical branches (cardio-thoracic, abdominal, etc.) and in the anaesthesiological field. These are sources that we orthopaedists too must finally take as an example and develop in our research, always relying on the 5 fundamental principles of D.A. Rogers: **'awareness, interest, evaluation, trial and adoption'** [57].

Bibliography

1. Aantaa R, Scheinin M. Alpha 2-adrenergic agents in anaesthesia. Acta Anaesthesiol Scand. 1993;37(5):433-448.

2. Absalom A, Pledger D, Kong A. Adrenocortical function in critically ill patients 24 h after a single dose of etomidate. Anaesthesia. 1999;54(9):861-867.

3. Allvin R, Berg K, Idvall E, Nilsson U. Postoperative recovery: a concept analysis. J Adv Nurs. 2007;57(5):552-558.

4. Amengual O, Atsumi T, Khamashta MA, Hughes GR. The role of the tissue factor pathway in the hypercoagulable state in patients with the antiphospholipid syndrome. Thromb Haemost. 1998;79(2):276-281.

5. Askanazi J, Rosenbaum SH, Hyman AI, Silverberg PA, Milic-Emili J, Kinney JM. Respiratory changes induced by the large glucose loads of total parenteral nutrition. JAMA. 1980;243(14):1444-1447.

6. Baigrie RJ, Lamont PM, Kwiatkowski D, Dallman MJ, Morris PJ. Systemic cytokine response after major surgery. Br J Surg. 1992;79(8):757-760.

7. Ballantyne JC, Carr DB, deFerranti S, et al. The comparative effects of postoperative analgesic therapies on pulmonary outcome: cumulative meta-analyses of randomized, controlled trials. Anesth Analg. 1998;86(3):598-612.

8. Bauer AJ, Boeckxstaens GE. Mechanisms of postoperative ileus. Neurogastroenterol Motil. 2004;16 Suppl 2:54-60.

9. Beilin B, Shavit Y, Dekeyser F, Itzik A, Weidenfeld J. The involvement of glucocorticoids and interleukin-1 in the regulation of brain prostaglandin production in response to surgical stress. Neuroimmunomodulation. 2006;13(1):36-42.

10. Bisgaard T, Klarskov B, Rosenberg J, Kehlet H. Factors determining convalescence after uncomplicated laparoscopic cholecystectomy. Arch Surg. 2001;136(8):917-921.

11. Bisgaard T, Støckel M, Klarskov B, Kehlet H, Rosenberg J. Prospective analysis of convalescence and early pain after uncomplicated laparoscopic fundoplication. Br J Surg. 2004;91(11):1473-1478.

12. Boelens PG, Heesakkers FF, Luyer MD, et al. Reduction of postoperative ileus by early enteral nutrition in patients undergoing major rectal surgery: prospective, randomized, controlled trial. Ann Surg. 2014;259(4):649-655.

13. Brandstrup B, Svendsen PE, Rasmussen M, et al. Which goal for fluid therapy during colorectal surgery is followed by the best outcome: near-maximal stroke volume or zero fluid balance?. Br J Anaesth. 2012;109(2):191-199.

14. Carli F. Physiologic considerations of Enhanced Recovery After Surgery (ERAS) programs: implications of the stress response. Can J Anaesth. 2015;62(2):110-119.

15. Chan JK, Roth J, Oppenheim JJ, et al. Alarmins: awaiting a clinical response. J Clin Invest. 2012;122(8):2711-2719.

16. Chowdhury AH, Lobo DN. Fluids and gastrointestinal function. Curr Opin Clin Nutr Metab Care. 2011;14(5):469-476.

17. Crowe PJ, Dennison A, Royle GT. The effect of pre-operative glucose loading on postoperative nitrogen metabolism. Br J Surg. 1984;71(8):635-637.

18. Cruzat V, Macedo Rogero M, Noel Keane K, Curi R, Newsholme P. Glutamine: Metabolism and Immune Function, Supplementation and Clinical Translation. Nutrients. 2018;10(11):1564.

19. Cuadrado MJ, López-Pedrera C, Khamashta MA, et al. Thrombosis in primary antiphospholipid syndrome: a pivotal role for monocyte tissue factor expression. Arthritis Rheum. 1997;40(5):834-841.

20. Curi R, Lagranha CJ, Doi SQ, et al. Molecular mechanisms of glutamine action. J Cell Physiol. 2005;204(2):392-401.

21. Degos V, Vacas S, Han Z, et al. Depletion of bone marrow-derived macrophages perturbs the innate immune response to surgery and reduces postoperative memory dysfunction. Anesthesiology. 2013;118(3):527-536.

22. Desborough JP. The stress response to trauma and surgery. Br J Anaesth. 2000;85(1):109-117.

23. Desborough JP, Hall GM: Endocrine response to surgery. In: Kaufman L. Anaesthesia Review, vol. 10. Edimburgh: Churchill Livingstone, 1993; 131-48.

24. DeCherney AH, Bachmann G, Isaacson K, Gall S. Postoperative fatigue negatively impacts the daily lives of patients recovering from hysterectomy. Obstet Gynecol. 2002;99(1):51-57.

25. Engquist A, Brandt MR, Fernandes A, Kehlet H. The blocking effect of epidural analgesia on the adrenocortical and hyperglycemic responses to surgery. Acta Anaesthesiol Scand. 1977;21(4):330-335.

26. Feldheiser A, Aziz O, Baldini G, et al. Enhanced Recovery After Surgery (ERAS) for gastrointestinal surgery, part 2: consensus state-

ment for anaesthesia practice. Acta Anaesthesiol Scand. 2016;60(3):289-334.
27. Fink B, Mittelstaedt A, Schulz MS, Sebena P, Singer J. Comparison of a minimally invasive posterior approach and the standard posterior approach for total hip arthroplasty A prospective and comparative study. J Orthop Surg Res. 2010;5:46.
28. Fragiadakis GK, Gaudillière B, Ganio EA, et al. Patient-specific Immune States before Surgery Are Strong Correlates of Surgical Recovery. Anesthesiology. 2015;123(6):1241-1255.
29. Gaudillière B, Fragiadakis GK, Bruggner RV, et al. Clinical recovery from surgery correlates with single-cell immune signatures. Sci Transl Med. 2014;6(255):255ra131.
30. Goulding K, Beaulé PE, Kim PR, Fazekas A. Incidence of lateral femoral cutaneous nerve neuropraxia after anterior approach hip arthroplasty. Clin Orthop Relat Res. 2010;468(9):2397-2404.
31. Grignani G, Maiolo A. Cytokines and hemostasis. Haematologica. 2000;85(9):967-972.
32. Hall GM, Young C, Holdcroft A, Alaghband-Zadeh H. Substrate mobilisation during surgery. Anaesthesia 1978;33:924-930.
33. Hatzakorzian R, Bui H, Carvalho G, Shan WL, Sidhu S, Schricker T. Fasting blood glucose levels in patients presenting for elective surgery. Nutrition. 2011;27(3):298-301.
34. Helander EM, Webb MP, Menard B, et al. Metabolic and the Surgical Stress Response Considerations to Improve Postoperative Recovery. Curr Pain Headache Rep. 2019;23(5):33.
35. Holte K, Kehlet H. Epidural anaesthesia and analgesia - effects on surgical stress responses and implications for postoperative nutrition. Clin Nutr. 2002;21(3):199-206.
36. Horber FF, Krayer S, Miles J, Cryer P, Rehder K, Haymond MW. Isoflurane and whole body leucine, glucose, and fatty acid metabolism in dogs. Anesthesiology. 1990;73(1):82-92.
37. Hozack WJ, Krismer M, Nogler M, Bonutti PM, Rachbauer F, Schaffer JL, Donnely WJ. Minimally Invasive Total Joint Arthroplasty. Springer, Berlin, Heidelberg, 2004.
38. Jakeways MS, Chadwick SJ, Carli F. A prospective comparison of laparoscopic versus open cholecystectomy. Ann R Coll Surg Engl. 1993;75(2):142.
39. Jameson P, Desborough JP, Bryant AE, Hall GM. The effect of cortisol suppression on interleukin-6 and white blood cell responses to surgery. Acta Anaesthesiol Scand. 1997;41(2):304-308.
40. Kehlet H. Multimodal approach to control postoperative pathophysiology and rehabilitation. Br J Anaesth. 1997;78(5):606-617.
41. Kehlet H. Acute pain control and accelerated postoperative surgical recovery. Surg Clin North Am. 1999;79(2):431-443.
42. Kehlet H, Dahl JB. Anaesthesia, surgery, and challenges in postoperative recovery. Lancet. 2003;362(9399):1921-1928.
43. Kim TK, Yoon JR. Comparison of the neuroendocrine and inflammatory responses after laparoscopic and abdominal hysterectomy. Korean J Anesthesiol. 2010;59(4):265-269.
44. Kinney JM, Elwyn DH. Protein metabolism and injury. Annu Rev Nutr. 1983;3:433-466.
45. Lacoumenta S, Yeo TH, Burrin JM, Bloom SR, Paterson JL, Hall GM. Fentanyl and the beta-endorphin, ACTH and glucoregulatory hormonal response to surgery. Br J Anaesth. 1987;59(6):713-720.
46. Lee L, Tran T, Mayo NE, Carli F, Feldman LS. What does it really mean to "recover" from an operation?. Surgery. 2014;155(2):211-216.
47. Liu S, Carpenter RL, Neal JM. Epidural anesthesia and analgesia. Their role in postoperative outcome. Anesthesiology. 1995;82(6):1474-1506.
48. Miniello S. Il Trauma. Una malattia sistemica. CIC, Roma, 2002.
49. Møiniche S, Bülow S, Hesselfeldt P, Hestbaek A, Kehlet H. Convalescence and hospital stay after colonic surgery with balanced analgesia, early oral feeding, and enforced mobilisation. Eur J Surg. 1995;161(4):283-288.
50. Nesargikar PN, Jaunoo SS: Natural Orifice translumenal endoscopicic surgery (N.O.T.E.S). Inter J of Surg, 2009;7:232-236.
51. Panchal SJ, Müller-Schwefe P, Wurzelmann JI. Opioid-induced bowel dysfunction: prevalence, pathophysiology and burden. Int J Clin Pract. 2007;61(7):1181-1187.
52. Podgoreanu MV, Michelotti GA, Sato Y, et al. Differential cardiac gene expression during cardiopulmonary bypass: ischemia-independent upregulation of proinflammatory genes. J Thorac Cardiovasc Surg. 2005;130(2):330-339.
53. Ranawat CS, Ranawat AS. Minimally invasive total joint arthroplasty: Where are we going?J Bone Joint Surg Am. 2003;85-A(11):2070–2071.
54. Rasmussen LS, Steentoft A, Rasmussen H, Kris-

tensen PA, Moller JT. Benzodiazepines and postoperative cognitive dysfunction in the elderly. ISPOCD Group. International Study of Postoperative Cognitive Dysfunction. Br J Anaesth. 1999;83(4):585-589.
55. Rasmussen LS, Johnson T, Kuipers HM, et al. Does anaesthesia cause postoperative cognitive dysfunction? A randomised study of regional versus general anaesthesia in 438 elderly patients. Acta Anaesthesiol Scand. 2003;47(3):260-266.
56. Risnes I, Ueland T, Lundblad R, et al. Changes in the cytokine network and complement parameters during open heart surgery. Interact Cardiovasc Thorac Surg. 2003;2(1):19-24.
57. Rogers DA. Ethical and educational considerations in minimally invasive surgery training for practicing surgeons. Semin Laparosc Surg. 2002;9(4):206-211.
58. Salmon P, Hall GM. A theory of postoperative fatigue. J R Soc Med. 1997;90(12):661-664.
59. Schricker T, Gougeon R, Eberhart L, et al. Type 2 diabetes mellitus and the catabolic response to surgery. Anesthesiology. 2005;102(2):320-326.
60. Schricker T, Lattermann R. Perioperative catabolism. Can J Anaesth. 2015;62(2):182-193.
61. Scott MJ, Miller TE. Pathophysiology of major surgery and the role of enhanced recovery pathways and the anesthesiologist to improve outcomes. Anesthesiol Clin. 2015;33(1):79-91.
62. Sheeran P, Hall GM. Cytokines in anaesthesia. Br J Anaesth. 1997;78(2):201-219.
63. Sies H, Jones DP. Reactive oxygen species (ROS) as pleiotropic physiological signalling agents. Nat Rev Mol Cell Biol. 2020;21(7):363-383.
64. Simon HU, Haj-Yehia A, Levi-Schaffer F. Role of reactive oxygen species (ROS) in apoptosis induction. Apoptosis. 2000;5(5):415-418.
65. Smit MJ, Beelen RH, Eijsbouts QA, Meijer S, Cuesta MA. Immunological response in laparoscopic surgery. Acta Gastroenterol Belg. 1996;59(4):245-247.
66. Snezhkina AV, et al. ROS Generation and Antioxidant Defense Systems in Normal and Malignant Cells. Oxid Med Cell Longev. 2019;2019:6175804.
67. Steinbrook RA. Epidural anesthesia and gastrointestinal motility. Anesth Analg. 1998;86(4):837-844.
68. Stephan RN, Kupper TS, Geha AS, Baue AE, Chaudry IH. Hemorrhage without tissue trauma produces immunosuppression and enhances susceptibility to sepsis. Arch Surg. 1987;122(1):62-68.
69. Stoecklein VM, Osuka A, Lederer JA. Trauma equals danger--damage control by the immune system. J Leukoc Biol. 2012;92(3):539-551.
70. Suzuki K, Kawachi S, Sakai H, Nanke H, Morita S. Mini-incision total hip arthroplasty: a quantitative assessment of laboratory data and clinical outcomes. J Orthop Sci. 2004;9(6):571-575.
71. Thorell A, Loftenius A, Andersson B, Ljungqvist O. Postoperative insulin resistance and circulating concentrations of stress hormones and cytokines. Clin Nutr. 1996;15(2):75-79.
72. Thorell A, Nygren J, Ljungqvist O. Insulin resistance: a marker of surgical stress. Curr Opin Clin Nutr Metab Care. 1999;2(1):69-78.
73. van den Berghe G, Wouters P, Weekers F, et al. Intensive insulin therapy in critically ill patients. N Engl J Med. 2001;345(19):1359-1367.
74. Wang C, Chan V, Yeung RT. Effect of surgical stress on pituitary-testicular function. Clin Endocrinol (Oxf). 1978;9(3):255-266.
75. Watt DG, Horgan PG, McMillan DC. Routine clinical markers of the magnitude of the systemic inflammatory response after elective operation: a systematic review. Surgery. 2015;157(2):362-380.
76. Weiser TG, Regenbogen SE, Thompson KD, et al. An estimation of the global volume of surgery: a modelling strategy based on available data. Lancet. 2008;372(9633):139-144.
77. Yagci G, Can MF, Ozturk E, et al. Effects of preoperative carbohydrate loading on glucose metabolism and gastric contents in patients undergoing moderate surgery: a randomized, controlled trial. Nutrition. 2008;24(3):212-216.
78. Zachary S Buchwald, Kiesel JR, Yang C, DiPaolo R, Novack DV, Aurora R. Osteoclast-induced Foxp3+ CD8 T-cells limit bone loss in mice. Bone. 2013;56(1):163-173.
79. Zorov DB, Juhaszova M, Sollott SJ. Mitochondrial reactive oxygen species (ROS) and ROS-induced ROS release. Physiol Rev. 2014;94(3):909-950.

CHAPTER 2

Surgical anatomy considerations for minimally invasive approaches to the hip

Carla Stecco, Raffaele De Caro

Institute of Normal Anatomy, University of Padova, Italy

Introduction

The hip is the most proximal joint of the lower limb. It belongs to the family of the enarthrosis (spherical joints): it has an articular cavity, the articular surfaces are covered with articular cartilage, it has a synovial membrane, that produces synovial fluid, and it is surrounded by a capsule, reinforced by thickenings identified as ligaments. The bony components are the acetabulum, an almost hemispherical joint cavity, and the femur with the femoral head which is about 2/3 of a solid sphere 4-5 cm in diameter. The articular ends have a complementary geometry: the femoral head has a convex surface, the acetabular cavity a concave surface. This creates a ball-in-socket joint with a high primary stability and at the same time a high degree of joint mobility in all three spatial axes. The structure of the hip ensures that the movements of the head inside the acetabulum occur with a homogeneous dispersion of the load over the entire joint surface, facilitating the action of the muscles. The hip is surrounded by powerful and well-balanced muscles, allowing a wide range of actions in the three planes of space granted. This delicate balance between mobility and stability, combined with significant loads, results in the hip joint being inevitably exposed to continuous and progressive wear of its osteoarticular surfaces. In the past, initial lesions of this type were often unrecognised due to the difficulty of diagnosing them early. The pathological processes that develop in the hip and their evolutionary potential have only recently been better understood. This has been made possible by the advent of the latest generation of MRI and even more so by arthro-RMN and arthroscopy. In addition to the new diagnostic potential, it is necessary to consider a renewed joint knowledge of anatomy, biomechanics and the minimal changes, hitherto underestimated, which can delay or avoid recourse to prosthetic surgery, if detected in time and adequately treated.

Osteology

Cotyle or acetabulum

The concave part of the coxo-femoral joint is called the cotyle. This is a word of Greek origin (Kotylé). due to its resemblance to a bowl, that was used later to identify a unit of measurement of capacity for liquids. Its absolute value varied from place to place between 0.21 and 0.33 litres. Alternatively, the cotyle is also identified with the term acetabulum,

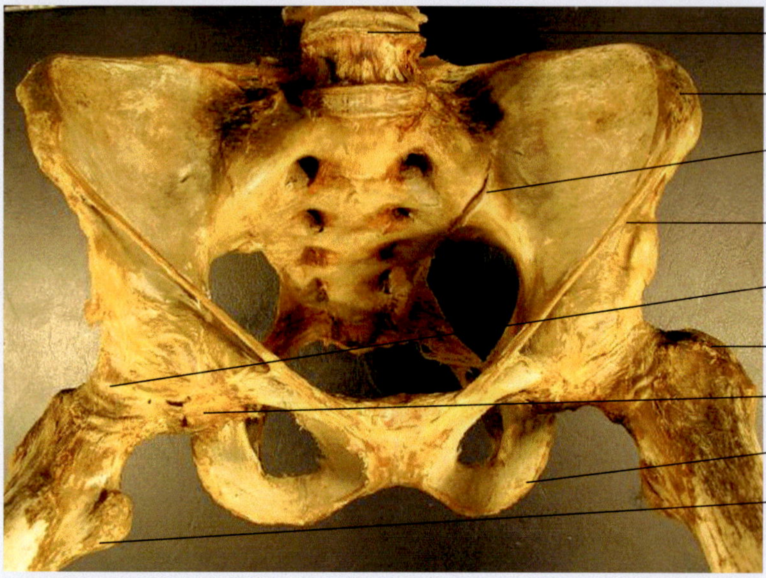

Figure 1 Human pelvis with the main ligaments

which in ancient Rome was a container (acetabulum) used to hold liquids, vinegar in most cases, of a certain capacity.

In general, the acetabulum identifies a socket into which the condyle of a nearby mobile bone fits. The cup is formed by the fusion of the ileum (about 40% of the acetabulum), ischium (40%) and pubis (20%). In the child these three bones are separated by triradiate cartilage. Their fusion begins to occur around 14-16 years of age and usually completes by the age of 23. The fusion point between ischium and pubis is clearly visible as the notch of the acetabulum. This is converted into a hole by the transverse acetabular ligament, which connects the two ends of the acetabular lip as a bridge (fig. 1).

The articular surface of the acetabulum consists of the half-moon surface, which together constitutes approximately ¾ of a circumference, interrupted by the underlying acetabular notch. Its surface is smooth and covered with hyaline articular cartilage, which is thicker where the pressure of body weight in an upright position is greater. This articular cartilage protrudes from the edge of the acetabulum to form the acetabular labrum. Not all of the acetabular cavity is directly involved in the joint. In fact, the fossa of the acetabulum, which is located in its centre, is a quadrilateral depression not covered by articular cartilage but by periosteum. This space contains a fibroelastic fat pad covered by the synovial membrane. The ligamentum teres femoris is inserted into this fossa and connects to the fovea capitis of the femoral head.

The acetabular labrum is a triangular-section fibrocartilage that surrounds the bony portion of the C-shaped acetabulum and continues with the transverse ligament to complete the ring surrounding the acetabulum. The acetabular labrum contributes to joint stability by increasing the joint surface by 22% and the volume of the cotyloid cavity by 33%. Unlike the glenoid labrum of the scapulohumeral joint, which has no other function than to widen the corresponding cavity, the acetabular labrum plays an important role in containing the joint. In fact, the edge of the acetabular labrum is slightly bent inwards. This narrows the diameter of the acetabular cavity and makes the coxo-femoral joint deeper than the bony joint surfaces alone would allow. It has also been suggested that it may play a role in controlling the movement of synovial fluid in the peripheral compartment of the hip. This would help to exert a negative pressure effect within the hip, like a gasket. The labrum has been carefully studied especially since the advent of arthroscopy. This technique has succeeded in giving us 'closed surgery' images of both its normal appearance and, more importantly, its pathological lesions. To

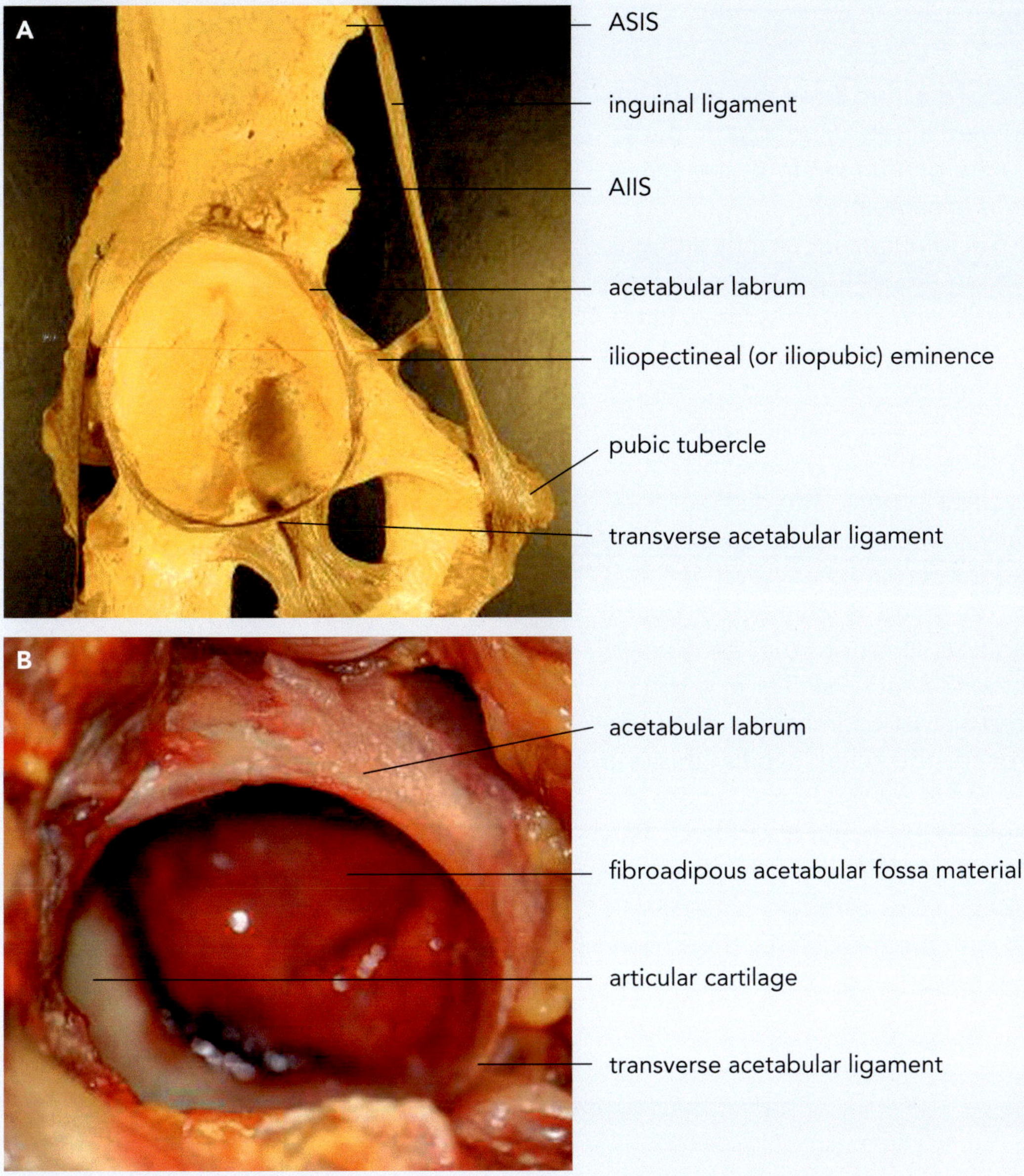

Figure 2 Acetabulum. A) Bone model, note the shape of the articular surface and the acetabular labrum. B) Dissection of a fresh specimen. Note the acetabular labrum and the acetabular fossa filled with fibroadipous material

date, labrum pathology is the most common indication for hip arthroscopy (fig. 2).

The labrum is relatively securely fixed to the edge of the acetabulum, while the transverse acetabular ligament is firmly attached to the two acetabular pillars. The acetabular labrum fuses on the capsular side with the acetabulum and on the articular side with the hyaline cartilage. However, it remains separated from the capsule by the capsular recess.

The attachment of the collagen fibres of the labrum to the acetabulum is different between the anterior and posterior portions. In the anterior aspect, the collagen fibres of the rim are parallel to those of the bony edge and therefore easily subject to separation when subjected to shear forces. In contrast, in the posterior portion, the fibres develop perpendicular to the rim before merging with the collagen fibres of the bony edge and are therefore resistant to shear forces. This may explain why the attachment of the labrum to the bone is stronger in the postero-inferior quadrants and consequently why labrum injuries are more frequent in the anterosuperior region.

The femur

The femur (fig. 3) is a long bone that is oblique inferiorly and medially in an upright. In the female, due to the greater width of the pelvis, this obliquity is accentuated.
The body of the femur is not exactly straight, but curved in an arc with posterior concavity. It is prismatic and has three faces (anterior, postero-medial and postero-lateral) and three margins (medial, lateral and posterior). The medial and lateral margins are blunt, while the posterior margin is thick and rough and is called linea aspera. The nutrient foramen is usually found along its course. The upper end of the femur has a head and two trochanters. The head is connected to the femoral diaphysis through the anatomical neck. The femoral head is similar to a sphere and is covered almost entirely by hyaline cartilage, except for the fovea capitis (this is a small groove in the femoral head where the round ligament of the femur is inserted. This ligament connects the femoral head to the acetabular fossa). The cartilage is thicker in the centre than at the margins, as this is generally where it takes the greatest load. Often the most proximal part of the femoral neck is also covered with cartilage (fig. 4).
The anatomical neck is a rectangular prismatic bone segment whose axis is aligned with that of the head and forms an angle of approximately 130° with the axis of the body of the femur. At the base of the anatomical neck are two strong eminences, the trochanters, connected by a pronounced intertrochanteric crest. The greater trochanter is located superiorly and laterally, while medially and inferiorly there is the lesser trochanter. Immediately below the small trochanter is the surgical neck, which marks the boundary between the diaphysis and the epiphysis. There are characteristic angles of the proximal epiphysis of the femur. When these angles are abnormal they can alter the normal femoroacetabular joint with femoro-acetabular impingement syndromes which in time can lead to labrum injuries and arthrosis.
The cervical-diaphyseal angle is formed between the diaphyseal axis of the femur and the neck. It is usually 125 +/- 5° in the normal adult hip. When it exceeds 130° it is called coxa valga, if it is less than 120° it is called coxa vara. These conditions are considered

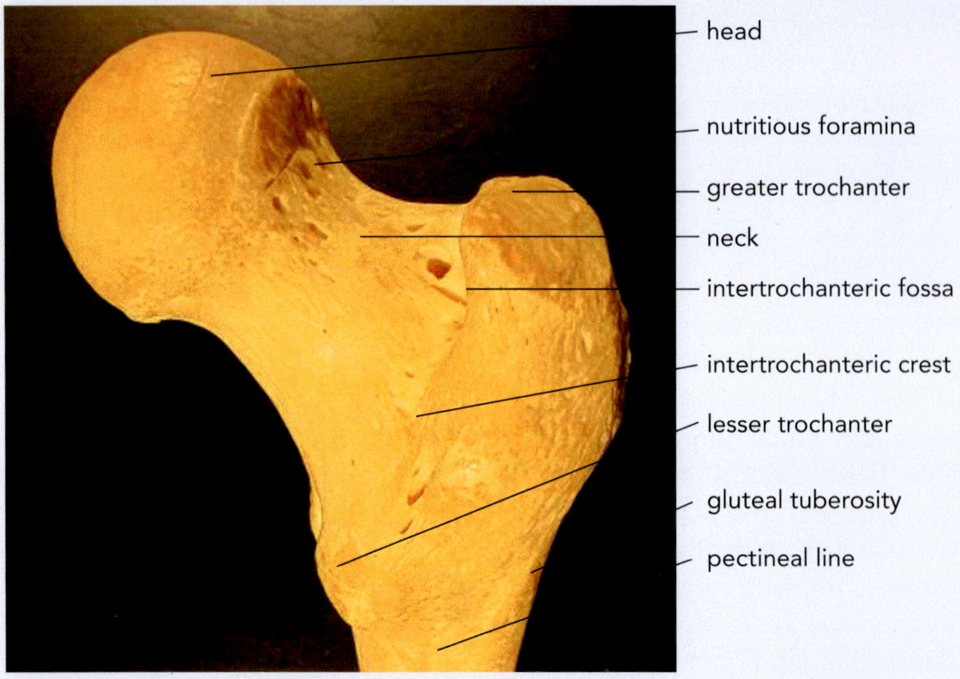

Figure 3 Proximal right femur portion, in a posterior view. Note the various nutritious foramina located mainly in the posterosuperior neck portion

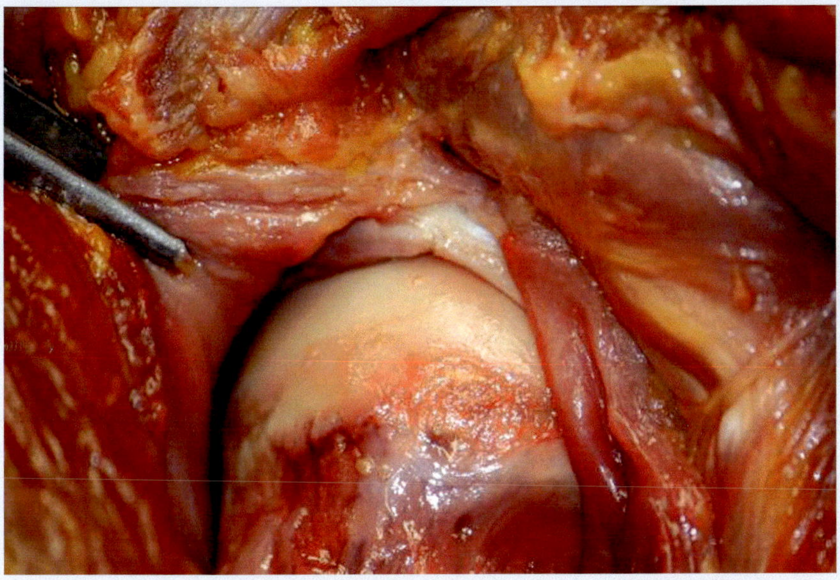

Figure 4 Femoral head inside the acetabulum. Dissection of a fresh specimen. Note the articular cartilage, the acetabular labrum and the capsule

pathological because they change the lever arms used for movement through the adductor muscles. The cervical-diaphyseal angle gradually decreases from 150° after birth to 125° in an adult due to bone remodelling in response to changing stress patterns.
The femoral anteversion angle indicates the forward rotation of the femoral neck. The anteversion angle is measured as the angle between the axis passing between the femoral condyles and the line passing through the femoral head. The average range of femoral anteversion is 15-20°.

The capsule and the ligaments

The capsule of the coxofemoral joint is a thick, strong fibrous sleeve. It originates half a centimetre medial to the acetabular margin, mostly following its profile both anteriorly and posteriorly. The exception are a few fibres that merge inferiorly to the acetabulum with the transverse acetabular ligament and with the superior margin of the obturator membrane. Distally it inserts at the intertrochanteric line on the anterior aspect of the femur, while it ends at the middle of the neck posteriorly. As a result, the anterior aspect of the anatomical neck of the femur is intracapsular, while the posterior aspect is intracapsular only in the medial two-thirds. The joint capsule is made up of both longitudinal and circular fibres. The longitudinal fibres are generally thicker in the antero-superior part of the capsule than in the posterior part. They often fuse with the ileofemoral ligament. The circular, or orbicular, fibres are internal to the longitudinal fibres and attach around the neck of the femur. They envelop it and partially fuse with the pubofemoral and ischiofemoral ligaments.
Although the capsule is very solid and reinforced by three ligaments, it has two weak areas. The first is anteriorly between the iliofemoral and pubofemoral ligaments and the second posteriorly between the iliofemoral and ischiofemoral ligaments. Dislocation episodes are more frequent precisely in these two areas of weakness (fig. 5).
Some muscle fibres from the gluteus minimus and rectus femoris insert into the capsule. These insertions are often overlooked in anatomy textbooks or considered anatomical variations. In reality, they are always present and are fundamental in tensioning the capsule during hip movements [1,29]. In particular, the gluteus minimus is able to tension the capsule posteriorly during hip extension and the rectus femoris, with its reflected tendon, tensions the capsule anteriorly during hip flexion. It is therefore possible that a dysfunction or fatigue of these two muscles may reduce the capsule protection

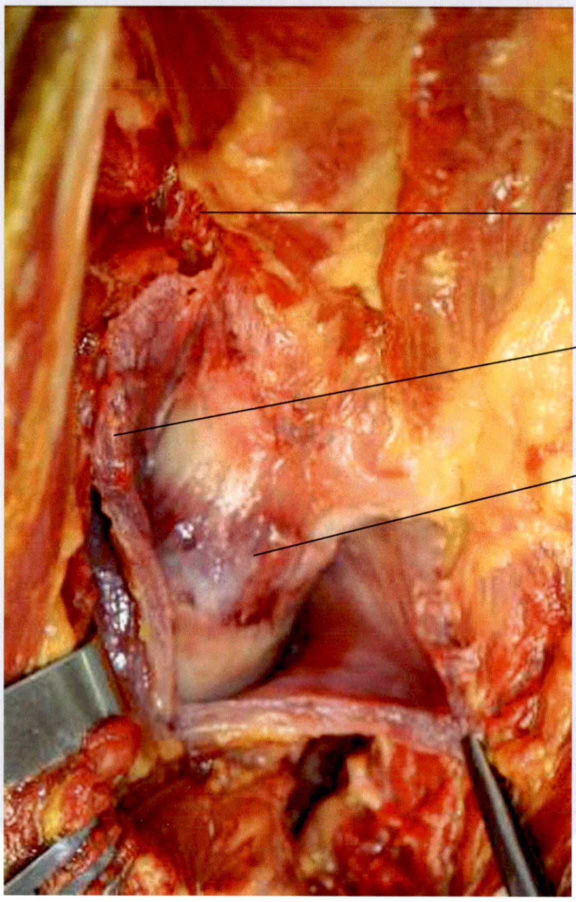

Figure 5 Joint capsule and ligaments, fresh dissection, anterior view. The capsule has been incised to reveal the femur neck. Note the thickness of the capsule

mechanism, causing episodes of capsule impingement between the articular ends and therefore pain during movement (fig. 6).

The synovial membrane has the characteristic pattern that it has in diarthrosis. It covers the inner surface of the capsule and, reached its insertions, reflects to cover the intracapsular portions of the bony ends up to the limits of the articular cartilages. In addition, the synovium forms a complete sheath around the round ligament.

The iliofemoral, or of Bigelow, or of Bertin, ligament is the most extensive and robust of the joint. It originates below the antero-inferior iliac spine and extends spirally until it attaches along the intertrochanteric line of the femur. Passing anterior to the joint capsule, this ligament joins it in several points and reinforces it, especially in its antero-superior portion. The iliofemoral ligament is sometimes referred to as the Y-shaped ligament because of its characteristic upturned Y shape. Sometimes it also has a fan-like '/\' shape. The 'stem' of the Y, which constitutes the apex, it laterally attaches to the antero-inferior iliac spine and medially to the acetabular margin. The medial bundle descends infero-medially toward the intertrochanteric line, while the lateral bundle descends infero-laterally toward the inferior part of the greater trochanter. The central portion of the ligament is therefore the weakest part. The iliofemoral ligament is stretched in extension and relaxed in flexion. It is the strongest ligament in the body with a tensile strength greater than 350N.

The pubofemoral ligament lies inferior and posterior to the ileofemoral ligament and is continuous with its medial border. It has a triangular shape: the base originates from the ileopectine eminence and the obturator crest, then the fibers continue inferolaterally until they merge with the medial portion of the ileofemoral ligament. The pubofemoral ligament contributes to the strength of the anteroinferior portion of the capsule, although it is the least mechanically resistant ligament.

The ischiofemoral ligament is located posteriorly. It consists of a central part that origi-

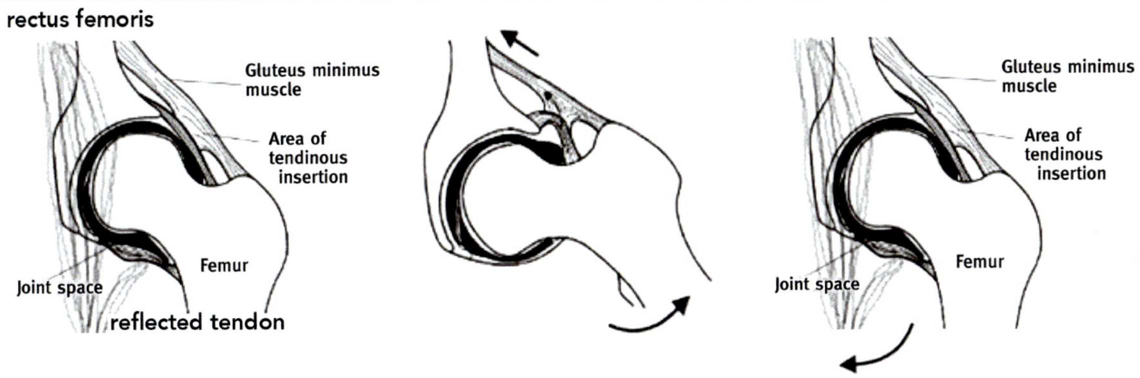

Figure 6 Role of the capsular insertions of the gluteus minimus and rectus femoris

nates above the ischial tuberosity and continues spirally to the great trochanter of the femur, partially merging with the iliofemoral ligament. The medial and lateral parts surround the femoral neck posteriorly, thickening the joint capsule.

The orbicular or angular zone surrounds the femur neck. It is placed deeper than the previous ligaments. It starts at the edge of the acetabulum and the acetabular labrum, passing behind the neck of the femur, reattaches to its point of origin.

The transverse acetabular ligament is a short band of collagen that bridges the two ends of the acetabular labrum. This closes the acetabular incisura, forming the lower margin of the acetabular fossa in vivo. It possesses foramina that allow branches of the obturator nerve and obturator artery to pass through.

The round ligament of the femur originates from the inferior part of the acetabular fossa, just above the transverse ligament (with which some fibers fuse), and attaches to the head of the femur at the fovea capitis. The ligament stretches during hip adduction and relaxes during abduction. It is completely enveloped by the synovial membrane, so it is intra-articular but extra-synovial. The round ligament contributes little in terms of stability for the hip and can be torn in traumatic dislocations. Some propose that it plays a role in the nutrition of the femoral head, as the round ligament is joined by the homonymous artery that continues to the femoral head.

The iliopectoral bursa is the main bursa of the coxo-femoral joint. This is located anterior to the ileopectineal ligament and is in communication with the rest of the hip joint through a cavity located between the ileopectineal and pubofemoral ligaments. This bursa creates a pad between the capsule and tendon of the iliopsoas, the main thigh flexor on the pelvis, which attaches to the small trochanter.

Hip vascularity

The vascular supply of the labrum is intimately interconnected with the hip as a whole. All of the vessels that nourish the labrum originate from the adjacent capsule and run through the body of the labrum to the articular side. None of the vessels cross the chondro-labral junction to reach the bony part of the acetabulum. The total number of blood vessels is significantly higher in the capsular zone than in the articular zone.

The hip vascularity is maintained by the two lateral and medial circumflex arteries of the femoral head, originating from the deep femoral artery, and the femoral head artery (obturator artery). In addition, there is a medullary canal supply.

The vascular supply to the femoral head has been well studied because of the risk of vascular necrosis of the head following femoral neck fractures or hip dislocation. Furthermore, the vascularisation of the femoral head is one of the crucial points of many hip joint diseases occurring in both paediatric

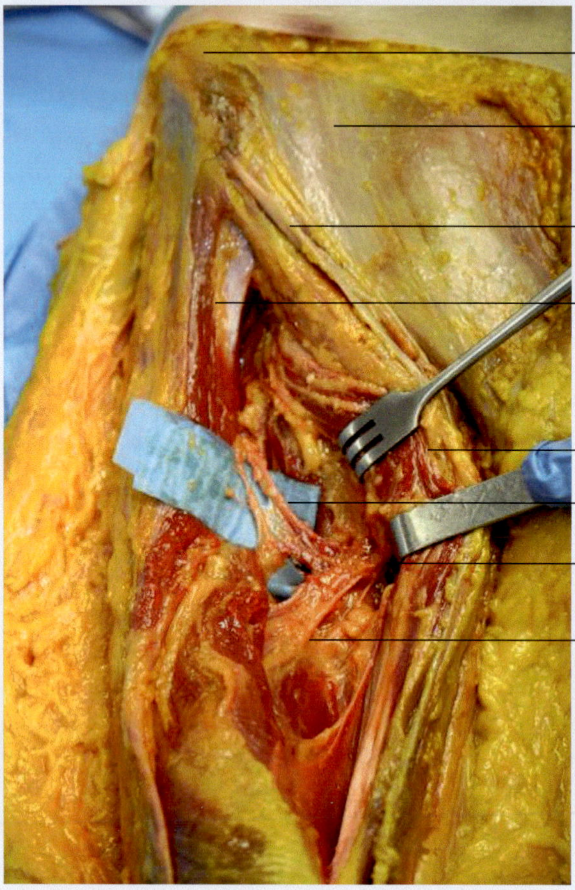

Figure 7 Anterior right hip region, fresh specimen. The dissection shows the lateral circumflex artery of the femur with its ascending and descending branches

and adult populations. The medial and lateral circumflex arteries can be damaged by retractors placed at the femoral neck during surgery (fig. 7).

The lateral circumflex artery originates from the deep femoral artery. It runs between branches of the femoral nerve, behind the sartorius muscle and the rectus femoris muscle, and divides into an ascending and a descending branch. It supplies most of the greater trochanter and the antero-medial part of the femoral head. The ascending branch of this artery runs along the intertrochanteric line and anastomoses with the superior gluteal and deep iliac circumflex arteries. It supplies muscular branches and joint of the hip. The descending branch distributes to the quadriceps femoris muscle and anastomoses with the third perforating artery and the lateral superior genicular artery of the knee. Lastly, the oblique branches penetrate at the level of the capsule insertion on the intertrochanteric crest.

The medial circumflex artery is the main artery for the head of the femur. It runs between the iliopsoas and pectineus muscles, surrounding the anterior part of the femoral neck. It is divided into a descending and an ascending branch. The first contributes to the posterior muscles of the thigh. The latter forms the posterior superior nutrient arteries, which enter the femoral head at the level of the nutritious foramina located in the postero-superior and antero-superior quadrants of the head and neck. Approximately 80% of all the nutritious foramina of the femoral head are located in these two quadrants.

The femoral head (or round ligament) artery originates from the medial circumflex artery or the obturator artery. It irrigates a small area of the femoral head. It is present in 80% of the population.

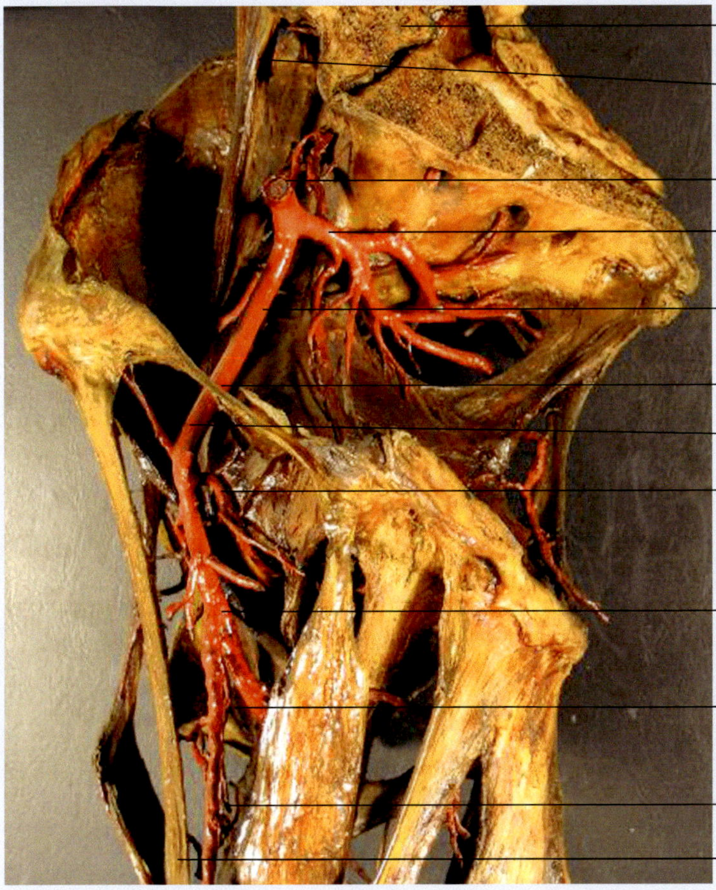

Figure 8 Hip vascularization, embalmed human specimen. The common iliac artery originates at L5-S1 and divides into the internal and external iliac artery. The latter, after passing the inguinal canal, becomes the femoral artery

Small arteries also run into the joint capsule, but these play no role in the blood supply to the femoral head. Therefore, a capsulotomy does not damage the vascularity of the femoral head unless the capsular incision reaches the intertrochanteric crest (fig. 8).
When hip surgery is performed, attention must still be paid to other vessels in the area: the internal and external iliac vessels, the internal pudendal artery, the obturator artery, the superior and inferior gluteal vessels. Damage to any of these causes massive haemorrhages.
The external iliac artery becomes the femoral artery when it passes below the inguinal ligament. The external iliac artery and its corresponding vein run adherent to the pelvis, and are poorly mobile. In particular, the vein is the structure most at risk. It runs 7mm from the bony plane at the level of the anterior inferior iliac spine and 4mm at the level of the anterior column of the acetabulum. The external iliac artery is less at risk because it has a thicker wall and runs 10 mm from the bone at the anterior inferior iliac spine level and 7mm at the level of the acetabulum.
The common femoral artery originates from the external iliac artery. The distinction between the two occurs at the inguinal ligament, which the artery crosses posteriorly at the level of the femoral head. The artery runs anterior and medial to the joint capsule. The iliopsoas alone lies between the vessels and the capsule at this level. The artery is covered by the skin, the subcutaneous tissue, in which the superficial inguinal lymph nodes are located, and the superficial layer of the fascia lata. The artery lays on the deep layer of the fascia lata enveloping the iliopsoas and pectoralis muscles. The femoral nerve, which divides into its terminal branches, lies lateral to it.

The femoral vein runs medial to the artery wrapped in the same vascular sheath. At the exit of Scarpa's triangle it divides into two branches: superficial (often considered only the continuation of the common artery, so much so that many authors make no difference between these two portions, calling them simply 'femoral artery') and deep. Other branches (in craniocaudal direction) are the pudendal, the superficial epigastric, the superficial circumflex iliac artery and the highest genicular artery.
The superficial femoral artery runs behind the sartorius muscle in the space formed by the vastus medialis and adductor longus muscles. In the adductor canal it is covered by the skin, the fascia lata, and the sartorius muscle. It rests on the adductor longus and adductor magnus muscles. The femoral vein is located behind the artery. The saphenous nerve runs next to the artery but then diverges, crossing the inferior part of the adductor canal together with the highest genicular artery.
The deep femoral artery originates 3-4 cm below the inguinal ligament and runs behind the trunk of the femoral artery until it reaches the medial surface of the femur.
It descends between the pectineus and adductor longus muscles and then passes between the adductor longus and adductor magnus muscles. Passing through the latter, the artery ends as the 3rd perforating artery, anastomosing with the superior articular branches of the popliteal artery. Its collateral branches are the medial and lateral circumflex arteries of the femur and the three perforating arteries.
The perforating arteries of the deep femoral artery pass through the tendons of the adductor muscles to the linea aspera of the femur until they reach the back of the thigh. At this point each artery divides into an ascending and a descending branch, which anastomose to each other. The ascending branch of the perforating artery extends proximally beneath the quadratus femoris muscle, issuing a branch to that muscle. It also anastomoses with the medial femoral circumflex artery and the inferior gluteal artery behind the short rotator muscles of the hip.
The internal iliac artery divides into two branches. A posterior branch from which the superior gluteal artery will originate. An anterior branch, which will be the source of the obturator artery, before splitting into the inferior gluteal artery and internal pudendal artery. The obturator vessels are at risk during hip surgery because they run within 1 mm of the bony surface at the level of the quadrilateral plate. Their only protection is provided by the interposition of the internal obturator muscle.
The superior gluteal artery extends below the gluteus minimus and the tensor fascia lata to anastomose anteriorly with the lateral circumflex femoral artery. The capsule, labrum and acetabulum are vascularised by the retinacular complex and the perforating branches of these vessels. The terminal blood supply to the labrum is provided by the retinacular vessels which are mainly derived from the superior and inferior gluteal arteries. The superior gluteal vessels are most at risk at the level of the greater sciatic notch, running on average 5 mm from the bone. The superior gluteal artery can cause profuse bleeding if injured, for example during posterior hip access.
At the level of the ischial spine, the inferior gluteal vessels run on average 6 mm from the posterior hip column, while the pudendal vessels run at 12 mm. However, at this level, both are protected by adipose tissue and are largely mobile, and therefore at low risk.
The anastomotic circle of the hip is essential, formed by the numerous anastomoses between the branches of the internal iliac, external iliac and femoral arteries. This structure allows the setting up of multiple collateral circles, ensuring the blood supply to the anterior and posterior labrum, the capsule, and the bony structures of the hip even under pathological conditions. However, in severe femoral artery obstructions, the only reliable anastomoses for an effective vascular supply are those between the inferior gluteal artery and the perforating arteries, branches of the deep femoral artery.

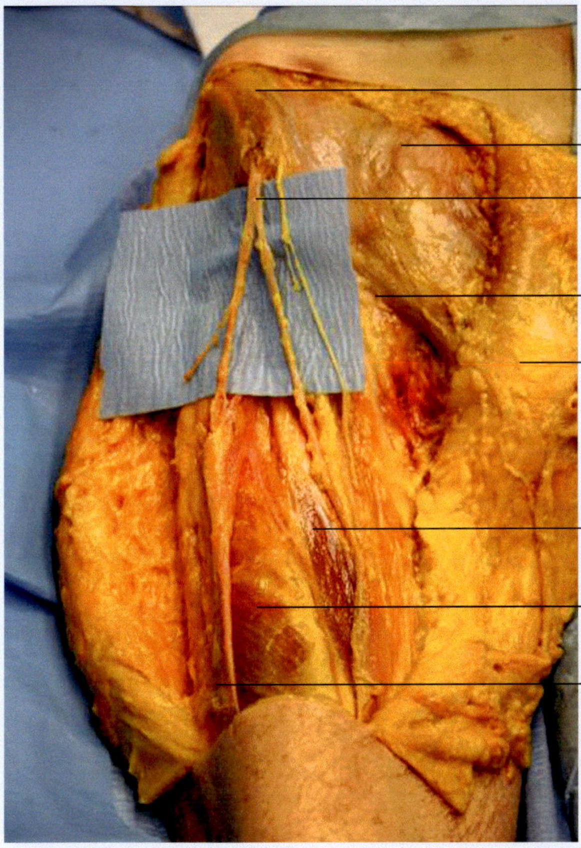

Figure 9 Anterior thigh region, fresh specimen dissection. The lateral femoral cutaneous nerve of the thigh has been isolated. Note the branched structure of this nerve

The innervation of the hip

In the area, the main nerves are the sciatic nerve, the femoral nerve, the superior and inferior gluteal nerves, the obturator nerve and the lateral femoro-cutaneous nerve of the leg. Depending on the surgical approach, these nerves may be subject to more or less frequent damage.

The anterior and posterior portions of the hip have separate innervations. The anterior aspect is innervated by the femoral nerve branches and the articular branches of the obturator nerve medially. The posterior aspect is innervated laterally by the superior gluteal nerve and medially by the articular branches of the sciatic nerve and the posterior branch of the obturator nerve (fig. 9).

The sciatic nerve originates from the lumbosacral plexus, emerges from the pelvis below the piriformis and enters the leg passing between the greater trochanter laterally and the ischium medially. It passes on average 9 mm from the posterior column at the level of the acetabular apex. This is where it is most frequently damaged. However, it is better protected at the level of the ischial spine, where the external rotator muscles of the hip interpose themselves between the nerve and the bone. Therefore, the nerve passes on average 15 mm from the ischial spine. The sciatic nerve consists of a tibial portion and a peroneal portion, which are clearly distinguishable at the origin. In 11% of subjects the peroneal portion of the sciatic nerve passes through the piriformis and the tibial portion anteriorly. In 3% of subjects the peroneal portion of the sciatic nerve passes over and behind the piriformis and the tibial portion anteriorly. While in 1% of cases the sciatic nerve passes through the piriformis muscle. This varying anatomical relationship may explain different individual susceptibility to sciatic compression, but there are no studies to support the idea that the sciatic nerve is at greater risk of compression when it passes through the belly of the piriformis.

Another nerve that needs to be considered during hip surgery, especially when performing anterior approach, is the lateral femoral-cutaneous nerve of the upper leg. It originates from the lumbosacral plexus and emerges from the pelvis passing under the inguinal ligament near the ASIS (Anterior Superior Iliac Spine). According to a study by Martins et al. [15], the lateral cutaneous nerve of the upper leg passes below the inguinal ligament in 80% of cases and lateral to the ASIS in the other cases. On average, the nerve passes 1.31 cm from the ASIS on the right, 1.22 cm on the left. However, there is a wide variability, ranging from 0 (immediately medial to the ASIS) to 5 cm. In 70% of cases, at the level of the inguinal ligament, the nerve is present with a single trunk, in other cases it is already divided into several branches. This nerve can also be damaged by improperly placed arthroscopic portals. It can also be subject to damage from nerve entrapment or external compression, giving the so-called meralgia paresthetica. Meralgia paresthetica is a condition characterised by a tingling, numbness and burning pain in the lateral part of the upper leg.

The femoral nerve is the most lateral structure within the femoral triangle (of Scarpa). It runs over the muscular belly of the iliopsoas, approximately midway between the anterosuperior iliac spine and the pubic tubercle. It relates to the anterior portion of the acetabulum, and therefore may be at risk during capsulotomy.

The superior gluteal nerve passes through the space between the gluteus medius and gluteus minimus. It is generally protected because it passes more than 5 cm from the greater trochanter and penetrates the gluteus maximus muscle proximal and medial to the incision usually made during a posterior access to the acetabulum.

The obturator nerve runs together with the homonymous vessels.

Myology

The hip geometry allows rotational movements in all directions, requiring a large number of muscles. The 22 muscles that act on the hip joint not only contribute to stability, but also provide the forces necessary for hip movement. Depending on the position of the hip, the same muscle can contribute to movement in different planes. This is due to a change in the relationship between the line of action of a muscle and the axis of rotation of the hip. This is referred to as 'reversal of muscle action'. For example, the gluteus medius and gluteus minimus act as external rotators when the hip is extended and as internal rotators when the hip is flexed. The adductor longus muscle acts as a flexor at 50° of hip flexion, and as an extensor at 70°. The main hip flexor is the iliopsoas, assisted by the sartorius, the rectus femoris and the tensor fascia lata. These muscles are all connected by the innominate fascia (or deep fascia lata layer). The tensor fascia lata is also a flexor and internal rotator of the hip joint. The sartorius also contributes to abduction and external rotation.

The most powerful hip extensor is the gluteus maximus. 80% of the fibres of the great gluteus do not have a bone insertion. These insert on the lateral intermuscular septum, the ilium tibial tract and the fascia lata. In particular, these fascial insertions imbricate perfectly with the proximal fascial insertions of the vastus lateralis muscle. As a result, there is a direct anatomical connection between the main extensor muscle of the upper leg (gluteus maximus) and the main extensor muscle of the knee (quadriceps femoris, in particular with the vastus lateralis). If this fascial continuity is interrupted or adhesions are created that limit the action of the fascia lata in its lateral portion, coordination between hip and knee may be affected. This would particularly involve movements such as getting up from a seated position. The gluteus maximus muscle is also considered a pivotal element for coordination between the lumbar region and the lower limbs. This is because, with its superficial fibres inserted simultaneously into the thoracolumbar fascia and the fascia lata, it can stretch them distally and proximally respectively. Therefore, excessive tension in the gluteus maximus may also irritate the nerve endings in the thora-

columbar fascia and the fascia lata. In this case the pain distribution may mimic that of a lumbar radiculopathy (crural pain, L2-L3).
The main external rotators of the hip are the gluteus medius and gluteus minimus, assisted by the piriformis muscle (which also has an extension function) and the short hip rotator muscles: the superior and inferior twin, the internal obturator, the quadratus femoris. In addition to playing a role in external rotation, these muscles are also hip adductors. The main adductors of the upper leg all originate on the pubic bone and insert distally on the femur below the level of the small trochanter or, in the case of the gracilis muscle, in the medial portion of the tibia (where it collaborates in the formation of the pes anserinus).
In proximal-distal order, the adductor muscles are: the pectineus and the adductor longus, and deeper the adductor brevis muscle and finally the adductor magnus muscle. The latter is a deeply situated flat muscle. It originates from the anterior aspect of the ischiopubic branch and the ischial tuberosity, and ends by attaching to the medial edge of the linea aspera up to almost the medial condyle. The insertion of the adductor magnus is interrupted by a series of openings which give passage to the perforating vessels. The last of these is called the adductor magnus hiatus and gives passage to the femoral artery which at this level continues as the popliteal artery. All the adductor muscles are innervated by the obturator nerve.

Fasciae

The hip muscles and upper leg are wrapped in a fibrous sheath called the fascia lata. The fascia lata inserts proximally to the inguinal ligament, the iliac crest lip, the posterior aspect of the sacrum, the ischial tuberosity, the body of the pubis and the pubic tubercle. Distally it continues into the crural fascia, proximally with the fasciae of the abdominal wall.
The fascia lata is thicker laterally than medially, in fact laterally it has a longitudinal reinforcement called the iliotibial band (or tract). The iliotibial band can also be considered the conjoint tendon of the tensor fascia lata and the gluteus maximus. It has an extensive insertion on the lateral intermuscular septum, and distally inserts into the Gerdy tubercle. The iliotibial tract significantly affects the lateral hip and knee stability by reducing shear forces at the level of the femur [28]. It is also frequently involved in overuse syndromes, especially in cyclists and runners.
Symptoms are usually referred to the lateral region of the knee, and were previously attributed to the band friction on the lateral condyle of the femur. However, Fairclough et al. [8] demonstrated that the iliotibial tract can only increase its tension during flexion-extension movements of the knee. This is because, being the iliotibial band part of the fascia lata that wraps around the whole leg and closely connected to the lateral intermuscular septum, it cannot be involved in friction movements in an antero-posterior direction. In fact, it has been demonstrated [24] that the fascia lata is maintained in a basal tension by a series of myofascial expansions. Among the most important ones that stretch the fascia lata proximally are those of the gluteus maximus (it is estimated that about 80% of the fibres of the gluteus maximus insert directly or via the lateral intermuscular septum onto the fascia lata) and the tensor fascia lata (which inserts entirely onto the fascia lata). While those of the vastus medialis and lateralis stretch the fascia distally. The fascia lata also receives myofascial expansions from the abdominal muscles. In particular, the contralateral external oblique gives an oblique expansion that crosses the pubic symphysis to proximally stretch the antero-medial part of the contralateral fascia lata.
The sartorius and tensor fascia lata muscles are wrapped in their own sheath, derived from the fascia lata. This allows them to contract independently from the surrounding muscles. In particular, the sartorius muscle, having a very oblique course, is free to slide within its sheath (sartorius sheath) thanks to the presence of abundant loose connective tissue rich in hyaluronic acid.

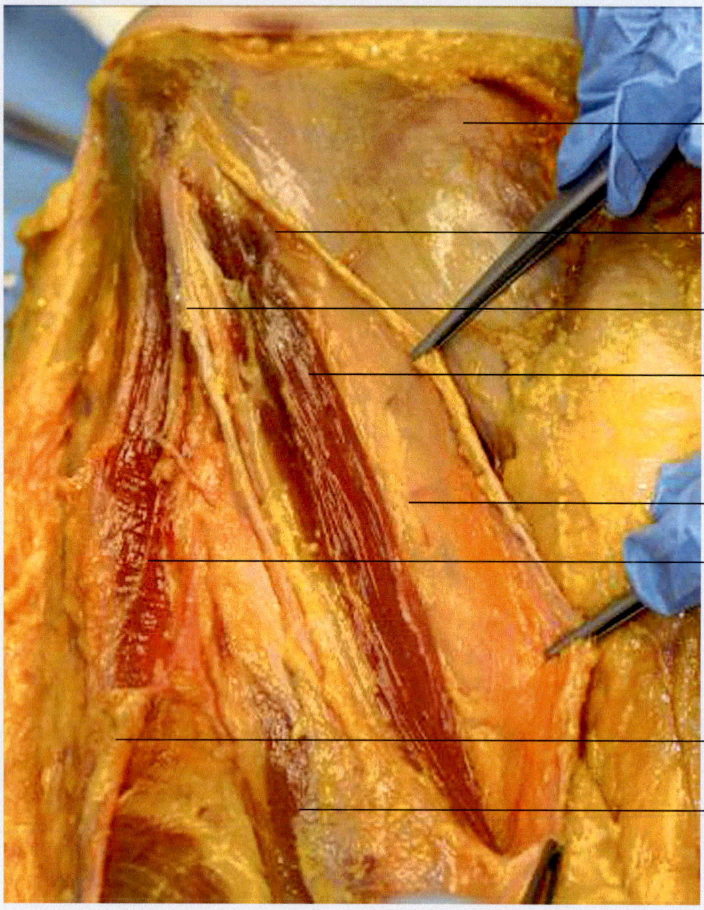

Figure 10 Anterior thigh region, fresh specimen dissection. The sartorius fascia was incised to show the sartorius muscle enveloped by its epimysium. Between the muscle and the fascial sheath there is always some loose connective tissue which facilitates the sliding between muscle and fascia. Note the close relationship between the lateral femoral cutaneous nerve of the thigh and the sartorius sheath

The innominate fascia or deep fascia lata sheet is located below the rectus femoris. This is a thick quadrangular fibrous sheet that connects the deep part of the tensor fascia lata and the rectus femoris muscle. Below this fascial plane runs the lateral circumflex artery of the femur.

In recent years, numerous functions have been attributed to the muscle fasciae. In particular, being a scarcely elastic tissue, they are able to limit the enlargement of the thigh muscles during their contraction, thus improving the efficiency of their contractions. They also facilitate venous return, especially in the lower limbs, by assisting the muscle pump. Yaman et al. [30] also showed that only 65% of muscle fibres insert at the tendon insertion. The other 35 % insert into the perimuscular connective tissue. The fasciae can therefore be considered as an element that assists the tendon in the transmission of muscle forces at a distance, limiting the concentration of mechanical forces at the enthesis [2].

Fasciae are a well innervated tissue [26], with a predominantly proprioceptive innervation (including Pacini and Ruffini corpuscles). Therefore, they can be considered as the key organ responsible for the body's proprioception, both static and dynamic (Stecco et al, 2007). However, for this action to take place, it is essential that the fasciae have adequate basal tension. This derives from the presence of various muscle expansions. These muscle insertions on the fascia are always present and have a specific spatial arrangement. This allows the underlying muscles to selectively stretch the fascia ac-

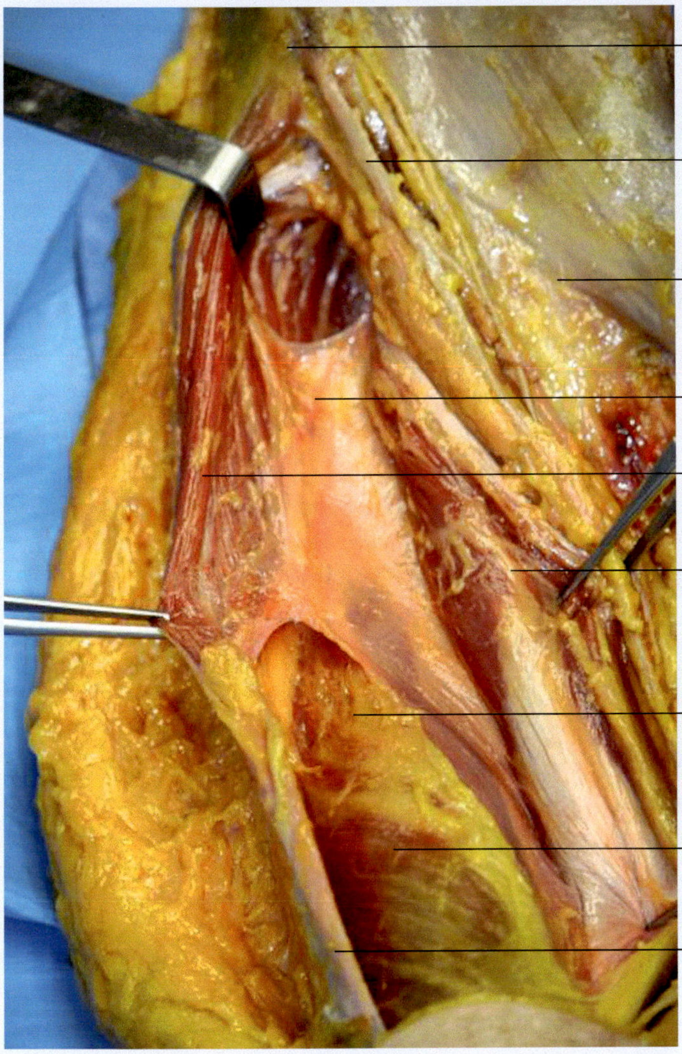

Figure 11 Dissection of the anterior region of the thigh, fresh specimen. The fascia lata has been incised, the sartorius and rectus femoris muscles have been retracted medially and the tensor fascia lata laterally, to show the innominate fascia (or deep fascia lata sheet). Note how this fascia allows a strong connection between these three muscles, which are all involved in hip flexion. If the coordinating role of these fasciae is confirmed, an interruption of this fascia could alter the peripheral motor coordination between these three muscles

cording to the activated muscle fibres. As a result, the stretching receptors within the fascia are activated, helping the CNS to perceive movement correctly. If the fascia becomes fibrous or adherent, or if the fascial continuity is interrupted, the receptors may give abnormal signals, from altered proprioception to pain. Pathological changes in the innervation of the fascia have been described by Sanchis-Alfonso & Rosello-Sastre (2000). They reported an increase in nociceptive fibres, reactive to substance P, in the fascia lata and retinaculum of the knee in subjects with patellofemoral syndrome.

Finally, the fascia lata seems to play a role in peripheral motor coordination. This is because it connects several synergistic muscles and, at the same time, separates antagonistic muscles. Being a connective tissue, the fascia is very much affected by the mechanical forces acting on it, and if damaged it quickly develops scarring processes. However, in order to recover its coordinating and proprioceptive role, it is essential that the fascia heals in its correct basal tension and length.

Hip joint kinematics

The pelvis bears most of the body's weight. For this reason, the coxofemoral joint is a much less free-moving enarthrosis than the scapulohumeral joint. The two femurs, through their respective heads, articulate deeply in their acetabula with a medial inclination that, together with the pelvis, forms an exceptional dynamic bridge. In addition, this joint is surrounded by large, powerful muscles, which dynamically stabilise the joint. The combined effect of body weight and muscular forces results in the femoral head being subjected to a force of approximately four times the body weight in the single limb stance phase. In normal locomotion, the hip is subject to wide fluctuations in compression load. The factors that influence the magnitude and direction of the compressive forces acting on the femoral head, are mainly the position of the centre of gravity and the lever arm of the abductor muscles (small and medium gluteus in primis). A reduction in the lever arm of the abductor muscles (an example would be the coxa valga) results in an increase in muscle activity and thus in the resulting force on the joint. The loads acting on the hip also vary according to body weight, body position and external forces applied.

The pelvis is placed at the centre of the kinematic chain of the body. An alteration of the hip joint kinematics is biomechanically reflected in both the superior and inferior skeleton areas. Equally, alterations in the spine kinematics or knee negatively affect the hip. For example, when walking with stiff knees, the pelvis would move parallel to itself, the body's centre of gravity would describe a very undulating path. This would result in a jerky and energy-consuming walk. In reality, the human walks using coordinated movements of the hip and knee joints, the ankle and the pelvis. This keeps his centre of gravity on a horizontal plane. The reduction of vertical oscillations is achieved by rotating the pelvis around an axis passing through the lumbar region of the spine. Seen from above, one side of the pelvis moves forward along with the limb that swings forward. Therefore, in the sagittal plane, the angle between the pelvis and the leg is reduced, as well as the angle between the limb and the ground. At the same time, on the frontal plane, the pelvis is lowered on the swinging limb side and the knee of the supporting limb is flexed. The centre of gravity shifts so that its perpendicular falls within the base of support. The lateral displacement of the centre of gravity is approximately 20 mm per side. This gait increases stride length without increasing the degree of hip flexion and extension. As people age, walking changes because the range of motion of the joints is reduced. If the strength of the hip abductor muscles (primarily the gluteus medius) is reduced, the force of gravity is no longer balanced in single-leg stance. Therefore, a lateral displacement of the trunk towards the side of weakness occurs. The centre of gravity is shifted so that the body is balanced on the limb with minimal muscular support at the hip. In order to prevent the fall, the trunk moves towards the side in support (Duchenne-Trendelenburg sign).

Bibliography

1. Beck M, Sledge JB, Gautier E, Dora CF, Ganz R. The anatomy and function of the gluteus minimus muscle. J Bone Joint Surg Br. 2000, 82:358-63.
2. Benjamin M. The fascia of the limbs and back a review. J Anat. 2009;214:1-18.
3. Birnbaum K, Prescher A, Hessler S, Heller KD. The sensory innervation of the hip joint an anatomical study. Surg Radiol Anat. 1997;19:371-5.
4. Byrd JW. Hip arthroscopy utilizing the supine position. Arthroscopy. 1994;10:275-80.
5. Byrd JW. Indications and contraindications. In: Byrd JW. Operative Hip Arthroscopy, 2nd ed, Springer Science + Business Media, 2005.
6. Campbell JD, Higgs R, Wright K, Leaver-Dunn D, Pevis, Guskiewicz KM, Holmes CF, Schenck RC. Hip and thigh injuries. Athletic Training and Sports Medicine. Rosemount: American Academy of Orthopaedic Surgeons, 399.
7. Edelson JG, Nathan H. Meralgia paresthetica, An anatomical interpretation. Clin Orthop Relat Res. 1997;122:255-62.
8. Fairclough J, Hayashi K, Toumi H, Lyons K, By-

dder G, et al. The functional anatomy of the iliotibial band during flexion and extension of the knee: implications for understanding iliotibial band syndrome. J Anat. 2006;208:309-16.
9. Ferguson SJ, Bryant JT, Ganz R, Ito K. An in vitro investigation of the acetabular labral seal in hip joint mechanics. J Biomech. 2003;36:171-8.
10. Grant JCB. An atlas of anatomy. 3rd ed., London: Bailliere, Tindall and Cox, 1951.
11. Gray AJ, Villar RN. The ligamentum teres of the hip: an arthroscopic classification of its pathology. Arthroscopy.1997;13:575-8.
12. Grose AW, Gardner MJ, Sussmann PS, Helfet DL, Lorich DG. The surgical anatomy of the blood supply to the femoral head: description of the anastomosis between the medial femoral circumflex and inferior gluteal arteries at the hip. J Bone Joint Surg Br. 2008;90:1298-1303.
13. Hoppenfeld S, deBoer P. Surgical Exposures in Orthopaedics. Philadelphia: Lippincott Williams and Wilkins, 2003.
14. Kim YH. Acetabular dysplasia and osteoarthritis developed by an eversion of the acetabular labrum. Clin Orthop Relat Res. 1987;215:289-95.
15. Martins RS, Siqueira MG, Silva FC Jr, Heise CO, Teixeira MJ. A practical approach to the lateral cutaneous nerve of the thigh: an anatomical study. Clin Neurol Neurosurg. 2011;113:868-71.
16. McCarthy J, Barsoum W, Puri L et al. The role of hip arthroscopy in the elite athlete. Clin Orthop Relat Res. 2003;406:71-4.
17. Moore K. Clinically Oriented Anatomy. 3rd ed, Baltimore: Williams and Wilkins, 1992.
18. Philippon M, Schenker M, Briggs K, Kuppersmith D. Femoroacetabular impingement in 45 professional athletes: associated pathologies and return to sport following arthroscopic decompression. Knee Surg Sports Traumatol Arthrosc. 2007;15:908-14.
19. Schuenke M, Schulte E, Schumacher U, Ross L, Lamperti E. Atlas of Anatomy, General Anatomy of the Musculoskeletal System. New York: Thieme, 2006.
20. Seldes RM, Tan V, Hunt J, Katz M, Winiarsky R, Fitzgerald RH Jr. Anatomy, histologic features and vascularity of the adult acetabular labrum. Clin Orthop Relat Res. 2001;382:232-240.
21. Stecco C, Gagey O, Belloni A, Pozzuoli A, Porzionato A, Macchi V, Aldegheri R, De Caro R, Delmas V. Anatomy of the deep fascia of the upper limb. Second part: study of innervation. Morphologie. 2007;91:38-43.
22. Stecco C, Gagey O, Macchi V, Porzionato A, De Caro R, Aldegheri R, Delmas V. Tendinous muscular insertions onto the deep fascia of the upper limb. First part: anatomical study. Morphologie. 2007;91:29-37.
23. Stecco C, Porzionato A, Macchi V, Stecco A, Vigato E, Parenti A, Delmas V, Aldegheri R, De Caro R. The expansions of the pectoral girdle muscles onto the brachial fascia: morphological aspects and spatial disposition. Cells Tissues Organs. 2008;188:320-9.
24. Stecco A, Gillard W, Robert H, Fullerton B, Stecco C. The anatomical and functional relation between gluteus maximus and fascia lata. J Bodyw Mov Ther. 2013;17:512-7.
25. Tanabe H. Aging process of the acetabular labrum an electron microscopic study. Nippon Seikeigeka Gakkai Zasshi. 1991;65:18-25.
26. Tesarz J, Hoheisel U, Wiedenhöfer B, Mense S. Sensory innervation of the thoracolumbar fascia in rats and humans. Neuroscience. 2011;194:302-8.
27. Türker M, Kılıçoğlu Ö, Göksan B, Bilgiç B. Vascularity and histology of fetal labrum and chondrolabral junction: its relevance to chondrolabral detachment tears. Knee Surg Sports Traumatol Arthrosc. 2012;20:381-6.
28. Vieira EL, Vieira EA, da Silva RT, Berlfein PA, et al. An anatomic study of the iliotibial tract. Arthroscopy. 2007;23(3):269-74.
29. Walters J, Solomons M, Davies J. Gluteus minimus: observations on its insertion. J Anat. 2001;198:239-242.
30. Yaman A, Ozturk C, Huijing PA, Yucesoy CA. Magnetic resonance imaging assessment of mechanical interactions between human lower leg muscles in vivo. J Biomech Eng. 2013;135(9):91003.

3

Surgical anatomy and minimally invasive approaches in hip arthroplasty

Sergio Candiotto*, Antonio Camporese*, Elisa Pala**, Pietro Ruggieri**

*Hip and Shoulder Surgery Unit, Abano Terme General Hospital, Padua, Italy
**Department of Orthopaedics and Orthopaedic Oncology, University of Padova, Italy

Introduction

Minimally invasive surgical approaches replicate the steps of traditional approaches except for the advantages concerning the extent of the skin incision and the severity of muscle damage ('muscle sparing, not muscle splitting or muscle detachment' Franz Rauchbauer). The anterior minimally invasive approach is quite similar to Carl Hueter's original version, while the variations introduced in the other minimally invasive approaches (anterolateral, lateral and posterior) are more elaborate. Figure 1 shows schematically the sites of the different surgical incisions proposed for the minimally invasive surgical approaches to the hip.

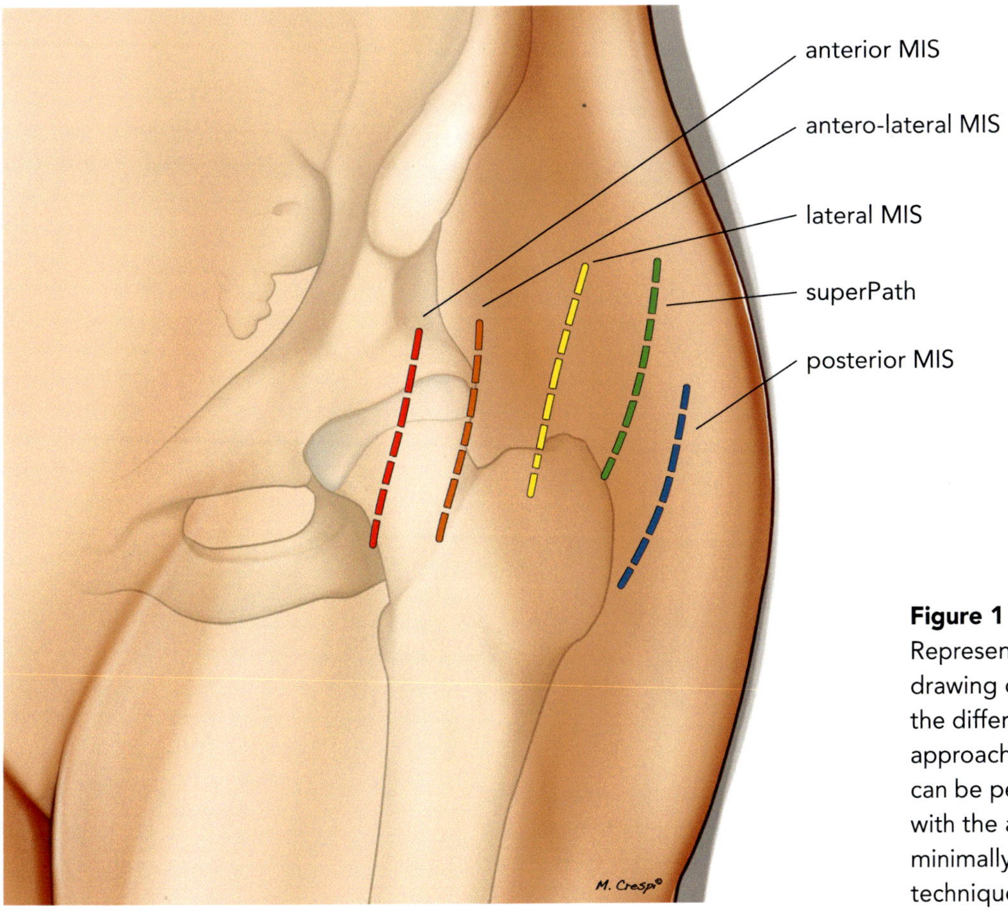

Figure 1
Representative drawing of the different approaches that can be performed with the anterior minimally invasive technique

Minimally invasive anterior approach

This surgical approach actually replicates Carl Hueter's historic anterior approach, but reduces its extent (fig. 3). It uses the same pathway between the superficial and deep nerve and muscle structures to perform the joint exposure. It is known by the acronym DAA ('direct anterior approach') and does not involve muscle-tendon detachment from the bone. It also does not violate the integrity of delicate lateral structures such as the iliotibial band, the greater trochanter and the abductor muscle-tendon complex represented by the gluteal muscles.

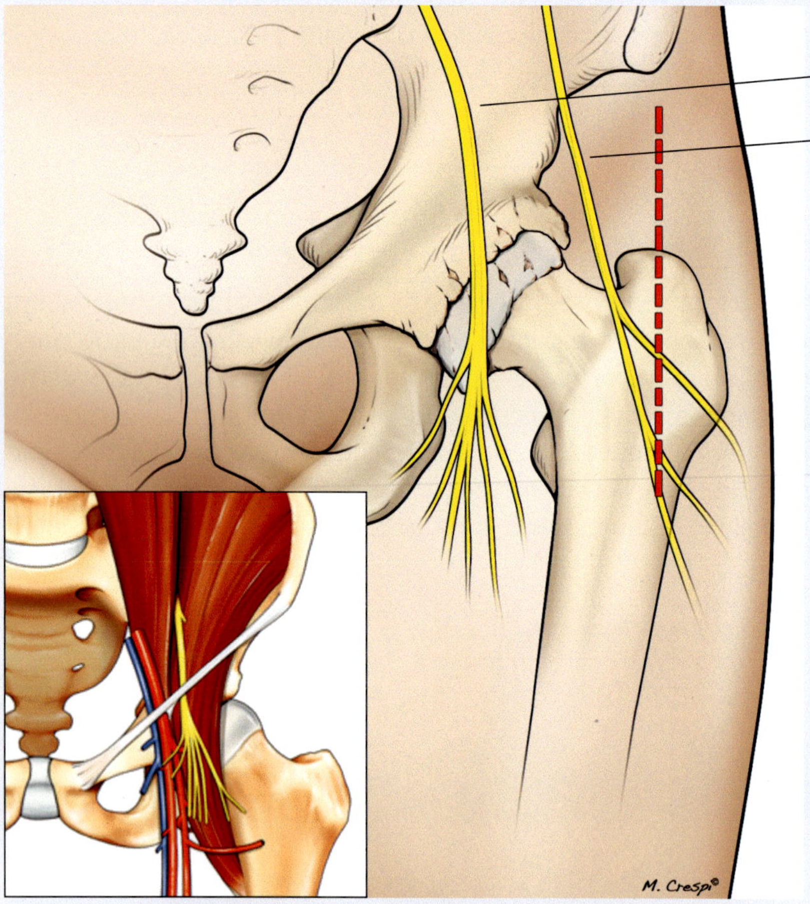

Figure 2 Anatomical landmarks to be considered in the minimally invasive anterior approach and the relationships with the femoral vascular-nerve bundle and the lateral femoral cutaneous nerve

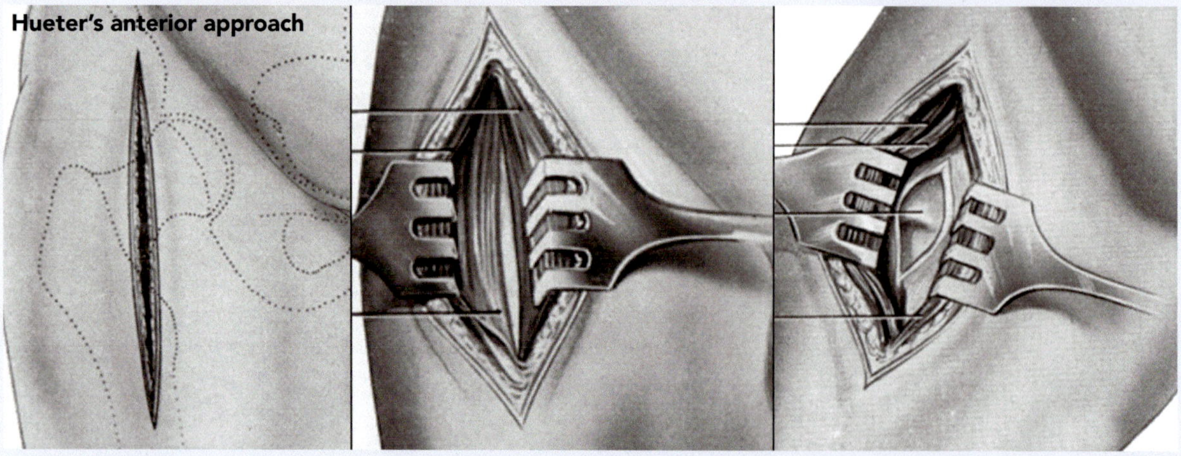

Figure 3 Scheme of the original anterior surgical approach, proposed in 1881 by Carl Hueter in Magdeburg, from which the currently used minimally invasive anterior approaches were also derived. From Stefano Teneff: Tecnica Chirurgica Ortopedica e Traumatologica (Orthopaedic and Traumatological Surgical Technique). Courtesy of Società Editrice Universo, Rome 1966.

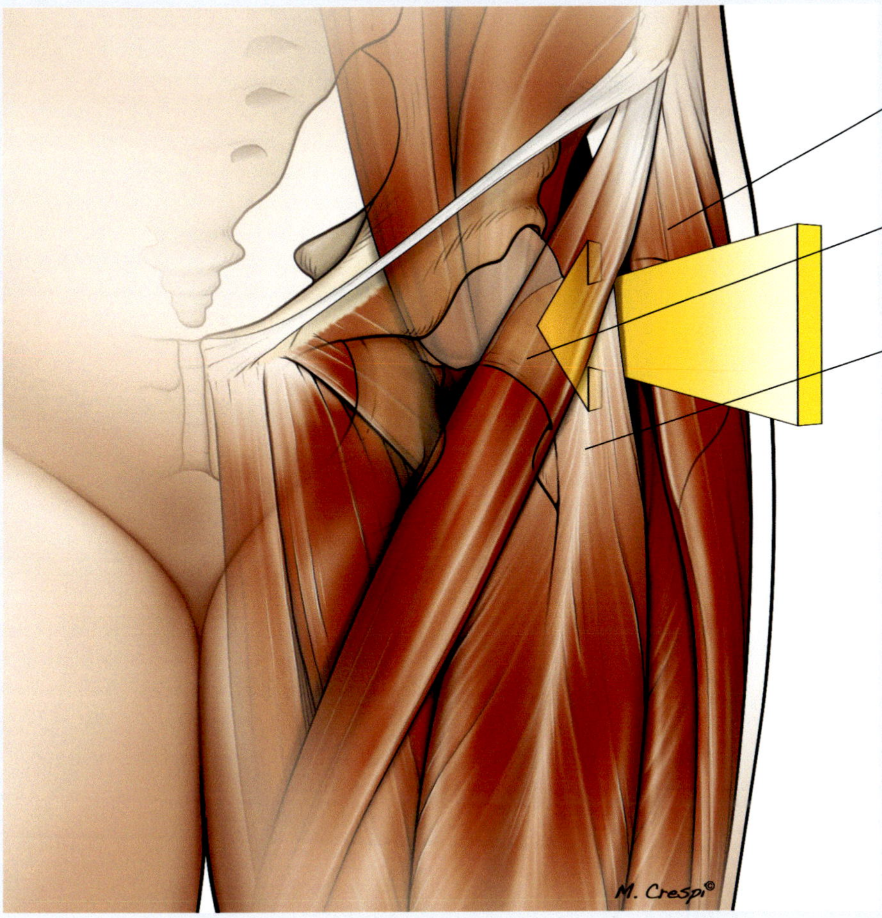

Figure 4A
A) Anatomical layers on the frontal plane.

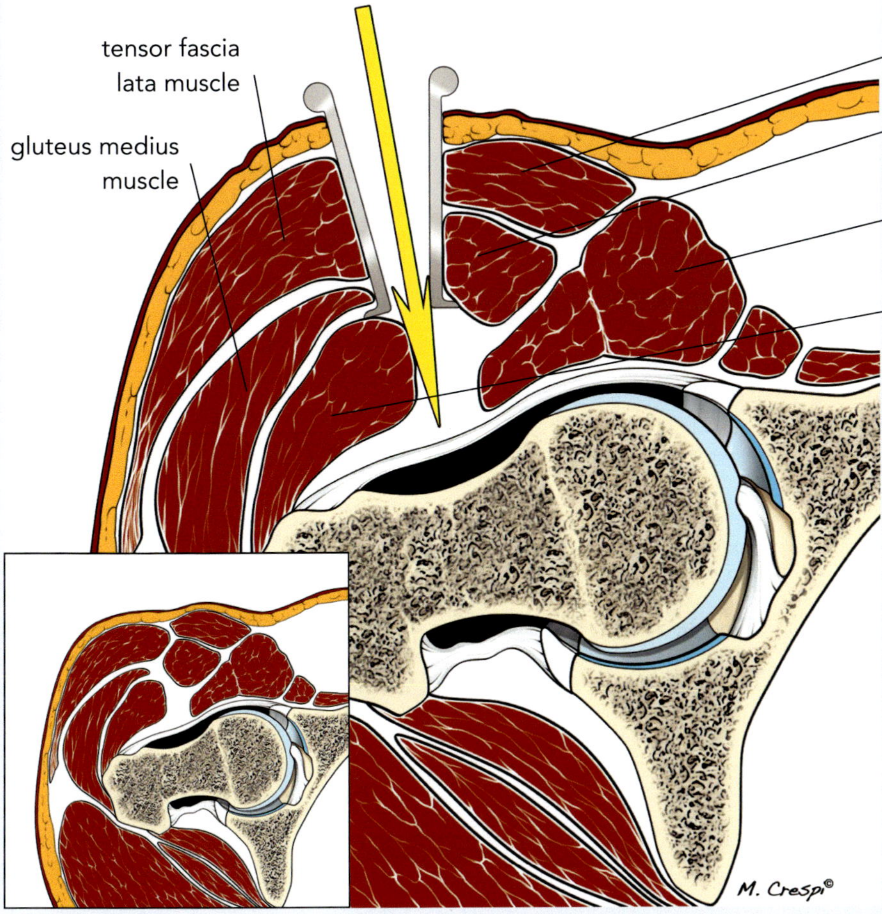

Figure 4B
B) Anatomical planes in the transverse plane. In the superficial layer the muscle space between the sartorius and tensor fascia lata muscles is used. In a deeper layer the space is between the gluteus medius/minimus and rectus femoris

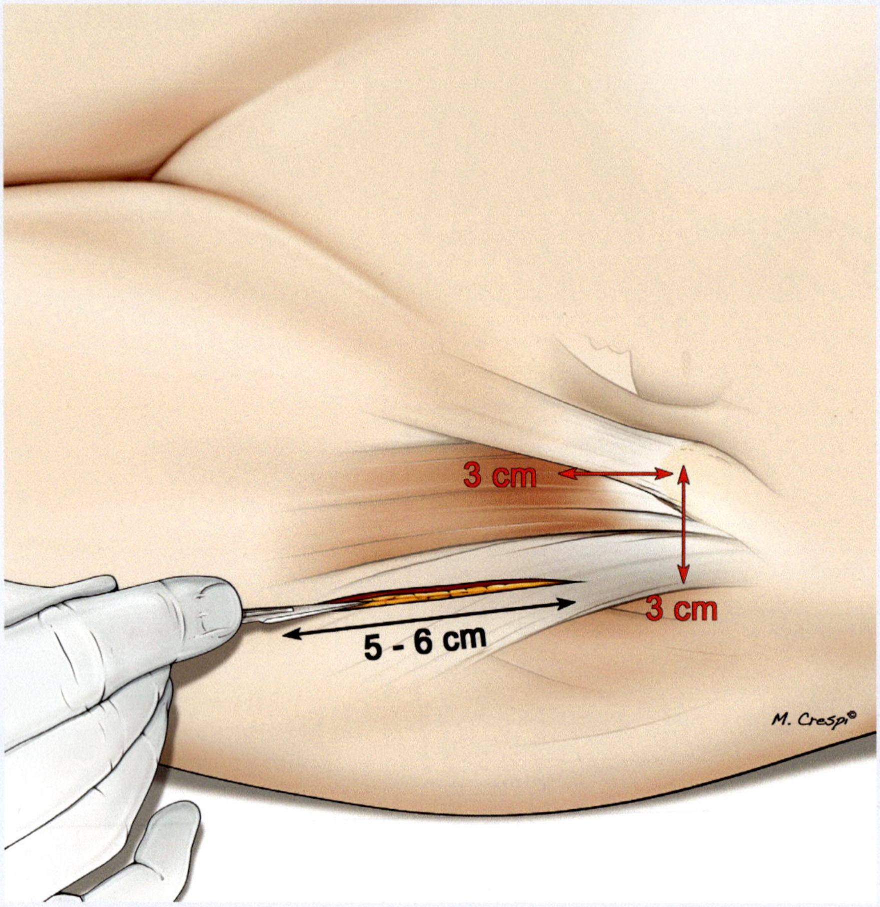

Figure 5
The skin incision is straight/longitudinal, starting two centimetres distal/lateral to the anterior superior iliac spine and extending 5-6 cm towards the external patellar margin

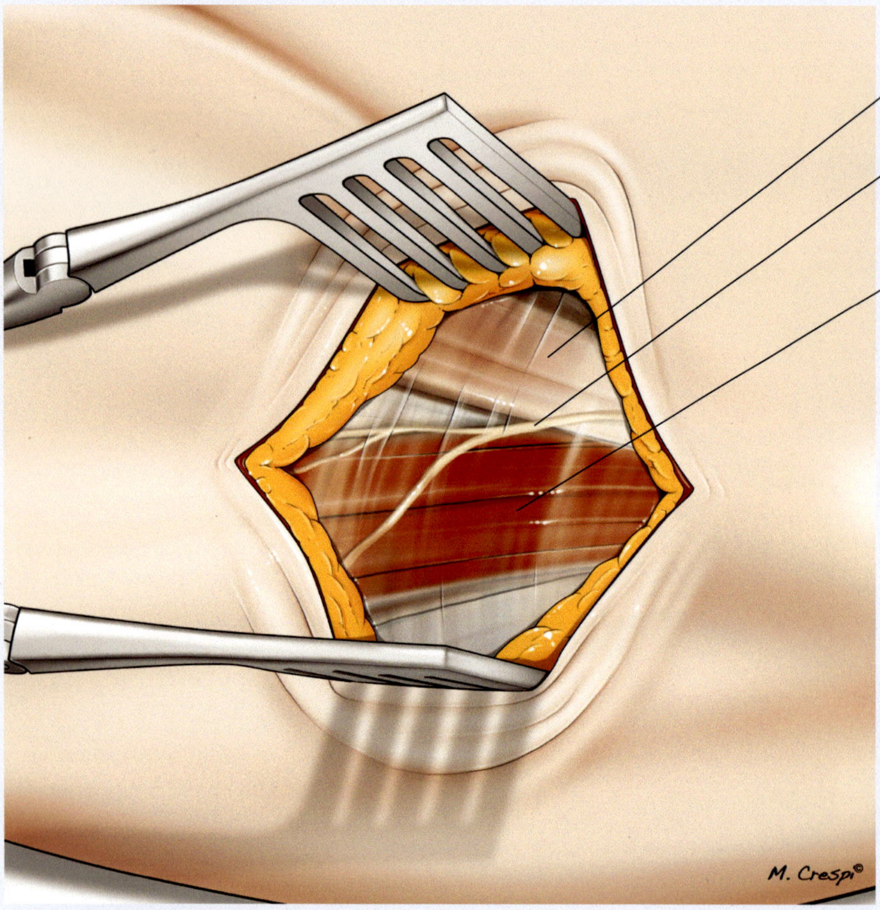

sartorius muscle

lateral cutaneous nerve of thigh

tensor fascia lata muscle

Figure 6
When the skin flaps are retracted, the fascia lata is exposed and the lateral cutaneous nerve of the thigh and some of its lateral branches can be identified. The nerve is usually located between the sartorius muscle and the tensor fascia lata muscle

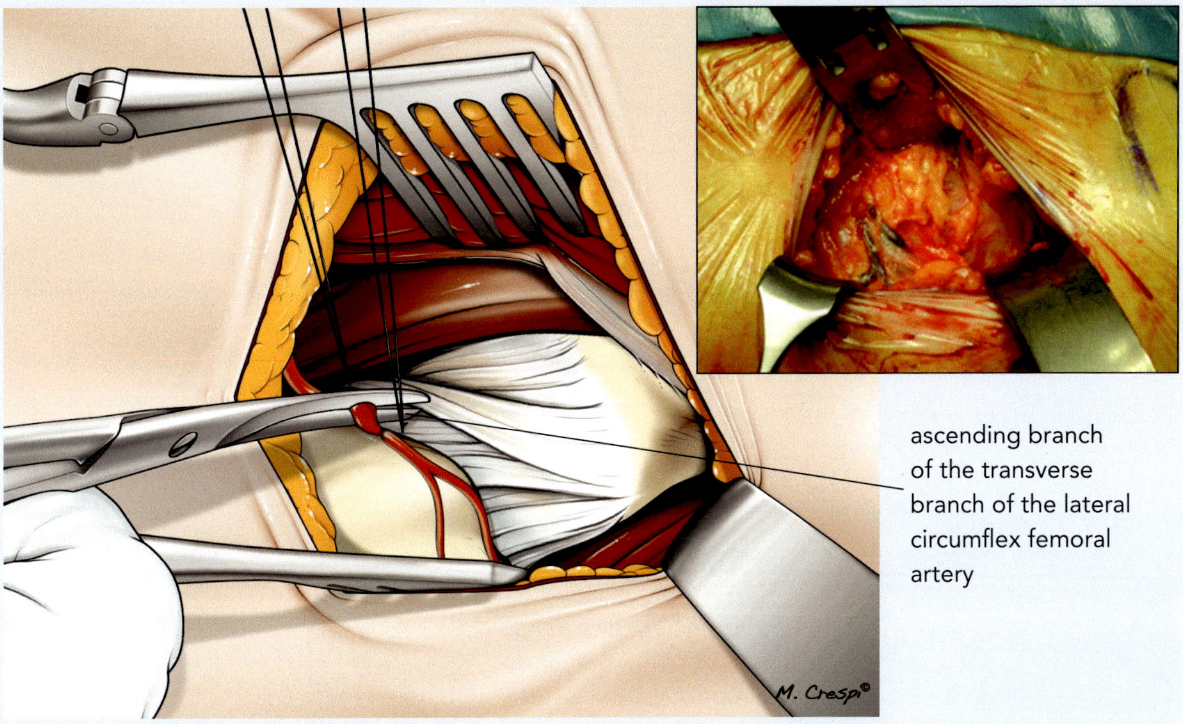

Figure 7 The surgical approach to the joint involves the separation and retraction of the sartorius and the tensor fascia lata superficially, and of the gluteus medius and rectus femoris in depth. The transverse arterial branch of the ascending artery should always be identified and ligated. This is derived from the lateral femoral circumflex artery which originates from the deep femoral. Ligation is necessary to avoid the risk of significant post-operative haematomas due to reopening of the vessels after electrocoagulation alone

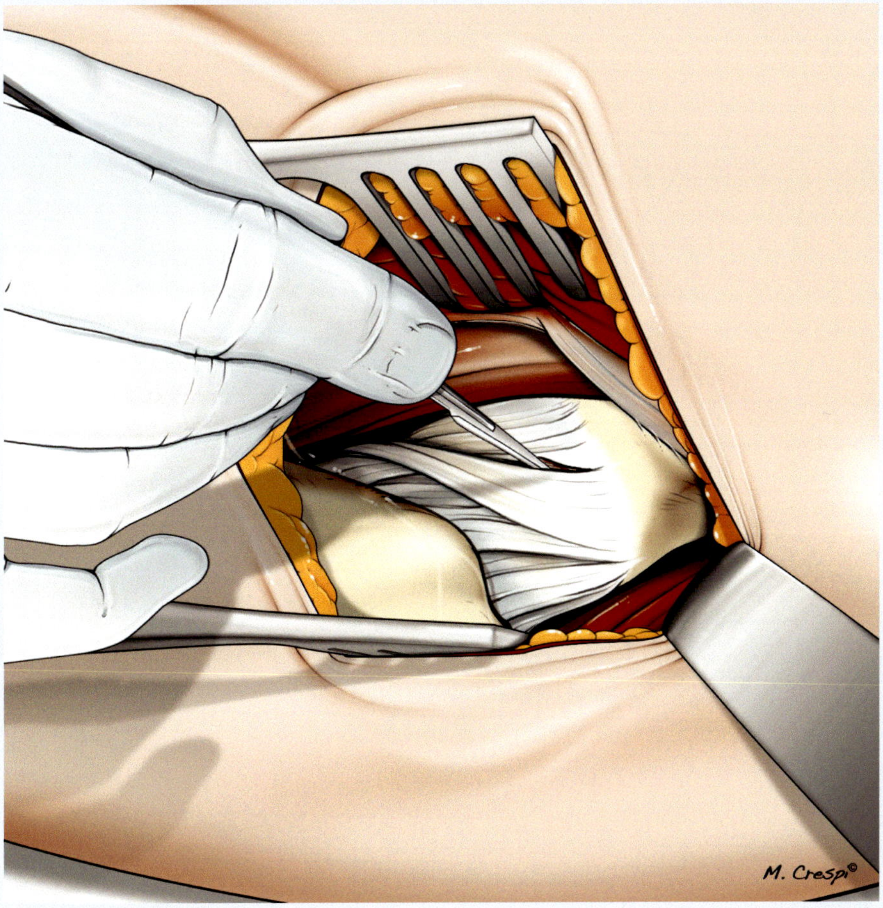

Figure 8
Complete exposure of the articular layer and anterior capsulotomy

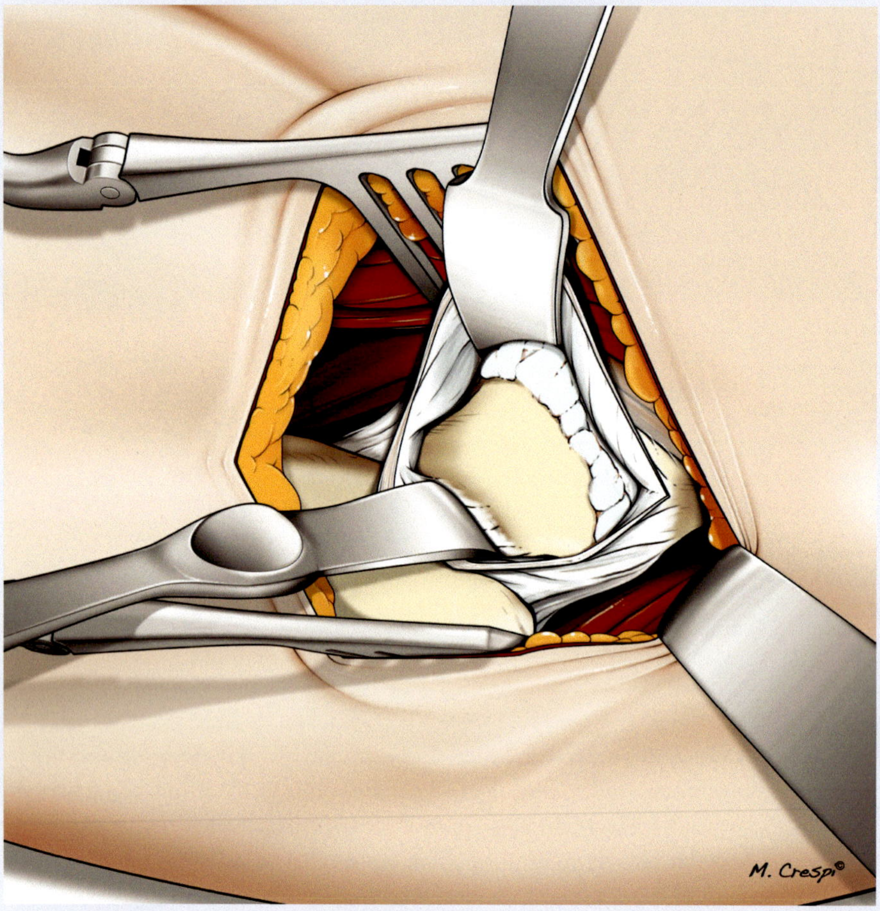

Figure 9
Incision and retraction of the capsule, with hip arthrotomy

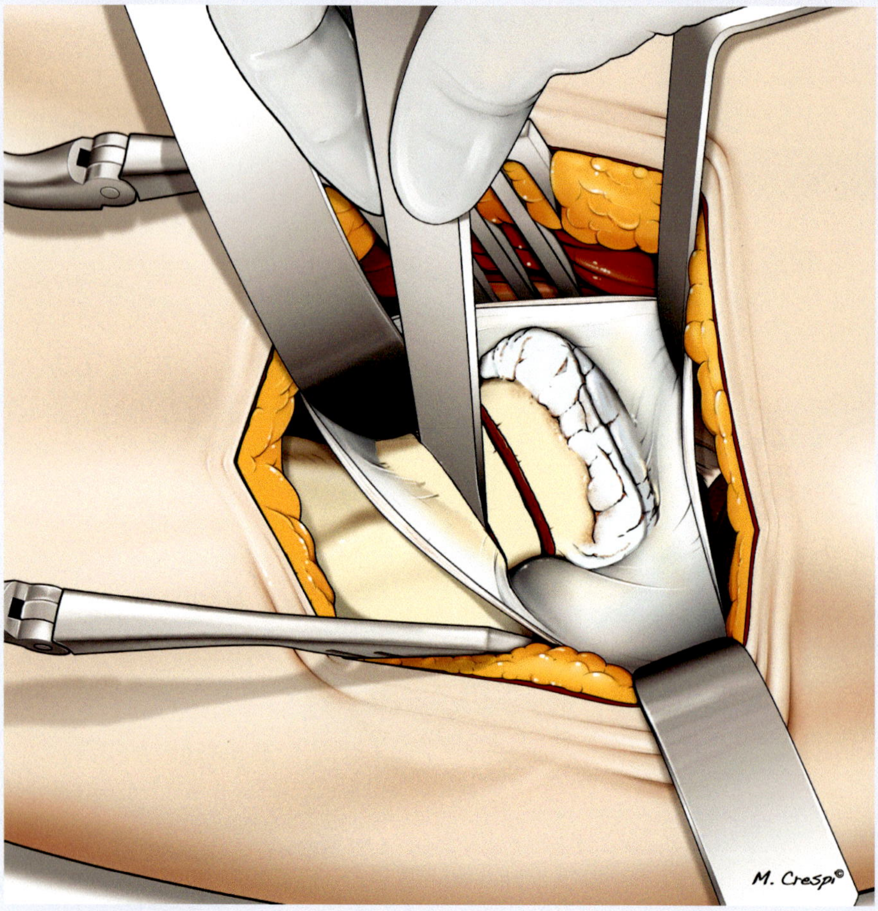

Figure 10
Osteotomy of the femoral neck and removal of the dissected bone portion ('wafer technique') to create space and thus facilitate the subsequent extraction of the femoral head

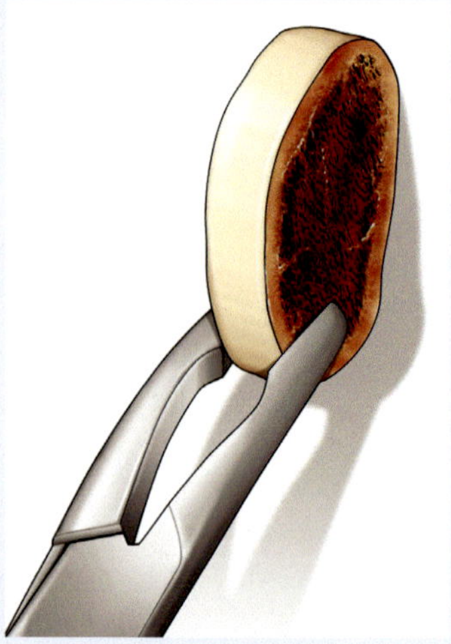

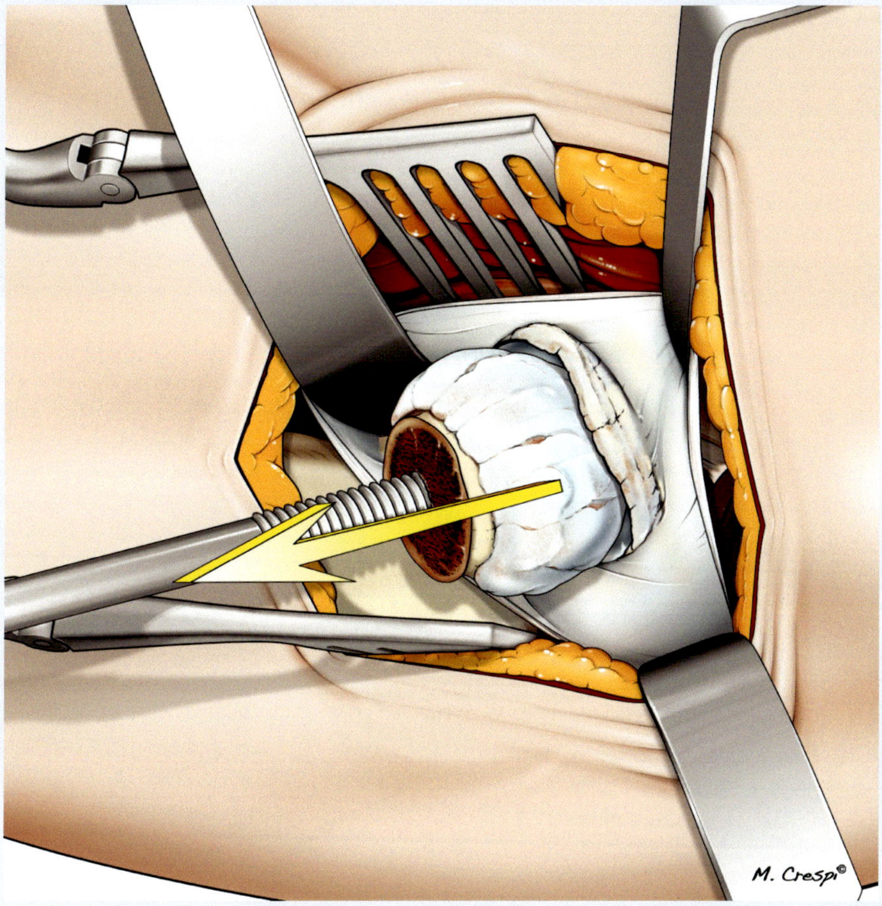

Figure 11 The femoral head is removed using the appropriate extractor

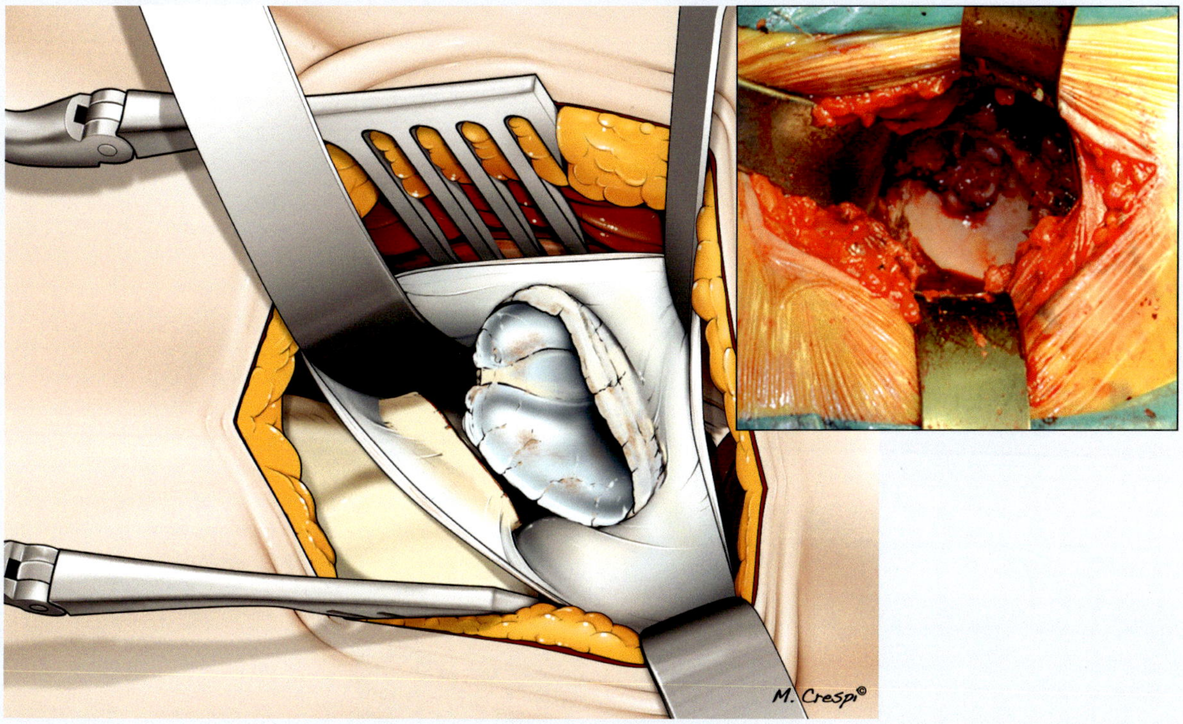

Figure 12 Exposure of the acetabulum. This is easy with this minimally invasive anterior approach. To avoid vascular and nerve damage the levers (modified Hohmann) should always be placed in close contact with the acetabular bone. They should not be placed in excessive traction and should be released appropriately and frequently during the acetabular preparation phase. We do not use the Charnley retractor to reduce the tension on the soft tissues

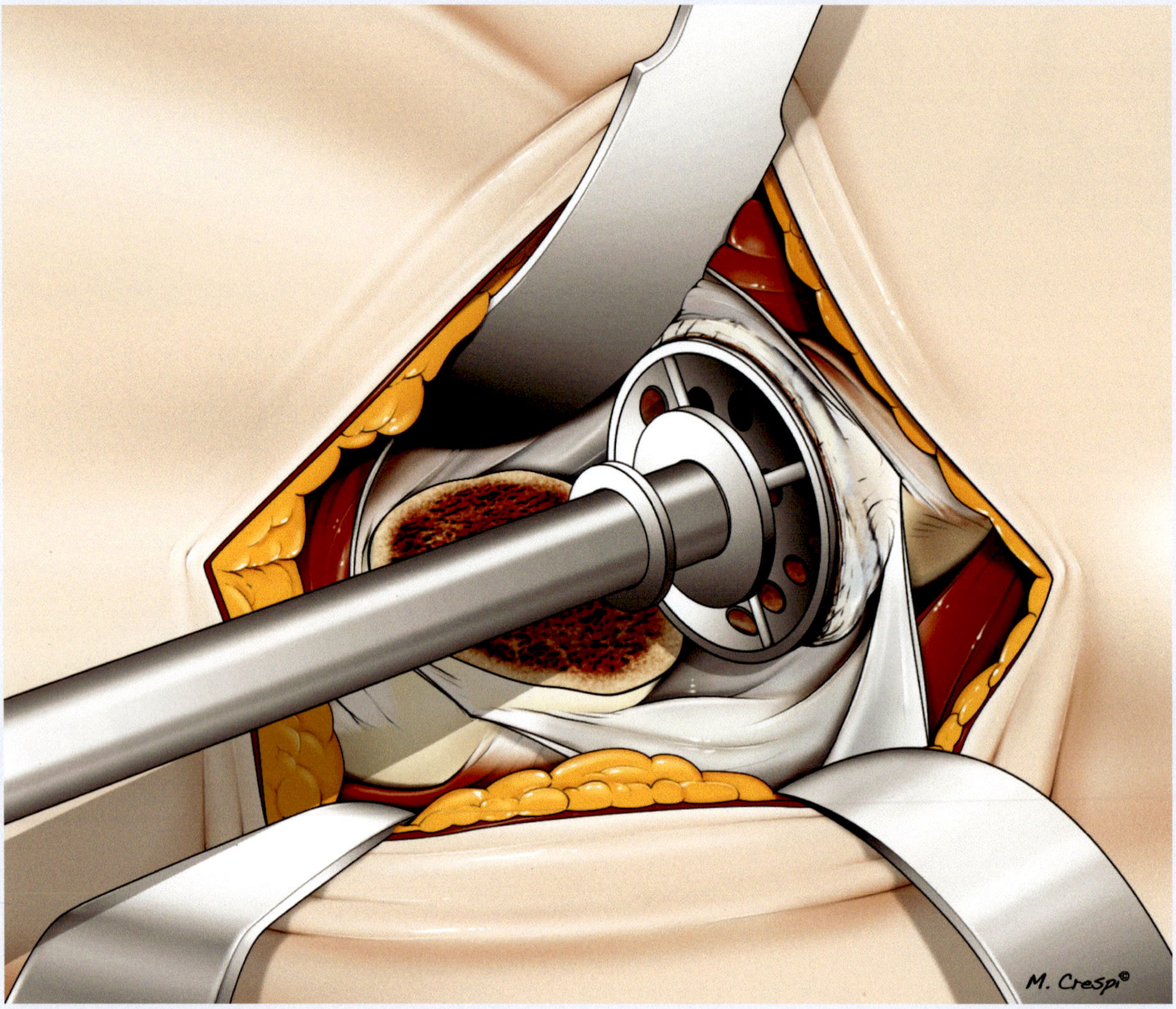

Figure 13 Preparation with hemispherical reamers of the acetabulum

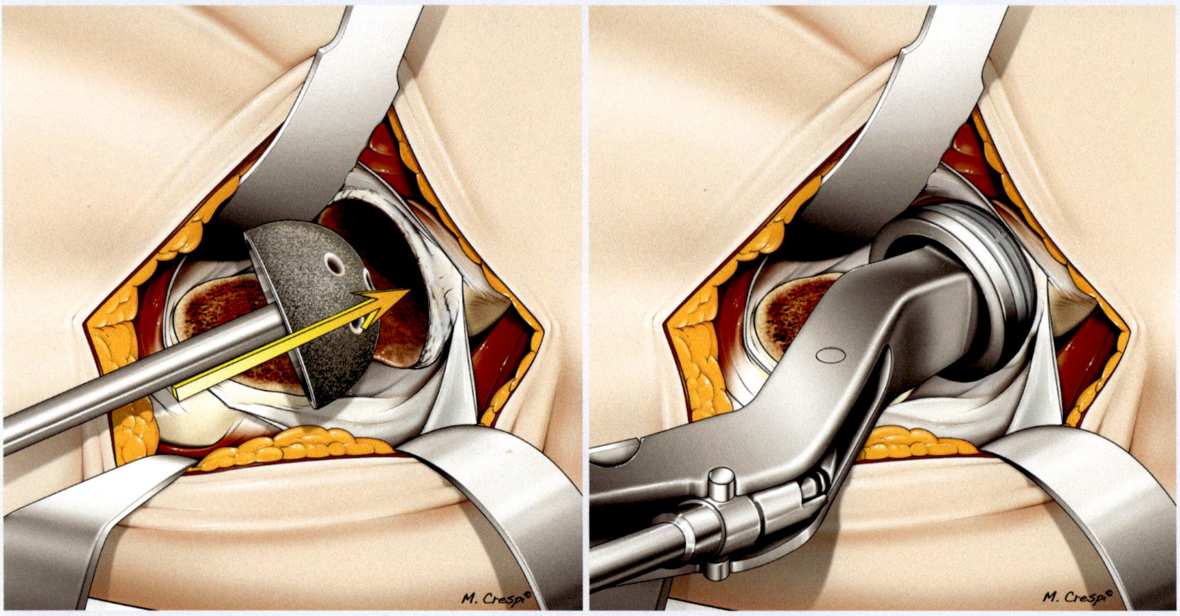

Figure 14 Insertion of the cup by applying pressure. The diameter of the cup is closely related to the diameter of the hemispherical reamer used for preparation. Both offset and straight handles can be used for cup insertion

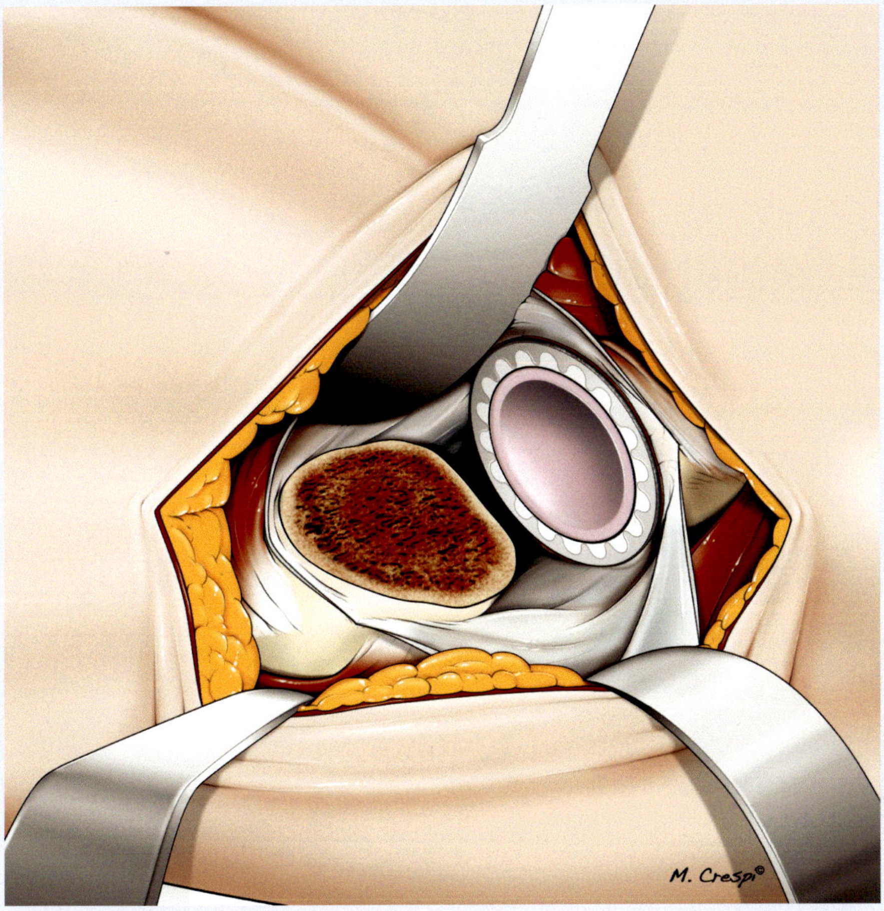

Figure 15
Metal cup and ceramic insert are placed with the appropriate abduction and anteversion angles

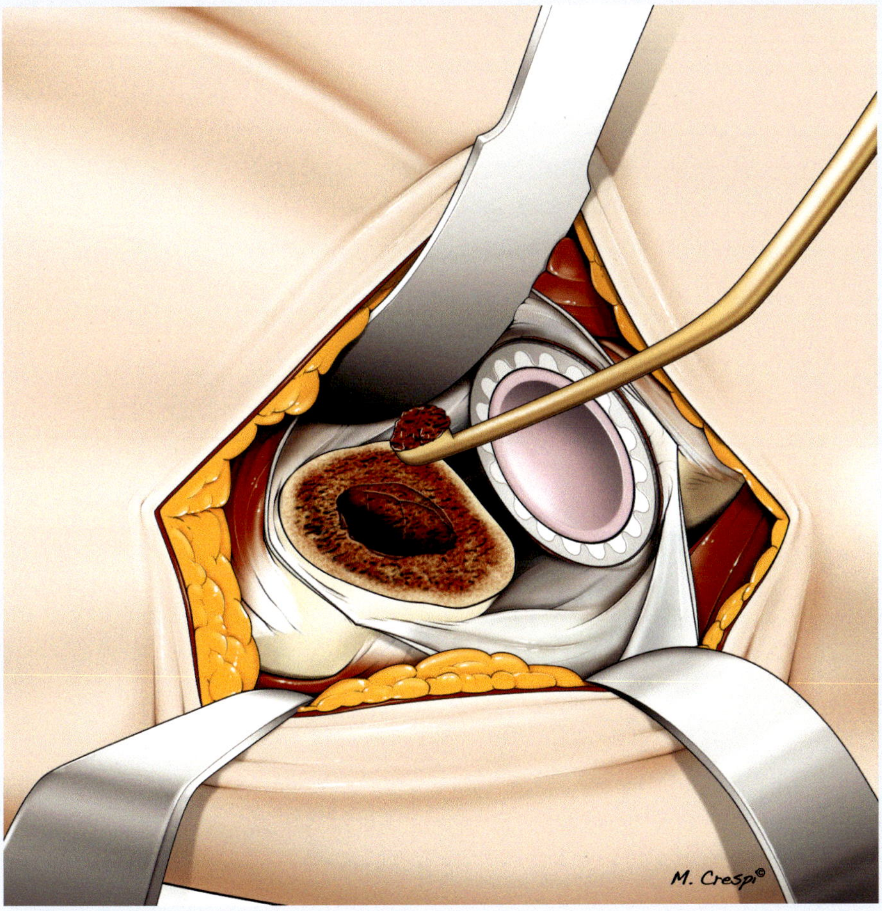

Figure 16
A curved spoon is used to access the femoral diaphyseal canal

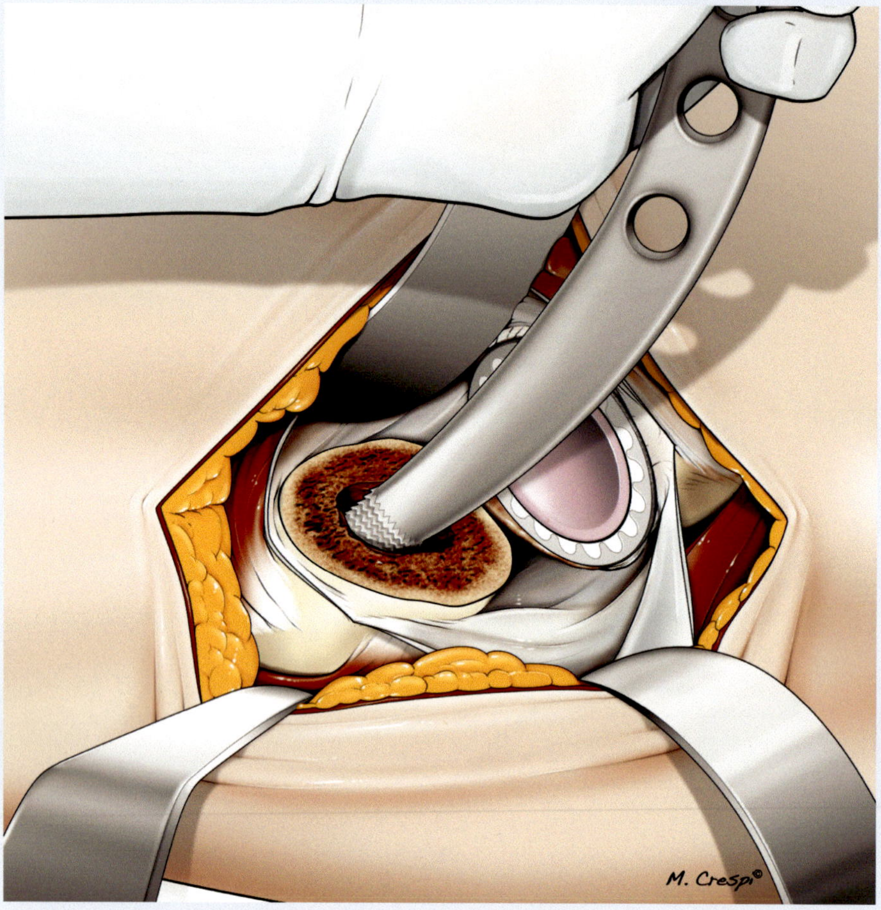

Figure 17
The curved ('banana') rasp widens the access to the diaphyseal canal, reducing the risk of a wrong direction when inserting the broaches

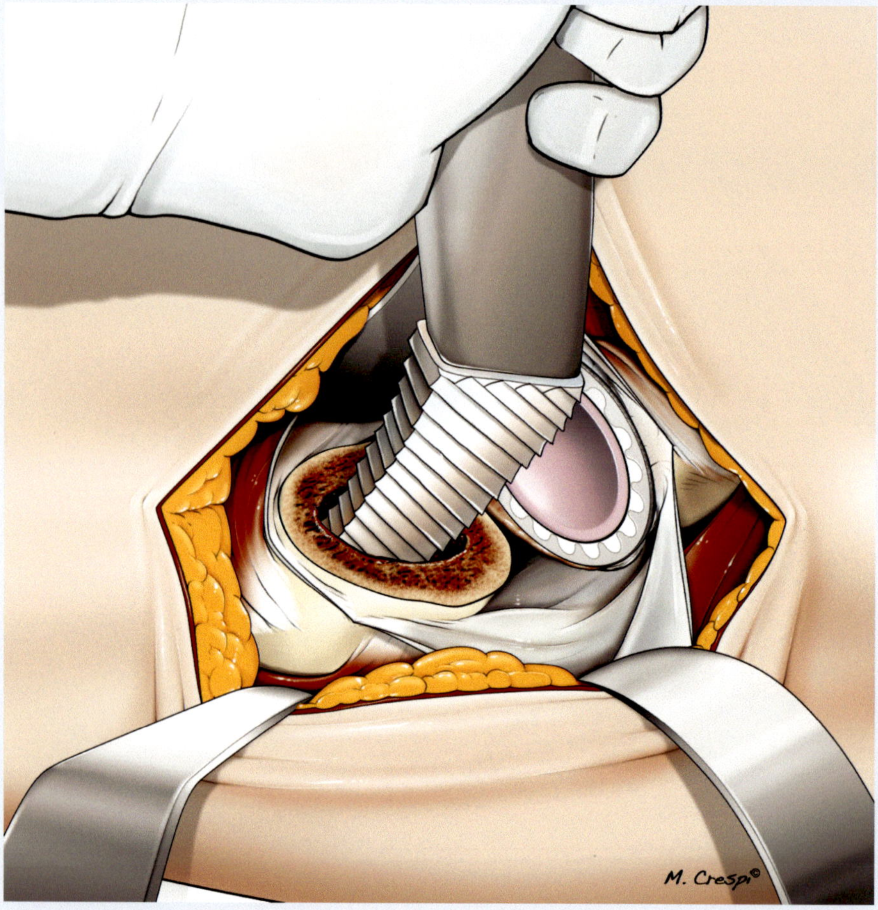

Figure 18
Completion of the diaphyseal canal preparation with the broaches

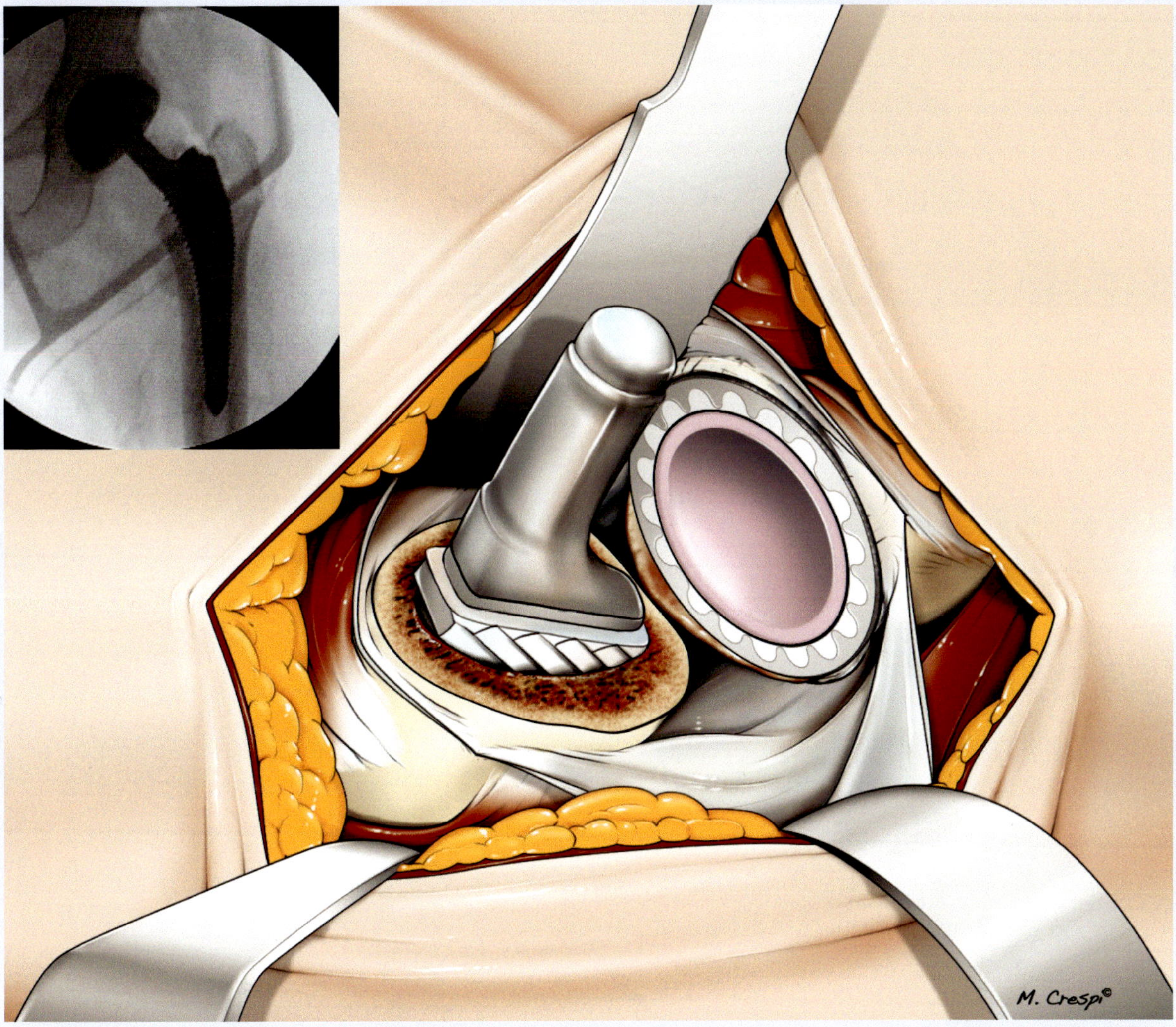

Figure 19 The broach considered suitable for implantation is left in place for the radiographic evaluation and the execution of prosthetic stability tests after the application of trial components (neck and head)

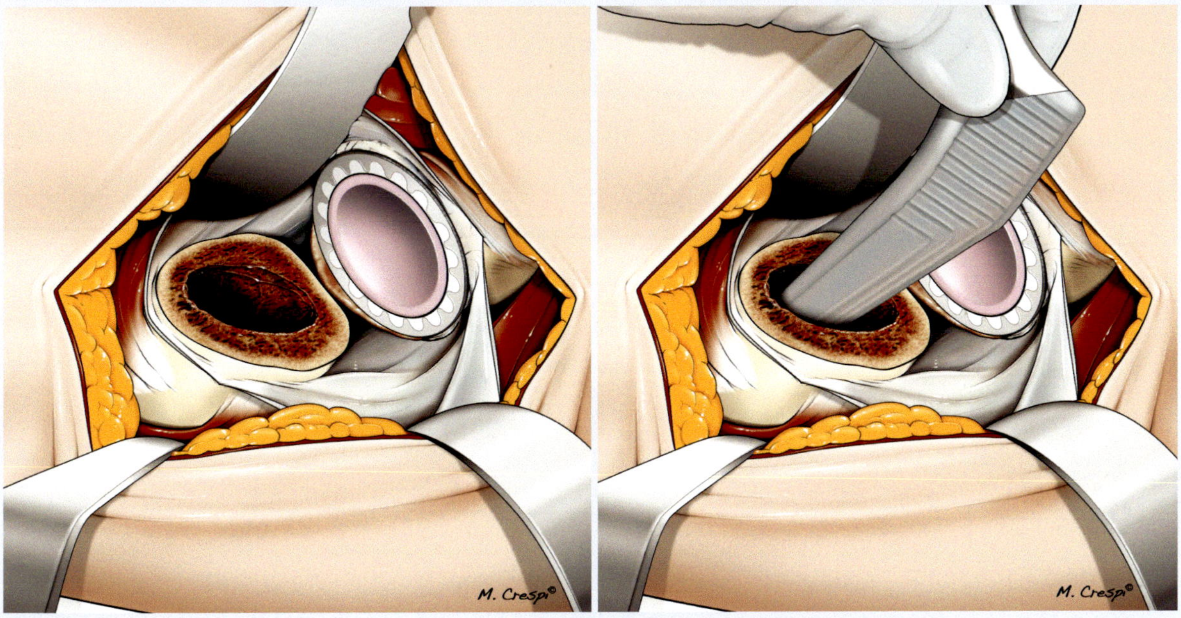

Figure 20 After radiographic confirmation of the correct prosthetic alignment and the positive stability tests, the final stem of the correct size is applied

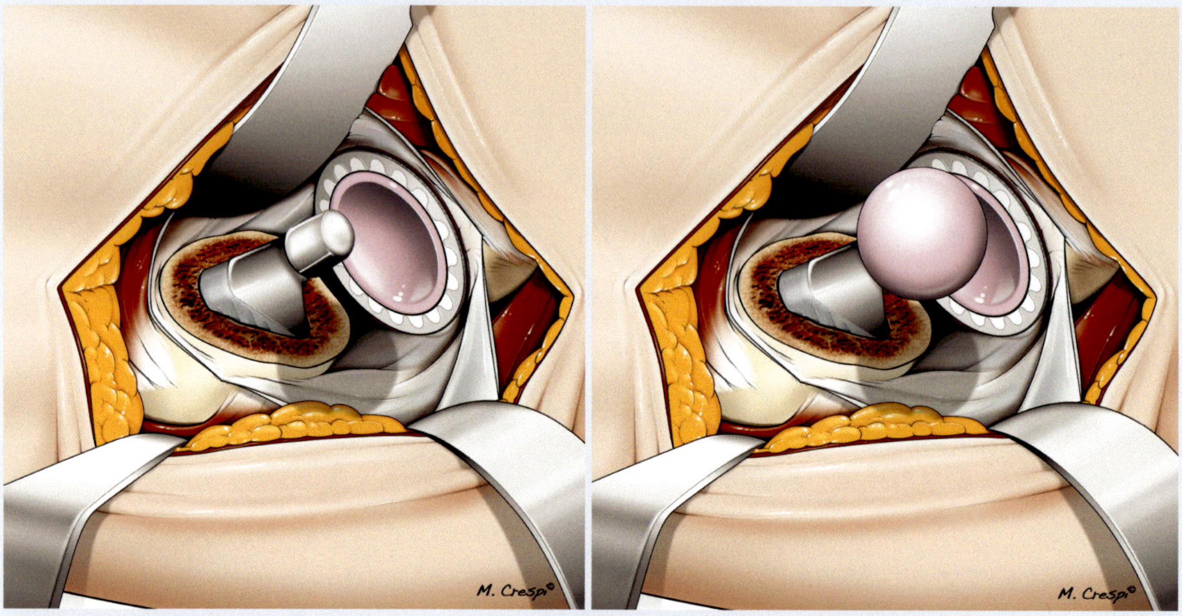

Figure 21 Completion of the femoral prosthetic device with application of the ceramic head

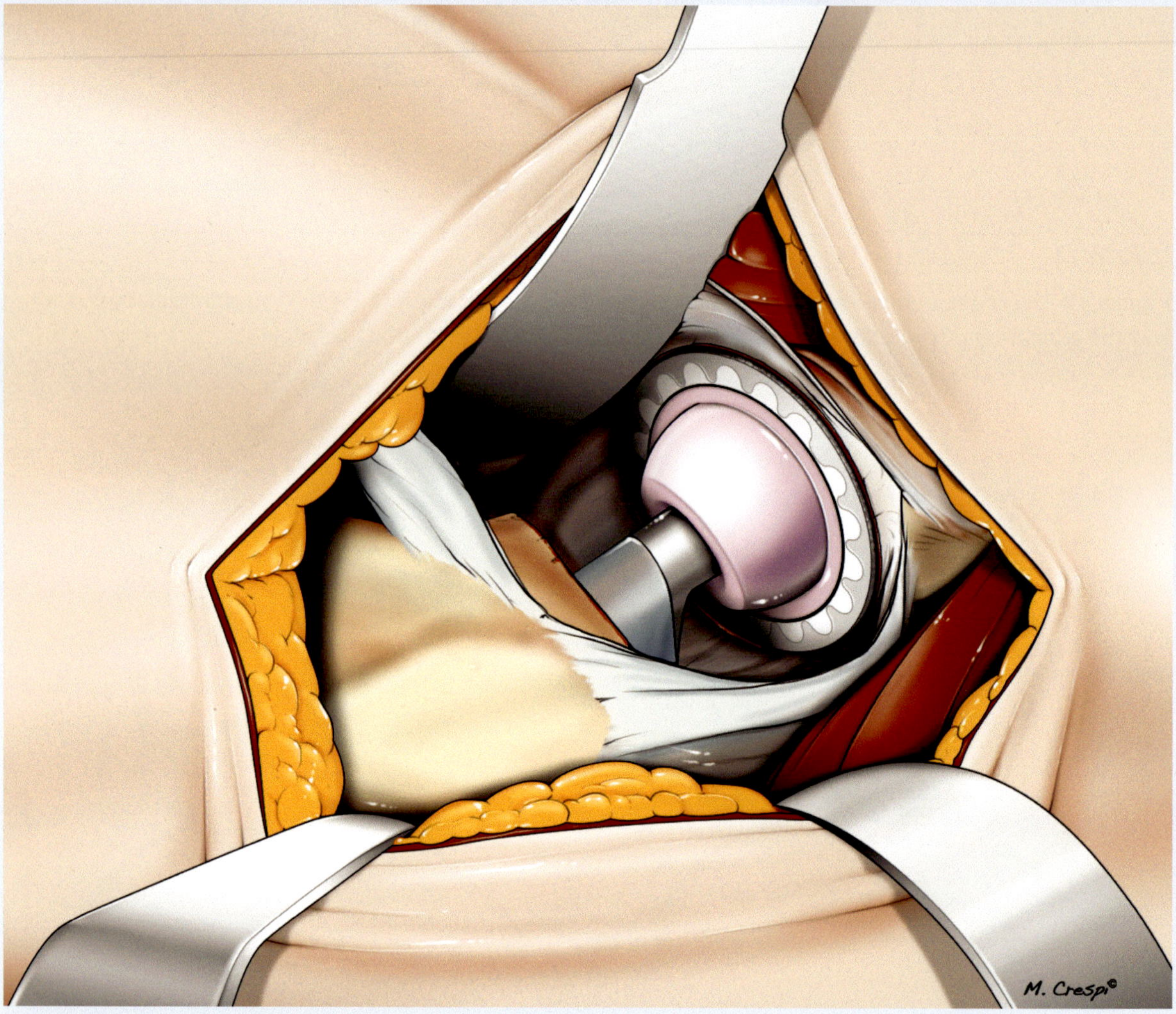

Figure 22 The prosthesis is then reduced and the stability tests are repeated. In case of doubt, another X-ray examination should be repeated for confirmation

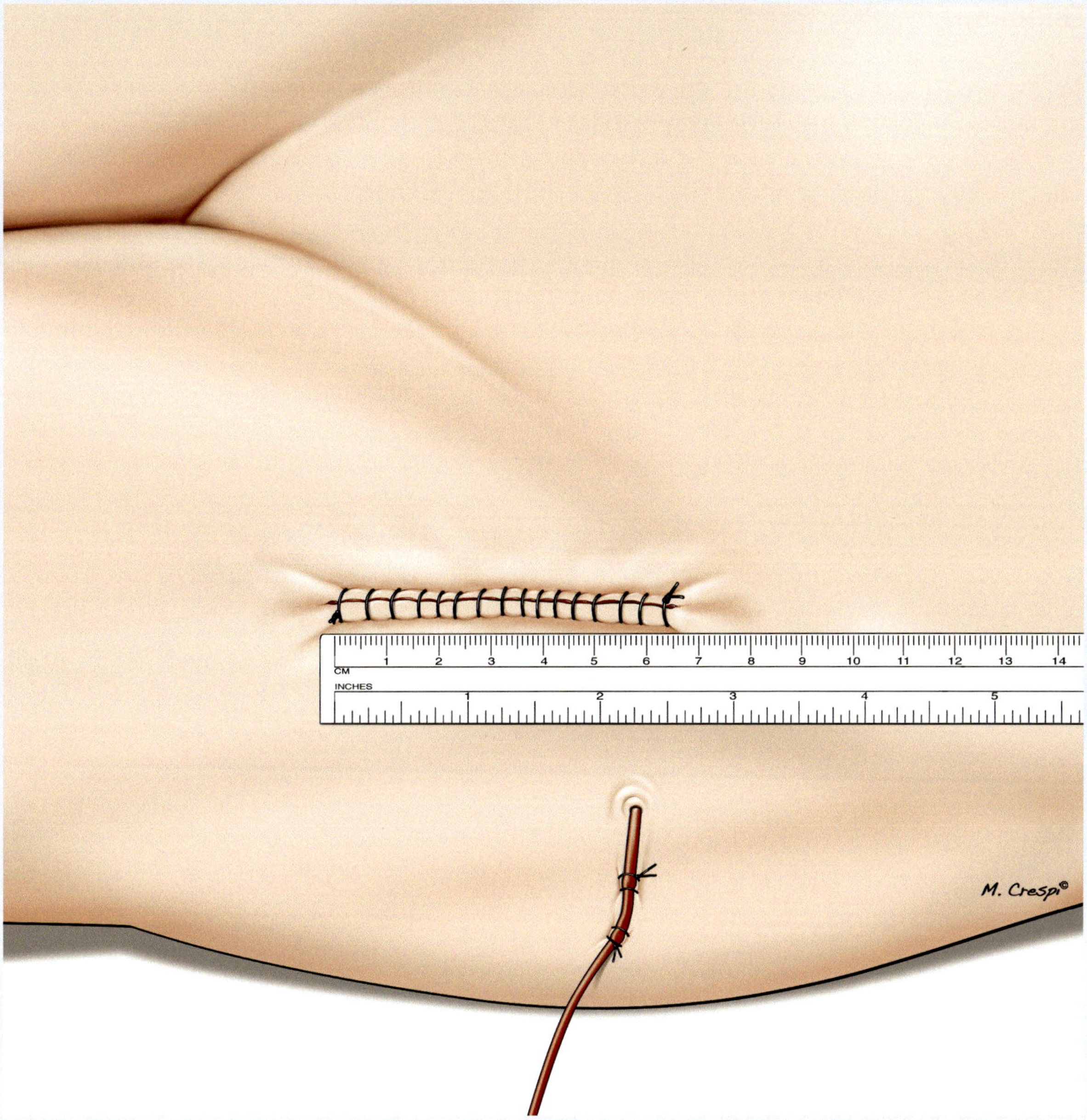

Figure 23 Suture of the surgical wound

Bikini approach

This approach is a repetition of the minimally invasive anterior approach. The path between the muscle units in the superficial (tensor fascia lata and sartorius) and deep (gluteus medius and rectus femoris) layers is the same, as is the respect for the lateral anatomical structures of the hip (iliotibial band, gran trochanter, and abductor muscles). However, a different surgical skin incision is performed. This time it is transverse-oblique, so that it is less noticeable and can even be concealed under clothing. Due to the intrinsic characteristics of the skin, the scarring results are also aesthetically better with this approach. This minimally invasive approach can be performed either with the patient positioned on the usual traction bed or with the free limbs managed in the various manoeuvres by the surgeons.

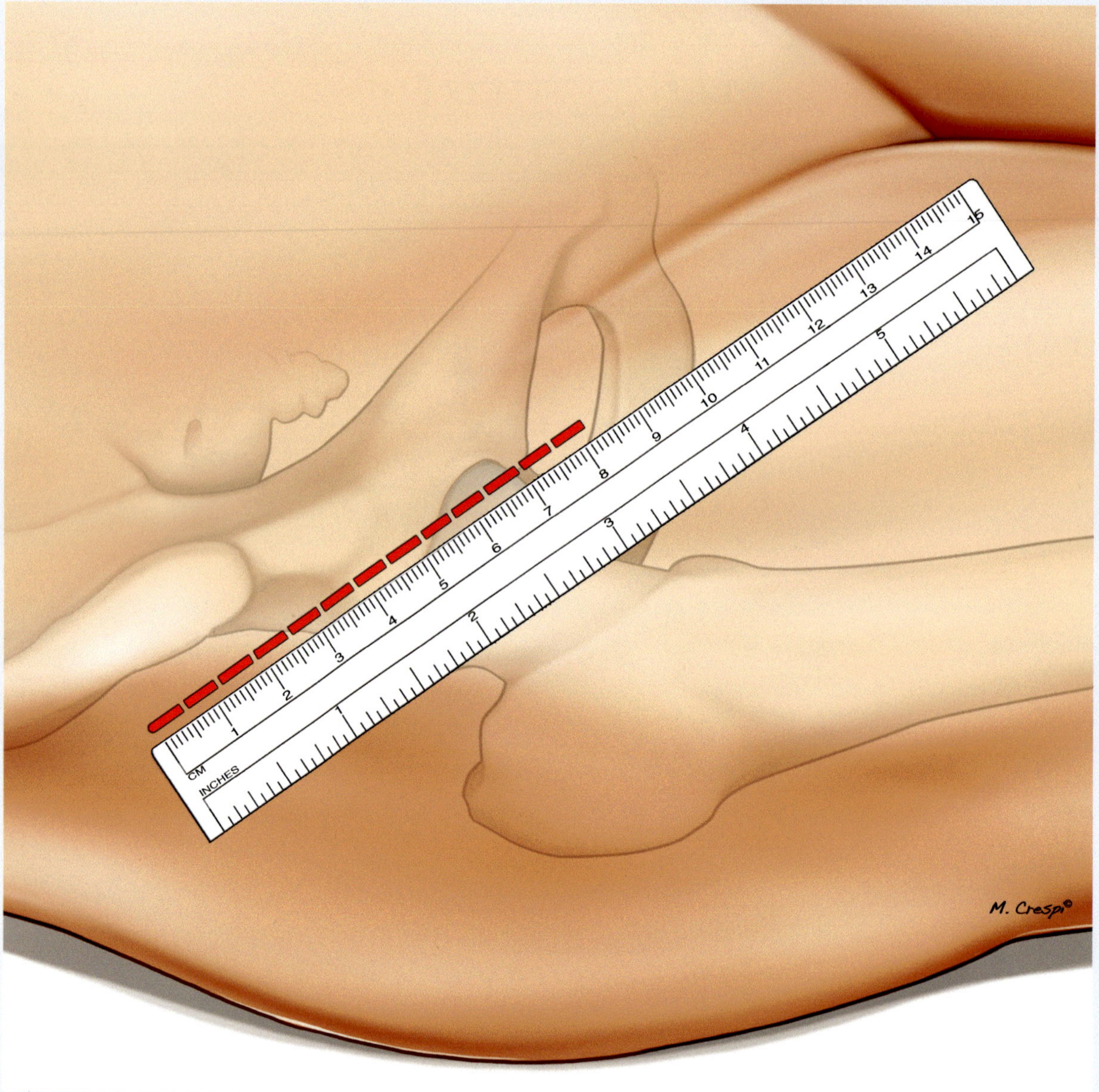

Figure 24 Patient is supine on surgical bed, either regular or with a traction device. The 7-8 cm long incision line starts 2 cm laterally and 2 cm distal to the anterior-superior iliac spine. It runs obliquely and medially just below the inguinal fold

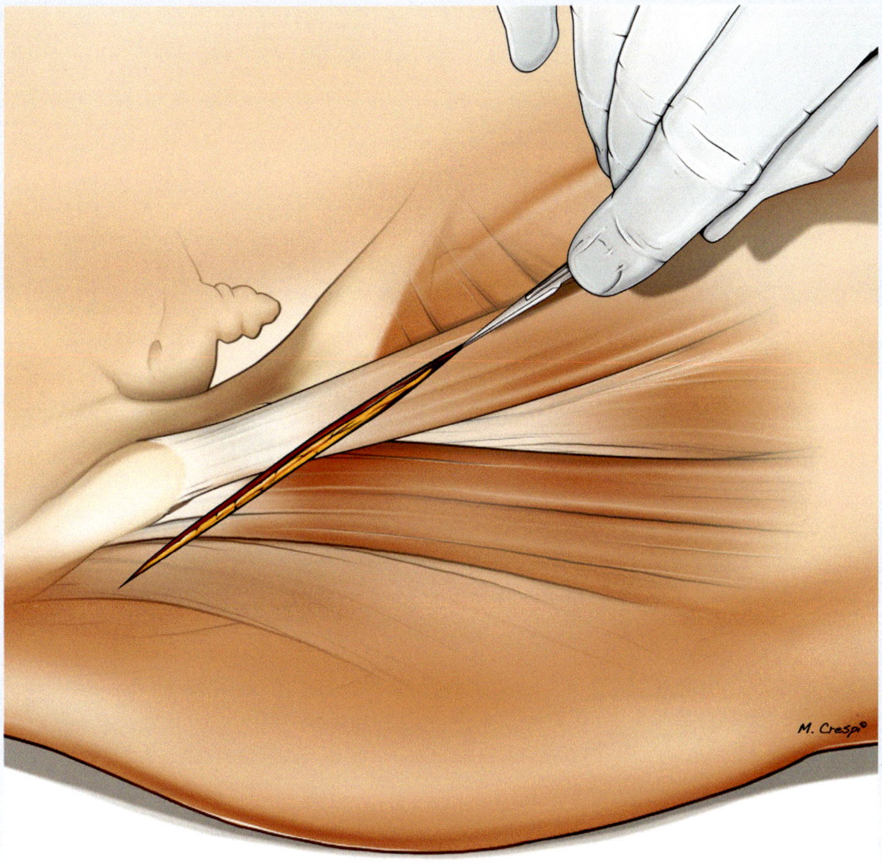

Figure 25
Skin incision

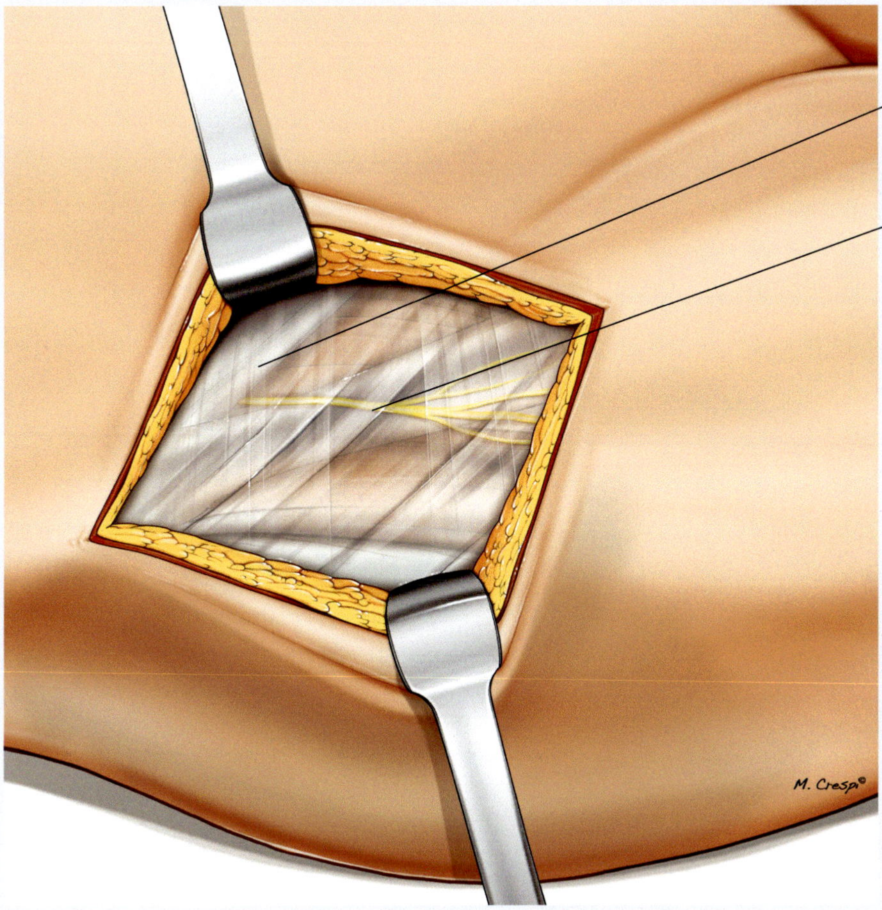

Figure 26
The fascia lata is reached and the lateral cutaneous nerve with its branches is identified. The nerve is located between the sartorius and tensor muscles of the fascia lata

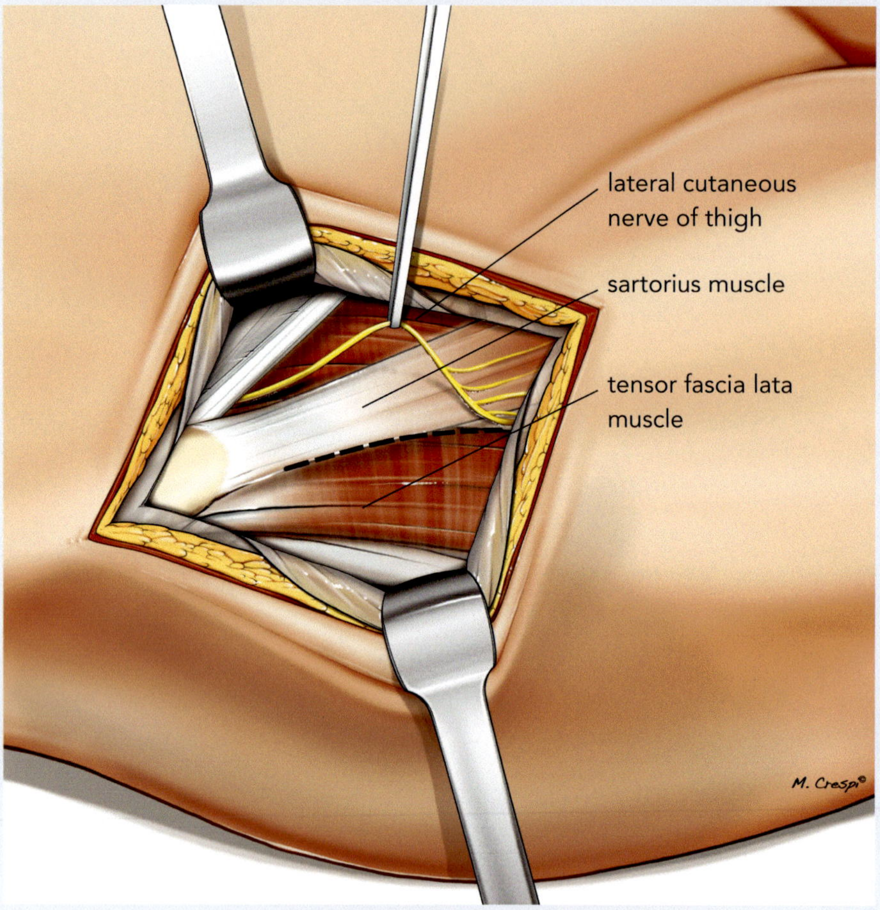

Figure 27
Isolation and protection of the lateral cutaneous nerve (LCN), which is retracted medially. The space between the tensor fascia lata muscle and the sartorius muscle is identified. This muscle interspace should be retracted just lateral to the ASIS in order not to injure (directly or by excessive traction) the LCN itself. As in the other anterior approaches, much attention should be paid to the LCN, its branches (especially laterally) or some variants of its course

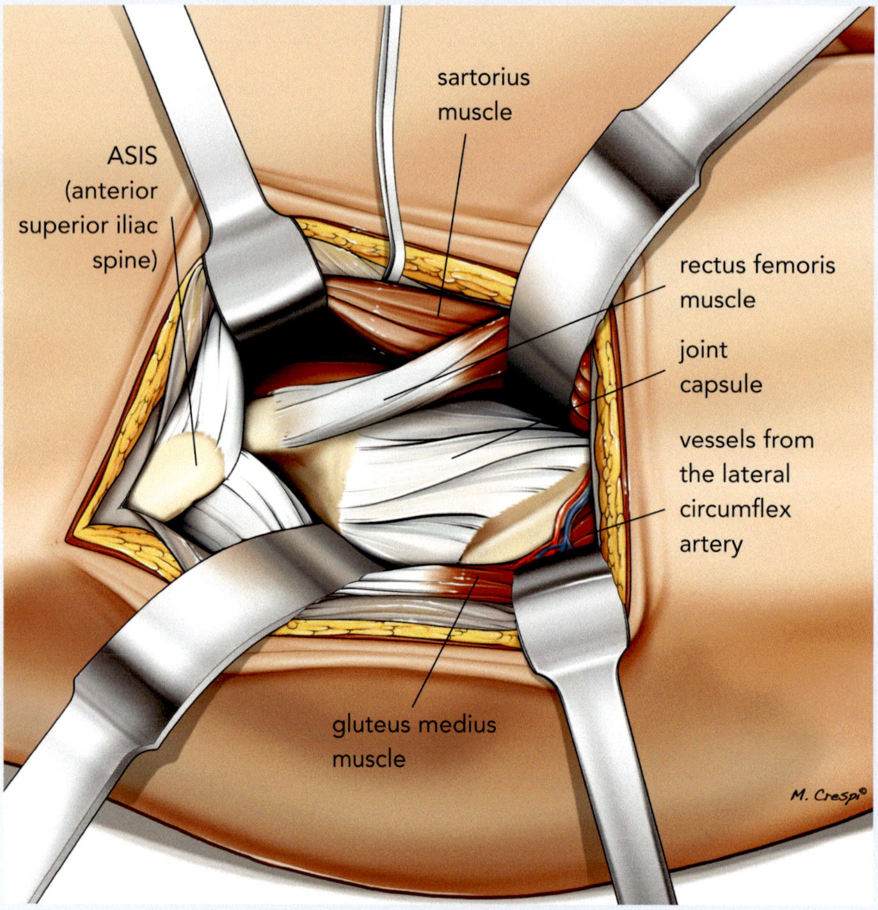

Figure 28
Retraction of the muscles and transition to the joint plane. The deeper muscles, rectus femoris and iliopsoas are retracted medially while the gluteus medius and minimus are retracted laterally. By properly positioning the Hohmann levers the joint capsule is exposed

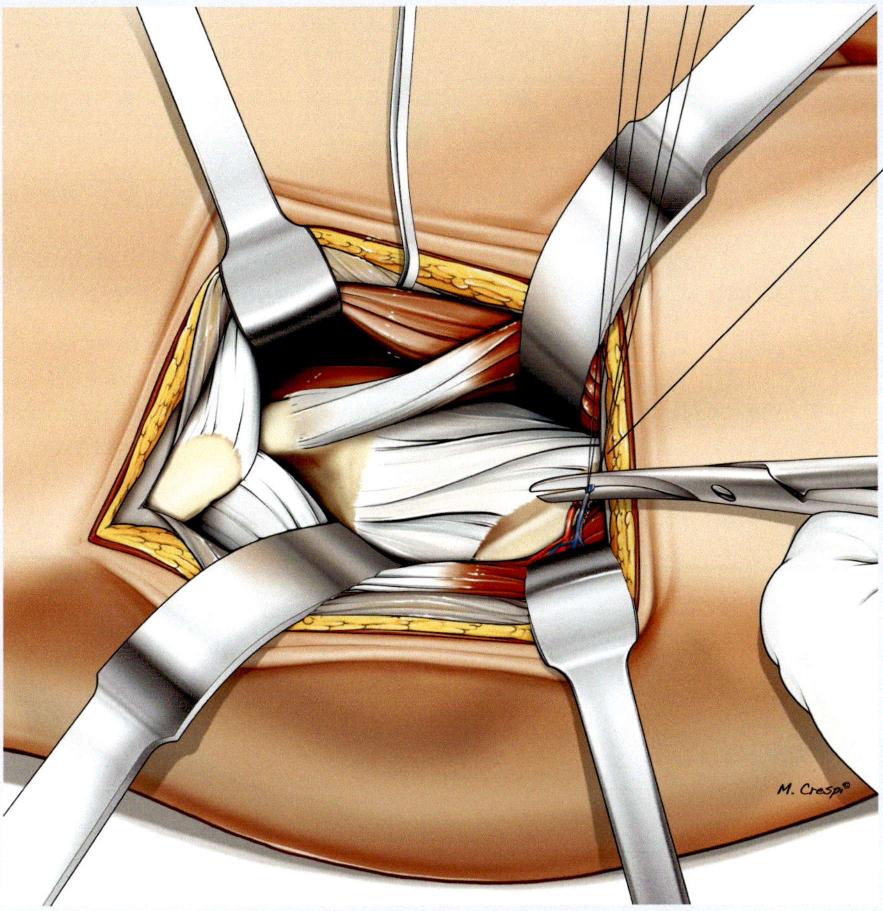

Figure 29
Identification, isolation and ligation of the ascending branch of the transverse trunk originating from the lateral circumflex artery of the femur. In fact, we do not consider the sole electrocoagulation of these vessels reliable, due to the high risk of post-operative haematoma formation

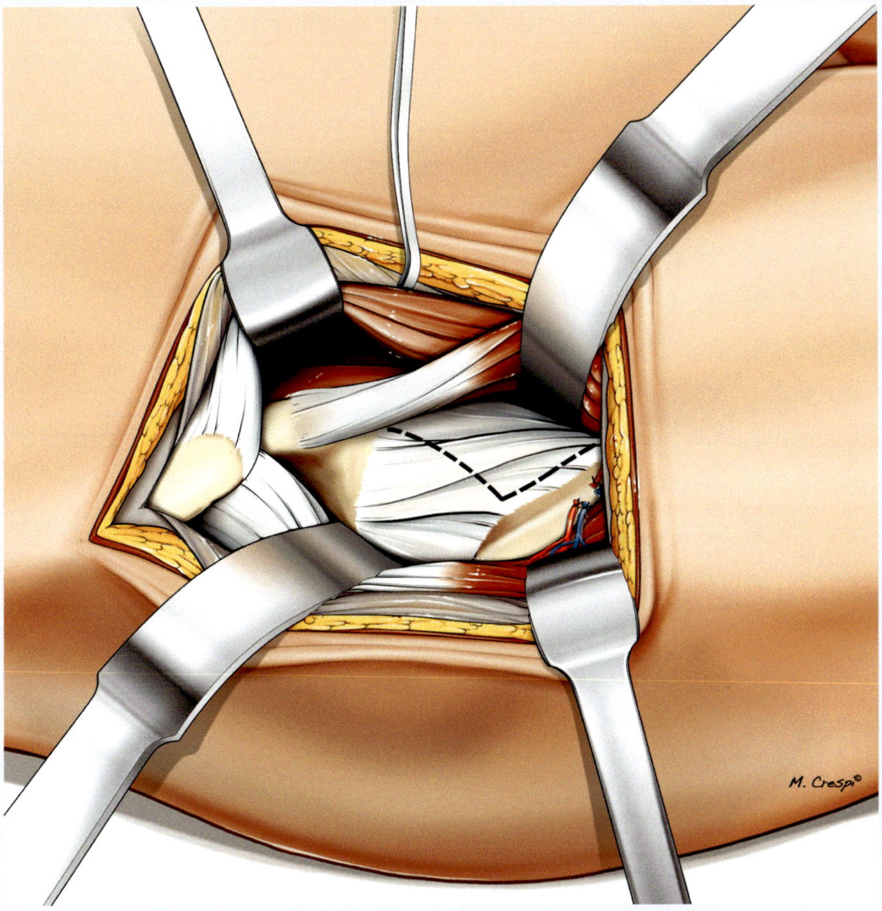

Figure 30
L-shaped anterior capsulotomy, which proximally involves the insertion of the rectus femoris and distally reaches the trochanteric tubercle

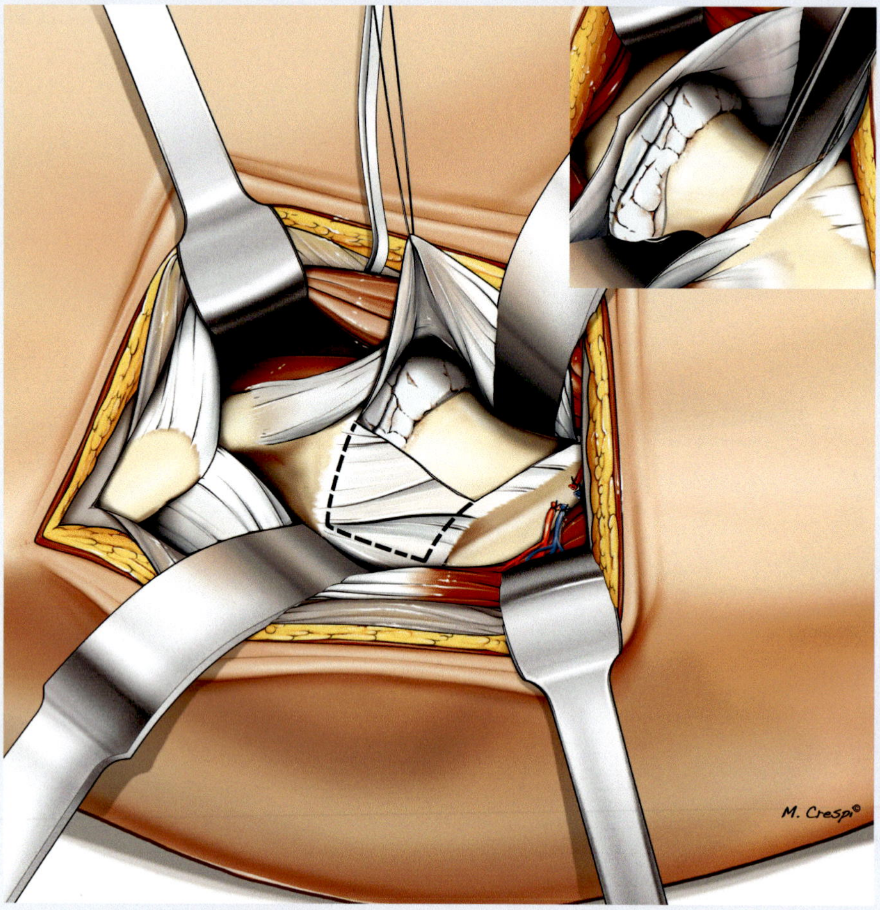

Figure 31
The capsulotomy is completed and the joint exposed, with the Hohmann levers safely positioned below the capsule. This allows the femoral neck and head to be exposed without risk of neurovascular damage (from traction, compression and tearing). It is very important not to move medial to the rectus femoris so as not to jeopardise the femoral neurovascular bundle

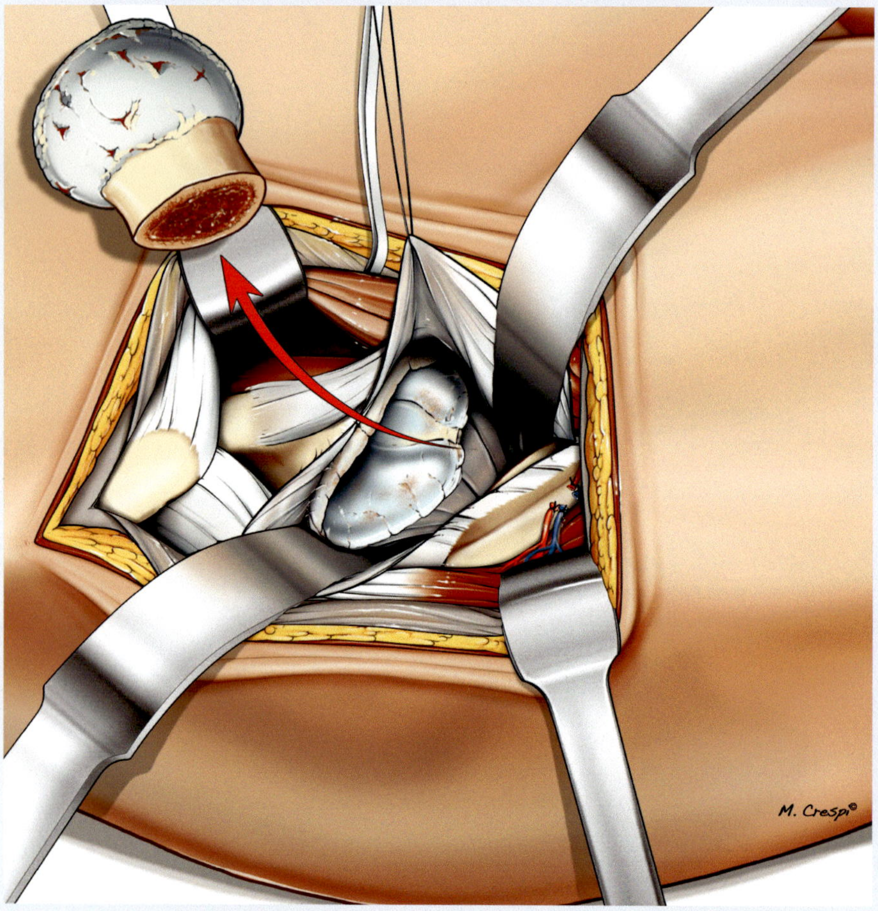

Figure 32
Resection of the femoral neck and removal of the femoral head

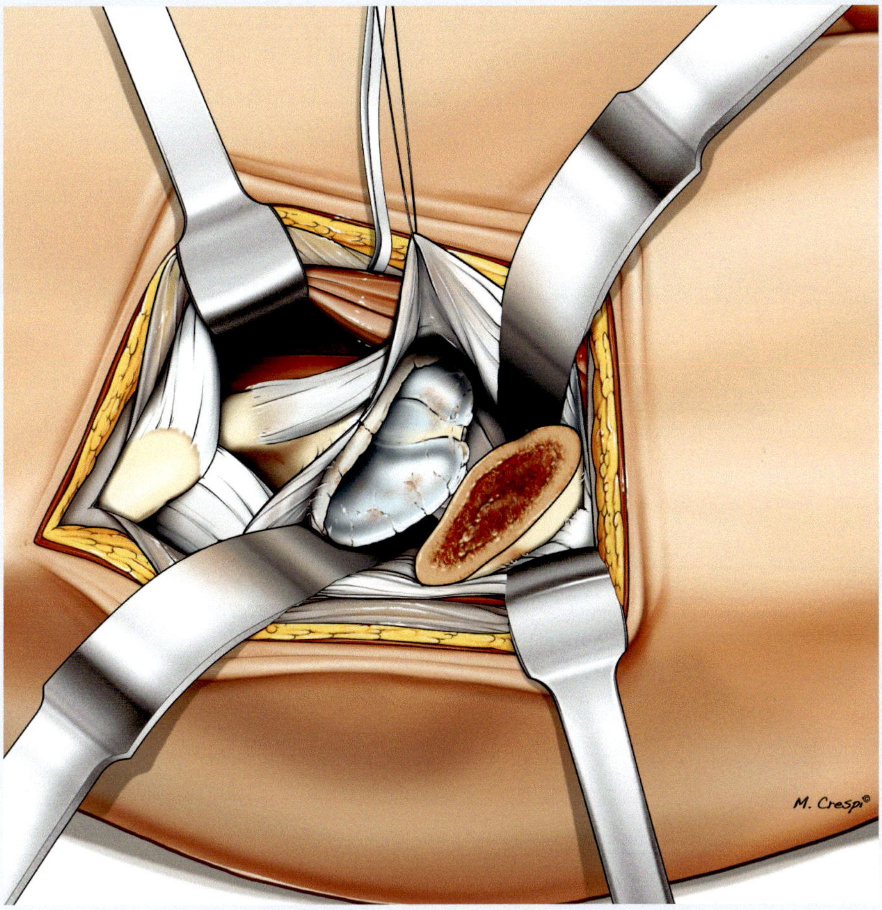

Figure 33
Illustration of the cup and femoral neck position. These will be prepared with the appropriate instruments (hemispherical burs and broaches) for the subsequent press&fit fit of the prosthetic components

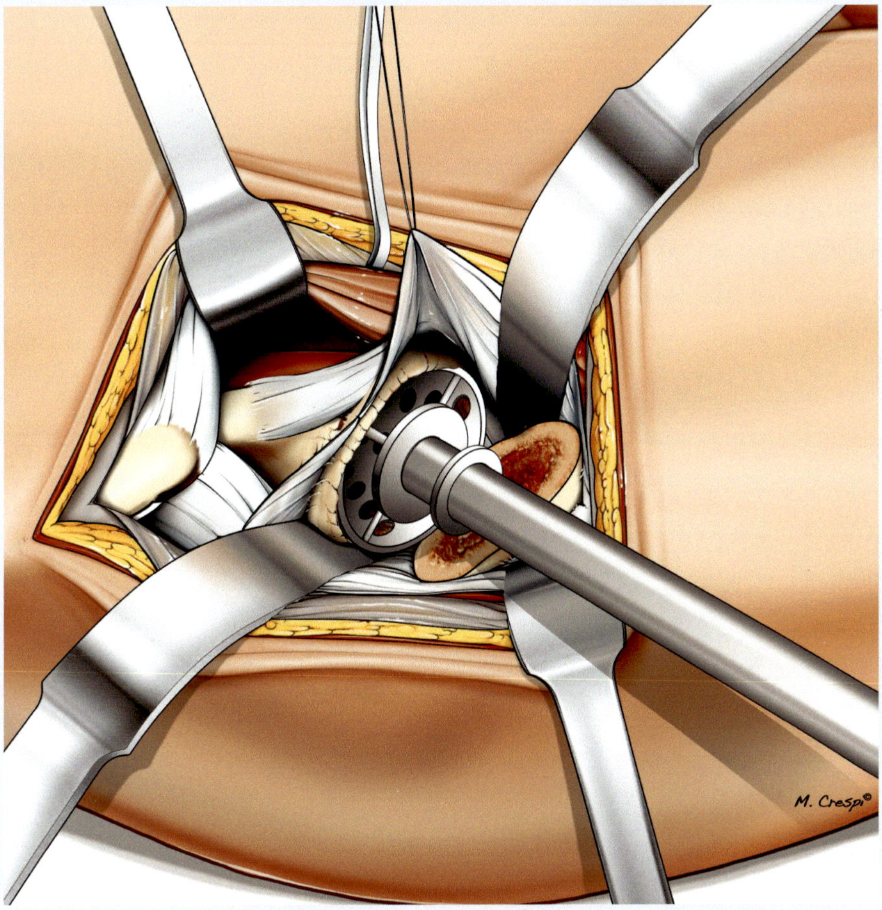

Figure 34
Preparation of the cup with the hemispherical burs. The diameter reached is the one determined with the pre-operative planning or derived from the surgeon's perception of adequacy (using the classical landmarks of the technique, acetabular floor, lateral edge of the cup, etc.)

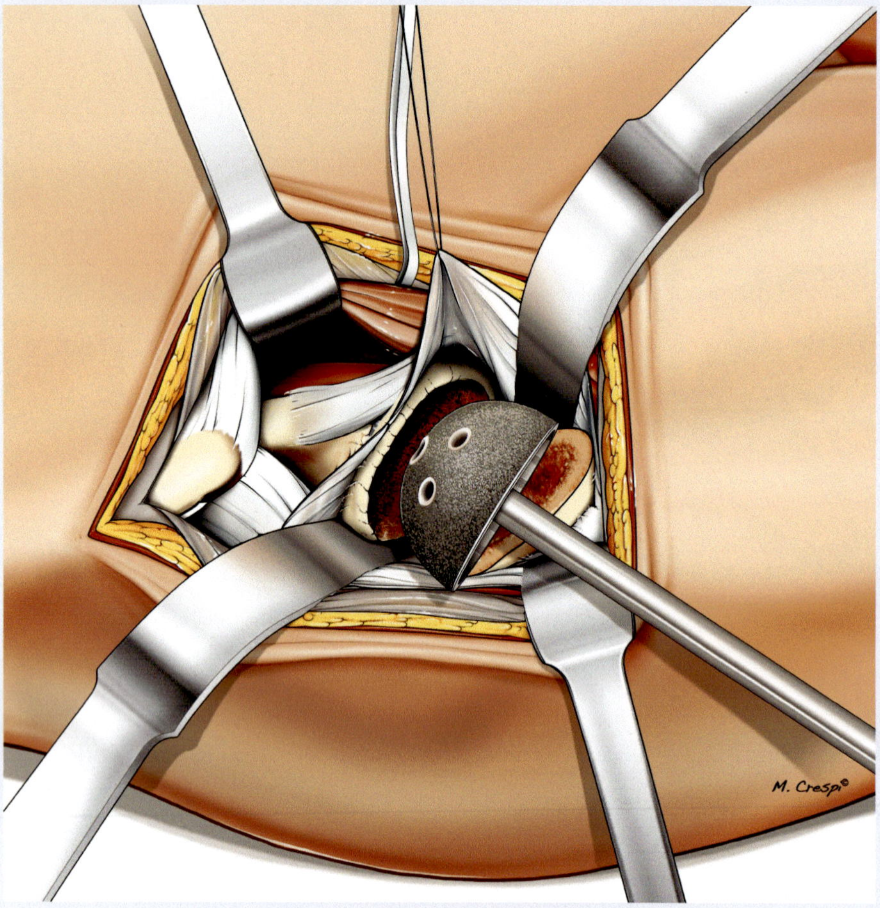

Figure 35
Insertion of the cup is possible with either the straight or offset handle, depending on the correct management of the anatomical spaces allowed by the minimally invasive anterior access

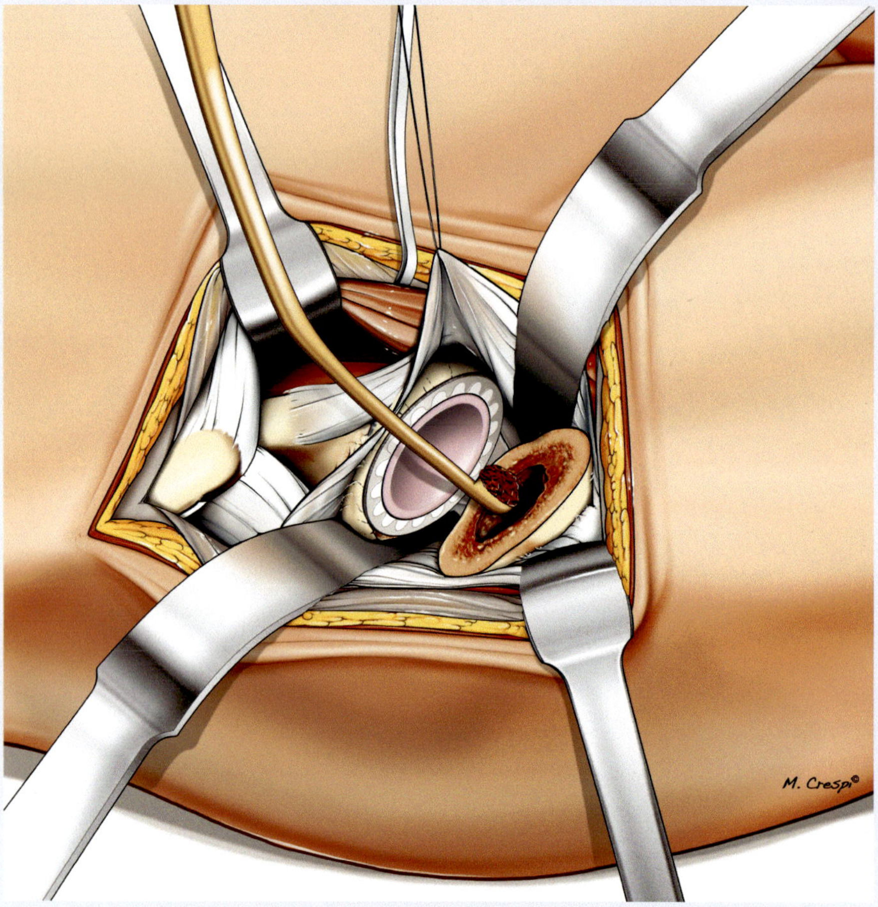

Figure 36
Opening of the femoral diaphyseal canal with a curved spoon

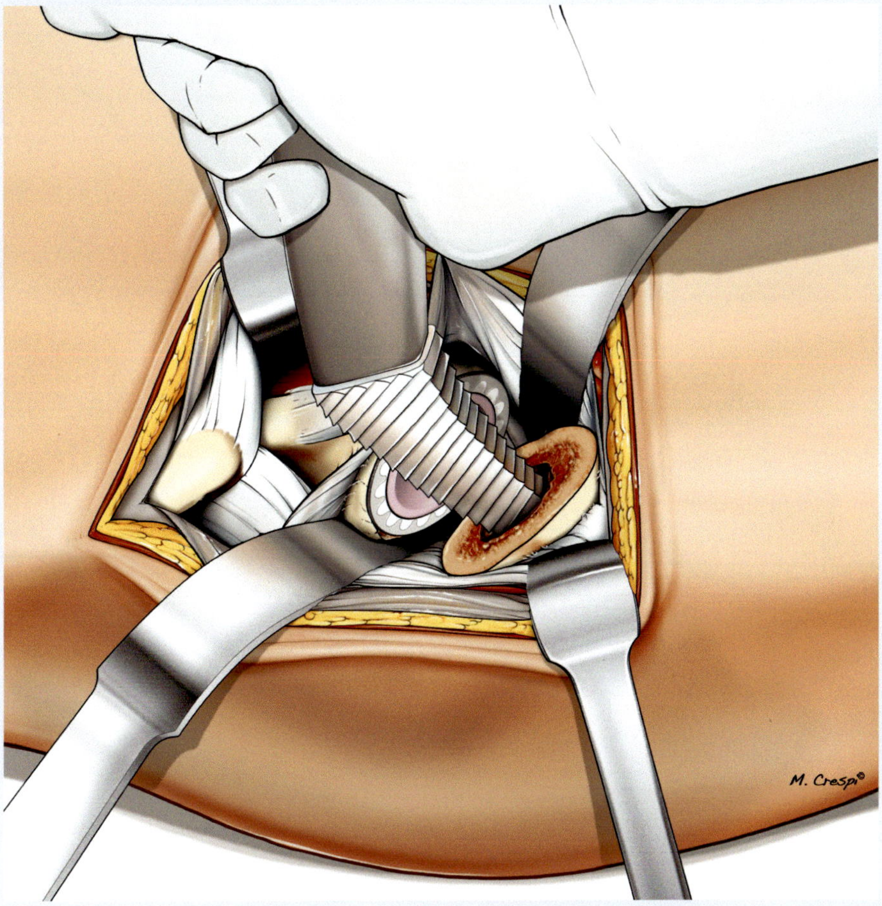

Figure 37
Preparation of the femoral diaphyseal canal with the broaches (up to the size established with the pre-operative planning or with the manual perception of filling and stability). With the rasp and the implantation of a trial neck and head it is possible to conduct stability tests, check the length of the limbs and verify the implant with an X-ray

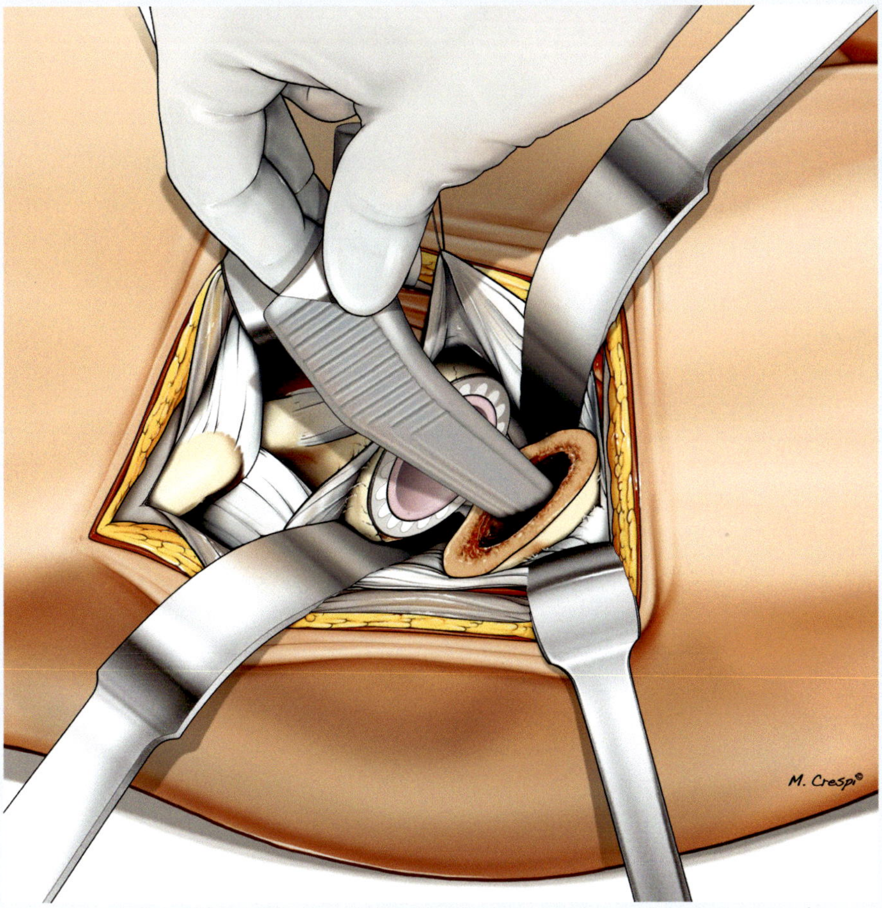

Figure 38
Implantation of the final uncemented stem

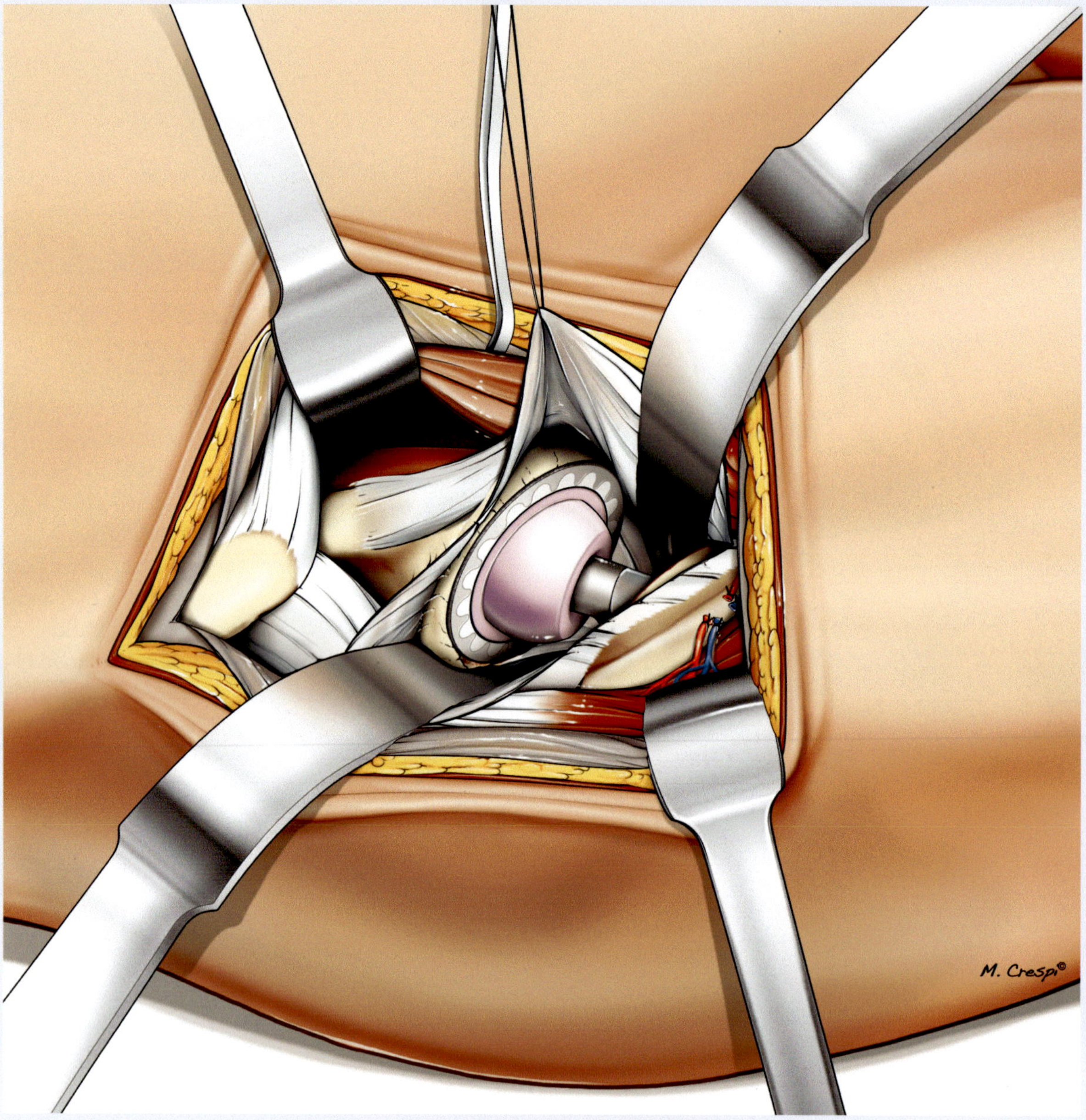

Figure 39 Reduction of the prosthesis. Stability tests are performed and the length of the lower limbs is checked

Posterior minimally invasive approach

This surgical approach, albeit with a different and smaller skin incision, replicates the original approach described by von Langenbeck and later partly modified by Kocher, Gibson and Moore. This approach, however, requires cutting and retracting the tendons of the deep planes (piriformis, short external rotators), conflicting with the concept of minimally invasive surgery ('sparing surgery').

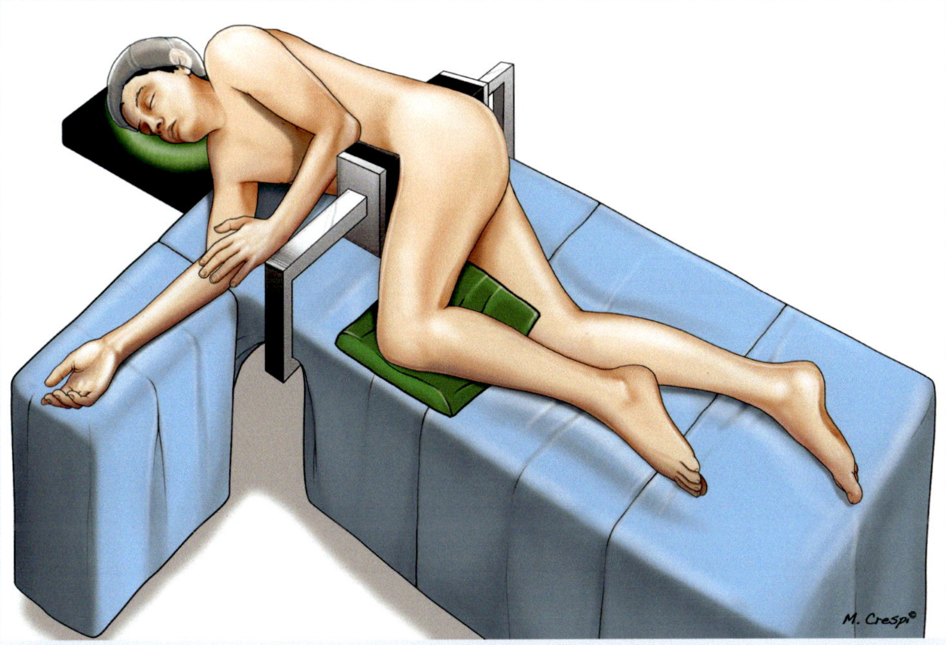

Figure 40 Patient in lateral decubitus, lying on the non-surgical side. The trunk is stabilised by pressors, applied in the appropriate places. The limb involved in the operation must remain free for the specific manoeuvres required during the surgical phase. In particular those required during the preparation of the femoral diaphyseal canal and the insertion of the prosthetic component

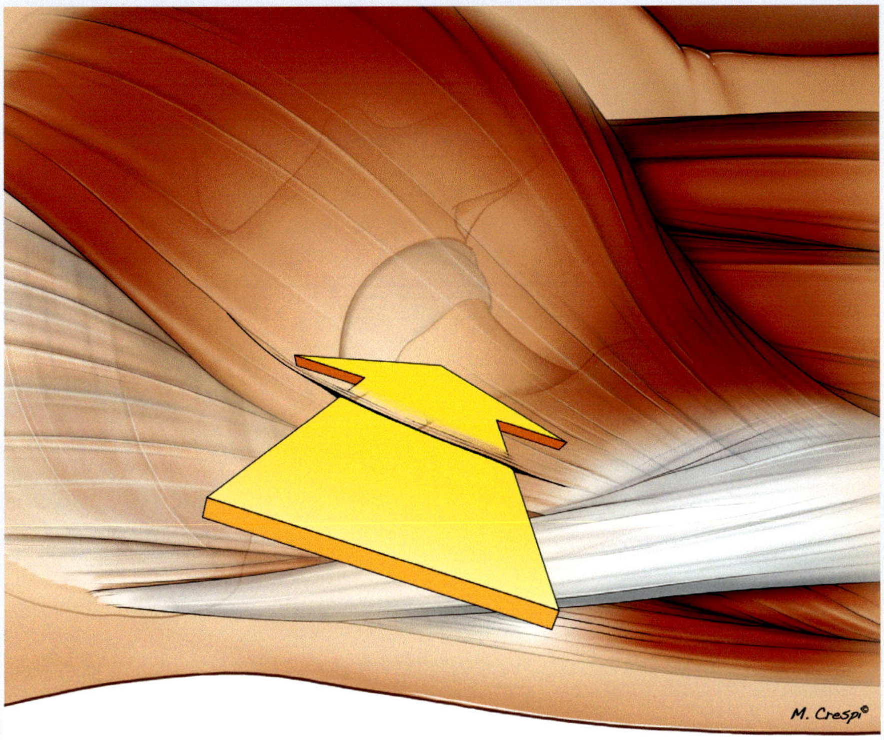

Figure 41 Anatomical overview of the gluteal region

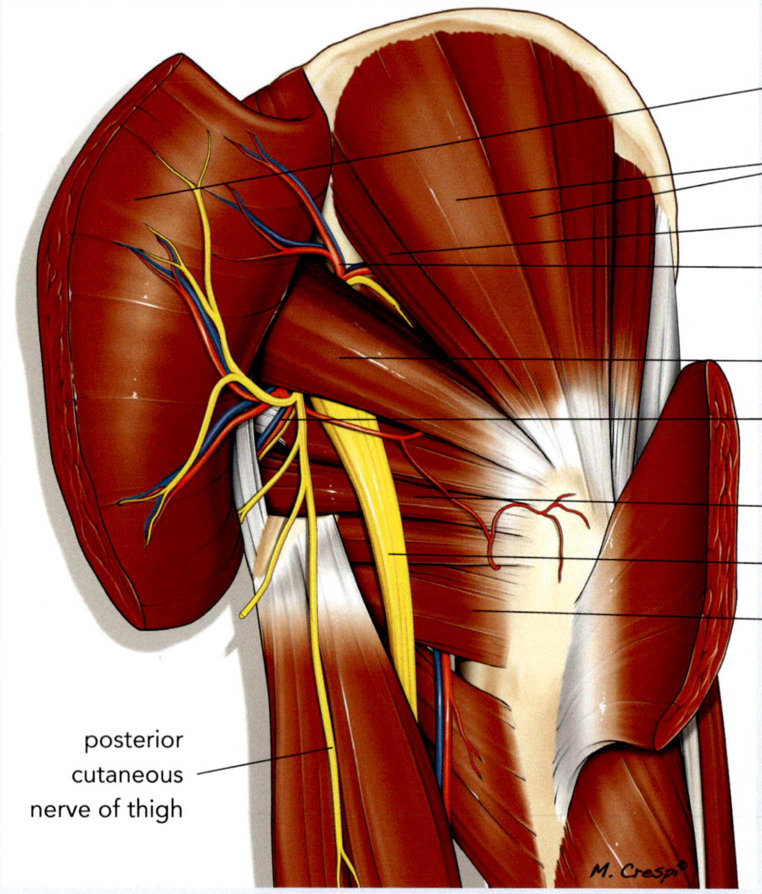

Figure 42
Anatomical detail view of the superficial and deep muscular, vascular and nervous structures that occupy the surgical field during hip replacement

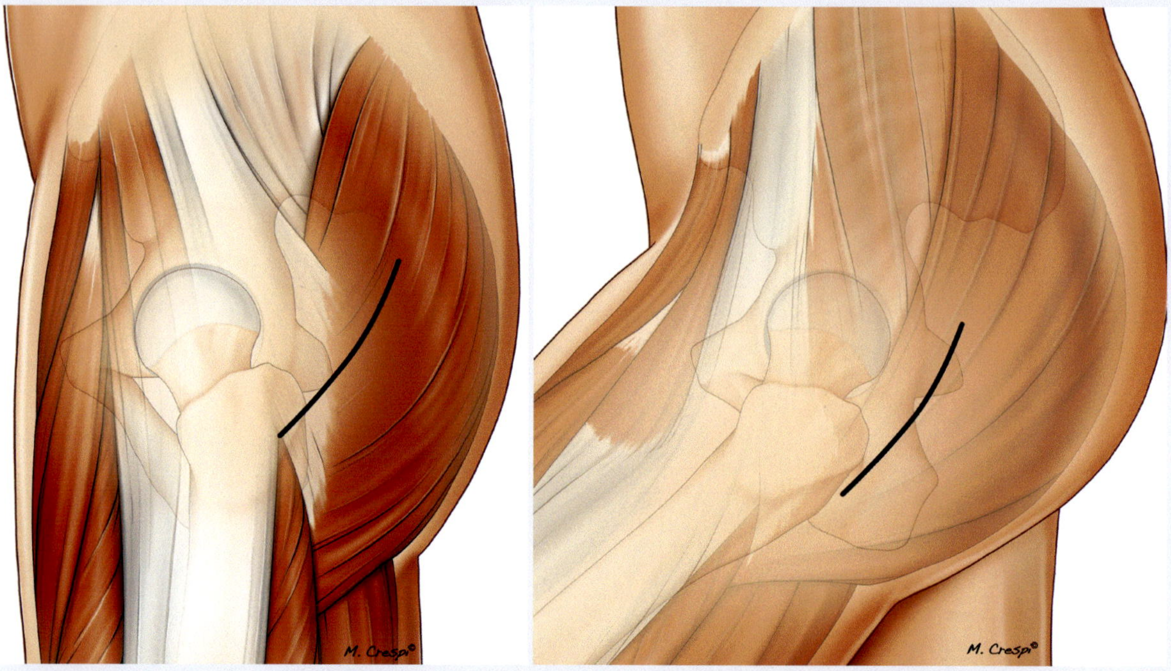

Figure 43 The 7-8 cm incision originates from the postero-superior margin of the greater trochanter and runs posteriorly in a straight or gently curved line. However, it follows the orientation of the fibres of the gluteus maximus

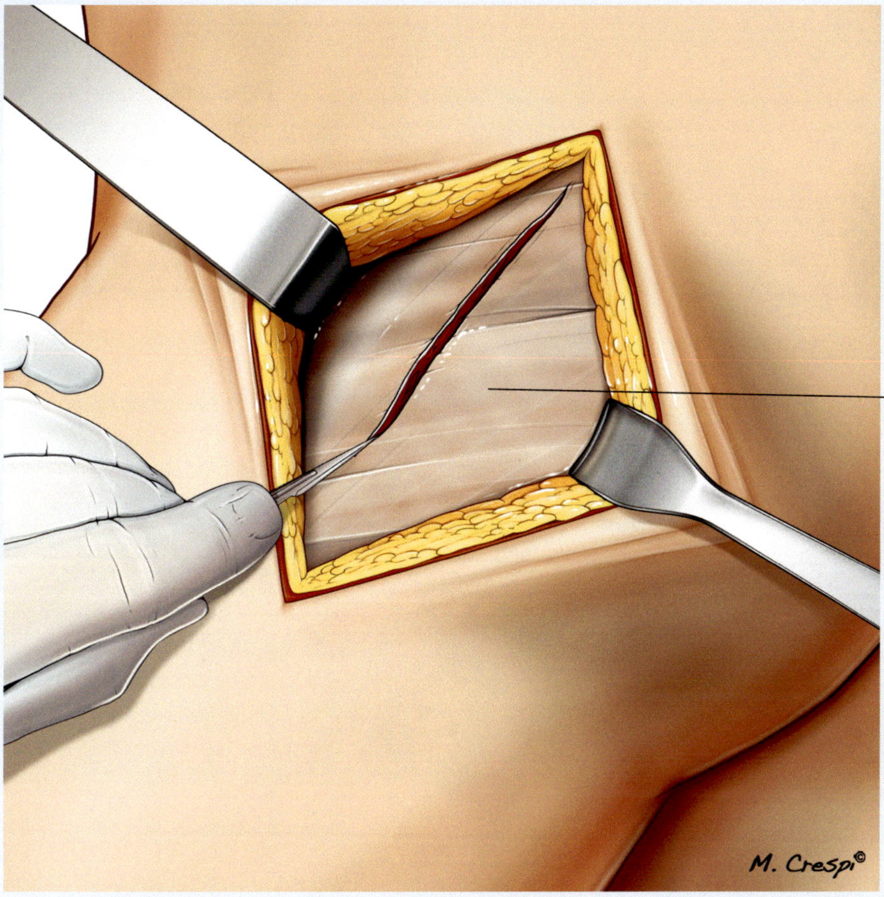

Figure 44
Incision of the gluteal fascia and splitting of the fibres of the gluteus maximus muscle in the direction of their length

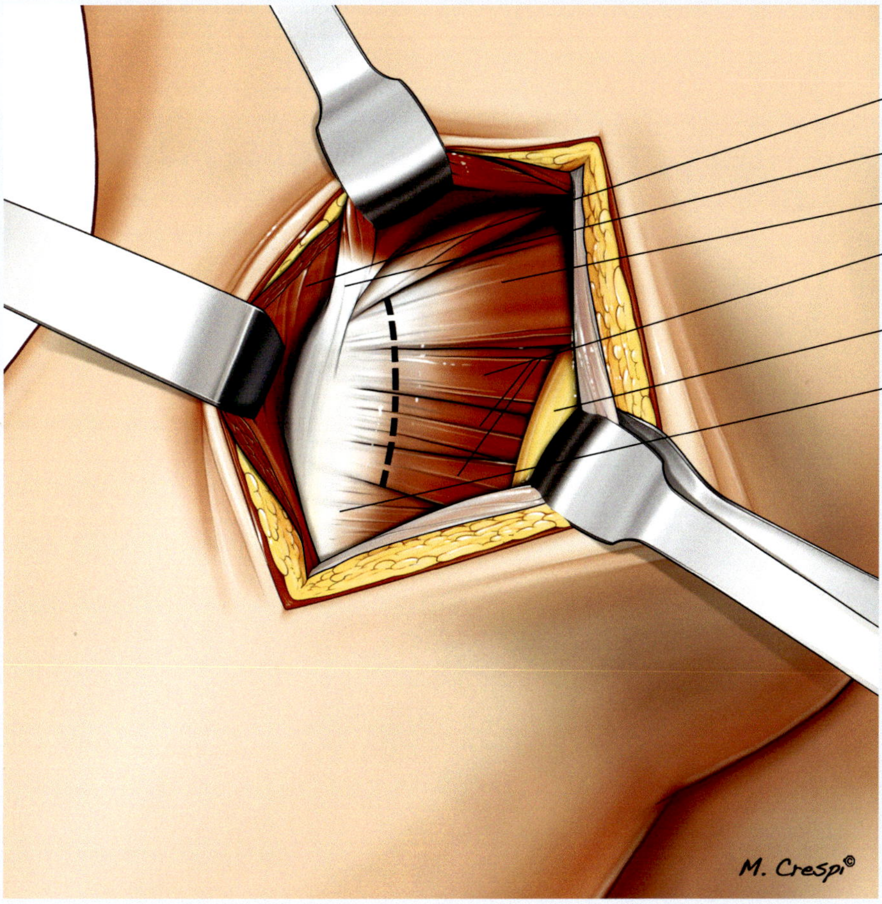

Figure 45
Exposure of the deep muscle layer and identification of the insertion of the short external rotator muscles to the femur. Attention is given to the sciatic nerve course, which is exposed below the piriformis muscle

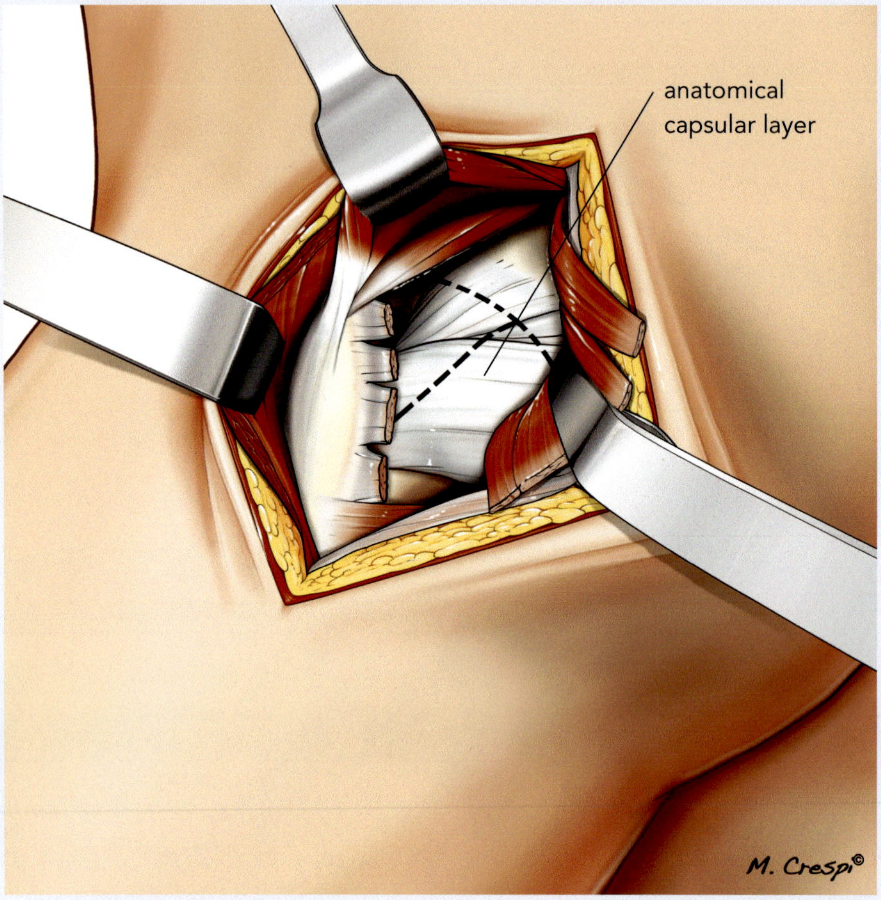

Figure 46
The tendon insertion to the femur of the short rotator muscles and, if necessary, of the piriformis is detached. These are then gently retracted backwards, avoiding excessive traction potentially damaging to the sciatic nerve. A residual part of tendon inserted on the femur should be spared to facilitate the subsequent reinsertion-reconstruction of the short rotator muscles (alternatively they should be reinserted with transosseous stitches). This is to avoid weakening the joint stability and the specific important function of these muscles. This exposes the capsular plane of the coxo-femoral joint

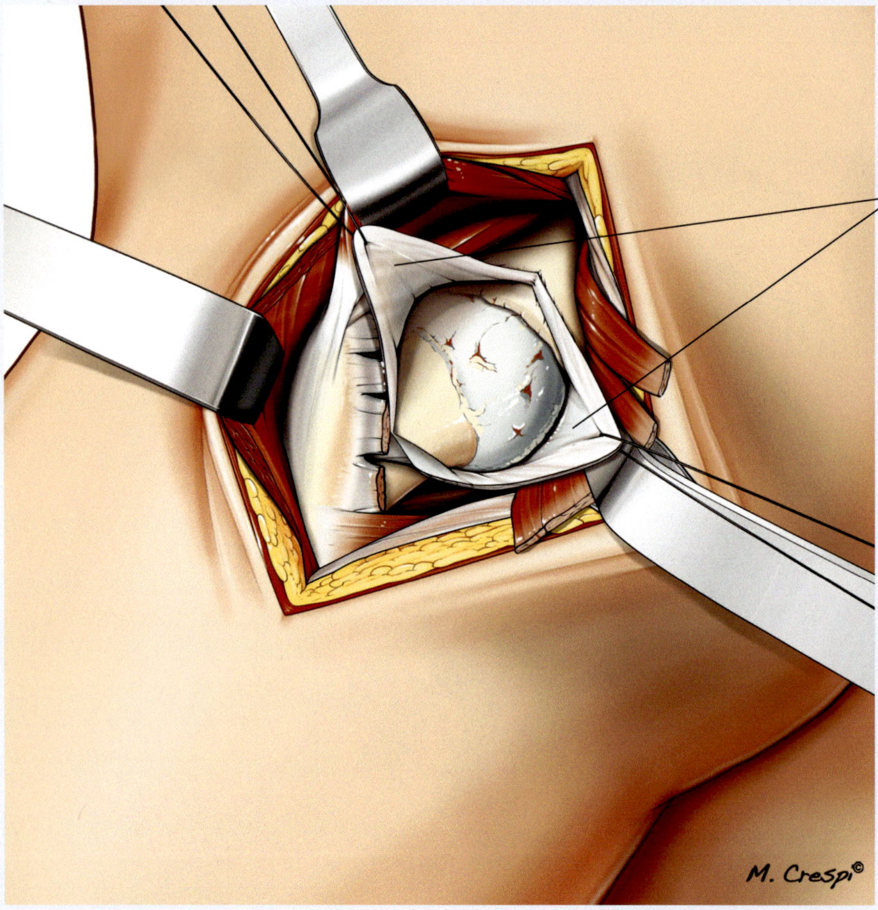

Figure 47
Posterior capsulotomy and exposure of the coxo-femoral joint

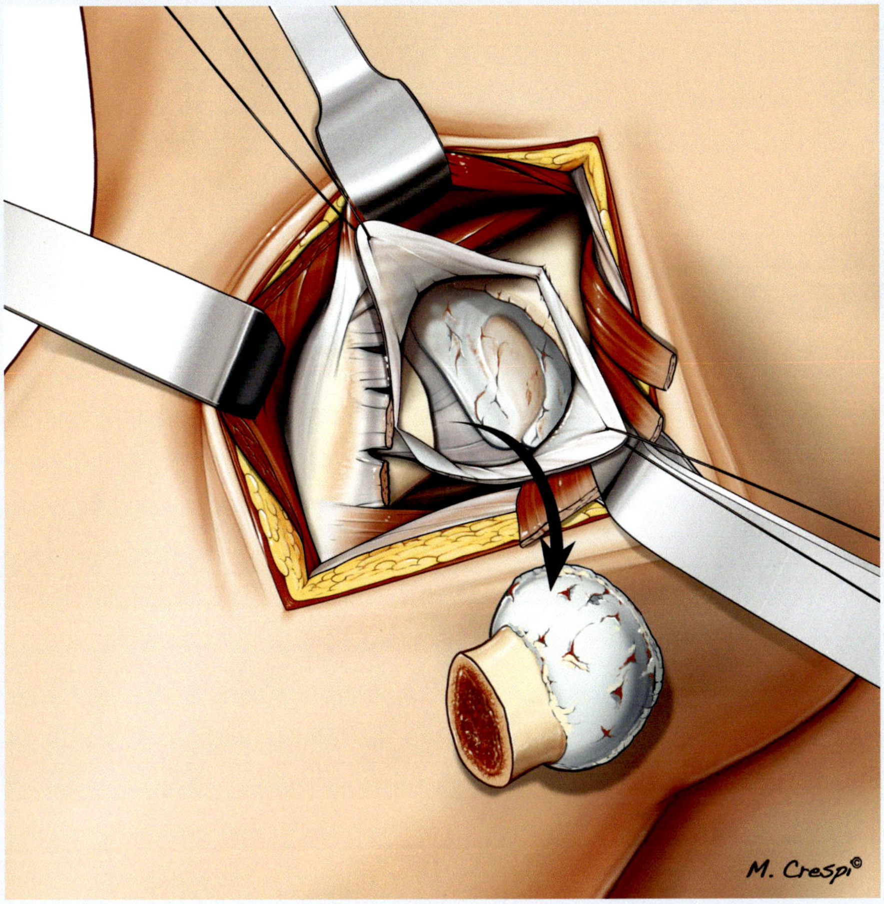

Figure 48
Resection of the femoral neck with oscillating saw at the planned site and femoral head removal

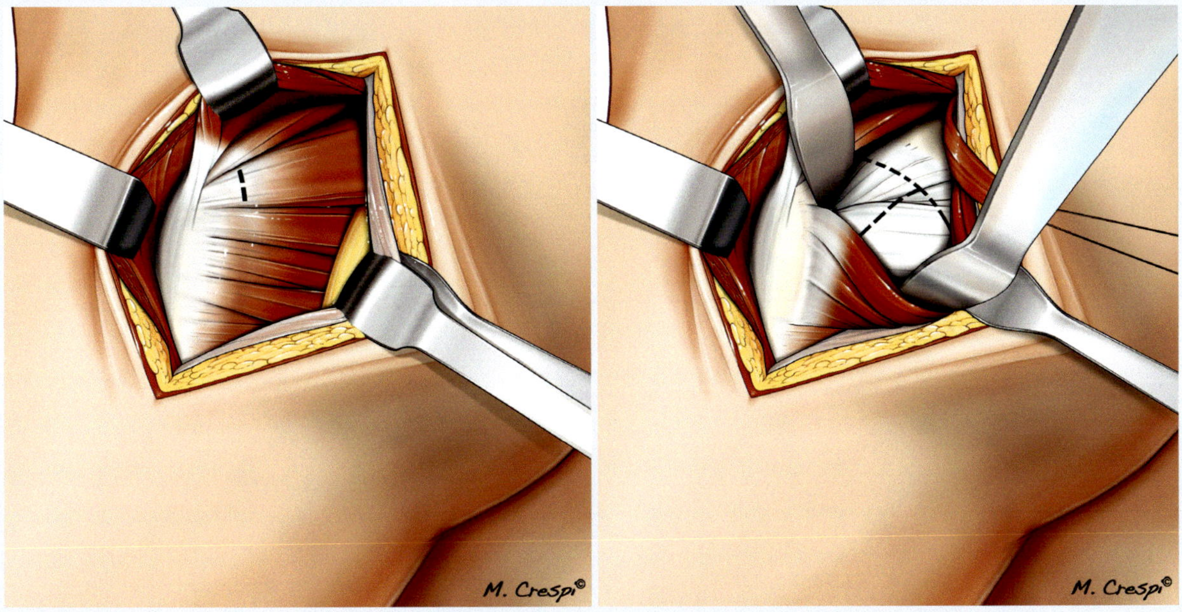

Figure 49 Alternatively, in selected cases, only the piriformis muscle is split and retracted posteriorly. Instead, the short rotator muscles can be split and retracted distally from the piriformis using Hohmann levers. In this way it is possible to expose the articular layer without sectioning the tendinous insertions to the femur

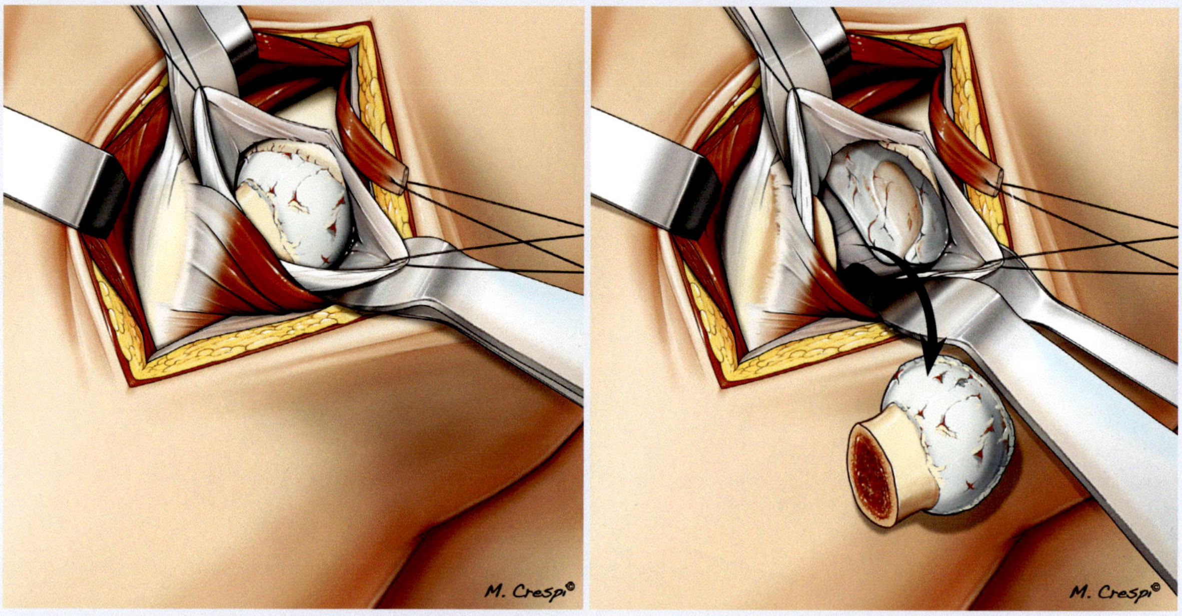

Figure 50 Coxo-femoral arthrotomy, osteotomy of the femoral neck at the planned level and removal of the femoral head with this surgical technique variant

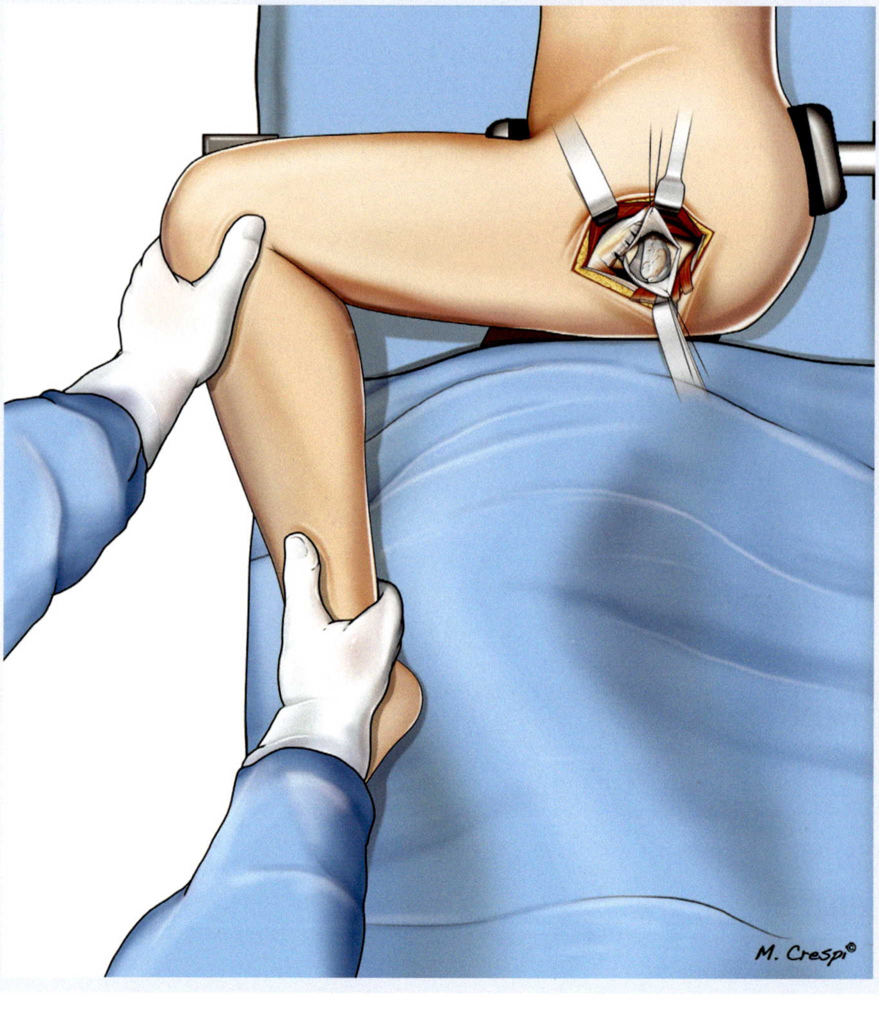

Figure 51
Control of passive limb movements in order to verify the adequacy of the spaces obtained. These are necessary for an easy preparation of the anatomical sites of prosthetic implantation. In particular it must be possible to flex, adduct and internally rotate the femur as the main difficulty is to expose the proximal part of the femur

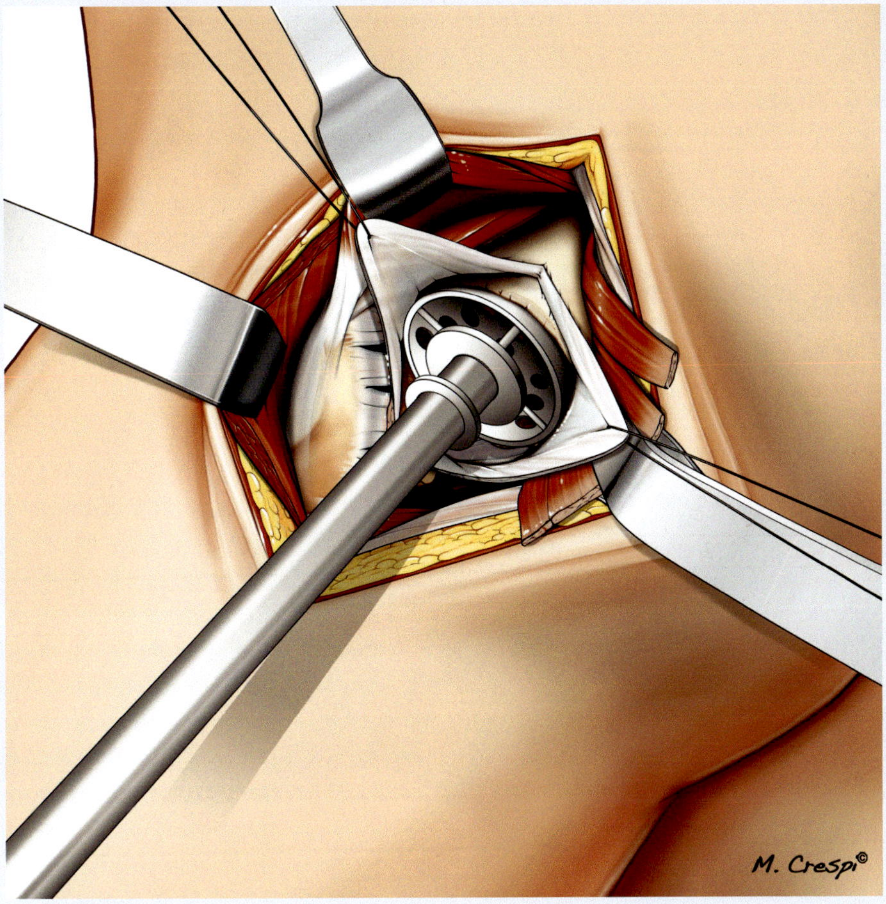

Figure 52
Preparation of the acetabulum with the hemispherical reamers. This step is performed up to the size established in the pre-operative planning. Alternatively, the size is determined by the surgeon's perception of the adequacy of the diameter, in relation to various factors (bone quality, sagittal and coronal cup diameters, matching the level of the acetabular fundus, etc.)

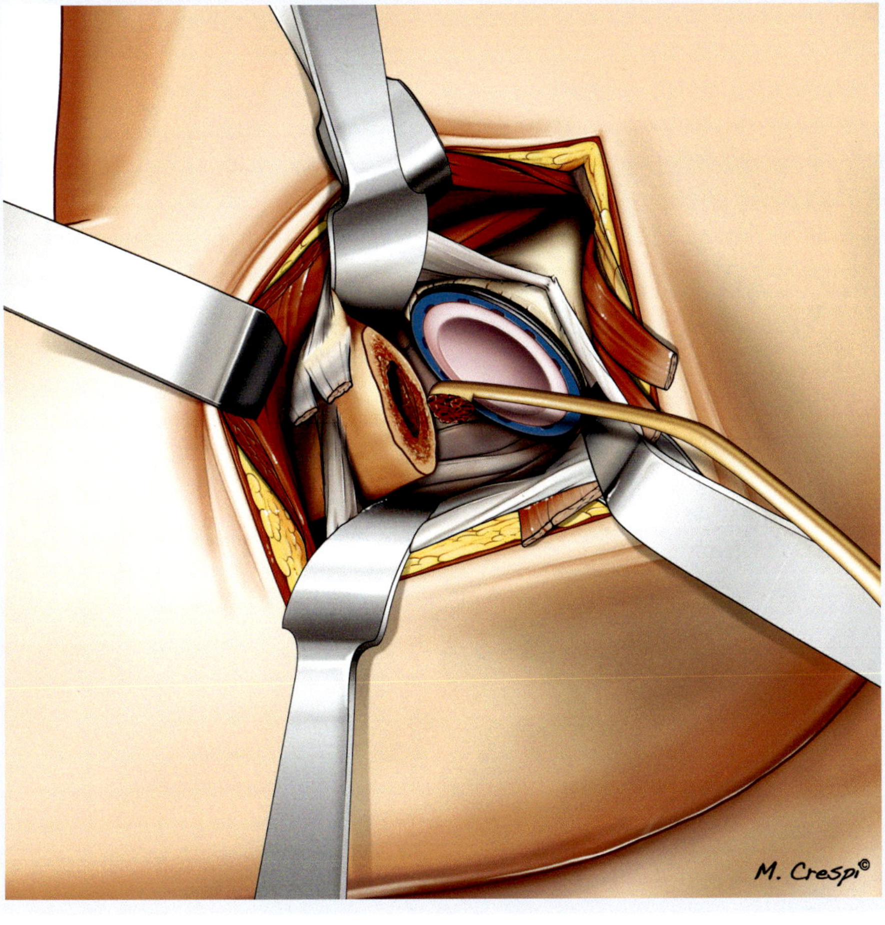

Figure 53
Application of cup and ceramic insert. Placing the limb in the appropriate position, the femoral diaphyseal canal is now approached with a curved instrument

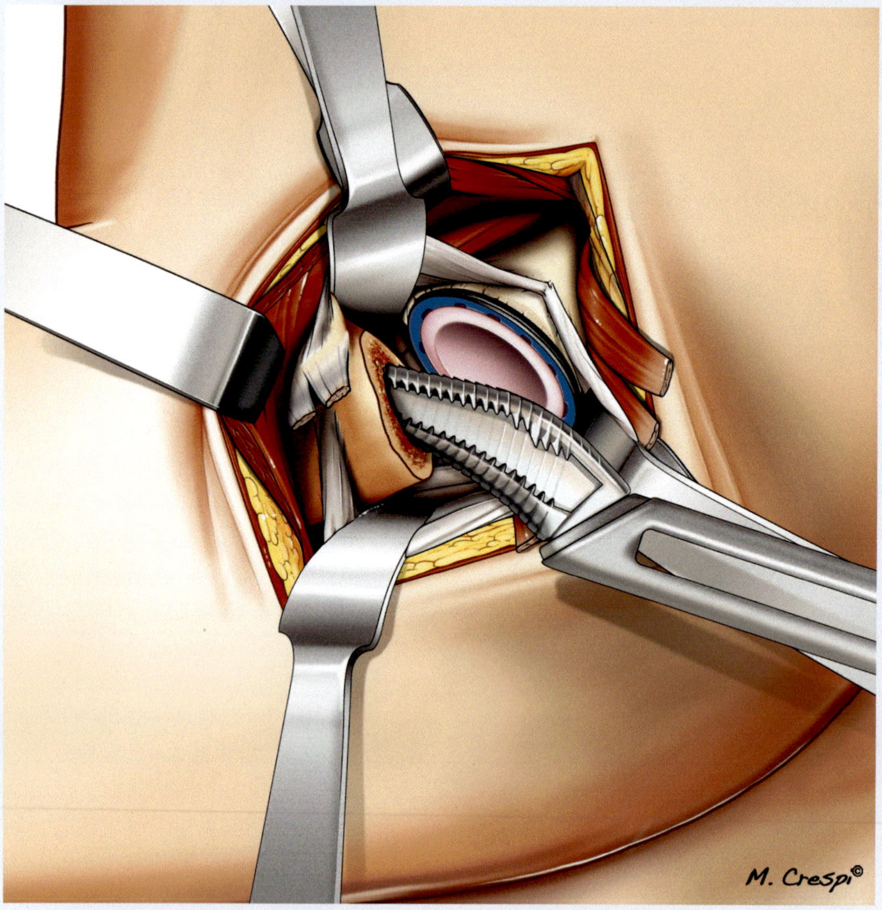

Figure 54
The diaphyseal canal is prepared with the broaches. The choice of the size is based on the indications of the pre-operative planning, but it is always balanced by the surgeon's perception of filling and stability. Once the stable size has been reached, the assembly is carried out with trial neck and head. The prosthesis is reduced and the stability tests are performed. It is also possible to perform an X-ray evaluation to judge the adequacy of the prosthetic size, the position of the implant and the possible presence of fractures

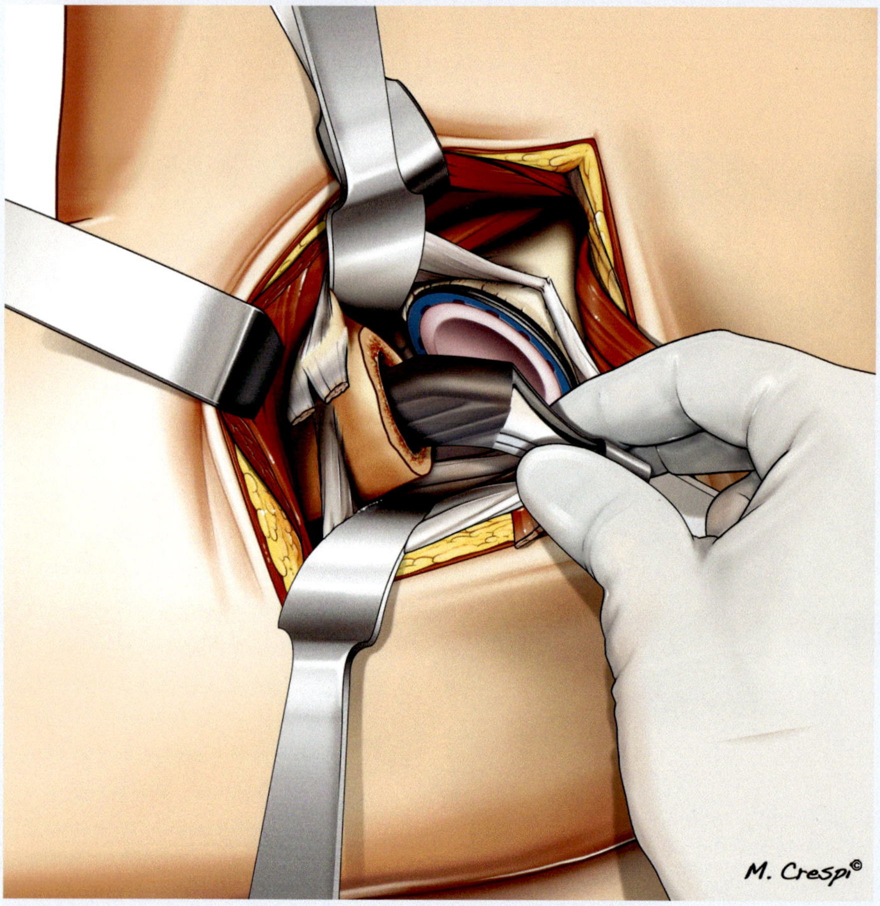

Figure 55
Application of definitive stem using the press-fit&fill technique

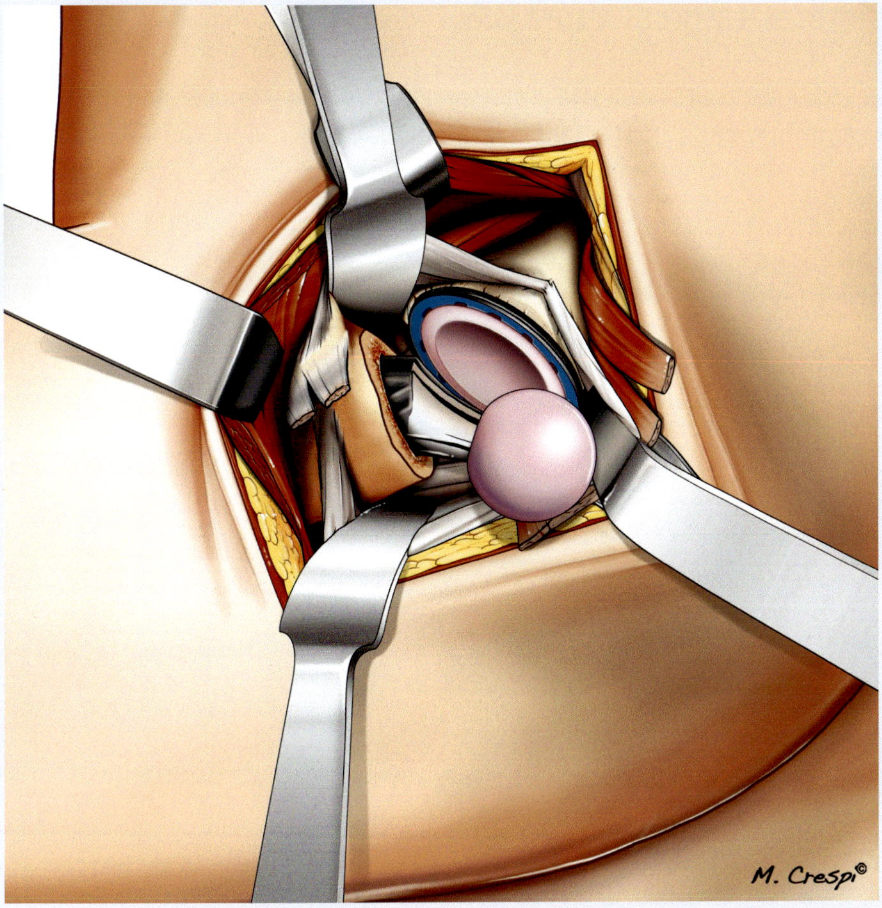

Figure 56
Application of the prosthetic head

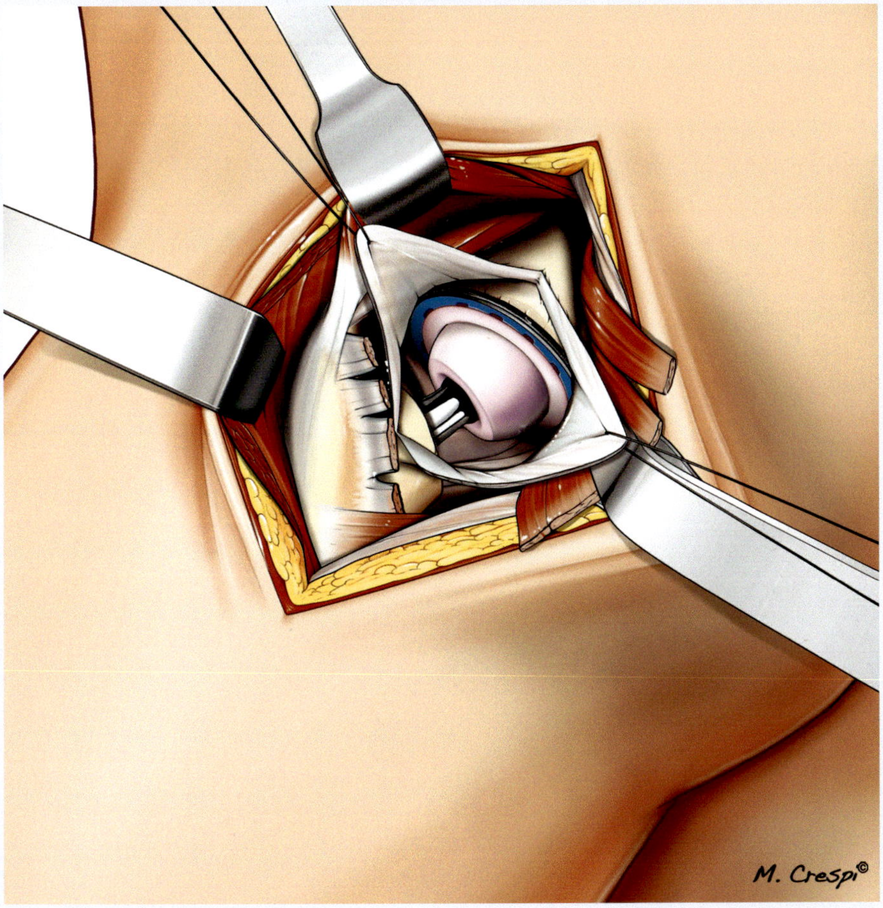

Figure 57
Final reduction of the prosthesis and further evaluation of implant stability. It should be remembered that it is imperative to reconstruct the deep muscle layer (piriformis and external rotators) to ensure the stability of the prosthetic implant and the recovery of joint function

Minimally invasive lateral surgical approach

This surgical technique actually replicates the one proposed by Watson-Jones, but significantly reduces the skin incision, the section of the fascia lata and the extension of the intermuscular deepening between the tensor fascia lata and the gluteus medius to reach the anterior capsular layer.

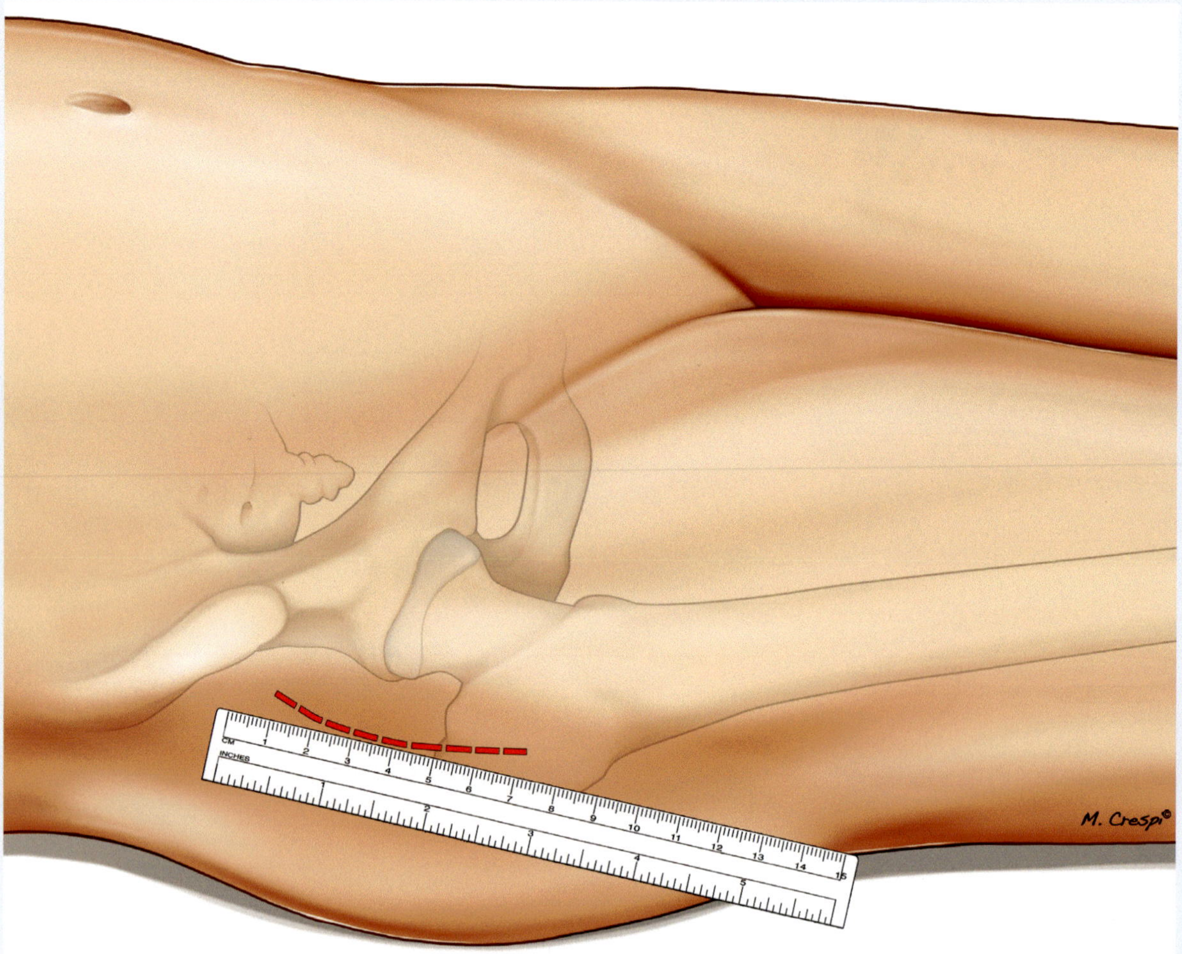

Figure 58 Patient in supine decubitus, with a support underneath the ipsilateral gluteus to slightly incline the hip. The 7-8 cm skin incision line, slightly curved posteriorly, between the great trochanter and the antero-superior iliac spine is marked

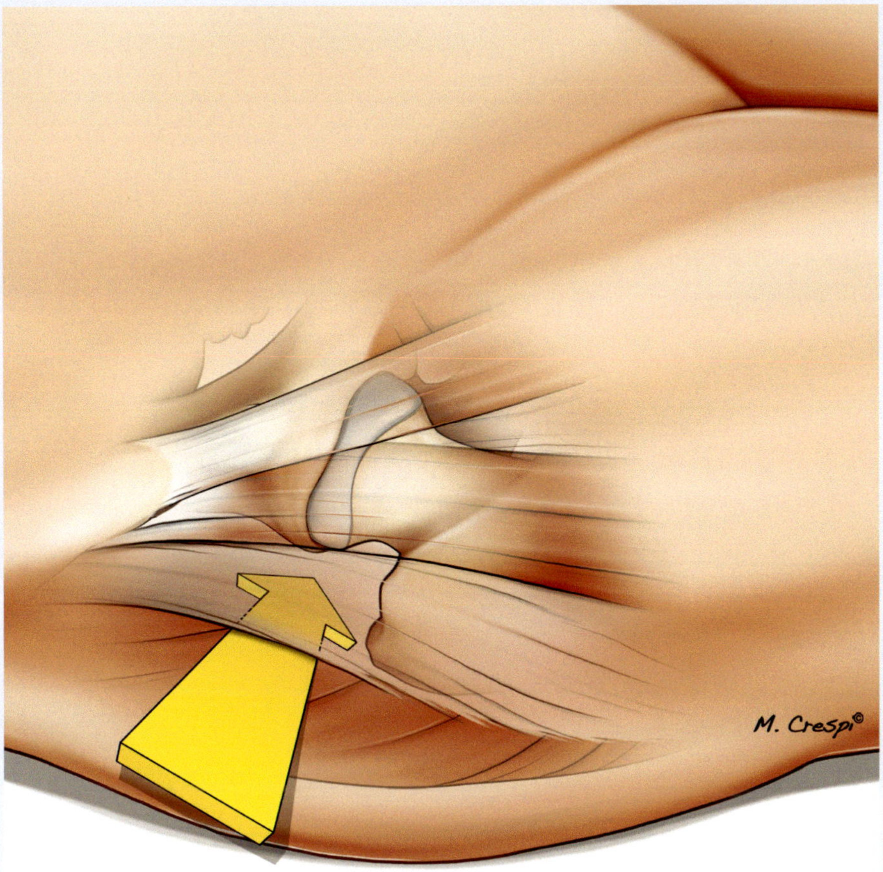

Figure 59
Anatomical overview. The yellow arrow indicates the direction of the intermuscular passage between the tensor fascia lata and the gluteus medius

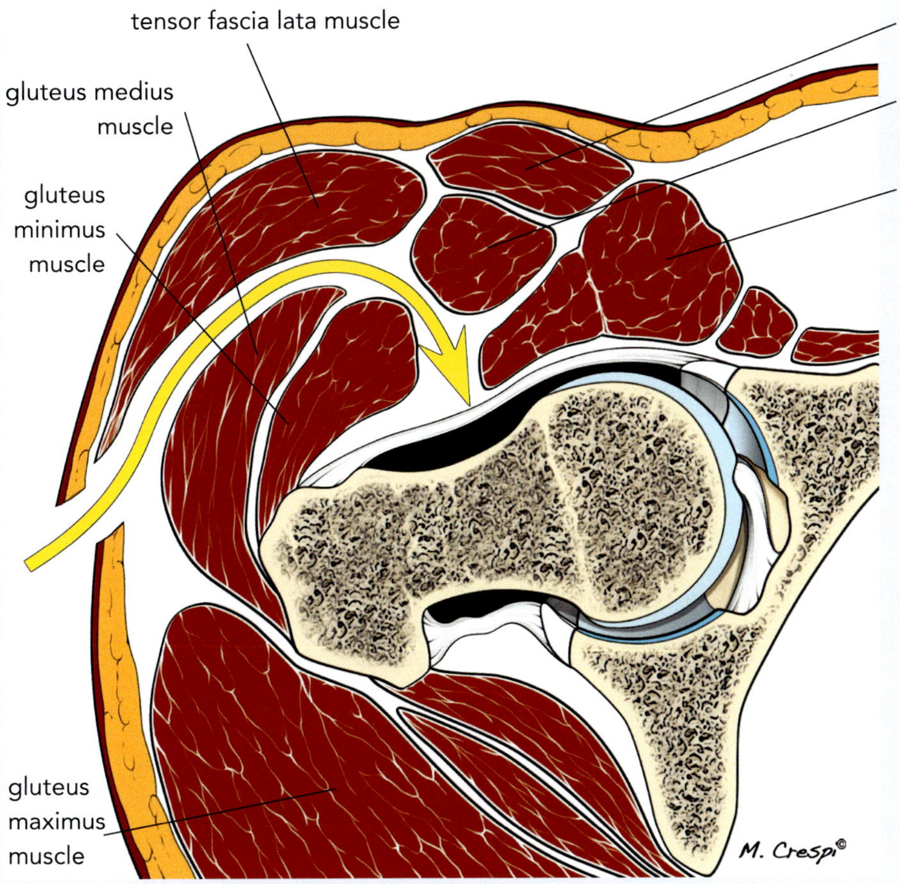

Figure 60
Reproduction of the anatomical scenario on the transverse plane. Despite starting from a more lateral skin incision, by splitting-separating the tensor fascia lata from the gluteus medius, we reach the capsular plane anteriorly. This approach is well represented by the yellow curved arrow

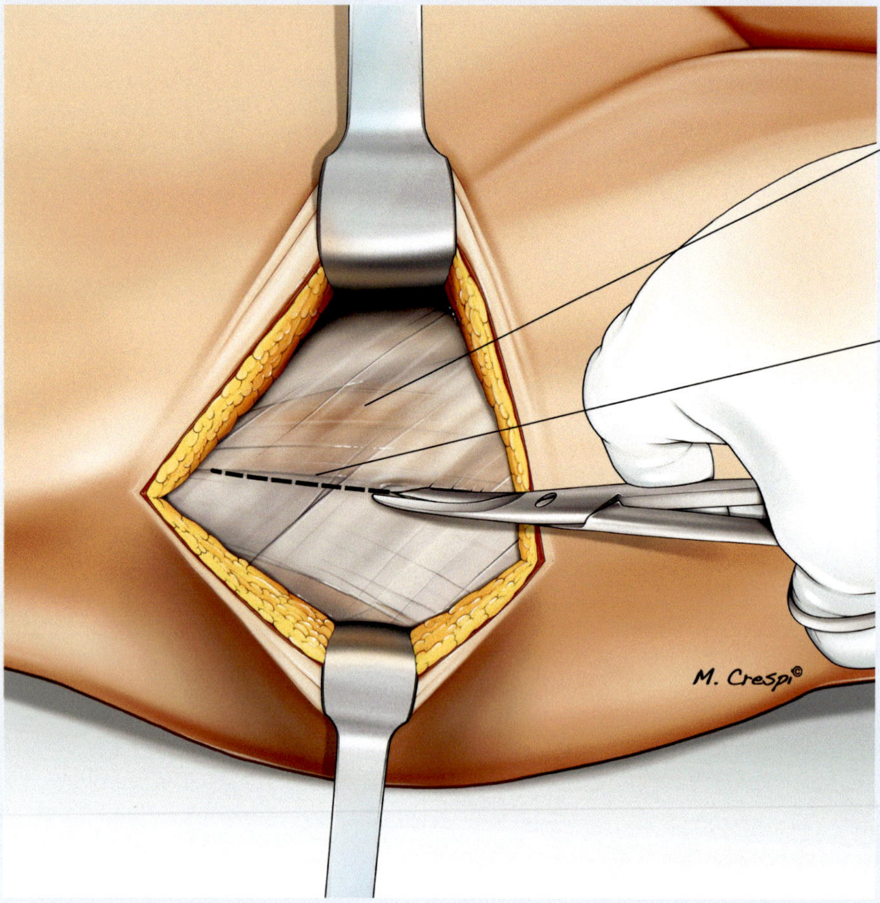

Figure 61 Retracting the layers (cutaneous and subcutaneous), the fascia lata is exposed. This is dissected longitudinally with scalpel or scissors above the muscular interstitium (palpable) between the tensor fascia lata and the gluteus medius

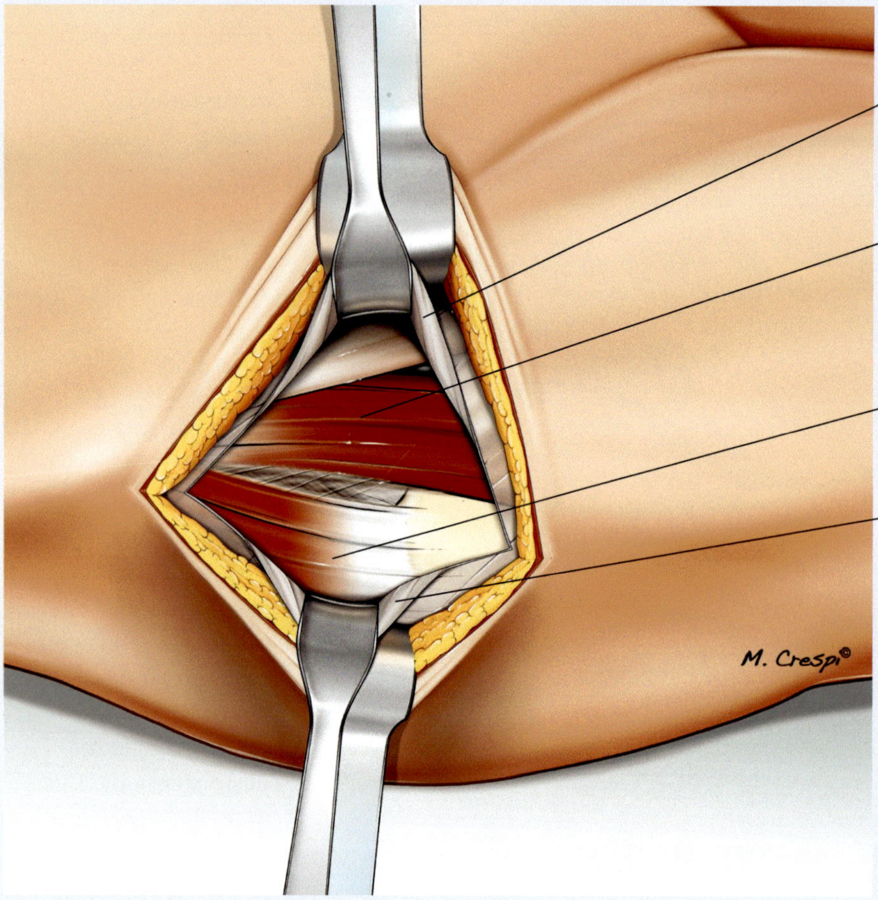

Figure 62 When the fascial flaps are retracted, the muscle bellies of the tensor fascia lata and the gluteus medius are exposed

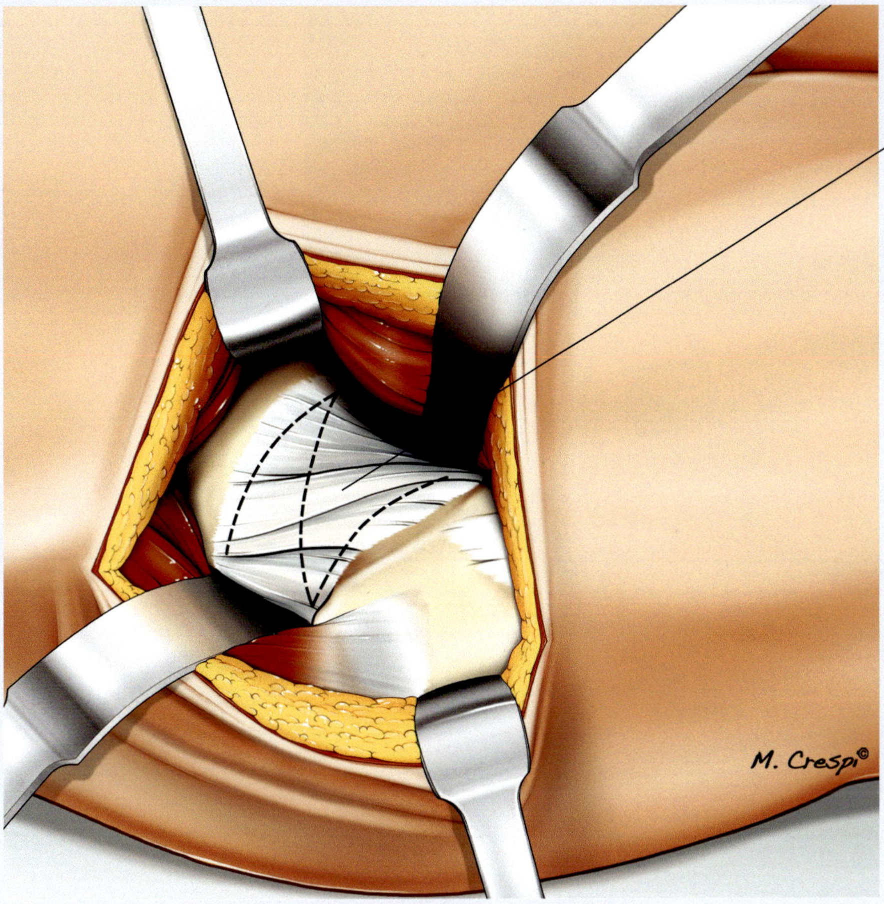

Figure 63
Splitting-retracting the muscular bellies of the tensor fascia lata and the gluteus medius we reach the anterior capsular layer

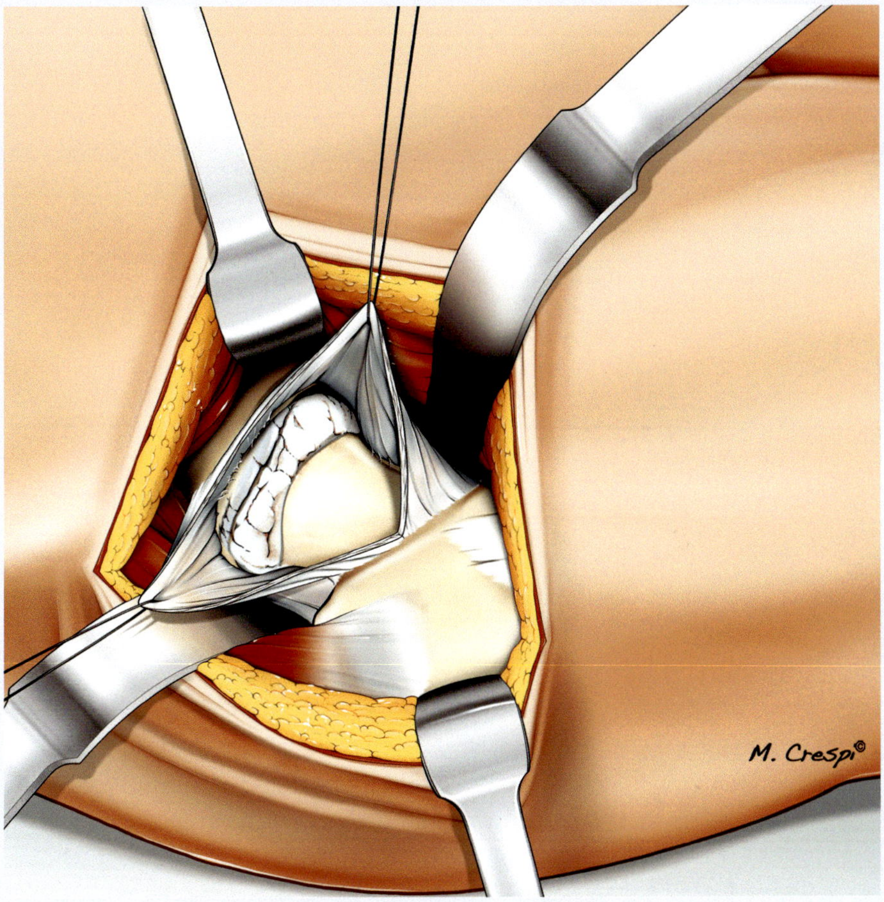

Figure 64
Capsulotomy and coxo-femoral arthrotomy

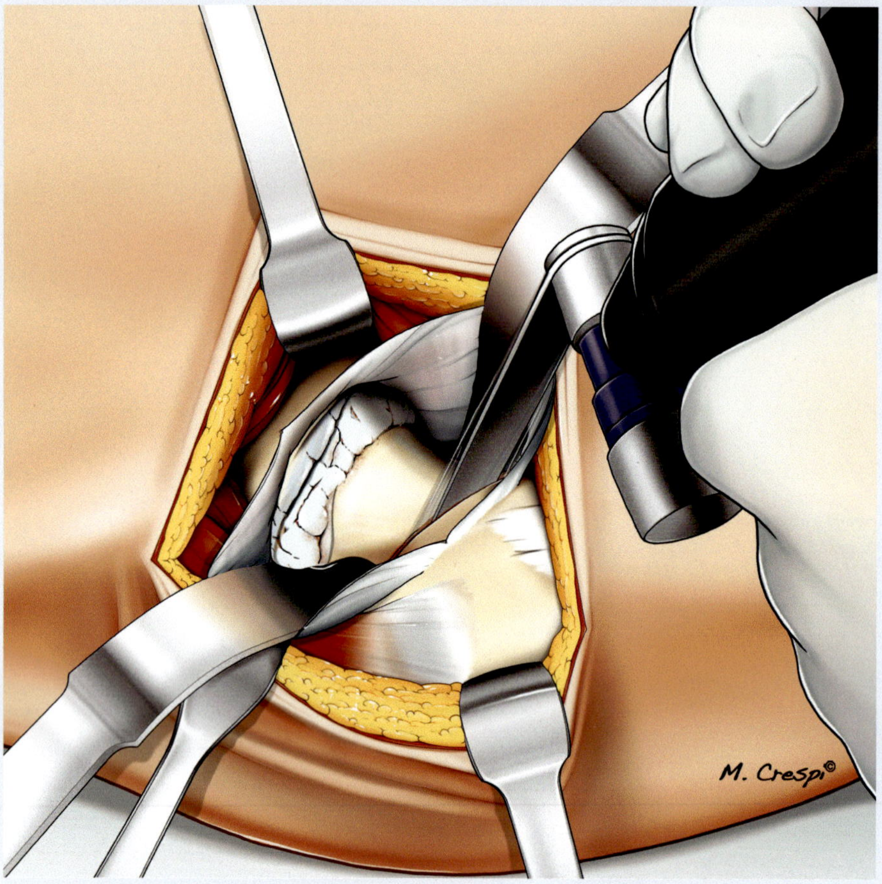

Figure 65
Osteotomy of the femoral neck at the level established by the pre-operative planning and removal of the femoral head

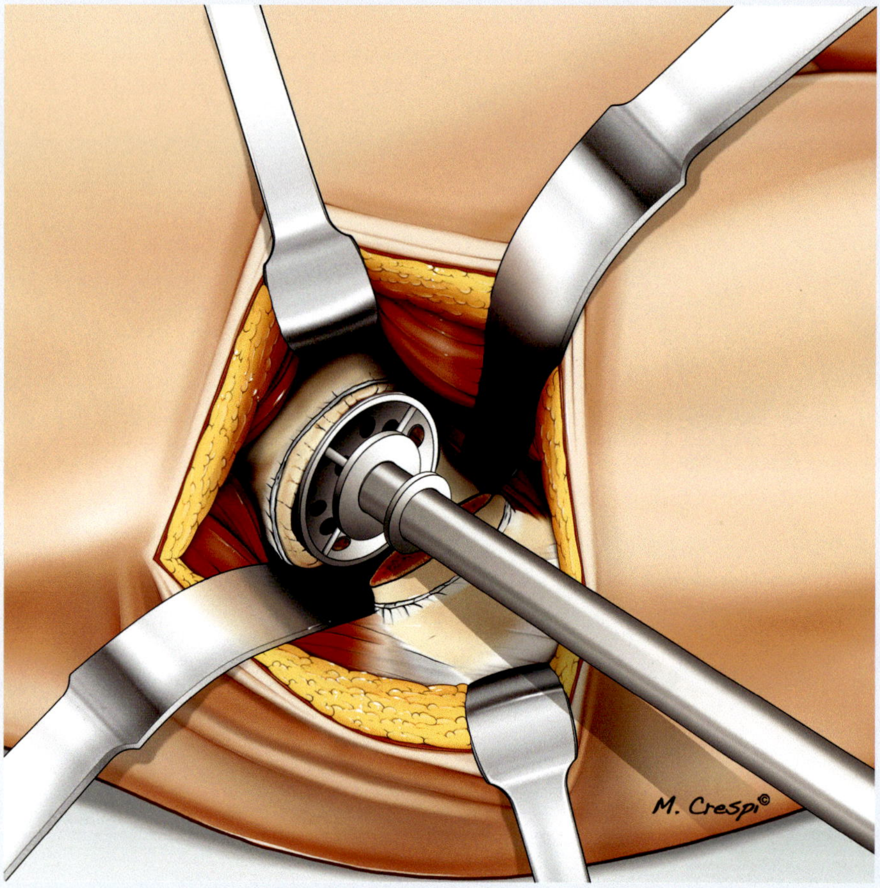

Figure 66
Preparation with hemispherical reamers of the acetabulum and application of the definitive cup and ceramic insert

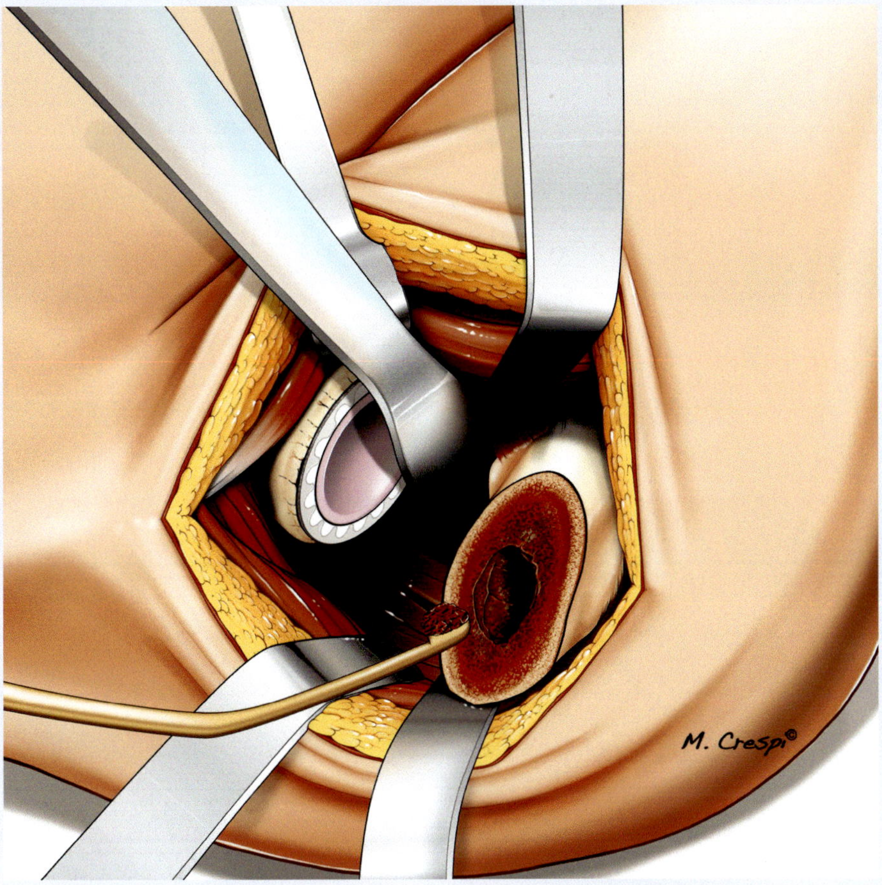

Figure 67
A curved instrument is used to penetrate the femoral diaphyseal canal

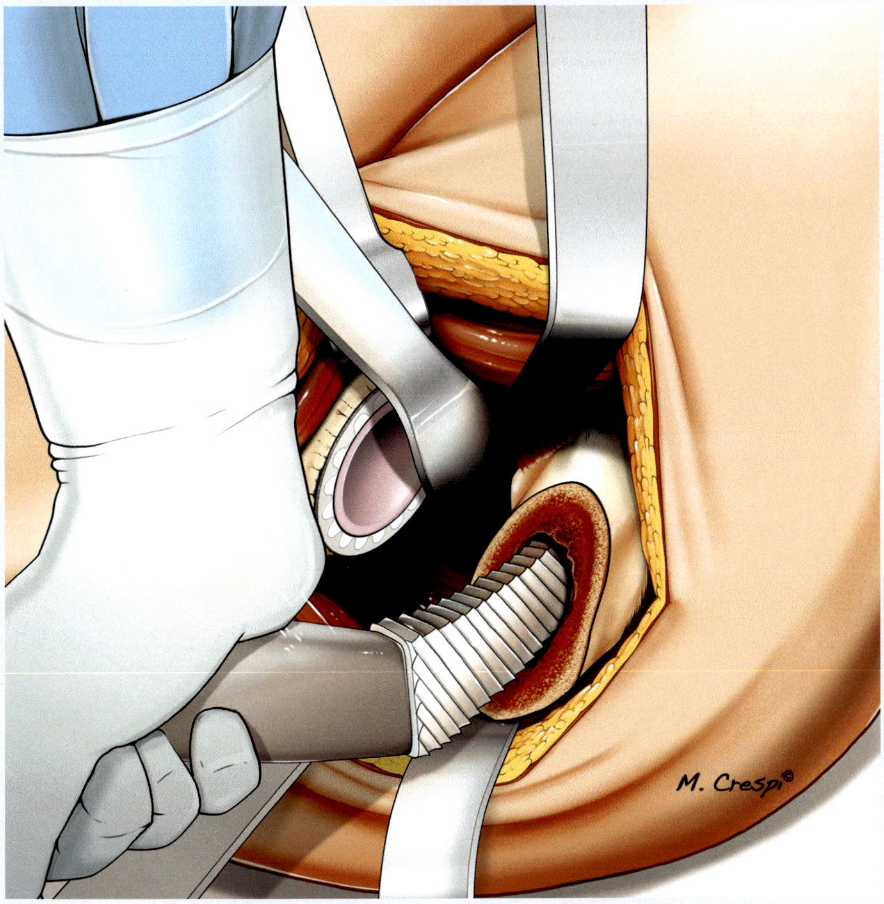

Figure 68
Preparation of the femoral diaphyseal canal with broaches of progressive sizes, according to the pre-operative planning and the perception of 'stable filling' of the device. A trial neck and head may be used to perform implant reduction and check its stability.
An X-ray evaluation can also be carried out to confirm the correct prosthetic alignment and the state of the periprosthetic bone (risk of fractures, etc.)

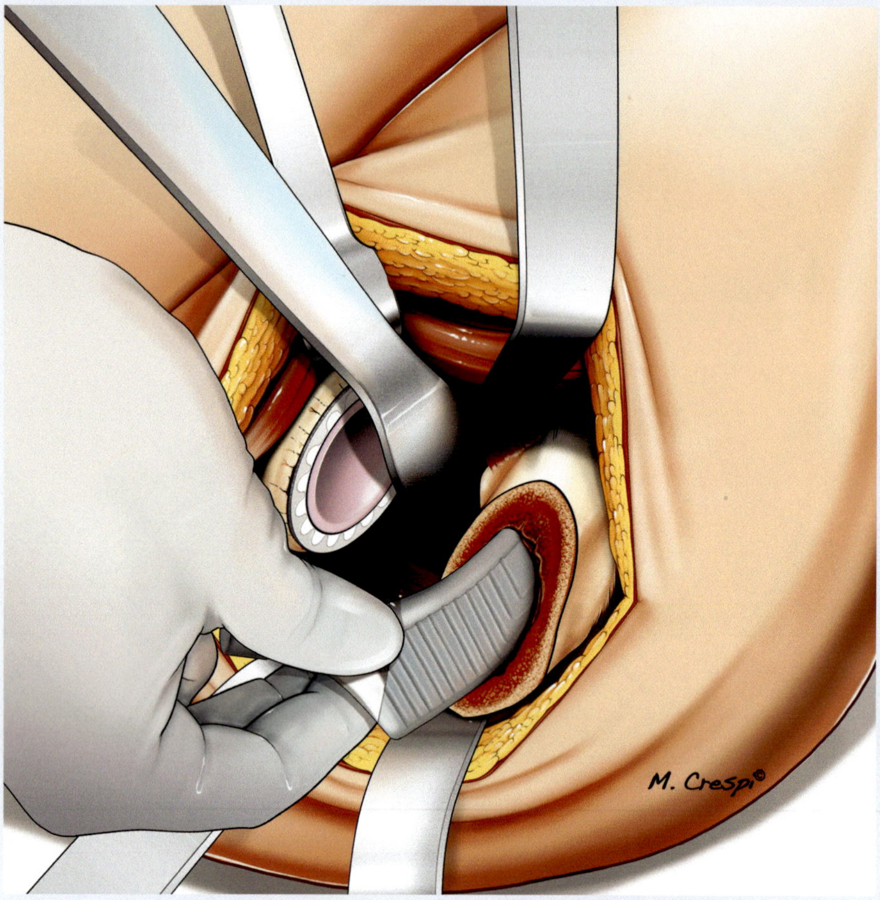

Figure 69
Application of the definitive stem

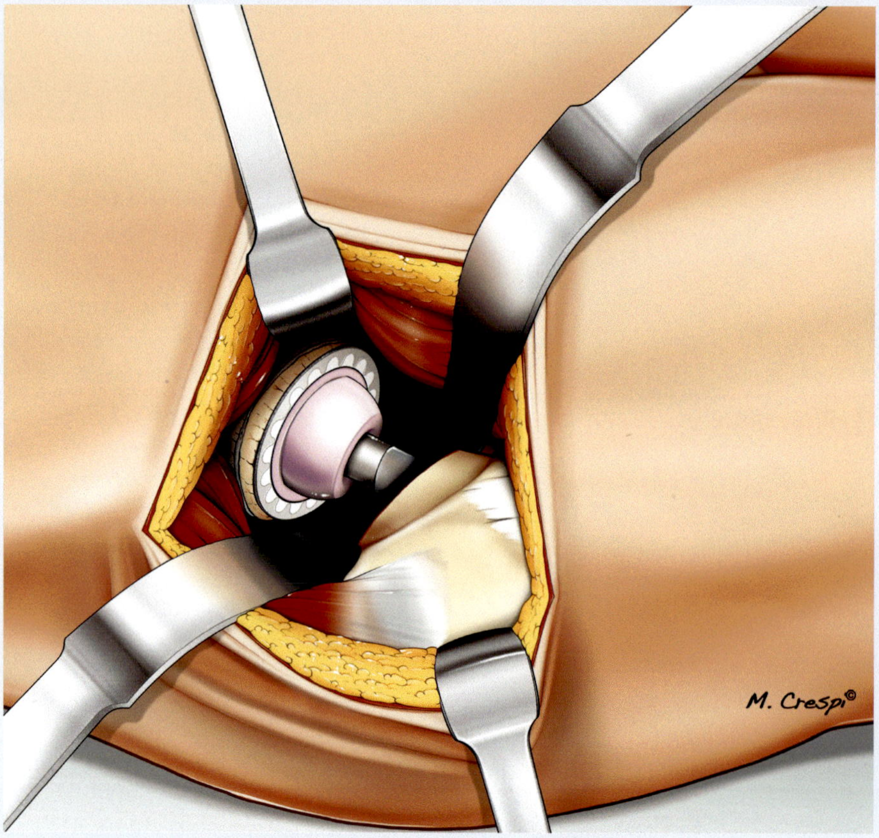

Figure 70
Application of the ceramic head, reduction of the prosthesis and execution of the implant stability tests

The lateral femoral cutaneous nerve in hip anterior surgical approaches: anatomical considerations

Sergio Candiotto*, Vittore Costa**, Antonio Camporese*, Giulio Edoardo Vigni***, Carla Stecco****, Raffaele De Caro****

*Hip and Shoulder Surgery Unit, Abano Terme General Hospital, Padua, Italy
**Hip and Prosthetic Surgery Unit, Humanitas Gavazzeni Hospital, Bergamo, Italy
***Department of Orthopaedics and Traumatology, University of Palermo, Italy
****Institute of Normal Anatomy, University of Padova, Italy

Introduction

Hip anterior surgical approaches have always required particular attention to the presence, course, and distribution of the lateral femoral cutaneous nerve (LCN). This occurred both in the first surgical approach provided in Germany by Carl Hueter in 1881 and in the subsequent revision by Marius Smith-Petersen, in the United States in the third decade of the twentieth century, involving a more extensive dissection. Then recently, it was also of great importance at the end of the last century when these surgical approaches were again revised and the minimally invasive anterior approach with a longitudinal or inguinal-oblique incision ('bikini approach') became popular. In fact, in all of these approaches, the muscle interstitium between sartorius and tensor fascia lata is split and branches of this nerve run on the corresponding suprafascial layer (fig. 1).
Letournell's ilioinguinal surgical approach, also puts the lateral femoral cutaneous nerve at risk. This approach is used for acetabular fractures or for certain prostheses (primary implants or revisions), when it is necessary to stabilize or reconstruct the anterior column of the acetabulum. In this case, the lateral femoral cutaneous nerve occupies the operative field when it emerges from the pelvis near the ASIS (Anterior Superior Iliac Spine). It has always been recognized that injury to the main trunk of the lateral femoral cutaneous nerve, whether direct (laceration) or indirect (compression, stretching, traction ischemia, or scar entrapment) could result in neuroapraxia of variable severity and transience. This may result in a particular clinical condition with numbness, tingling, itching and burning in the cutaneous distribution area of the nerve (lateral surface of the thigh). This scenario resembles in some aspects meralgia paresthetica or Roth's syndrome [18,23,28,35,39,40,41,53,55].
In any case, it is somewhat surprising to note the large number of scientific studies on this small and exclusively sensory nerve. Its variability in course and distribution has always been of great interest to anatomists and several surgical specialities.
Recent research has made it possible to modify the anatomical knowledge of the lateral femoral cutaneous nerve. This nerve affects four different areas: the vertebral area due to its origin from the nerve roots, the intrapelvic course, the inguinal emergence and the distribution on the thigh. Consequently, misconceptions about the anatomy of the nerve that had previously been perpetuated in the scientific literature and in the training of surgeons have been corrected.

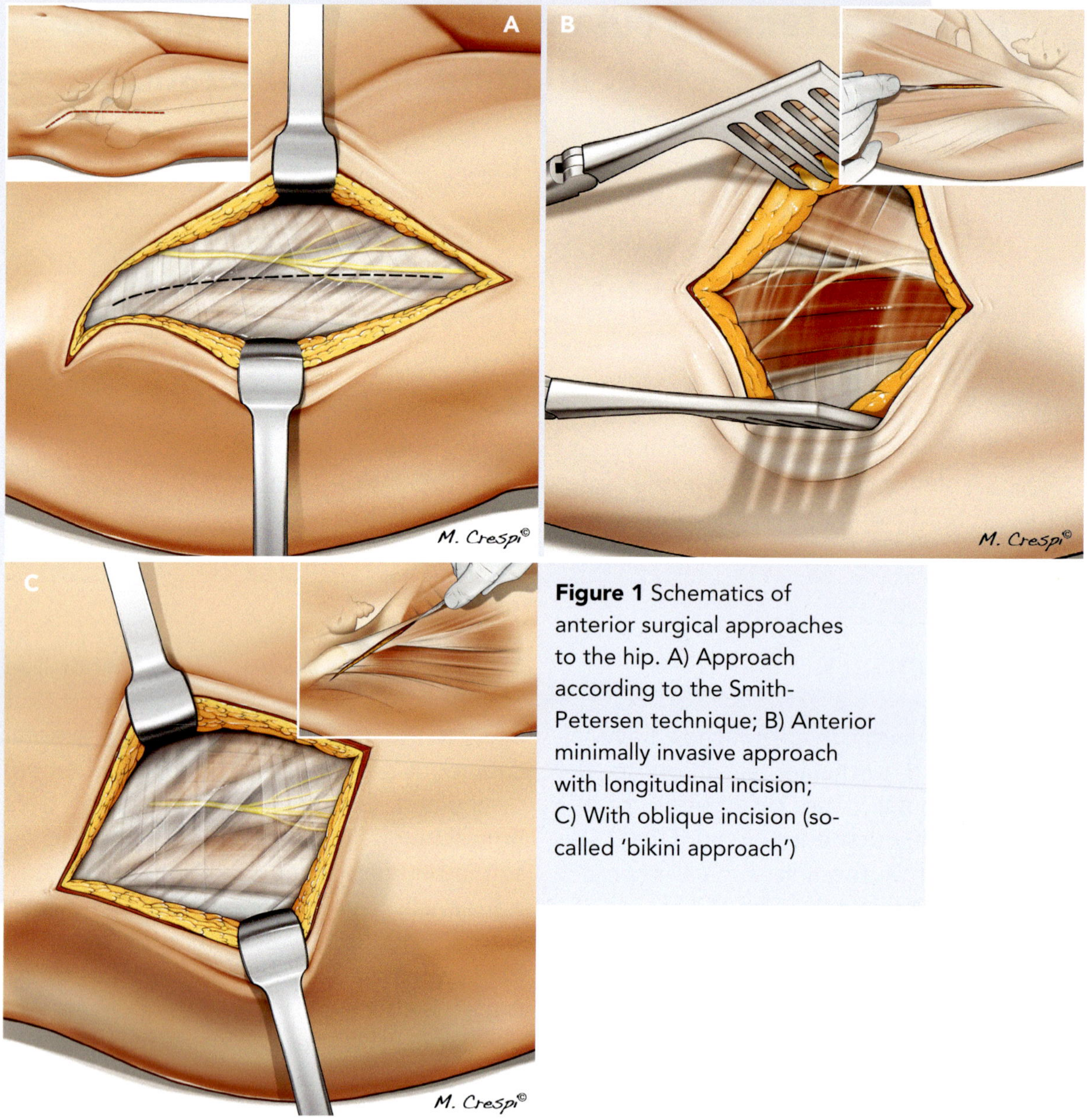

Figure 1 Schematics of anterior surgical approaches to the hip. A) Approach according to the Smith-Petersen technique; B) Anterior minimally invasive approach with longitudinal incision; C) With oblique incision (so-called 'bikini approach')

For example, maxillofacial surgeons and dentists are also interested in the lateral femoral cutaneous nerve. Bone grafts from the iliac crest, harvested near the ASIS, can frequently lead to possible local residual pain.

'Donor site pain' is partly related to the bone harvest itself, due to the interruption of the iliac crest and the injury of the muscles that insert into it. On the other hand, part of it is imputable to direct or indirect involvement of the lateral femoral cutaneous nerve.

Orthopaedic surgeons are interested in the lateral femoral cutaneous nerve because of its difficult identification and management in hip anterior approaches or in pelvic and femoral osteotomies. Its variable and partly unpredictable anatomical configuration, especially in its course distal to the inguinal ligament, can interfere with surgical approach and manoeuvres.

Portals from arthroscopic hip surgery can also lead to injuries to the lateral femoral cutaneous nerve or its branches.

Similarly, surgeons of the pelvis (whether open or laparoscopic surgery for the urogenital, vascular, and intestinal apparatus or for the correction of inguinal hernia), may be affected by painful outcomes resulting from injury to the nerve in its extraperitoneal pelvic course. For example, on the right side, the nerve establishes a close relationship with the ileum and cecum, while on the left with the sigma.

In laparoscopic extraperitoneal surgical repair of inguinal hernia, the **'trapezoid disaster'** and the **'triangle of Doom'** are reported by some authors. These are due to the possible risk of entrapment (entrapment neuropathies) of the spermatic vessels, vas deferens, external iliac vessels, and genitofemoral, lateral femoral cutaneous, and femoral nerves [15].

The conditions underlying the possible injury of the lateral femoral cutaneous nerve in different surgical areas are: the structure, the multiple branches and the variable course of the nerve, the need to extend the surgical dissection, the traction ischaemia, the entrapment of the nerve in scar tissue or in implanted devices (such as mesh for inguinal hernias) and the close contiguity of the nerve with the anatomical structures subject to surgery [2,9,10,26,30].

Current anatomical knowledge of the nerve in its intrapelvic course and its emergence from the pelvis can also explain its injury for non-surgical causes. For example, these may be direct trauma to the pelvis, the use of specific constricting clothing (belts, etc.), ascites, pregnancy, prolonged sitting in confined spaces (e.g. aircraft) and abdominal redundancy (especially in the not infrequent cases of ectopic nerve course, such as above the iliac crest).

Similarly, the presence of an intrapelvic mass could lead to a clinical onset similar to meralgia paresthesica. This mass could affect the lateral femoral cutaneous nerve due to compression or stretching in its retroperitoneal and pre-ligamentous inguinal course.

Anatomical considerations

In classic anatomical treatises, the lateral femoral cutaneous nerve generally originates from the dorsal branches of the second and third lumbar nerve roots. Other descriptions report a less frequent origin from the first and second roots or an origin from only the second or third nerve root [40,45,49].

The nerve emerges below the lateral margin of the psoas muscle, heads obliquely distal and lateral and infiltrates below the fascia of the iliac muscle, passing close to the iliac branch of the iliolumbar artery. It then heads towards the ASIS, crosses the deep iliac circumflex artery and with a single trunk runs below the inguinal ligament of Poupart, just medial to the anterior-superior iliac spine, where the ligament itself inserts (precisely in the angle between ASIS, ligament and insertion of the sartorius muscle. (figs. 2-3).

The nerve enters the thigh and runs in a canal (figs. 4-5) formed by the coalescence of the superficial fascia with the fascia lata [50,51,52]. For some authors [1,17,23,27,28] the fascial canal is formed by a splitting of the fascia lata.

In the thigh the nerve runs above the sartorius (figs. 6-7). At 2-3 centimetres from the inguinal ligament, the nerve divides into two main branches, the anterior branch and the posterior branch (gluteal branch).

The anterior branch heads distally and about 9-10 cm from the ASIS further divides into the medial and lateral branches. These continue in the subcutaneous layer up to the knee, creating numerous branches for the antero-lateral and lateral skin of the thigh (figs. 3, 7-10). The gluteal branch, on the other hand, heads posteriorly, becoming subcutaneous. It divides into branches that innervate the skin of the greater trochanter region and the lateral side of the superior half of the thigh.

The skin area pertaining to the lateral femoral cutaneous nerve can also be innervated by the following branches: genitofemoral, anterior cutaneous branches of femoral nerve, ileoinguinal and femoral. This complex nerve overlapping can make it difficult to correlate an eventual dysesthesia with a specific cause.

The classical anatomical description, which is essentially based on common clinical experience, however, proves inadequate in the light of more recent anatomical studies. In any case, even on a cadaver, it is particu-

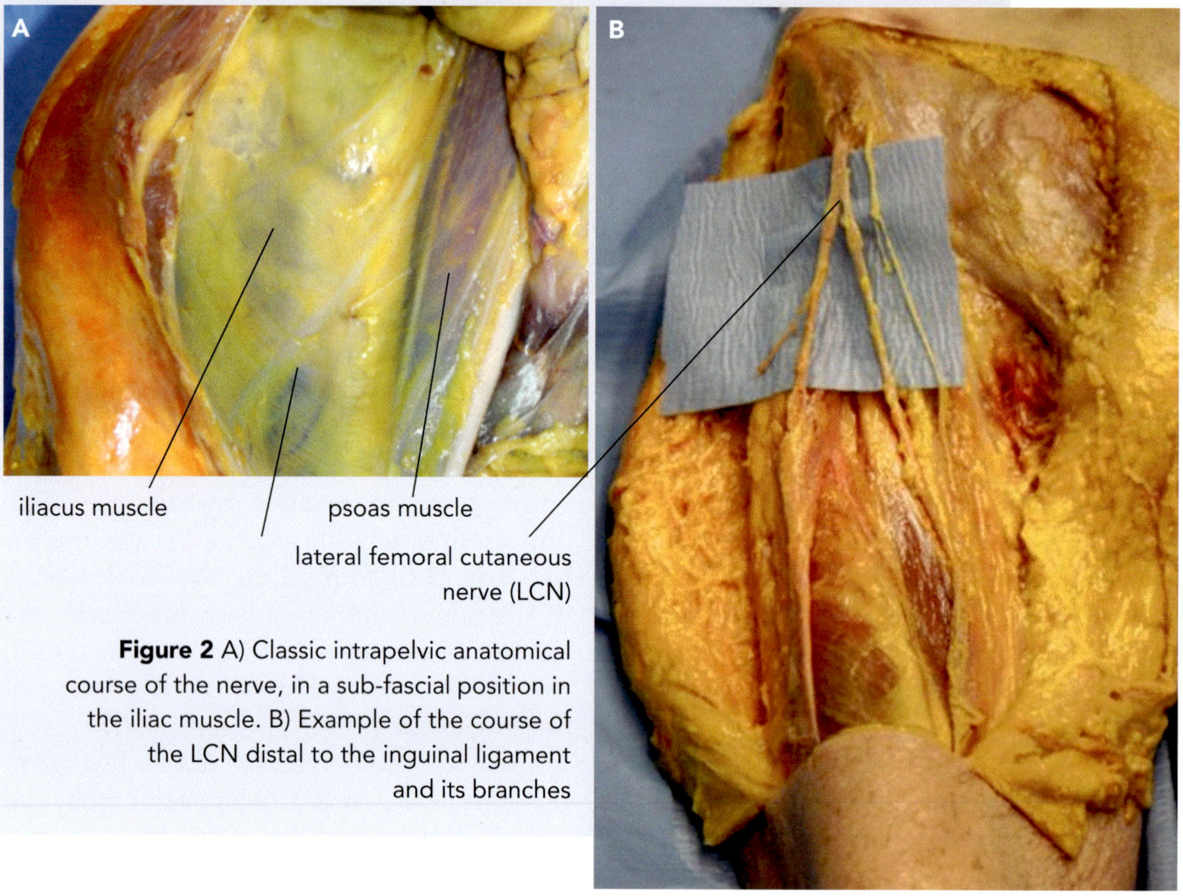

Figure 2 A) Classic intrapelvic anatomical course of the nerve, in a sub-fascial position in the iliac muscle. B) Example of the course of the LCN distal to the inguinal ligament and its branches

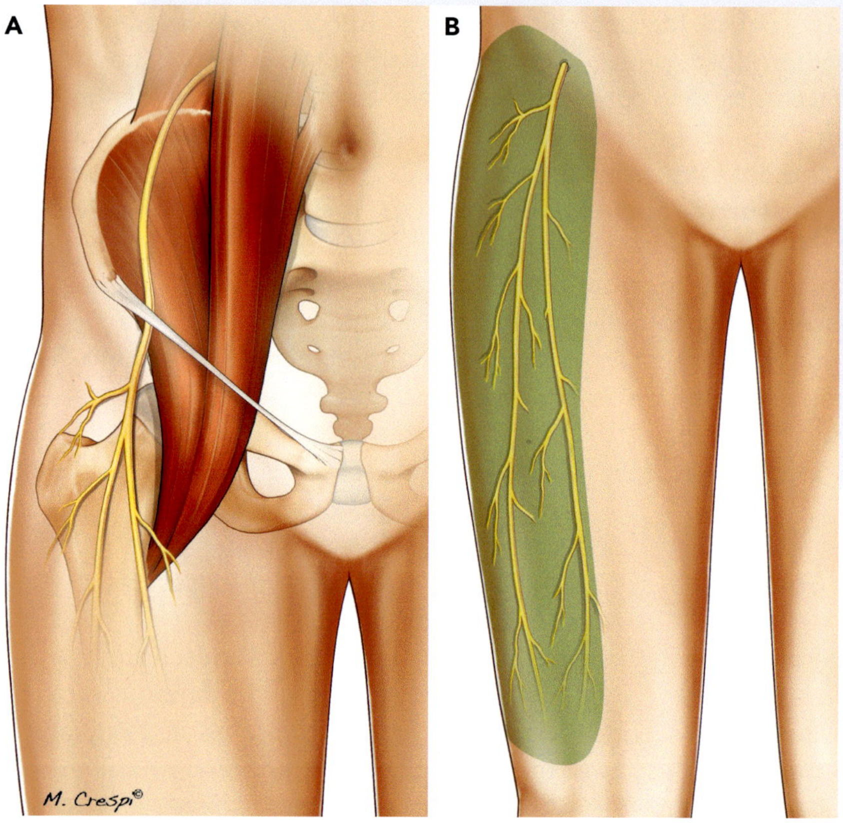

Figure 3 A) Classic anatomical diagram of the LCN, from the intrapelvic tract to the emergence below the inguinal ligament with its ramifications on the thigh. B) Area of cutaneous sensory innervation of the LCN

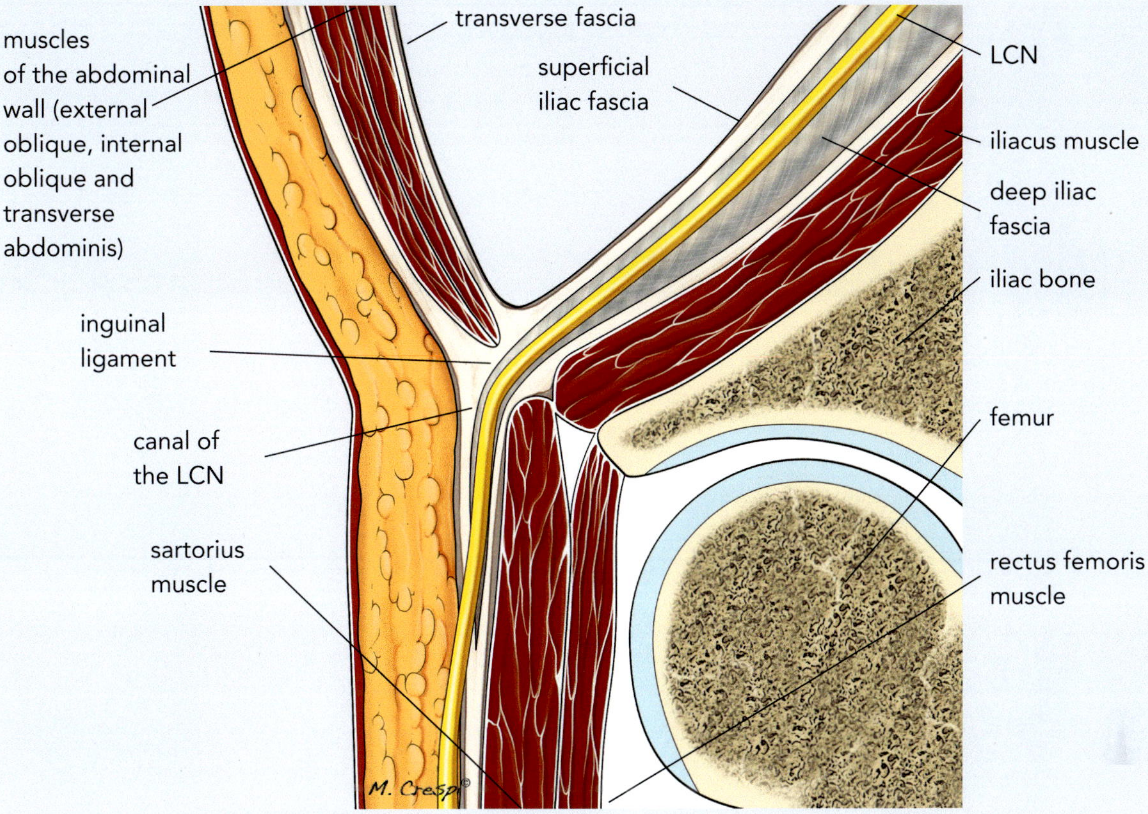

Figure 4 Representative diagram of the fascial canal in which the LCN runs and its relationship with the musculature and inguinal ligament

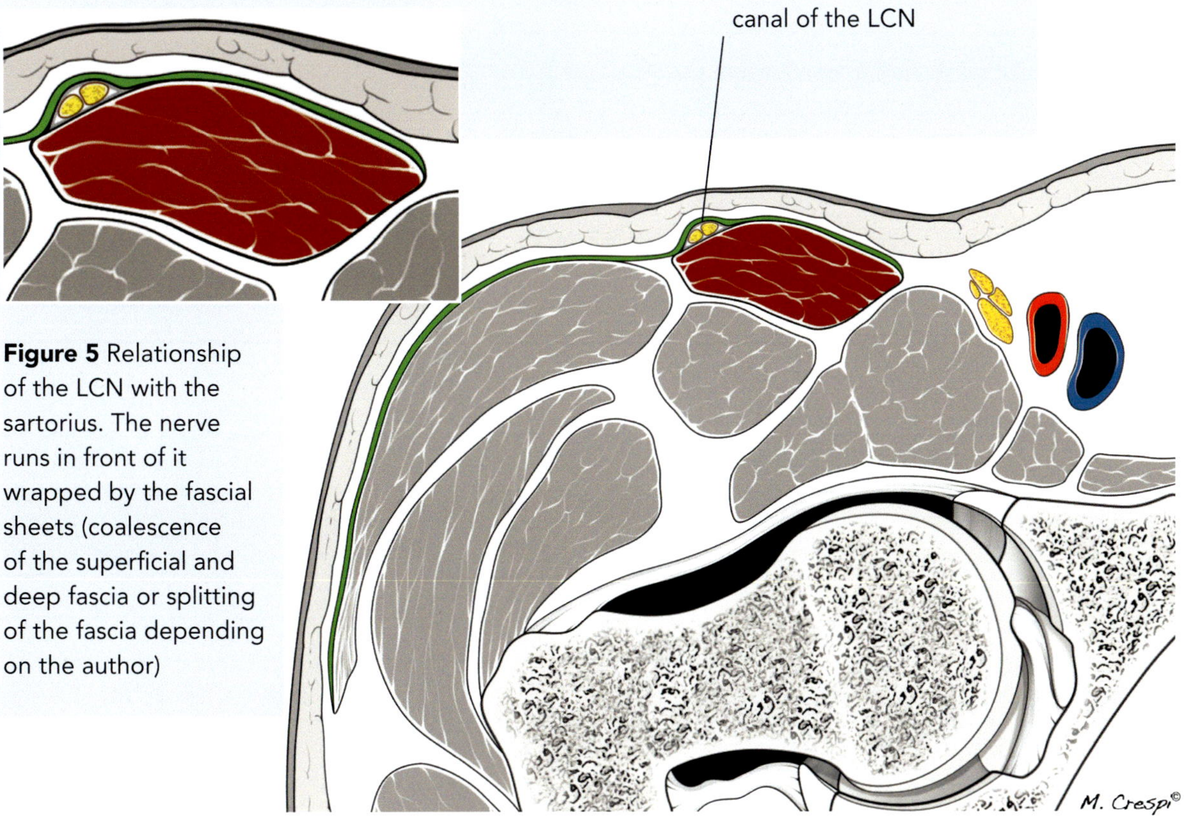

Figure 5 Relationship of the LCN with the sartorius. The nerve runs in front of it wrapped by the fascial sheets (coalescence of the superficial and deep fascia or splitting of the fascia depending on the author)

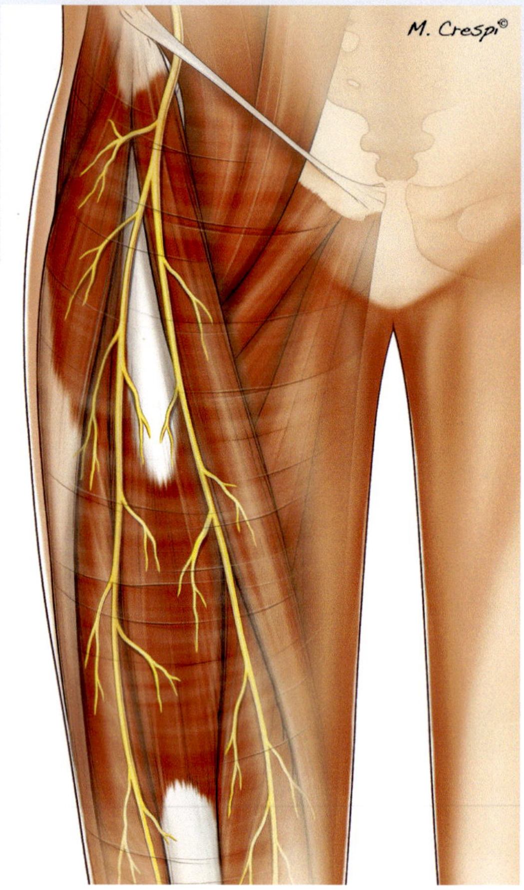

Figure 6 Diagram of the traditional course in the nerve on the thigh

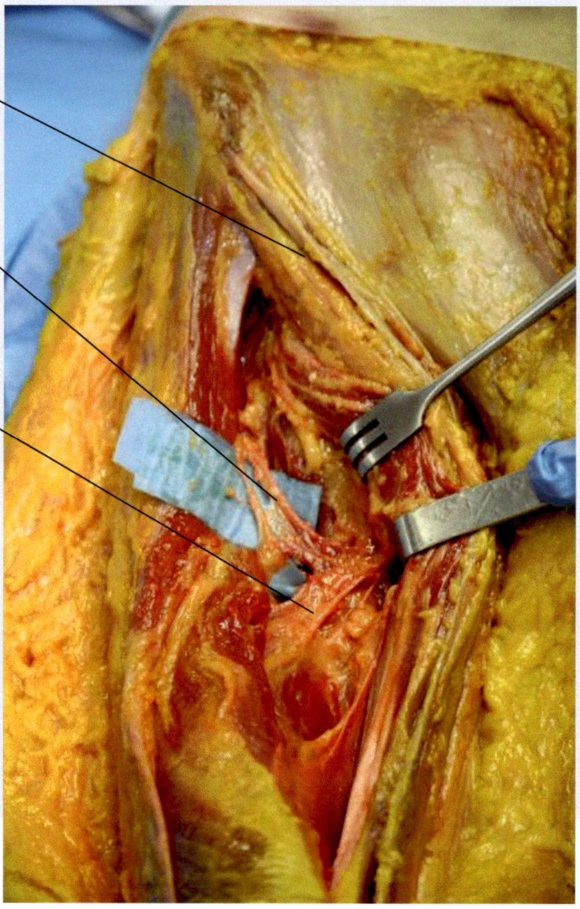

Figure 7 Cadaver study. The LCN is shown transiting medially to the sartorius. The ascending arterial branches of the lateral femoral circumflex are visible in depth

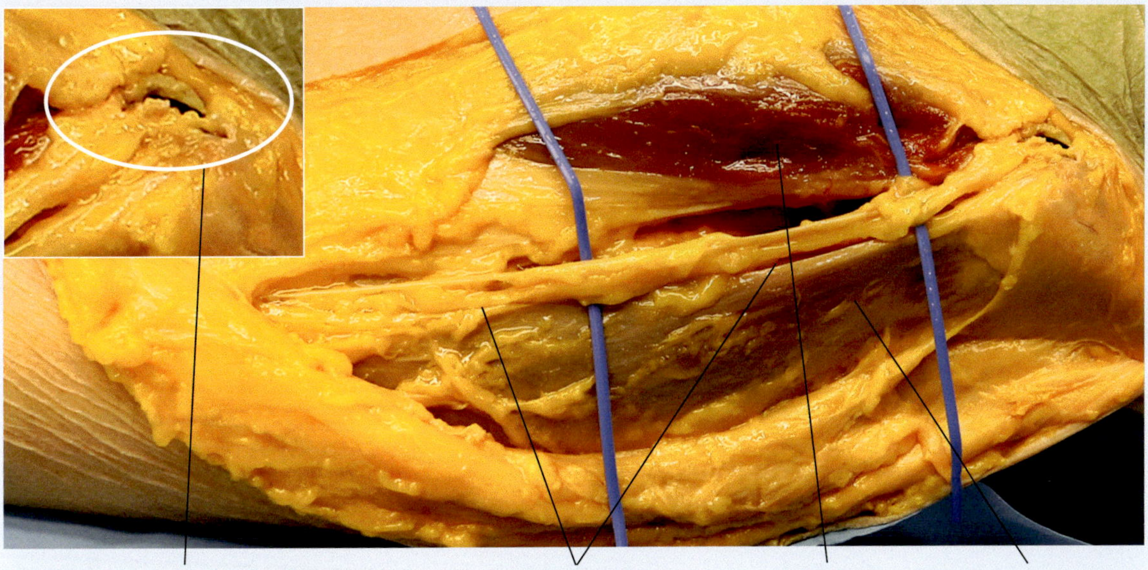

Figure 8 Cadaver study. Emergence of the nerve under the ligament and its course on the thigh, with splitting of the nerve

Figure 9
Distribution of the LCN on the thigh. Note in B the 'net-like' arrangement of the nerve. The branches appear increasingly thin and therefore difficult to isolate

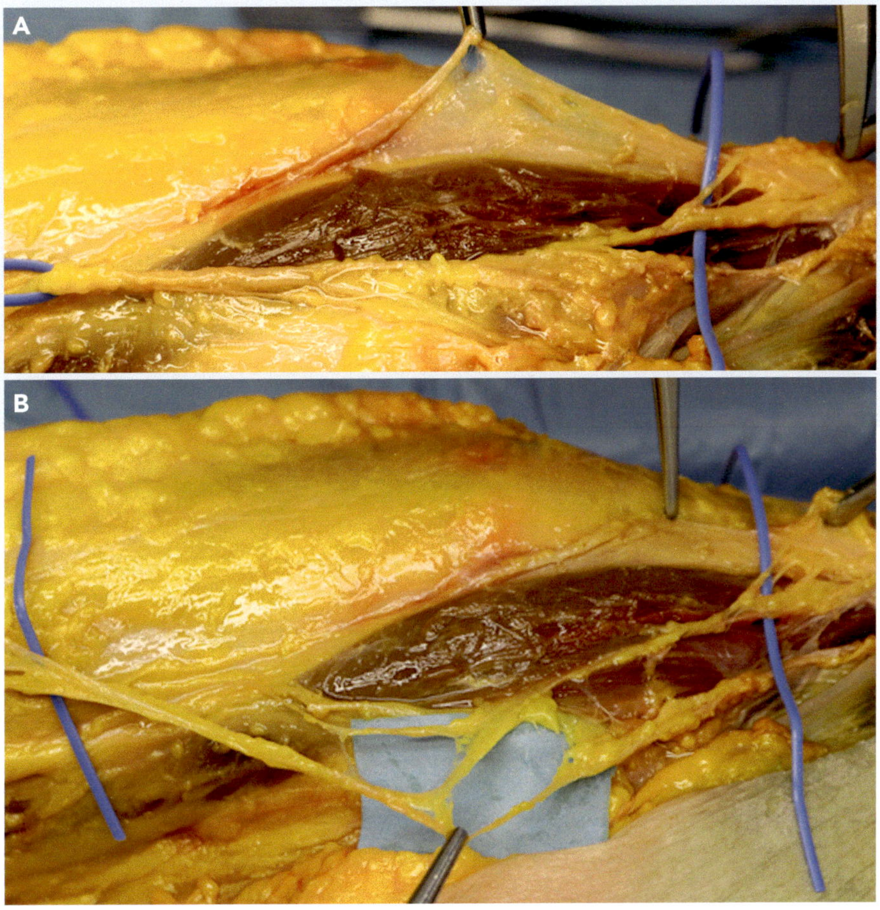

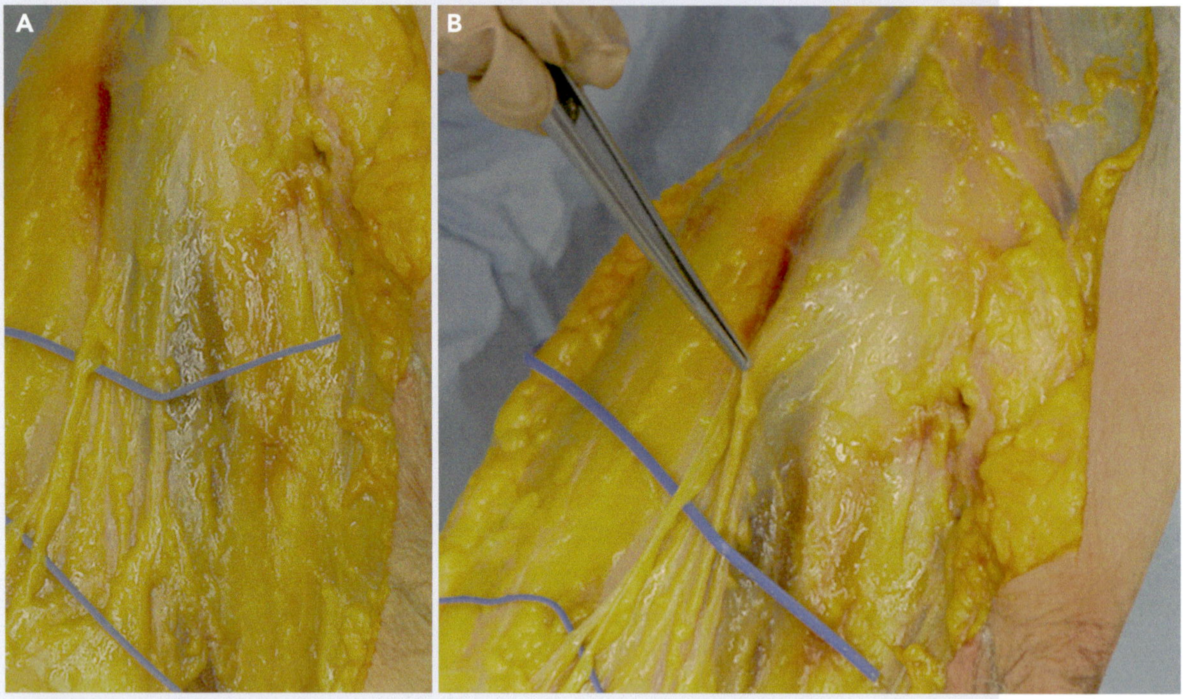

Figure 10 Branches and network distribution of nerve endings on the thigh

larly difficult to isolate and expose the entire nerve distribution, from the largest trunks to the extensive, thin branches to the terminal filaments.

The lateral femoral cutaneous nerve presents numerous variations in origin, course and distribution. Even 'aberrant' forms are described. In these, the nerve originates from other nerve trunks with distinct branches. For example, origins from the genitofemoral and femoral trunks are reported [1,23,28,40], resulting in significant variation in the nerve course.

In addition, even rarer forms have been described: duplicity of the lateral femoral cutaneous nerve [14], union with accessory branches from the femoral nerve [34] or absence/non-identifiability in between 5% and 8.8% [1,6,34].

The literature reports that the symmetry of the course and distribution of the nerve is not certain either, with possible differences between the two sides of the body [14].

More recent anatomical studies have changed our knowledge of the lateral femoral cutaneous nerve, especially in terms of its inguinal emergence and its distribution on the thigh.

The course of the lateral femoral cutaneous nerve in the haemibacinum varies in relation to the actual point of emergence from the pelvic ring.

Yasuaki Murata [36] in a cadaver study of 216 nerves classified nerve emergence from the pelvis into 4 categories (fig. 11): A when the nerve emerges behind the spine more than 2 cm from the ASIS (2%) or B less than 2 cm from the ASIS (10.8%); C when it passes above the ASIS (28.8%); D when the emergence is at the traditionally described location below the inguinal ligament and close to the spine (58.5%).

Therefore, the course within the pelvis will be different. In types A and B the nerve will run laterally towards the iliacus muscle (lateral iliac emergence). In contrast, in types C and D, the nerve will follow a subfascial curvilinear path inclined anteriorly and downwards towards the ASIS.

The authors also provide a further subdivision depending on the point of penetration into the iliac muscle below the fascia: within 3 cm posterior to the ASIS in the first type and more than 3 cm in the second type.

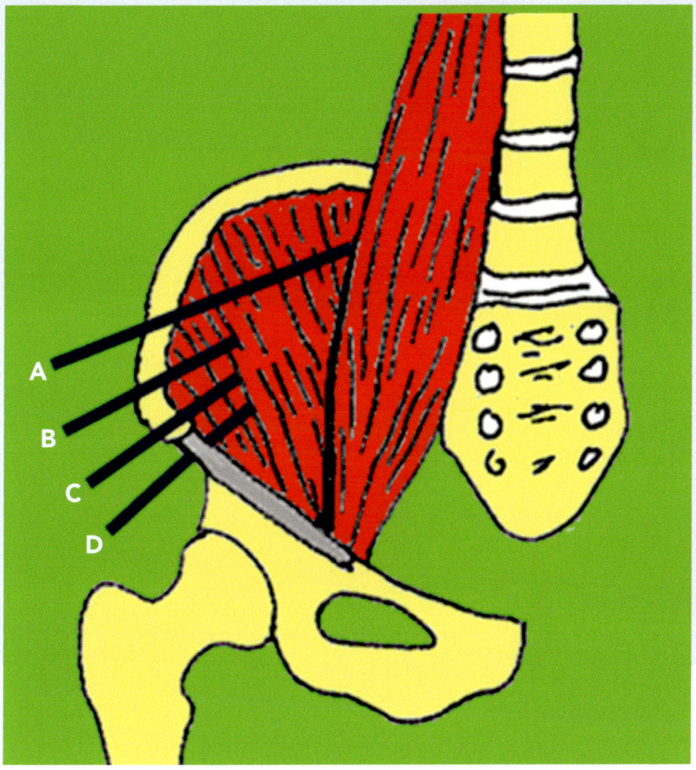

Figure 11 Yasuaki Murata diagram of the pelvic outlet of the LCN nerve. Type A (approx. 2% of cases): the nerve passes over the iliac crest more than 2 cm posterior to the ASIS. Type B (about 11% of cases): the nerve passes over the iliac crest but less than 2 cm posterior to the ASIS. Type C (29% of cases): the nerve passes over the ASIS. Type D (approximately 58% of cases): the nerve passes under the inguinal ligament close to the ASIS

In 2000, KS Tomaszewski [54] published a more complex classification, which the authors consider to be more in line with anatomical-surgical findings. Depending on the actual emergence from the pelvis, seven types were identified (fig. 12).
In the first type (86.8%) the nerve emerges below the inguinal ligament medial to the ASIS. In the second type (3.7%) the emergence is still medial but in the context of the ligament and in the third (0.9%) it is medial but above the ligament. In the fourth type (1.9%) the emergence is over the ASIS. In the fifth type (2.6%) the nerve is lateral or behind the spine. Finally, the nerve passes through the ASIS in the sixth type (2.4%) or the sartorius in the seventh type (1.7%).
Diana Rudin [47] distinguished the pelvic nerve outlet into only three types, based on the relationship with the ASIS: in 62% it is slightly medial, in 27% it is above and in 11% it is lateral (fig. 13).
Recent observations also describe the presence of more than one nerve trunk in the area anterior to the inguinal ligament. This is contrary to the prevailing opinion in the past that described a single trunk.
In his extensive study Rudin [47] identifies a single trunk in only 50% of the cases, while in the remaining cases 2 to 4 nerve branches were found. Other studies [21] confirm the presence of 2 to 5 branches in 27.6% of cases.
In the most common type of emergence from the pelvis, medial to the ASIS and beneath the ligament, studies have investigated the midpoint of nerve transit. Here too, significant variability was found, ranging from 0.5 cm to 7.3 cm [21,23], which was also correlated with race. In fact, significant variations were found between the South American population (average measurement 0.99 cm - range 0.43-1.55) and the North American and Eurasian population (2.31 cm - 1.83-2.81).
Analysing the number of nerve trunks emerging from beneath the ligament, a single trunk is described as most frequent (62.2 to 79.1% of cases) (Carai, Tomaszewsky). The presence of 2, 3 or 4 distinct trunks, which can be found in different percentages in studies from 20.9 to 37.8%, is less frequent [47].
Other cadaver studies [6,14,32,34,54], have even noted the absence of the nerve from

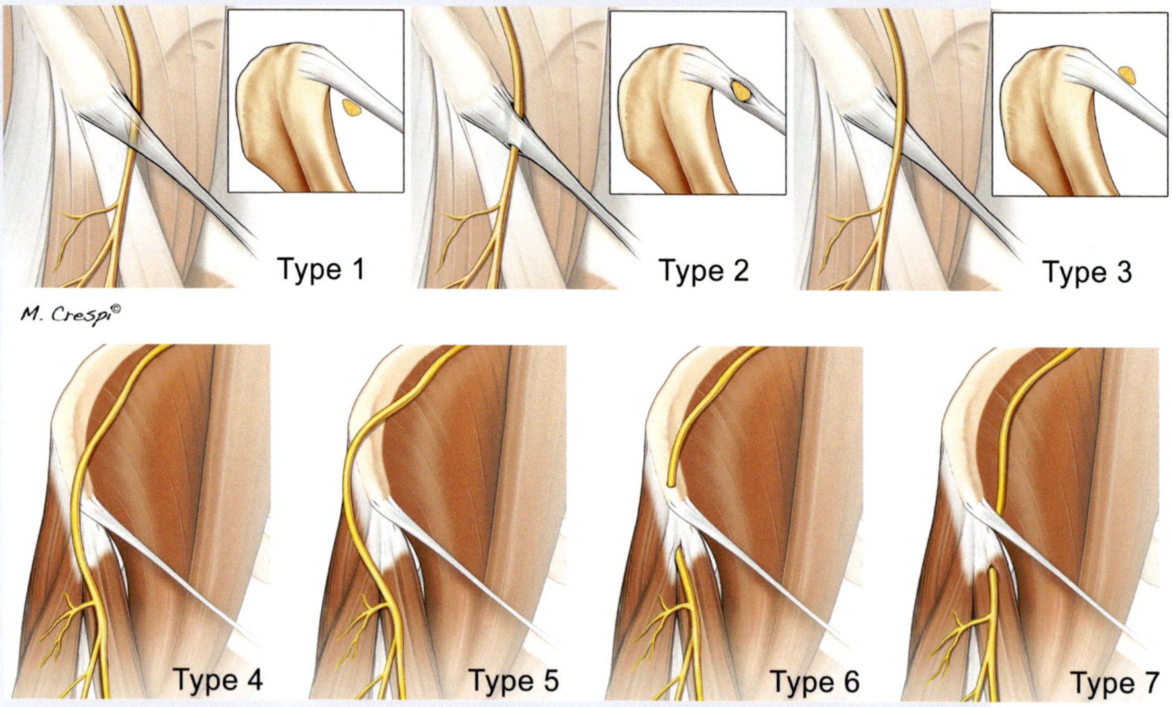

Figure 12 K.A. Tomaszewski's diagram of the nerve exit from the pelvis. Type 1 (86.8% of cases): medial to the ASIS and below the inguinal ligament. Type 2 (3.7% of cases): medial to the spine but within the inguinal ligament. Type 3 (0.9% of cases): medial to the spine but above the inguinal ligament. Type 4 (1.9%): above the ASIS. Type 5 (2.6%): lateral to or behind the ASIS. Type 6 (2.4%): crosses the ASIS with a bony canal. Type 7 (1.7%): through the sartorius muscle

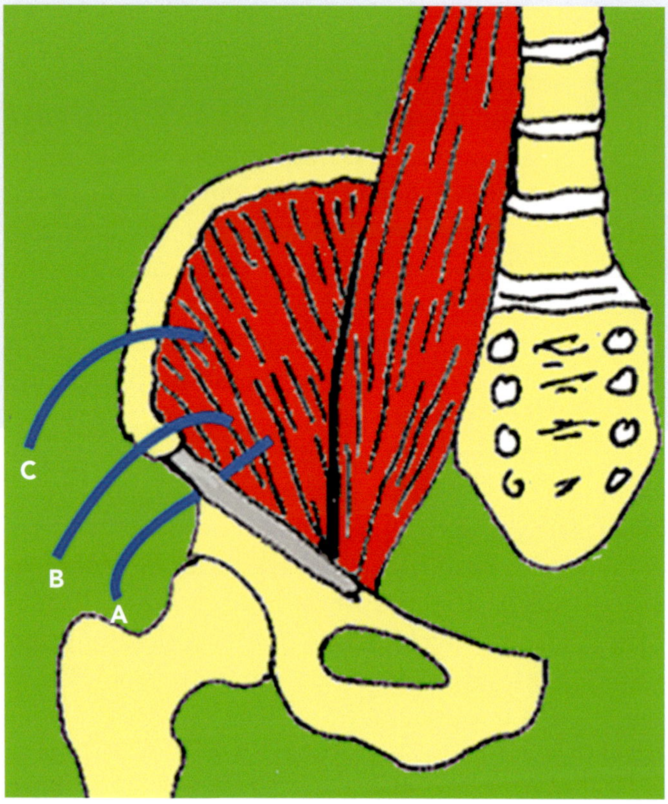

Figure 13 Schematic diagram of pelvic outlet of the LCN nerve according to D. Rudin. A) Passage of the nerve medial to the ASIS (62%). B) Passage over the ASIS (27%). C) Passage lateral to the ASIS (11%)

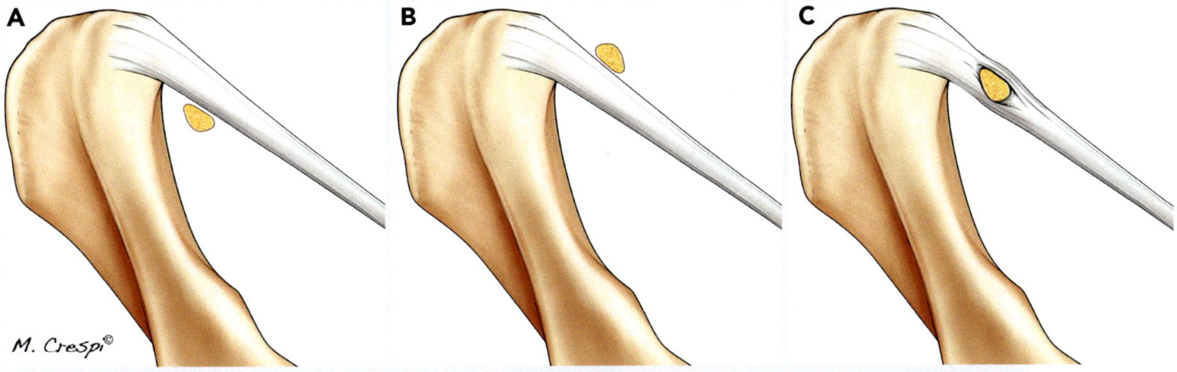

Figure 14 Relationship of the nerve to the ASIS and inguinal ligament.
A) Course below the ligament (76-86.8%). B) Course above the ligament (0.9-8.5%).
C) Intra-ligamentous course (3.7-13.9%)

the iuxtaspinous anatomical site described in the classical anatomy in 13-20% of cases. This is an indirect confirmation of the existence of nerve courses outside the spine or of its possible absence/unidentifiability.

In the most common cases of medial emergence with respect to ASIS (fig. 14), the emergence can be: sub ligamentous (a) from 76% to 86.8% [14,32,42,54], intraligamentous (b) from 3.7 to 13.9% and supraligamentous (c) (supra-iliac groove) from 0.9 to 8.5% of the cases [6,23].

In 2.4 to 4.4% of cases, a course through a distinct canal in the iliac bone (complete iliac bony canal) was even detected [6,14,23,2432,42,54].

Many authors [21,34] point out the importance of the angle of intersection of the lateral femoral cutaneous nerve with the inguinal ligament (IA = Internal Angle) (fig. 15). This has an average value of 63-69° [24, 34,45] but wide variations are reported: 40-120° on the right (av 66.92) and 40-130° (av 69.92) on the left.

Comparison between the sexes also showed differences, the angle has average values of 72.78 in females and 67.16 in males [54].

The wide variability (40-130°) of the IA (inguinal angle) also highlights the different course of the nerve distal to the inguinal ligament. The lateral femoral cutaneous nerve normally crosses the lateral margin of the sartorius about 54 mm from the ligament.

Lower values of the internal angle (IA) imply that its path is more lateral and inclined outwards, thus increasing the risk of iatrogenic damage.

In the anatomical area contiguous to the ASIS, the **'dangerous zone'** and the **'boxed area'** are identified. These areas are those related to the greater presence of the main branches, consequently at greater risk of surgical damage [21,54].

The dangerous zone is a circular area around the ASIS with a radius of approximately 3-4 cm, where the main trunk or the most important branches of the lateral femoral cutaneous nerve subdivision are most frequently detected (fig. 16).

The boxed area, on the other hand, is a rectangular-like surface that originates from the inguinal ligament (0.6 cm to 7.1 cm from the ASIS) and develops in the first 11.3 cm of the thigh. This area also includes the area with the trunks and main branches of the lateral femoral cutaneous nerve (fig. 17).

Finally, with regard to the distribution of the nerve on the thigh, the most recent studies [13,47] provide a much more complex anatomical scenario that is, however, more in line with the anatomical-surgical reality.

From the studies of Diana Rudin [47], branching patterns of the LCN in the thigh are divided into three types (fig. 18):

- sartorius type (type A) is present in 36% of cases. A dominant anterior branch of the LCN runs along the lateral border of the sartorius and innervates mainly the ante-

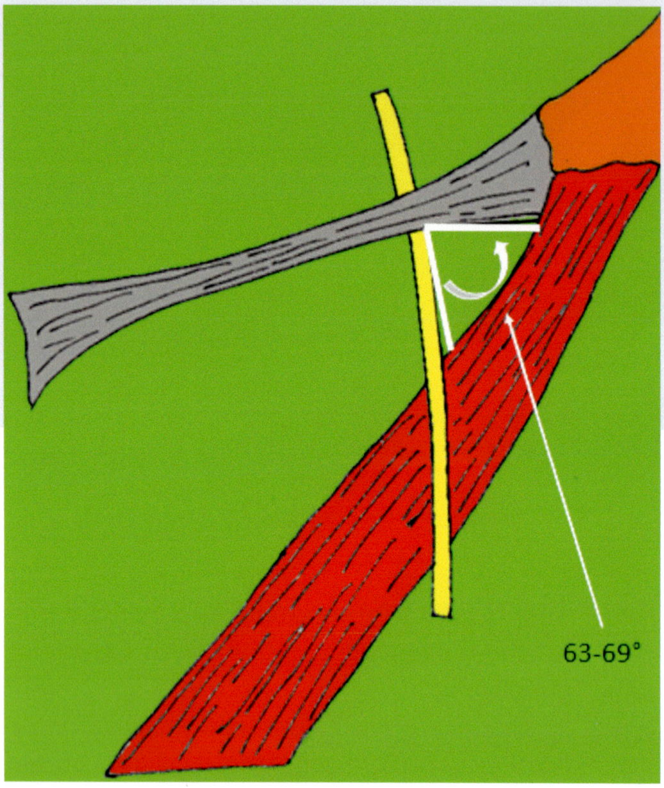

Figure 15 Internal angle (IA): angle formed at the intersection of the inguinal ligament with the LCN. This angle has average values of 63-69°

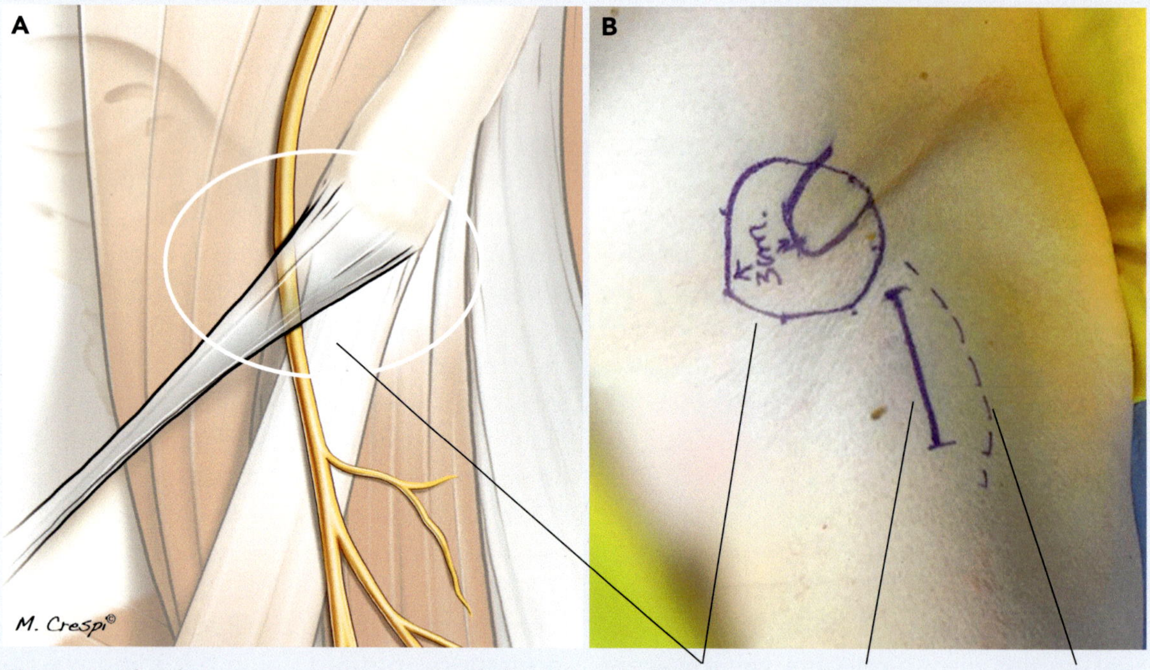

Figure 16 The dangerous zone (A) is a circular area of approximately 3 cm, centred on the ASIS. This includes, in a high percentage of cases, the main trunks of the LCN. Figure (B) shows the relationships with the cutaneous and fascial surgical incision lines

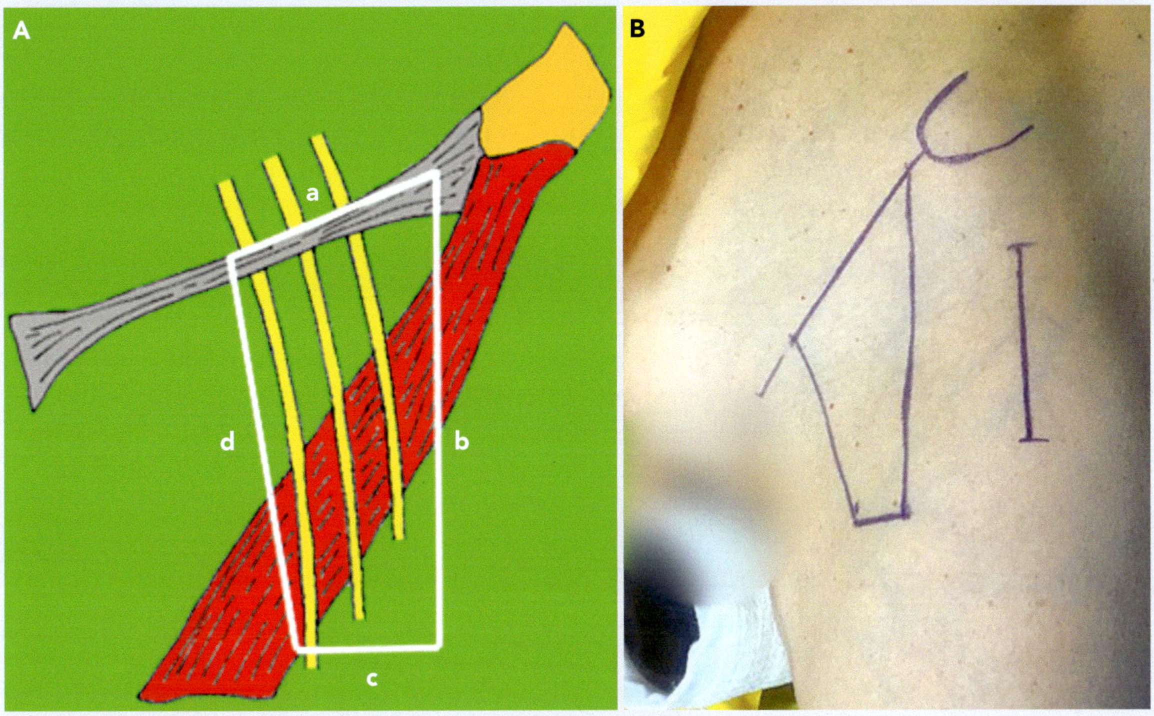

Figure 17 A) Diagram of the boxed zone. This area statistically includes the path of most of the main nerve trunks and branches of the LCN: a = line running from 0.6 cm from the ASIS and extending medially for 7.3 cm (distance considered to be the one most affected by the crossing of the LCN nerve); b = 11.3 cm line running distally from line a to the furthest point provided by the overlap of the nerve trunk with the sartorius; c = line connecting 'b' to the lateral margin of the sartorius; d = line connecting 'a' to 'c'. B) The boxed zone marked on the patient and its topographical relationship to the ASIS and the cutaneous surgical incision line

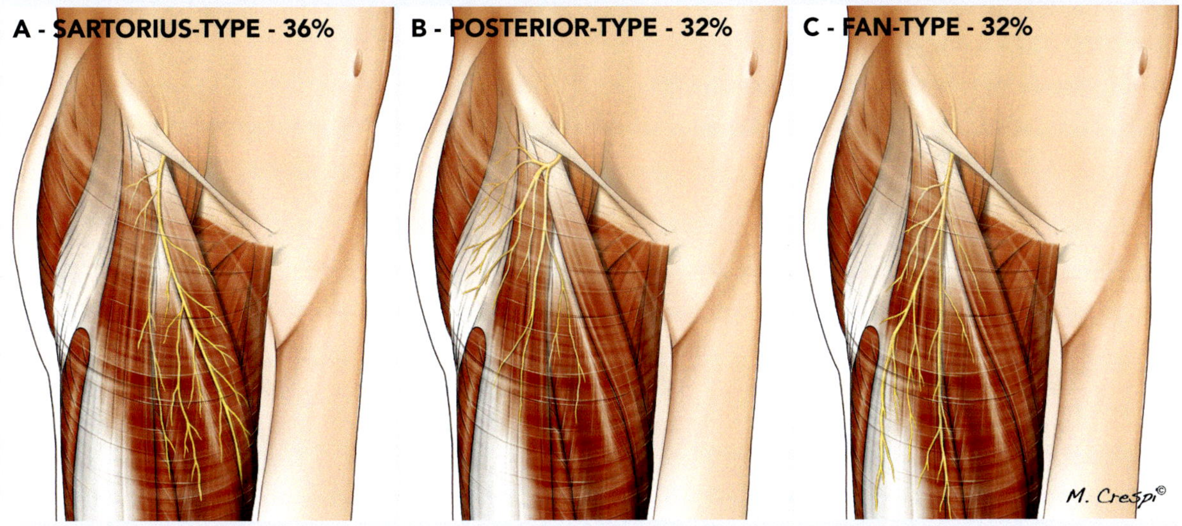

Figure 18 Anatomical diagrams of LCN distribution on the thigh according to D.F. Rudin.
A) Sartorius type, this type has a predominantly anterior distribution above the sartorius muscle.
B) Posterior type, in this type a posterior branch is added for the skin of the trochanteric era.
C) Fan type, in this type the arborization involves more extensively the surface of the tensor fascia lata muscle.

rior part of the thigh, sending only a few thin branches posteriorly;
- posterior type (type B) is found in 32% of cases. In this case there is also a posterior nerve branch, of equal or greater thickness than the anterior. This is directed laterally and crosses the medial edge of the tensor distributing itself on its suprafascial surface. In this variant, the nerve runs with 1 or 2 small vessels wrapped in a thin membrane separating them from the superficial or deep fat. This branch innervates the trochanteric region and the upper lateral part of the thigh;
- fan-type (type C) is observable in 32% of cases. This variant has numerous nerve branches of equal thickness that open into a mesh above the anterolateral region of the proximal part of the thigh. These branches run above the tensor and, to a lesser extent, on the lateral border of the sartorius. This type predominantly innervates the lateral skin of the thigh.

Considerations

The lateral femoral cutaneous nerve has a wide anatomical variability that makes it a singular and complex structure, sometimes difficult to identify and manage [4,6,16,33,40]. In fact, it can vary in the following aspects: the paravertebral formation from the roots, the intrapelvic course, the pelvic outlet, the number of pre and post ligamentous branches, the distribution on the thigh, the terminal filamentous network, the possible absence, the duplicity, the union with other regional nerve branches (ilioinguinal, genitofemoral, anterior femoral cutaneous), the cutaneous area of distribution in common with other nerves (genitofemoral and anterior femoral cutaneous) and the morphology in the pelvis.
In the literature, following hip arthroplasty operations with direct anterior surgical approach (DAA), complications of lateral femoral cutaneous nerve suffering are described with a wide variability (0.2-81%) [9,11,12,19,22,29,31]. This is a contradictory, unreliable and clinically unmanageable finding.
This wide difference is probably due to the following reasons survey methods used (subjective/objective), the type of verification (outpatient visit, in-house self-reported questionnaires), the study design (prospective or retrospective), the absence of reference to the surgical access technique (longitudinal minimally invasive, bikini approach, extended anterior according to Smith-Petersen), the level and extent of the skin incision and fascial incision, the duration of surgery, the surgical volume of the specialist centres and surgeons, the stage of the operators' learning curve, the possible coexistence with other neuropathic conditions [9,19,22,23,31,44,47].
According to more uniform and reliable criteria, on the other hand, signs of LCN nerve suffering in the early post-operative phase are 20-31.9% [37,38]. These are predominantly limited to cutaneous hypoesthesia, with a tendency to reversibility and without significant functional consequences. In these cases, only a small minority evolve to paresthetic meralgia.
Roth's (or Roth-Bernhardt) syndrome is known in common clinical experience. This was distinctly described by the authors in 1895 (after Hager's initial observations in 1885) and considered by many authors to be secondary to injury/compression of the main trunk of the lateral femoral cutaneous nerve proximally or at the inguinal ligament. [4,7,15,19,20,22,40,43]. It is characterised by numbness, tingling, itching and burning, affecting an anterolateral skin area of the thigh. Meralgia paresthesica is now often erroneously referred to as any involvement of the lateral femoral cutaneous nerve. Several studies suggest that neuroapraxia of the lateral femoral cutaneous nerve cannot be considered analogous to meralgia, having different pathogenetic bases and clinical behaviour.
In Lovell's series, in fact, less than 1% of his cases of post-surgical neuroparapraxia (in the various surgical branches studied) were within the scope of paresthetic meralgia [32,32].

The clinical-interpretative limit of this pathological entity was and is represented by the knowledge of the anatomy of this nerve. For a long time these were limited to the existence of the single trunk at the outlet (below the inguinal ligament just medial to the ASIS and its division with two branches on the thigh).
Current and more precise anatomical knowledge about the origin, intrapelvic course, pelvic outlet and complex distribution on the thigh, however, impose a profound distinction of the nerve anatomy and clinical disorders attributable to the suffering of this nerve. From a clinical point of view it appears more relevant and reliable to attribute the post-operative disorders to the condition of neurapraxia of the extensive truncular structure and secondary branching of this nerve, largely expressed by the sole 'numbness' of a circumscribed skin area. These are rarely able to recall the classical form of meralgia paresthesica, where instead the burning pain and paresthesias are dominant.
In our opinion, the most effective surgical measures capable of limiting the frequency and extent of damage to the lateral femoral cutaneous nerve are the following: reduced extension and more lateral location of the surgical incision, subfascial and intermuscular dissection, less tension on the soft tissue exerted by retractors, and shorter operating times.
Neuroapraxia of the lateral femoral cutaneous nerve has a multifactorial genesis and can be caused by compression, stretching, scarring, ischaemia [3,10,19,20]. However, it is to be considered overrepresented in current clinical experience and is not to be confused with the more common and generic peri-incisional pain and sensory disorders [19].
Particular morphologies of the hip joint may also predispose to LCN nerve pain. One example is the 'small femoral offset' condition, which results in medialisation of the surgical incision and increased retraction tension on the contiguous soft tissue [37]. Some authors have made a distinction between 'long hip' and 'short hip'. The position of the nerve varies in relation to the joint, and in 'short hips', precisely because of the reduced offset, it is subjected to greater tension during prosthetic surgery [16].
In our experience, post-surgical neuroapraxic damage is mostly represented by numbness alone, in the target skin area. Most of it turns out to be partial and transient, although usually slowly resolving [4,5,8,10,36,39,41,43,46,49,55]. Only 1% of this may result in the complete and definitive meralgesic form [19,32].
Among the anterior surgical approaches that can be used in orthopaedics, such as Hueter's (and its minimally invasive derivations that use the same intermuscular interval), Smith-Petersen's and Letournell's ileo-inguinal approaches, only the last two can lead to direct injuries of the main nerve trunk. This is because the nerve crosses the surgical field right at the ASIS below the ligament of Poupart, the obligatory passage of these two surgical approaches.
Anterior minimally invasive approaches should make it possible to avoid the area at risk, i.e. where the concentration and size of the nerve branches are greater. It is a good rule not to go deep into the muscle interstitium, incising the fascia lata above the interval, in order not to directly damage the nerve branches. Similarly, there should be no need to move the major trunks with the consequent inevitable sacrifice of the filiform branches that originate from them (fig. 19).
Above all, it is necessary to keep a proper distance from the ASIS, from whose medial profile, below the inguinal ligament, the lateral femoral cutaneous nerve exits in 80% of cases. Reference can be made to the so-called anterior superior 'dangerous zone' near the spine and the 'boxed area', where the larger nerve branches are more concentrated, even considering the different branching patterns.
The extent of the surgical skin incision, which must correspond to the extent of the dissection of the underlying planes, is in our opinion another very important factor. Experience gained from a significant number of operations allows us to limit tissue retraction to 6-8 cm to achieve the arthrotomy.
This results in a strong reduction of the inju-

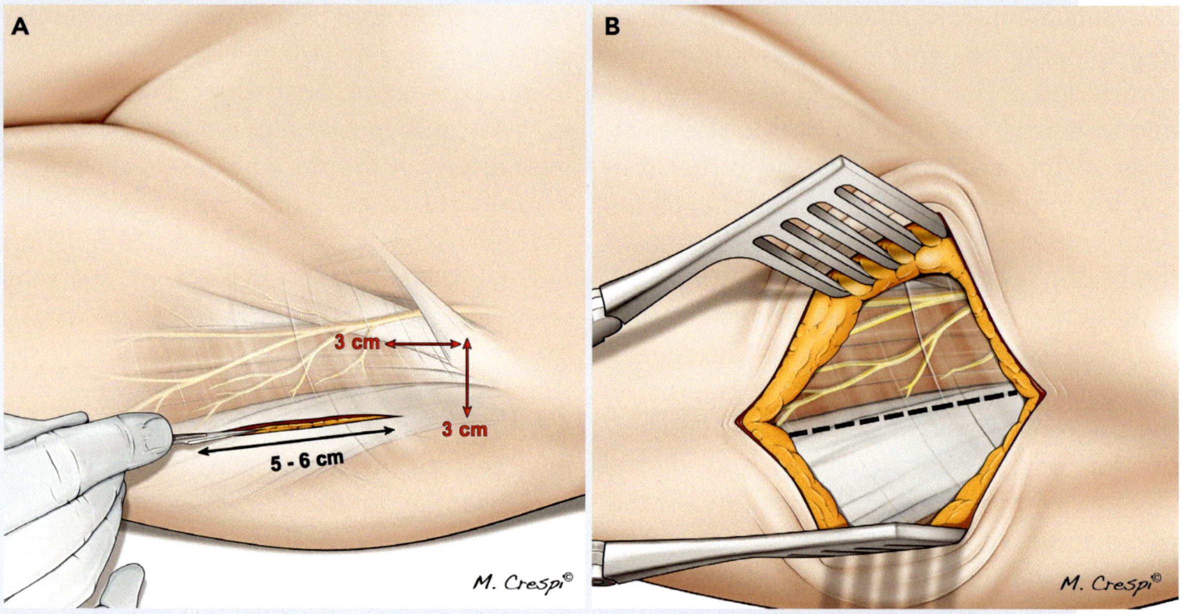

Figure 19 Schematic diagram of cutaneous (A) and fascial (B) incision. The incision is made approximately 3 cm distal and lateral to the ASIS. In order to retract the fascia lata to protect the nerve endings of the LCN, the limits of fusion with the gluteal fascia are sought

ry of the more peripheral and thinner nerve endings (arborization), therefore limited to the area of surgical dissection. Then, this translates into a reduction of the denervated skin area. However, this is destined to recovery for compensatory reinnervation by contiguity and for subjective adaptation by the patient.

In our daily clinical practice, the surgical incision is made as distal and lateral to the anterior superior iliac spine (3 cm distally and 3 cm laterally), following a line directed distally towards the peroneal head or the external patellar margin (fig. 20).

The underlying fascia lata is incised more laterally, close to its junction with the fascia glutea. It is then separated from the underlying epimysius of the tensor fascia lata and retracted. Below the fascia, the muscular interstice between the sartorius and tensor fascia is reached. After dividing these muscles, one arrives on the deeper plane for the arthrotomy (figs. 21-24).

The retracted fascial plane will also serve as protection for the overlying nerve branches and counteract the damaging action of the procedure.

In contrast, direct dissection of the transfascial intermuscular plane will result in difficult management of the lateral femoral cutaneous nerve. Its medial or lateral displacement, in order to allow for arthrotomy and operative manoeuvres, may result in damage to its lateral or medial branches (fig. 25).

We try to reduce the stretching-compression of the muscles involved in the dissection plane as much as possible, separating them carefully and avoiding excessive and prolonged tension with the retractors.

We also avoid 'stripping' the fascia lata or dissecting the adipose layer above so as not to injure the almost invisible nerve filaments running through it.

In addition, we take great care when retracting the rectus femoris and the sartorius during implantation of the prosthetic components to avoid excessive muscular stress [2,3,20].

In our opinion, the reduction of the operating time is crucial. This is a factor not only in the control of blood loss but also in the prolonged retraction tension on the muscles and other structures.

In this way, we are convinced that we significantly reduce the risk of direct or indirect traction injuries to the larger nerve branches of the lateral femoral cutaneous nerve. We

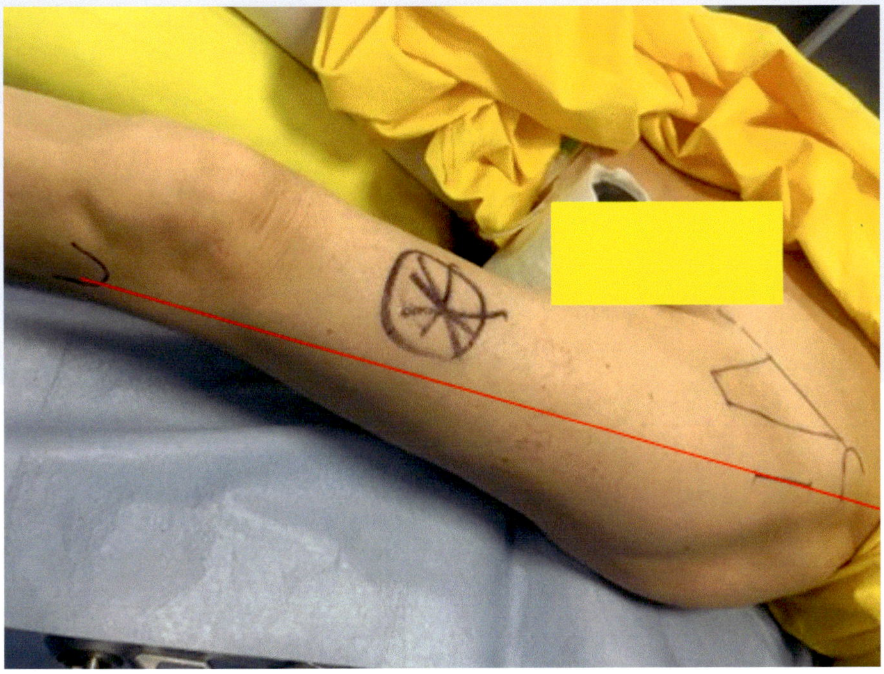

Figure 20 This figure shows the position of the surgical incision (directed towards the head of the fibula) and its relationship to the ASIS and the boxed zone

circumscribe possible nerve injuries to small lateral nerve branches only at the level of the short surgical incision. This limits the problem to milder, circumscribed and potentially transient neuroapraxic lesions [2,3,20].

The majority of our patients who presented with disorders of the lateral femoral cutaneous nerve identified a 'lanceolate' area of hypoesthesia ('numbness') on the lateral surface of the thigh, with a progressive tendency to reduce the extent and intensity of dysesthesia (fig. 26).

In our experience, after 8-9 months the area of hypoesthesia had disappeared or significantly reduced in extent. Almost always this area is no longer recognised subjectively by the patient, although it is sometimes detectable on clinical examination.

Spontaneous individual adaptation, progressive functional recovery of the apraxic nerve endings, and the substitutive action of some neighbouring nerves (femoral, ileofemoral and genitofemoral) usually lead to a reduction or resolution of the hypoesthesia (numbness).

On the other hand, in our experience, paresthesias and burning pain have represented a small minority of LCN-related complications in the anterior surgical approach.

In this context, however, one must consider what is currently referred to as **'PISC' (Peri-Incisional Sensorial Changes)**. This is a frequent clinical condition involving peri-incisional changes in the sensitivity and nociception of a skin area (of varying extent) around the surgical incision. PISC is not limited to the hip but can be found in any part of the body and for any type of surgery [19]. In knee surgery, for example, after an arthroplasty or an ACL reconstruction, there may be residual pain and tenderness in the anterolateral side. This occurs due to direct or indirect involvement of the saphenous nerve or the infrapatellar plexus that derives from it. The same can be said of other approaches to the hip (posterior lateral) or the shoulder [25,48].

This condition, which varies in extent and is potentially not entirely reversible, can also be found in other surgical branches.

We have also radically changed the use of retractors (fig. 27). In our opinion, the Charnley retractor, once applied and tensioned, excessively 'stiffens' the surgical field. This can result in strong, circumscribed and continuous pressure on the soft tissue. This oc-

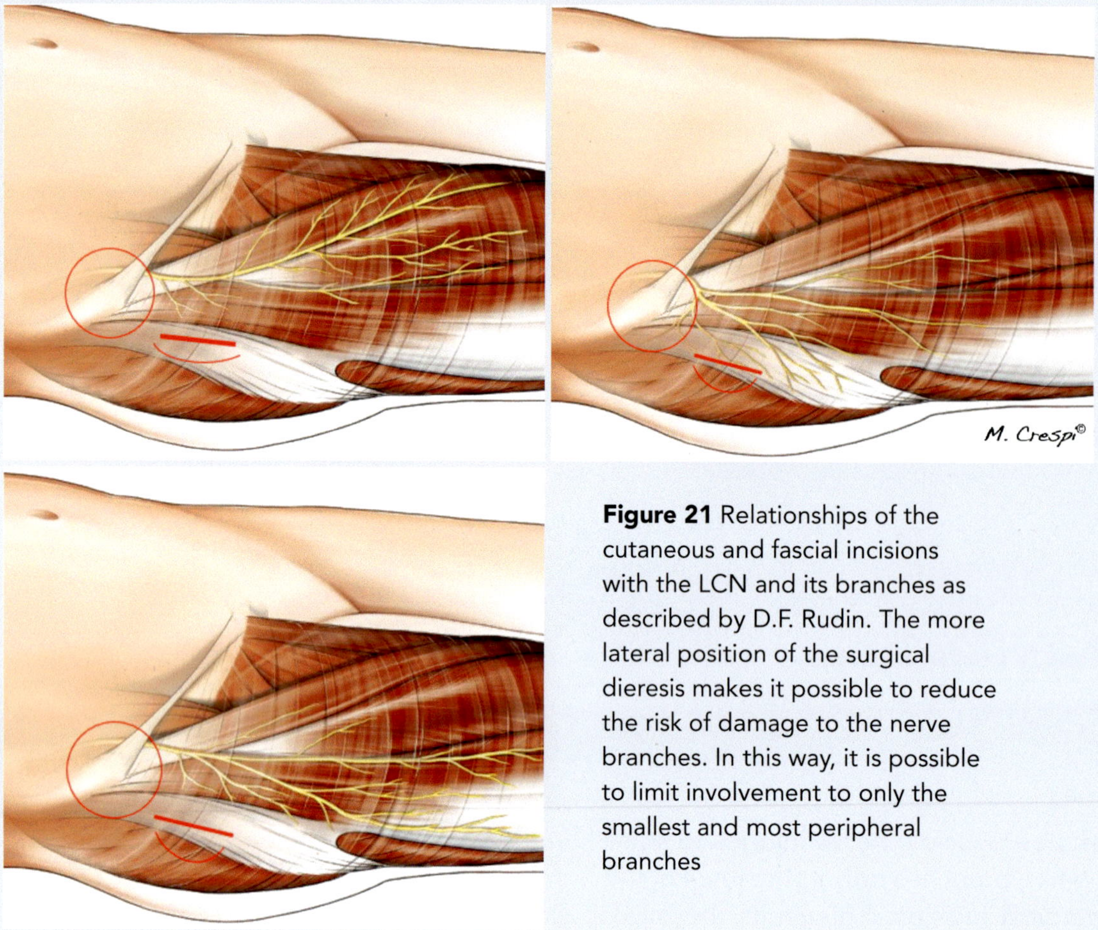

Figure 21 Relationships of the cutaneous and fascial incisions with the LCN and its branches as described by D.F. Rudin. The more lateral position of the surgical dieresis makes it possible to reduce the risk of damage to the nerve branches. In this way, it is possible to limit involvement to only the smallest and most peripheral branches

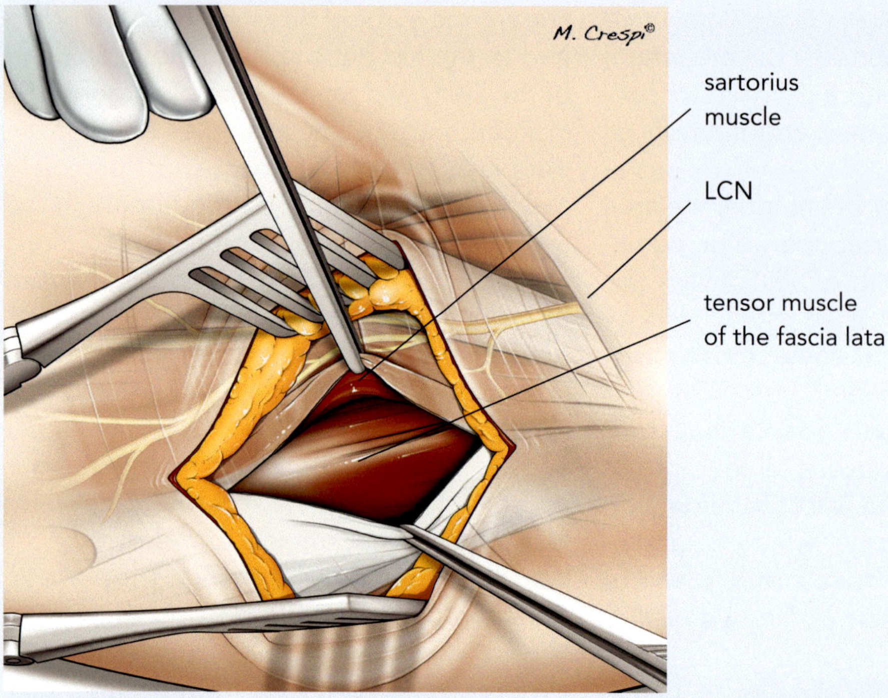

Figure 22 After the lateral incision of the fascia, the fascia is retracted to look for the gap between the tensor and sartorius. Thus, the fascia isolates and protects the overlying nerve branches of the LCN

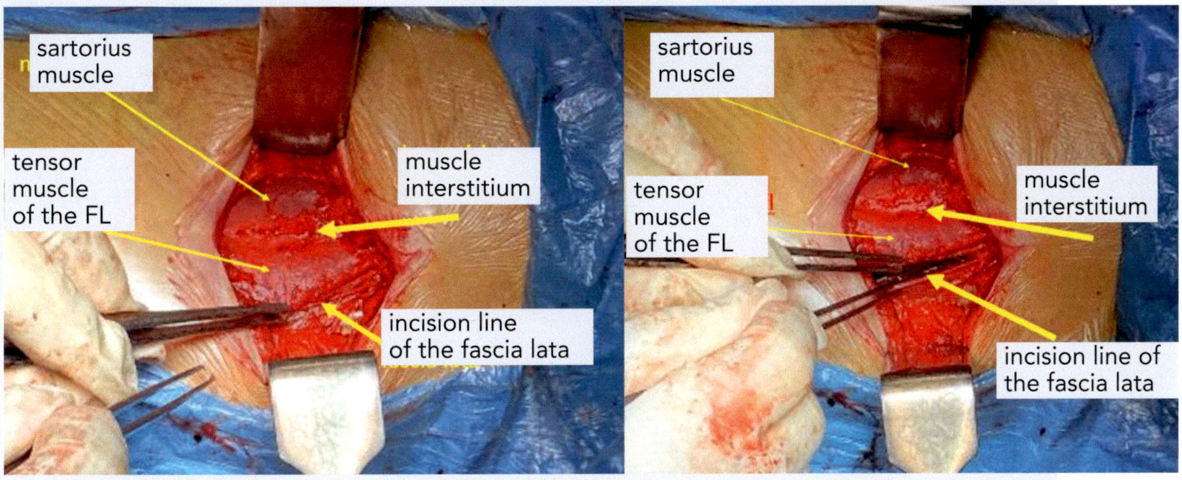

Figure 23 Intraoperative photo. The fascia lata is incised lateral to the tensor and retracted medially to protect the overlying nerve endings of the LCN

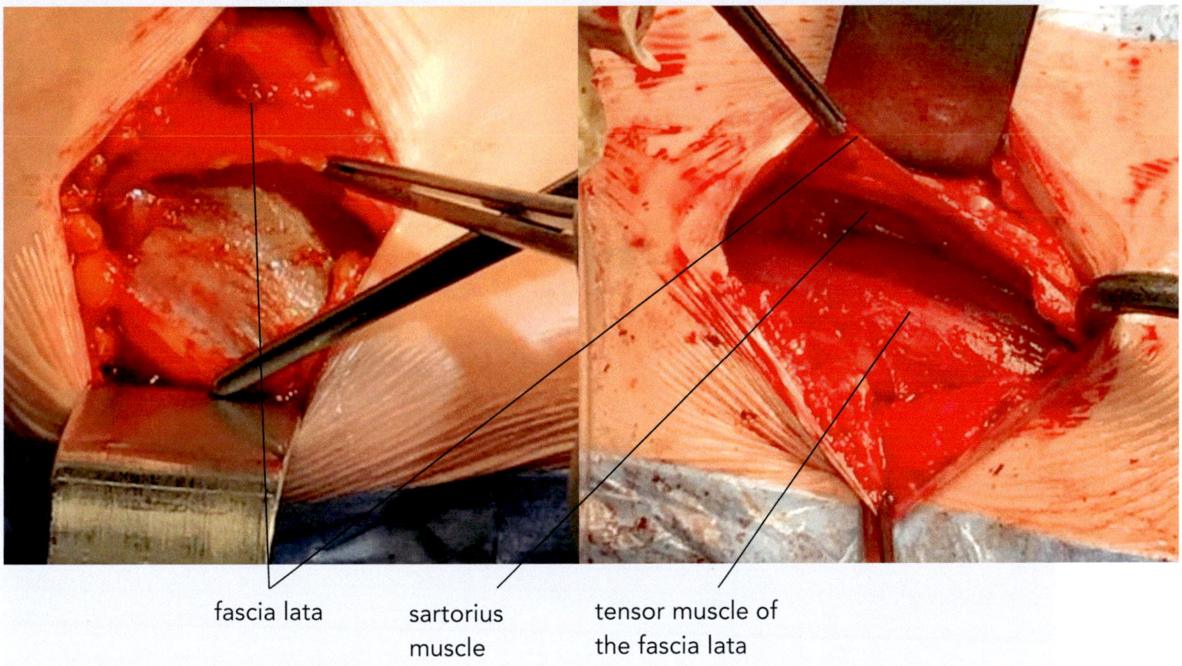

Figure 24 Intraoperative example of retraction of the fascia lata without overlying dissection and exposure of the muscle gap between the tensor fascia lata and sartorius. This space allows deepening for arthrotomy

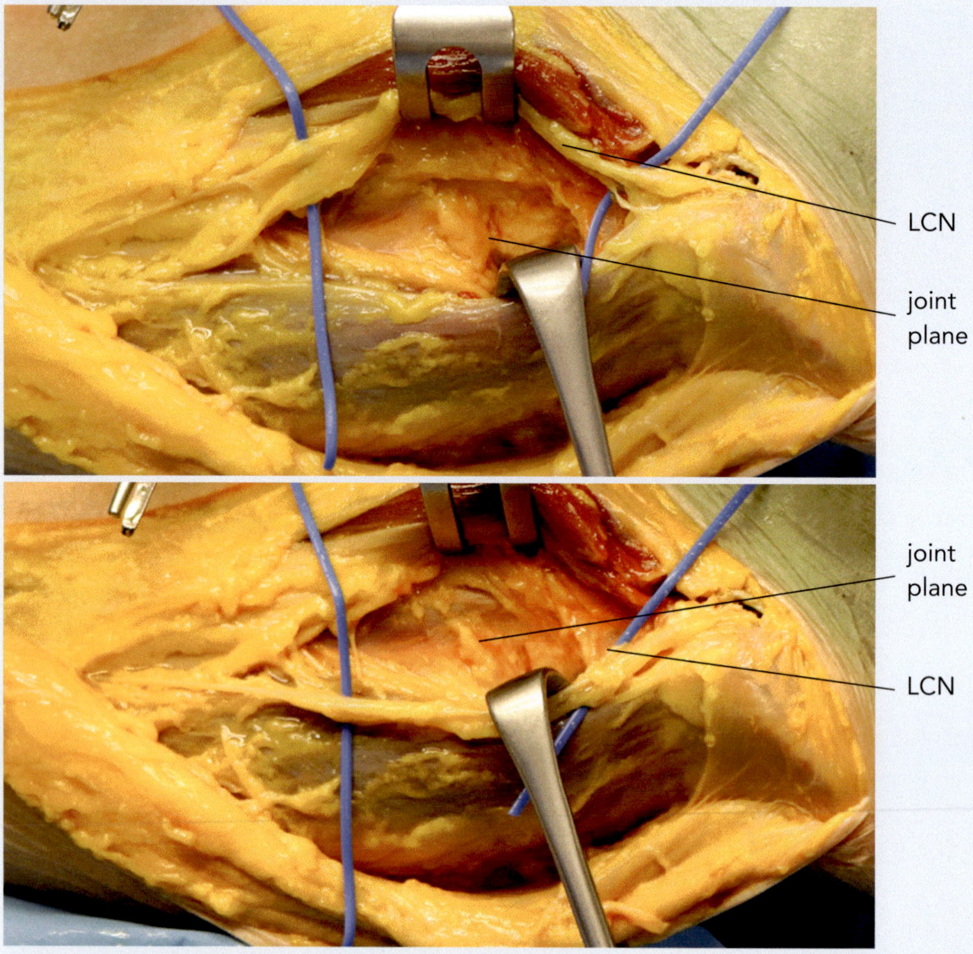

Figure 25 Anatomical study on cadaver. Directly reaching deep planes over the muscle interstitium inevitably results in (direct or indirect) damage to the main nerve endings of the LCN. The nerve is placed above the interstitium in a high percentage of cases, and damage can occur whether the nerve is moved medially or laterally

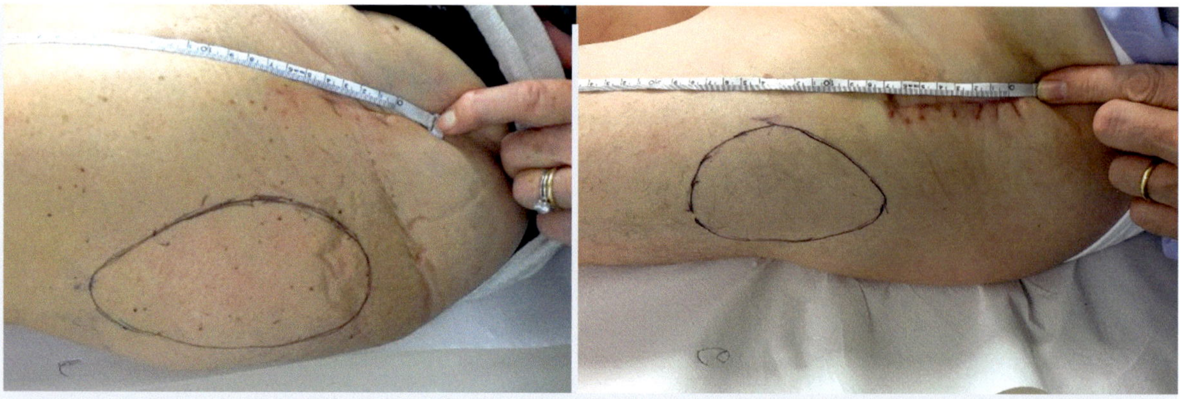

Figure 26 The area of cutaneous hypoesthesia of the lateral thigh as reported by the operated patients is shown. At 4 months after surgery, the hypoesthesia is reported to be regressing in both extent and magnitude

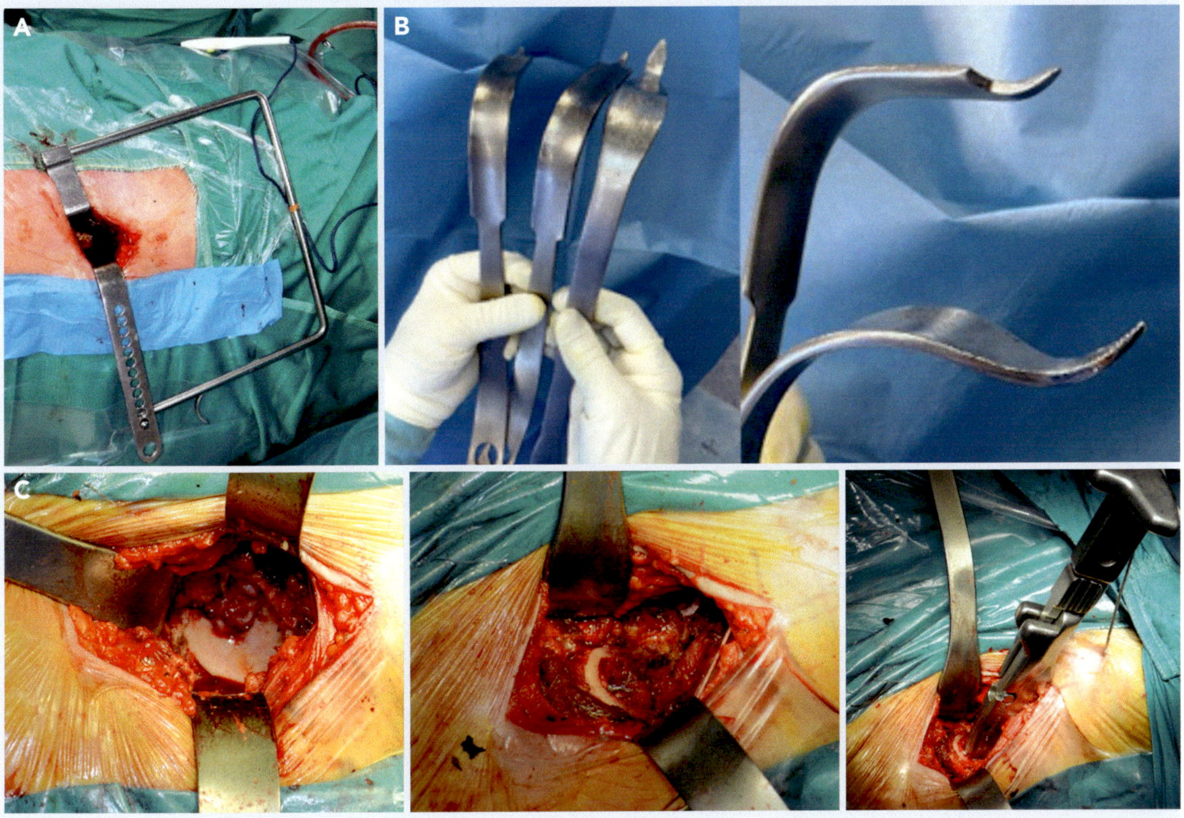

Figure 27 A) The use of the Charnley retractor. B) The retractors we use allow adequate exposure of the surgical field and a more controllable tension on the soft parts. C) Example of surgical field exposure for cup and femur preparation

curs mainly during the movements necessary for the surgical procedure, in particular extension, external rotation of the limb and adduction. The Charnley retractor can therefore exert a local injurious action, especially with its medial component.

We have been using retractors with a special design for a long time. These do not overstress the soft tissue, allowing continuous and gradual modulation of pressure, even with useful phases of reduced tension.

In a high percentage of cases, the lateral femoral cutaneous nerve is multiform in composition, course and distribution and can be difficult to recognise and complex to manage.

In Rudin's C/fan-type variant (32% of cases) for example, where the fine nerve arborization diffusely overlaps the tensor fascia lata, an inadequate incision and incorrect suprafascial surgical dissection can significantly damage the nerve branches.

For this reason, an ultrasound scan (fig. 28) can be a helpful measure. This can allow us to identify the type of nerve distribution, particularly in the case of the C/fan-type variant. The ultrasound investigation can also provide the surgeon with information that leads him to perform specific accessory surgical gestures. These may be a more lateral section of the fascia lata and the scrupulous subfascial (not transfascial) intermuscular deepening, or prefer a more lateral minimally invasive incision or even renounce to the anterior approach.

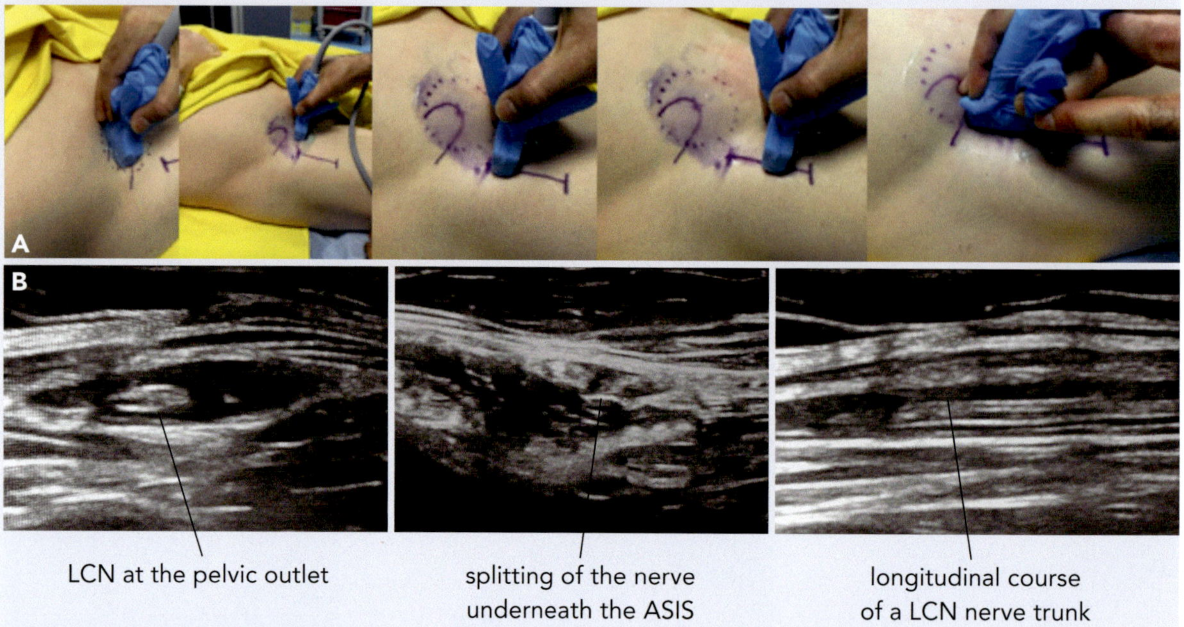

Figure 28 Pre-operative ultrasound study. A) Various phases of image acquisition of the course of the LCN. B) Images of the various anatomical planes studied

Conclusions

The great advantages of hip prosthetic surgery with the minimally invasive anterior surgical approach can be seen in a large number of patients and the comparison with numerous similar surgical experiences allows us to look with particular interest at modern tissue sparing surgery (TSS). The complete knowledge of the anatomy of the region allows us to perform the operation with proper efficiency and prudence. However, great care must always be taken with the thin lateral femoral cutaneous nerve, which is small and only sensitive. This is characterised in a relatively high percentage of cases by abnormalities of origin, course and distribution, especially in terms of the pelvic outlet and the 'network' distribution on the thigh.

Obviously, the surgical act must anticipate the presence of such abnormalities, identify and respect the nerve structures, limiting the risk of nerve damage as much as possible.

The following factors allowed us to avoid or limit nerve damage to the lateral femoral cutaneous nerve: the short incision and extension of the surgical approach allow only the smallest branches or terminal nerve filaments to be involved in the surgical field, and the reduction in surgical time limits the tension involved in the retraction of the muscles, which is in any case more prudent and gradual.

In our experience, most lateral femoral cutaneous nerve lesions have resulted in only transient numbness (not pain or burning) of a circumscribed lateral skin area of the thigh. However, there are anatomical variants (e.g. B and C type described by D.F. Rudin), with extensive lateral branching of the nerve, where it becomes difficult to avoid the involvement of certain nerve branches or filaments. This is a possible complication in any surgical field.

The largely positive clinical results and the actual extent of the complications observed, also considering the problems related to the anatomy of the lateral femoral cutaneous nerve, lead us to confirm our confidence in this minimally invasive anterior surgical technique. Furthermore, it encourages us to continue improving both anatomical knowledge and surgical techniques in order to respect each structure involved in the surgical act.

Bibliography

1. Aszmann OC, Dellon ES, Dellon AL. Anatomical course of the lateral femoral cutaneous nerve and its susceptibility to compression and injury. Plast Reconstr Surg. 1997;100(3):600-604.
2. Barton C, Kim PR. Complications of the direct anterior approach for total hip arthroplasty. Orthop Clin North Am. 2009;40(3):371-375.
3. Bender B, Nogler M, Hozack WJ. Direct anterior approach for total hip arthroplasty. Orthop Clin North Am. 2009;40(3):321-328.
4. Benezis I, Boutaud B, Leclerc J, Fabre T, Durandeau A. Lateral femoral cutaneous neuropathy and its surgical treatment: a report of 167 cases. Muscle Nerve. 2007;36(5):659-663.
5. Buch, KA, Campbell, J.Acute onset meralgia paresthetica after fracture of the anterior superior iliac spine. Injury 1993;24:569–70
6. Carai A, Fenu G, Sechi E, Crotti FM, Montella A. Anatomical variability of the lateral femoral cutaneous nerve: findings from a surgical series. Clin Anat. 2009;22(3):365-370.
7. Coert JH, Dellon AL. Documenting neuropathy of the lateral femoral cutaneous nerve using the Pressure-Specified Sensory Testing device. Ann Plast Surg. 2003;50(4):373-377.
8. Cordato DJ, Yiannikas C, Stroud J, et al. Evoked potentials elicited by stimulation of the lateral and anterior femoral cutaneous nerves in meralgia paresthetica. Muscle Nerve. 2004;29(1):139-142.
9. Corujo A, Franco CD, Williams JM. The sensory territory of the lateral cutaneous nerve of the thigh as determined by anatomic dissections and ultrasound-guided blocks. Reg Anesth Pain Med. 2012;37(5):561-564.
10. Dellon AL, Mont M, Ducic I. Involvement of the lateral femoral cutaneous nerve as source of persistent pain after total hip arthroplasty. J Arthroplasty. 2008;23(3):480-485.
11. den Hartog YM, Mathijssen NM, Peters SJ, Vehmeijer SB. The anterior supine intermuscular approach for total hip arthroplasty: reducing the complication rate by improving the procedure. Hip Int. 2015;25(1):28-33.
12. De Geest T, Fennema P, Lenaerts G, De Loore G. Adverse effects associated with the direct anterior approach for total hip arthroplasty: a Bayesian meta-analysis. Arch Orthop Trauma Surg. 2015;135(8):1183-1192.
13. de Ridder VA, de Lange S, Popta JV. Anatomical variations of the lateral femoral cutaneous nerve and the consequences for surgery. J Orthop Trauma. 1999;13(3):207-211.
14. Dias Filho LC, Valença MM, Guimarães Filho FA, et al. Lateral femoral cutaneous neuralgia: an anatomical insight. Clin Anat. 2003;16(4):309-316.
15. Dibenedetto LM, Lei Q, Gilroy AM, Hermey DC, Marks SC Jr, Page DW. Variations in the inferior pelvic pathway of the lateral femoral cutaneous nerve: implications for laparoscopic hernia repair. Clin Anat. 1996;9(4):232-236.
16. Doklamyai P, Agthong S, Chentanez V, et al. Anatomy of the lateral femoral cutaneous nerve related to inguinal ligament, adjacent bony landmarks, and femoral artery. Clin Anat. 2008;21(8):769-774.
17. Ecker AD, Woltman HW. Meralgia paresthetica: a report of one hundred and fifty cases. JAMA. 1938;110:1650-1652
18. GHENT WR. Further studies on meralgia paresthetica. Can Med Assoc J. 1961;85(16):871-875.
19. Goulding K, Beaulé PE, Kim PR, Fazekas A. Incidence of lateral femoral cutaneous nerve neuropraxia after anterior approach hip arthroplasty. Clin Orthop Relat Res. 2010;468(9):2397-2404.
20. Grossman MG, Ducey SA, Nadler SS, Levy AS. Meralgia paresthetica: diagnosis and treatment. J Am Acad Orthop Surg. 2001;9(5):336-344.
21. Grothaus MC, Holt M, Mekhail AO, Ebraheim NA, Yeasting RA. Lateral femoral cutaneous nerve: an anatomic study. Clin Orthop Relat Res. 2005;(437):164-168.
22. Hanna A. The lateral femoral cutaneous nerve canal. J Neurosurg. 2017;126(3):972-978.
23. Homma Y, Baba T, Sano K, et al. Lateral femoral cutaneous nerve injury with the direct anterior approach for total hip arthroplasty. Int Orthop. 2016;40(8):1587-1593.
24. Hospodar PP, Ashman ES, Traub JA. Anatomic study of the lateral femoral cutaneous nerve with respect to the ilioinguinal surgical dissection. J Orthop Trauma. 1999;13(1):17-19.
25. Hunter LY, Louis DS, et al. The saphenous nerve: its course and importance in medial arthrotomy. Am J Sports Med. 1979;7(4):227-230.
26. Jablecki CK. Postoperative lateral femoral cutaneous neuropathy. Muscle Nerve. 1999;22(8):1129-1131.
27. Jefferson D, Eames RA. Subclinical entrapment of the lateral femoral cutaneous nerve: an autopsy study. Muscle Nerve. 1979;2(2):145-154.

28. Keegan JJ, Holyoke EA. Meralgia paresthetica. An anatomical and surgical study. J Neurosurg. 1962;19:341-345.
29. Kennon RE, Keggi JM, Wetmore RS, Zatorski LE, Huo MH, Keggi KJ. Total hip arthroplasty through a minimally invasive anterior surgical approach. J Bone Joint Surg Am. 2003;85-A Suppl 4:39-48.
30. Kushnir M, Klein C, Kimiagar Y, Pollak L, Rabey JM. Distal lesion of the lateral femoral cutaneous nerve. Muscle Nerve. 2008;37(1):101-103.
31. Leunig M, Faas M, von Knoch F, Naal FD. Skin crease 'bikini' incision for anterior approach total hip arthroplasty: surgical technique and preliminary results. Clin Orthop Relat Res. 2013;471(7):2245-2252.
32. Lovell TP. Single-incision direct anterior approach for total hip arthroplasty using a standard operating table. J Arthroplasty. 2008;23(7 Suppl):64-68.
33. Majkrzak A, Johnston J, Kacey D, Zeller J. Variability of the lateral femoral cutaneous nerve: An anatomic basis for planning safe surgical approaches. Clin Anat. 2010;23(3):304-311.
34. Martins RS, M G Siqueira, Silva FC Jr, Heise CO, Teixeira MJ. A practical approach to the lateral cutaneous nerve of the thigh: an anatomical study. Clin Neurol Neurosurg. 2011;113(10):868-871.
35. Massey EW. Meralgia paresthetica secondary to trauma of bone graft. J Trauma. 1980;20(4):342-343.
36. Murata Y, Takahashi K, Yamagata M, Shimada Y, Moriya H. The anatomy of the lateral femoral cutaneous nerve, with special reference to the harvesting of iliac bone graft. J Bone Joint Surg Am. 2000;82(5):746-747
37. Nahabedian MY, Dellon AL. Meralgia paresthetica: etiology, diagnosis, and outcome of surgical decompression. Ann Plast Surg. 1995;35(6):590-594.
38. Ozaki Y, Homma Y, Sano K, et al. Small femoral offset is a risk factor for lateral femoral cutaneous nerve injury during total hip arthroplasty using a direct anterior approach. Orthop Traumatol Surg Res. 2016;102(8):1043-1047.
39. Ozaki Y, Baba T, Homma Y, et al. Preoperative ultrasound to identify distribution of the lateral femoral cutaneous nerve in total hip arthroplasty using the direct anterior approach. SICOT J. 2018;4:42.
40. Park JW, et al. Meralgia paresthetica caused by hip-huggers in a patient with aberrant course of the lateral femoral cutaneous nerve. Muscle Nerve. 2007;35(5):678-680.
41. Puig L, Alegro M, Moragas JM. Treatment of meralgia paraesthetica. Dermatology. 1995;191:73–74.
42. Ray B, D'Souza AS, Kumar B, et al. Variations in the course and microanatomical study of the lateral femoral cutaneous nerve and its clinical importance. Clin Anat. 2010;23(8):978-984.
43. Reid V, Cros D. Proximal sensory neuropathies of the Leg. Neurol Clin. 1999;17(3):655-viii.
44. Restrepo C, Parvizi J, Pour AE, Hozack WJ. Prospective randomized study of two surgical approaches for total hip arthroplasty. J Arthroplasty. 2010;25(5):671-9.e1.
45. Ropars M, Morandi X, Huten D, Thomazeau H, Berton E, Darnault P. Anatomical study of the lateral femoral cutaneous nerve with special reference to minimally invasive anterior approach for total hip replacement. Surg Radiol Anat. 2009;31(3):199-204.
46. Rosenquist RW, Lederhaas G. Femoral and lateral femoral cutaneous nerve block. Tech Reg Anesth Pain Manage 1999;3:33–38.
47. Rudin D, et al. The Anatomical Course of the Lateral Femoral Cutaneous Nerve with Special Attention to the Anterior Approach to the Hip Joint. J Bone Joint Surg Am. 2016;98(7):561-567.
48. Sanders B, Rolf R, McClelland W, Xerogeanes J. Prevalence of saphenous nerve injury after autogenous hamstring harvest: an anatomic and clinical study of sartorial branch injury. Arthroscopy. 2007;23(9):956-963.
49. Seddon HJ. Surgical disorders of the peripheral nerves. 2nd ed. Edinburgh: Churchill Livingstone, 1975.
50. Stecco C, Gagey O, Belloni A, et al. Anatomy of the deep fascia of the upper limb. Second part: study of innervation. Morphologie. 2007;91(292):38-43.
51. Stecco C, Pavan P, Pachera P, De Caro R, Natali A. Investigation of the mechanical properties of the human crural fascia and their possible clinical implications. Surg Radiol Anat. 2014;36(1):25-32.
52. Stecco C. Functional Atlas of the Human Fascial System. Churchill Livingstone, 2015.
53. Sunderland S. Lateral femoral cutaneous nerve. Meralgia paraesthetica. Nerves and nerve injuries. Churchill Livingstone, 1968, 1110-1113.
54. Tomaszewski KA, Popieluszko P, Henry BM, et al. The surgical anatomy of the lateral femoral cutaneous nerve in the inguinal region: a meta-analysis. Hernia. 2016;20(5):649-657.
55. Yang SH, Wu CC, Chen PQ. Postoperative meralgia paresthetica after posterior spine surgery: incidence, risk factors, and clinical outcomes. Spine (Phila Pa 1976). 2005;30(18):E547-E550.

CHAPTER 5

Physiopathology of minimally invasive surgery in hip arthroplasty. Histochemical, immunological and endocrinological aspects

Elisa Pala, Maria Chiara Cerchiaro, Pietro Ruggieri

Department of Orthopaedics and Orthopaedic Oncology, University of Padova, Italy

Introduction

Minimally invasive surgery is referred to a specific access strategy such as laparoscopy, robotic surgery or endoscopy. In minimally invasive surgery the following factors must be respected: the pathology must be treated with the best possible safety profile; improve surgical efficacy decreasing blood loss, post-operative pain, post-operative complications, surgical time, cosmetic outcome and length of hospital stay; improve surgical cosmesis and cost-effectiveness ratios; provide equivalent outcome to traditional open surgery.

"Scarless surgery" refers to a new minimally invasive treatment performed through the body's natural orifices without need for external incision for procedures that previously required abdominal incisions. Surgical stress activates a complex response, which includes the activation of the stress system, the hypothalamic-pituitary-adrenal (HPA) axis, the sympathetic nervous system and the renin-angiotensin axis. The systemic inflammatory response caused by surgical stress increases cytokines (TNF-a, IL-6 and IL-1) and suppresses lymphocytes, CD8+ T cells, CD4+ T cells and NK cells in the early post-operative period. IL-1, TNF and IL-6 are the major mediators of the acute-phase response caused by surgery and trauma.

In the early post-operative days (from day 1 to day 14 after surgery), after some surgical procedures such as cholecystectomies with, a significant level of cytokines (mostly IL-1, IL-6, IL-8, IL-10) in the blood can be found; in the meantime, there is a reduced secretion of IL-2, TNF and IL-4. In the late post-operative days, T-cell cytokine secretion returns to normal levels.

The main hormones that well correlated with the extent of the surgical trauma were cortisol and catecholamines. Clinical trials documented that post-operative inflammation and changes in immunologic parameters are less pronounced after laparoscopic approaches compared to open surgery. There is also evidence that the extent of the tissue trauma rather than the duration of surgery or anesthesia is the primary determinant of the IL-6 response.

The C-reactive proteins have also been found reduced in laparoscopic procedures compared with traditional laparotomy.

This less local cytokine production and C-reactive protein (CRP) during laparoscopic surgery results in less post-operative pain and infectious complications due to the reduction of the tissue trauma. Moreover, the duration of the cytokine secretion is different. For example, in one study comparing open vs laparoscopic cholecystectomy, the induced changes of the cytokines were normalized after 48 hours, whereas IL-6 and IL-8 still were elevated in the group who had conventional cholecystectomy.

Some of the benefits of minimally invasive surgery, such as less pain, more rapid recovery and a shorter hospital stay may be attributed to lower cytokine levels in comparison with those of conventional open surgery.

Also, the neuroendocrine response is more limited in laparoscopic than in open surgery; some studies reported the plasma adrenaline, noradrenaline and cortisol concentrations were significantly lower in both cholecystectomies and adrenalectomies during laparoscopic than during open surgery.

The serum inflammatory cytokine levels and CK are markers of muscle damage in orthopedic surgery. Some Authors have suggested that lower elevation of these serum markers is indicative of lower surgical invasiveness in orthopedic patient.

In total hip arthroplasty (THA) some studies compared the CK levels after different approaches. There is a significant increase in CK levels after THA by a posterior approach than when an anterior approach was used. Direct anterior approach can be considered to be minimally-invasive surgery because it was associated with the lowest increase in CK. There was also an overall trend toward lower levels of markers of inflammation in the anterior group, as compared with those in the posterior group.

In the meantime a relatively small difference was reported in levels of the general inflammatory cytokines. No difference was found in post-operative CRP levels comparing direct anterior approach with postero-lateral o direct lateral approach. Probably the inflammatory cascade in total hip arthroplasty is not greatly influenced by the surgical approach and is more related with bone removal and insertion of the implant than with the release of soft tissues.

Mjaaland et al. measured CK and CRP perioperatively (from day 1 to day 4) in patients undergoing THA by a direct anterior approach or direct lateral approach and found that post-operative CK levels were higher in the DAA group than in the direct lateral approach group at each measure. Rykov et al. found no difference in CK and CRP levels in patients undergoing THA by the direct anterior approach or posterolateral approach 2 hours, 1 day, 2 weeks and 6 weeks post- operatively. Monaghan et al. reported that patients treated by the mini-posterior approach had a greater rise in CK on post-operative days 1 and 2 than patients treated by direct anterior approach.

During direct anterior approach the muscles are mainly spared, but the tensor fascia latae, rectus femoris, sartorius, and gluteus medius are extensively stretched and might be damaged by the retractor. Moreover, the abovementioned muscles may be damaged during broaching and stem implantation. These intraoperative manipulations could lead to a greater increase in CK levels than when the muscle is detached or split during the posterior approach. During surgery, if important muscles are damaged, early rehabilitation after surgery may cause further damage to those muscles resulting in a delay in the return to normal CK levels. CK levels were higher in the 2 weeks after THA by a direct anterior approach than after the posterior approach indicating that direct anterior approach causes prolonged muscle damage.

The use of serum inflammatory cytokine levels and CK as marker of muscle damage are an objective method to evaluate the invasiveness of surgical procedures and defining the impact of surgical approaches in arthroplasty.

Conclusions

In conclusions, minimally invasive hip surgery, in the purpose, has all the advantages previously documented in less invasive surgical procedures for the immunological, histochemical and endocrinological standpoints. Moreover, the more conservative approach to muscles decreasing or minimizing dissection leads to a minimal inflammatory response and reduced CK level increase. Further correlation to these findings with clinical aspect are needed, including the examination of the capacity for regeneration of the damaged muscle tissue.

Bibliography

1. Bergin PF, Doppelt JD, Kephart CJ, et al. Comparison of minimally invasive direct anterior versus posterior total hip arthroplasty based on inflammation and muscle damage markers. J Bone Joint Surg Am. 2011;93(15):1392-1398.
2. Poehling-Monaghan KL, Taunton MJ, Kamath AF, Trousdale RT, Sierra RJ, Pagnano MW. No Correlation Between Serum Markers and Early Functional Outcome After Contemporary THA. Clin Orthop Relat Res. 2017;475(2):452-462.
3. Meneghini RM, Pagnano MW, Trousdale RT, Hozack WJ. Muscle damage during MIS total hip arthroplasty: Smith-Petersen versus posterior approach. Clin Orthop Relat Res. 2006;453:293-298.
4. Maezawa K, Nozawa M, Gomi M, Sugimoto M, Maruyama Y. Changes in serum creatine kinase and C-reactive protein after posterior and direct anterior approaches in total hip arthroplasty. Hip Int. 2022;32(5):591-595.
5. Mjaaland KE, Kivle K, Svenningsen S, Pripp AH, Nordsletten L. Comparison of markers for muscle damage, inflammation, and pain using minimally invasive direct anterior versus direct lateral approach in total hip arthroplasty: A prospective, randomized, controlled trial. J Orthop Res. 2015;33(9):1305-1310.
6. Reber PU, Sandberg A, Schmied B, Buchler MW. Cytokines in surgical trauma: cholecystectomy as an example. Dig Surg. 1998;15(2):92-101.
7. Udelsman R, Goldstein DS, Loriaux DL, Chrousos GP. Catecholamine-glucocorticoid interactions during surgical stress. J Surg Res. 1987;43(6):539-545.
8. Udelsman R, Norton JA, Jelenich SE, et al. Responses of the hypothalamic-pituitary-adrenal and renin-angiotensin axes and the sympathetic system during controlled surgical and anesthetic stress. J Clin Endocrinol Metab. 1987;64(5):986-994.
9. Donald RA, Perry EG, Wittert GA, et al. The plasma ACTH, AVP, CRH and catecholamine responses to conventional and laparoscopic cholecystectomy. Clin Endocrinol (Oxf). 1993;38(6):609-615.
10. Vittimberga FJ Jr, Foley DP, Meyers WC, Callery MP. Laparoscopic surgery and the systemic immune response. Ann Surg. 1998;227(3):326-334.
11. Jacobi CA, Ordemann J, Bohm B, et al. Increased tumor growth after laparotomy and laparoscopy with air versus CO2. Surg Endosc 1996;10:55.
12. Buunen M, Gholghesaei M, Veldkamp R, Meijer DW, Bonjer HJ, Bouvy ND. Stress response to laparoscopic surgery: a review. Surg Endosc. 2004;18(7):1022-1028.
13. Rykov K, Reininga IHF, Sietsma MS, Knobben BAS, Ten Have BLEF. Posterolateral vs Direct Anterior Approach in Total Hip Arthroplasty (POLADA Trial): A Randomized Controlled Trial to Assess Differences in Serum Markers. J Arthroplasty. 2017;32(12):3652-3658.e1.
14. Sietses C, Wiezer MJ, Eijsbouts QA, et al. A prospective randomized study of the systemic immune response after laparoscopic and conventional Nissen fundoplication. Surgery. 1999;126(1):5-9.
15. Landgraeber S, et al. A prospective randomized peri- and post-operative comparison of the minimally invasive anterolateral approach versus the lateral approach. Orthop Rev. 2013;5(3):e19.

CHAPTER 6

Pre-operative planning in primary hip surgery

Stefano Basso

Orthopaedics and Traumatology Unit, San Candido Hospital, Bolzano, Italy

Introduction

Pre-operative planning is a fundamental preliminary step in any orthopaedic surgery. It allows the surgeon to anticipate any problems he may face during surgery and to plan the most effective surgical strategies for overcoming them.

The theorisation of pre-operative planning in orthopaedics dates back to the 1960s by Maurice E. Müller. The following is what he wrote decades later, in 1989, about hip replacement surgery: '*This provides important information on choosing the correct model and the correct size of the prosthesis, the depth of the acetabulum preparation, the height of the neck resection, and the positioning and alignment of the pelvic and femoral components. It allows fast and systematic execution of the operation and thus minimises the risk of complications for the patient*' (Müller, M.E., Jaberg, 1989).

In hip replacement surgery, pre-operative planning is now considered an indispensable clinical practice even for the most experienced surgeon. This procedure allows the morphology of the hip and the length of the limbs to be assessed. It also helps to identify any congenital or acquired anatomical alterations (which are possible sources of intra-operative complications) and allows the planning of any complementary surgery (e.g. removal of osteophytes or trabecular bone grafting, etc.) [1]. Moreover, it permits to choose the prosthetic components that, for design and size, are most suitable to restore the joint geometry.

With an accurate radiological study and a correct pre-operative planning it is possible to reduce the time of surgery, prevent possible intraoperative complications and above all perform a correct joint reconstruction. This avoids, or at least limits as much as possible, errors in reproducing the femoral offset, restoring the exact limb length and orienting the cup.

Offset errors and limb length discrepancies, if significant, are always a cause of patient dissatisfaction [2], as they are related to clinical consequences. In addition, these can also lead to medico-legal issues for the surgeon.

Among the complications that can be generated by these two types of errors, the most relevant are: paralysis of the large nerve trunks such as the sciatic nerve and femoral nerve [3], low back pain [4], anserine gait [5] and an increased risk of dislocation [6].

An excessive increase in the femoral offset, increases, especially the lever arm of the abductor muscles. This results in an increase in load stress on the implant and thus on the interface between bone and prosthesis, with possible early aseptic loosening of the implant as a final outcome [7]. At the same time the excessive offset increases the contact stress between the trochanteric massif and the fascia lata, leading to painful bursitis [8].

Pre-operative planning is also critical in cup positioning. Revel and Kennedy identify improper cup placement as the most frequent cause of painful symptoms in the prosthetic hip. This is responsible for impingement, early loosening or abnormal wear of the liners [9-10].

Pre-operative planning therefore provides information that helps to minimise the complications listed above. These findings show that accurate planning is an effective weapon in lowering the risk of implant failure [11-12].

Pre-operative templating is traditionally performed on an AP-projected pelvis and lateral-projected hip x-ray at an average magnification of 15%. This enables two-dimensional planning with a sufficient degree of reliability and precision, as experience has shown for decades.

With computer technology it is now also possible to carry out three-dimensional planning based on the processing of tomographic scans (CT) by dedicated software.

In addition to providing more accurate preoperative measurements, 3D planning can also provide the surgeon with patient-specific guides that some industries have recently developed. This type of planning which is more elaborate but more efficient than traditional planning, can be extremely useful in difficult cases and revision surgeries.

Pre-operative planning must be carried out not only by studying the anatomical morphology of the pelvis and hip, but also by studying the patient's gait and movement in general.

Two-dimensional planning of total hip replacement

Two-dimensional planning is performed on standardised pre-operative radiographs: an anteroposterior (AP) projection of the pelvis in a standing position, a supine pelvis radiograph, an AP projection of the hip including the proximal third of the femur (with the patient supine on the radiographic table) and an axial or lateral ('frog-leg') projection of the same hip.

It is important to keep the hips rotated approximately 20° during standing radiographs. This is to compensate for the effect of the neck anteversion and thus to visualize the true length of the neck.

The X-ray beam should be perpendicular to the patient, centred on the pubic symphysis

The image should include the sacrum, the last lumbar vertebra, the iliac crests and the proximal third of the femoral diaphysis. The apex of the coccyx should be in line with the pubic symphysis. The X-ray tube must be rotated craniocaudally to achieve a distance in the image between the apex of the coccyx and the superior margin of the pubic symphysis of 1 cm in men and 2.5 cm in women [13-15].

All projections must be performed by placing a radiopaque reference of a known size at the height of the affected hip (approx. 1420 cm from the surface). This enables to determine the real geometric distortion caused by the X-ray beam and the real dimensions of the hip. This landmark becomes indispensable in two-dimensional digital planning.

The phases of correct planning are now reported in detail.

1) Morpho-functional observation of the patient's gait

It consists of observing the gait and movements of patients as they sit and stand up from their chairs and as they climb and descend stairs. This makes it possible to detect any dimorphisms, attitude defects, heterometries or other. Gait analysis in particular is fundamental to understand the patients' specific issues. Not only the pelvis but also the spine has to be examined, in particular to investigate the exact cause of any heterometry.

2) Morphological and anatomical observation of the hip

This consists of scrupulous observation of the pre-operative X-rays, in order to examine both the pelvis as a whole and the specific morphology of the hip to be operated on. The aim of this phase is to formulate a diagnosis, assess the severity of the anatomical-pathological alterations and the quality of the bone in order to prepare for possible difficulties. The detailed morphological assessment of the hip allows to visualise the morpho-structural changes in the joint heads (shape, size, bone quality) and the changes they induce in the geometry of the joint. The joint orientation, the position of the centre of rotation, the cervical-diaphyseal angle of the femur (varus-valgus), the anteversion of the femoral neck and the degree of lateralisation of the femur (offset) are analysed. All possible localised structural alterations that may cause intraoperative difficulties, such as geodesic cavities, bulky osteophytes or areas of osteosclerosis, must also be detected and noted. Simple observation provides some very important technical information. The state of the cotyloid cavity walls and their capacity to stably contain the prosthetic component can be assessed. In addition, the presence of axial deviations (femoral distortion or curvature), ossifications or marginal osteophytes can be assessed, as these will have to be removed to avoid phenomena of conflict with the prosthetic neck. These observations give a precise idea of the biomechanics of the affected hip. At the same time, they provide important indications for the choice of the prosthesis model and the optimal type of fixation (with or without cement) to be used in the case under consideration.

3) Radiographic measurement

What is detected visually is then evaluated quantitatively through radiographic measurements, of linear and angular type. These are obtained by constructing a system of lines on the X-ray from anatomical landmarks of the pelvis and femur. Implant simulations are then carried out by superimposing transparencies on the X-ray that reproduce the prosthetic models at the same scale of magnification. Nowadays, this procedure can be carried out not only in the traditional form (which is the subject of the following explanations), but also in digital form. This is done through the use of software dedicated to two-dimensional planning which will soon become a common procedure. The detailed procedure for planning in digital form is dependent on the specific software used. However, the principles and theoretical basis do not change and are those of the traditional form described, which remains the essential theoretical basis for this activity.

The final result of the measurement phase is the definition of a prosthetic implant hypothesis in terms of: model, size and position of the components, method of fixation and strategy for the reconstruction of the joint geometry.

There are various methods of radiographic measurement, but they all have in common the definition of the basal plane of the pelvis as a starting point. From this, depending on the specific geometric characteristics of the hip and the correction of any dysmetria, the following parameters are determined:

1. Centre of rotation
2. Limb dysmetria (if present)
3. Morphologic cortical index (MCI, fig. 1)
4. Canal bone ratio (CBR, fig. 1)
5. Canal-calcar ratio (CCR, fig. 1)
6. Canal-flair index (CFI, fig. 1)
7. Position and size of the acetabular component
8. Position, design and size of the femoral component
9. Femoral osteotomy orientation and level
10. Angle of inclination and ideal prosthetic neck length.

According to the classical method of Maurice E. Müller et al., the basal plane is described by the intersection of a line passing through the caudal ends of the two lacrimal figures, called the basal line, with the perpendicular line drawn through the midpoint of the pubic symphysis.

We then proceed to draw the line of the small trochanters, parallel to the basal line and passing through the most prominent point of the small trochanter of the healthy hip. Of great importance is the acetabular

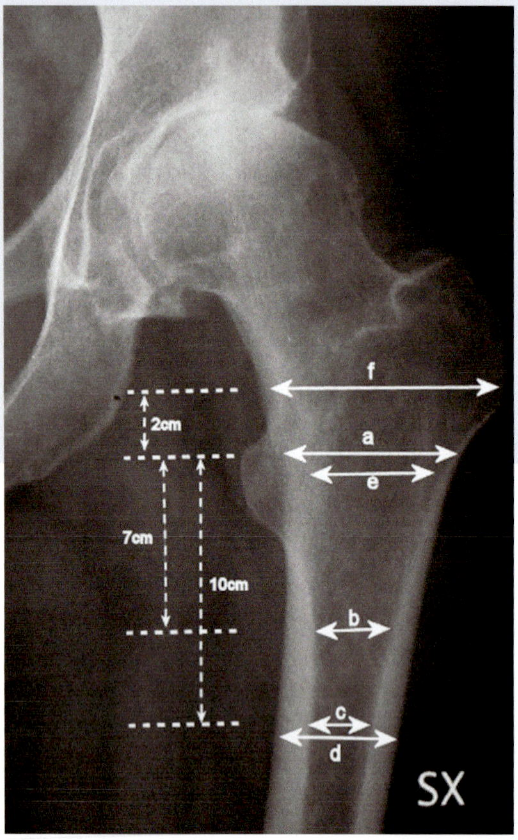

Figure 1 Radiological parameters of morphological analysis of the proximal femur

Morphological cortical index MCI = a/b
Canal bone index CBI = c/d
Canal calcar ratio CCR = c/e
Canal flair index CFI = f/c

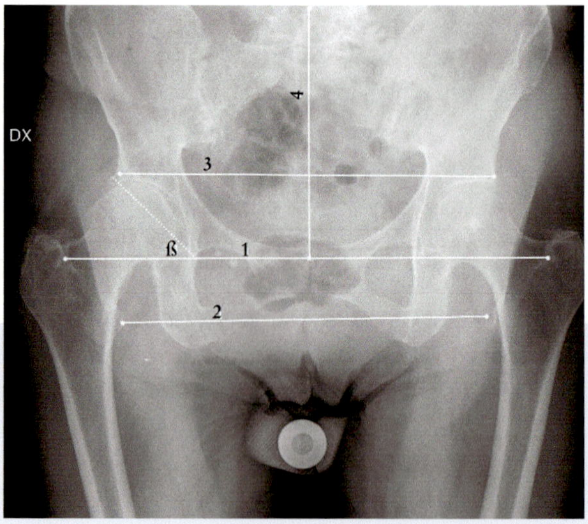

Figure 2 1) Basal line; 2) line of the lesser trochanters; ß) angle of acetabular inclination; 3) junction of the acetabular roofs; 4) longitudinal axis of the body

equator line, which defines the inclination of the acetabulum. This line originates at the superior margin of the acetabulum and ends at the lacrimal figure. At its intersection with the baseline, the acetabular inclination angle is measured (fig. 2).

4) The step-by-step measurement technique

1. The following lines (already defined in figure 2) are drawn on the standard radiographic plate of the pelvis:
   a) The basal line: the junction of the two tear shape figures;
   b) The junction of the acetabular roofs. If this line is parallel to the previous one, it means that there are no acetabular dysmetries;
   c) The longitudinal axis of the body, perpendicular to the junction of the two lacrimal figures and passing through the pubic symphysis: this, together with the basal line, defines the basal plane.
2. To determine the possible dysmetria of the limbs, a parallel line to the basal line is drawn starting from the apex of the small trochanter of the contralateral hip (line of the small trochanters). This is taken as a reference. The distance between the apex of the small trochanter of the pathological hip and this line determines the dysmetry (fig. 3, in green). The most caudal end of the tear shape figure on the pathological side will then be raised or lowered according to the length discrepancy measured and used as a sup-

port for the drawing sheet (see point 7).

3. The rotation center of the healthy hip is marked and mirrored on the pathological side using the longitudinal axis as the axis of symmetry (fig. 4).
4. The ideal rotation centre of the acetabular cup will coincide with the one that has been traced. If a compromise choice is necessary, it can be moved within the safety zone. This is along the continuous green line in figure 5 or within the quadrant defined by the two green lines, continuous and dotted, in the same figure. Going outside this zone would alter the biomechanics of the hip too much. The lines that define the safety zone are: the line passing through the ideal centre of rotation obtained in the previous point at an angle of 45° to the baseline in the supero-medial direction (the solid line in the picture) and the vertical (dashed) originating from the centre of rotation.
5. The outline of the pathological haemibacinum is drawn by holding the drawing sheet (a transparent glossy paper) over the radiograph and aligned with the longitudinal axis of the body.
6. Determine the estimated size of the acetabular cup (see also paragraph V) by overlaying the transparencies of the chosen prosthetic implant on the x-ray. This should be adapted to the acetabular cavity, taking into account the desired inclination and the position where its rotation center will be situated. The acetabular cup thus determined and positioned is then placed on the drawing sheet.
7. In order to determine the probable size of the stem (see also paragraph VI) the transparencies of the implant considered most suitable for the case are overlaid on the medullary canal. The size chosen is the one that best fills the canal by touching the medial and lateral corticals of the femur. At the same time the correct size must allow one of the head centres shown on the cone (representing the different head lengths available) to match the rotation centre of the acetabulum that has been indicated in the previous point on the drawing sheet. This must be placed on the sheet in such a way that the base of the tear-shaped figure on the sheet does not match the actual figure on the sheet but the one corrected as described in point 2, taking into account the dys-

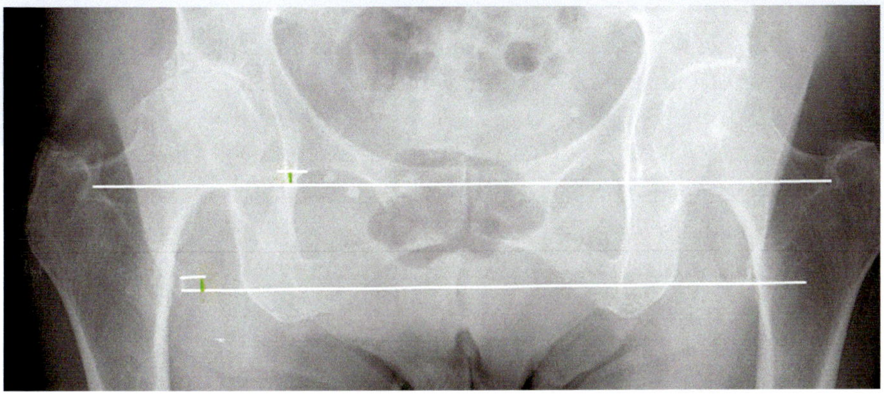

Figure 3 Determination of dysmetry

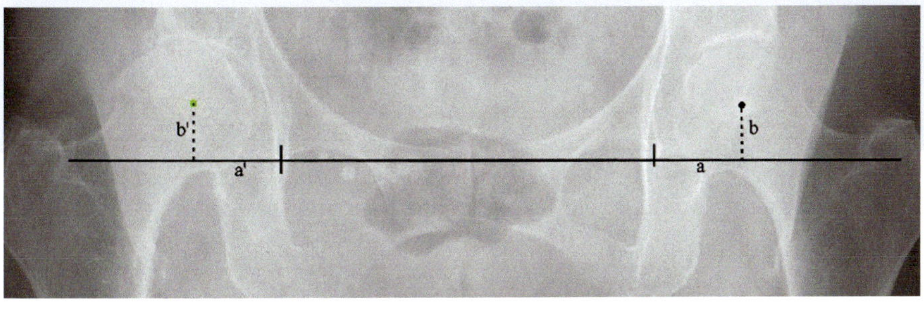

Figure 4 Centre of rotation

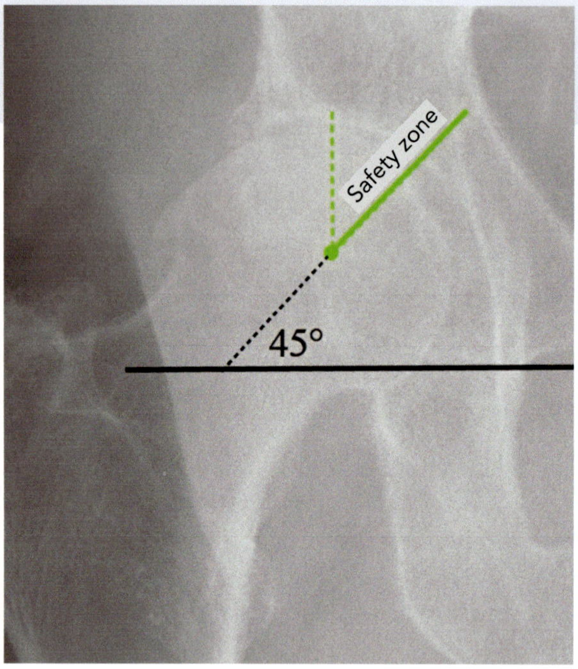

Figure 5
Safety zone

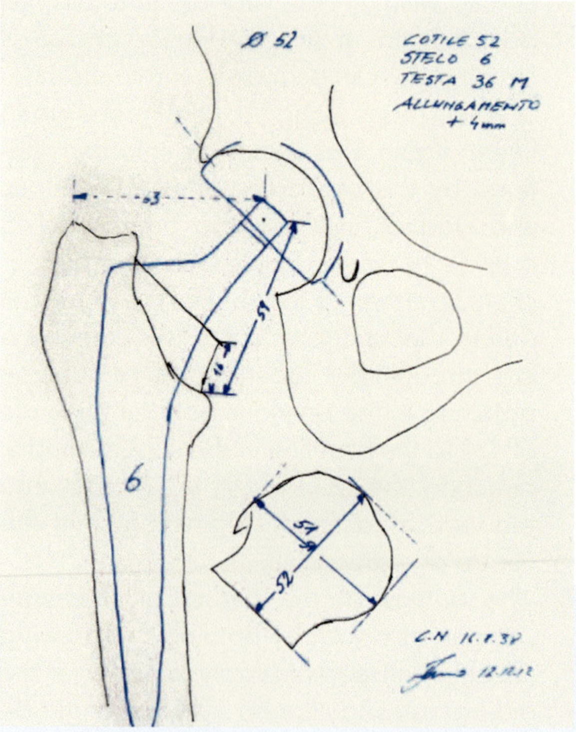

Figure 6
Drawing sheet (planning)

metria of the limbs. In this way, the correction of the dysmetria is achieved and the optimal stem depth and length of the prosthetic head are determined. The level of the femoral neck resection line is also determined at this stage. All this is recorded on the drawing sheet.

8. Once the position of the stem and consequently of the femoral neck cut line has been determined, the resected femoral head can be reproduced separately on the drawing sheet. The distance 'a' (between head apex and base of the cut) and 'b' (largest diameter of the head) are measured and reproduced on the drawing sheet (fig. 6). These distances will then be measured during surgery and will be used to check the congruity of the pre-operative plan. The correspondence between the actual femoral head diameter (measurable with a caliper) and the measured value 'b' is an important method for verifying the correct radiological magnification scale. The accuracy of the distance 'a', on the other hand, indicates a correct height of the neck cut.
9. The distances between:
   a) medial apex of stem cone and lesser trochanter;
   b) lateral apex of the stem cone and the greater trochanter.
   These measurements should be considered reliable if the checks described in paragraph 8 are positive.
10. Complete the drawing with all other useful data, if not already indicated, such as:
    a) type and size of acetabular cup,
    b) stem type and size;
    c) head size and neck length;
    d) extent of dysmetria;
    e) patient's biographical data;
    f) date of planning,

g) signature of the planning physician.

In the following two paragraphs, the selection methods for the acetabular and femoral component during planning in terms of size and position are discussed in more detail.

5) Positioning and selection of the acetabular cup size

To determine the position of the acetabular component, the cup template of the chosen model is overlayed on the radiograph of the pelvis. The rotation center indicated on the template must coincide with the desired one, as determined during the measurement phase (fig. 7A). The acetabular cup is oriented at an angle of 45° to the baseline. The permitted variation is +/-5° in order to optimally occupy the acetabulum. The measurement is correct when its image perfectly covers the bony borders of the acetabulum and its external profile coincides with the limit of the subchondral spongiosa. In accordance with the philosophy of maximum bone stock conservation, the bottom of the implanted acetabular cup should not be extended beyond the quadrilateral lamina of the pelvis. In addition, its inferior-medial border must not go beyond the point of intersection between the lateral end of the inferior margin of the iliopubic spine and the lateral end of the external margin of the ischiopubic spine. It must be underlined that the position and size chosen must guarantee a biomechanically ideal positioning of the centre of rotation (fig. 7B).

6) Positioning and choice of femoral stem design, size and position

At the femoral side, the morphologically most suitable prosthetic design must be chosen. The wide availability of designs on the market makes it possible to make an optimal choice even in the most difficult cases, such as in a dysplastic hip or one that has undergone previous surgery. The size and position of the femoral stem is determined by overlaying the templates corresponding to the chosen stem type on the radiographic image of the proximal femur, so that the medial side of the stem image corresponds

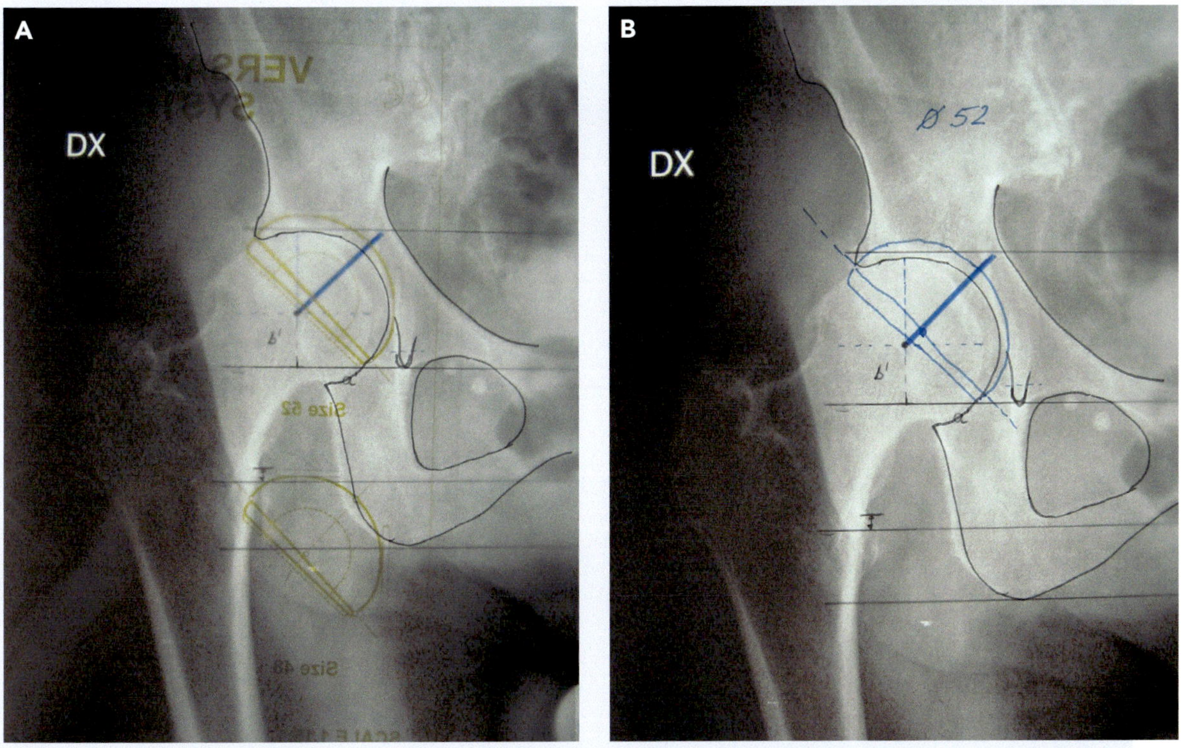

Figure 7 A) Placement of the tracing paper of the acetabular cup. B) Selected acetabular cup to be marked on the worksheet

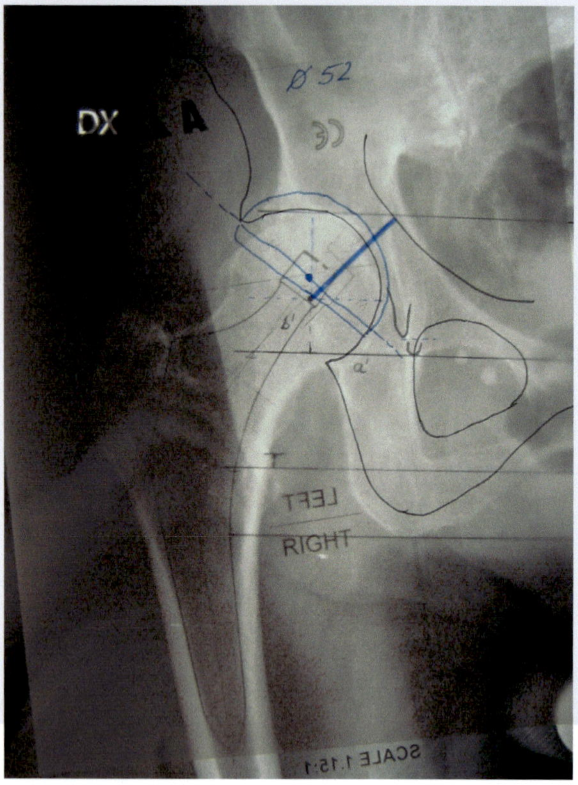

Figure 8 Choice of design, size and position of the femoral stem

to the medial margin of the medullary canal. The ideal size of an uncemented stem is the one that guarantees optimal contact between bone and prosthesis in relation to the prosthetic design. For example, classic press-fit prostheses must perfectly fill the proximal third of the femur, while with the new short stem models one must try to obtain support with the calcar and the lateral wall of the femoral metaphysis.
In addition to the correct centering in the mid-lateral canal, it is equally important to establish the correct position of the stem in the femur in the proximal-distal direction (sink level). On this depends the choice of level and orientation of the cervical osteotomy and the length of the prosthetic head. All these factors are fundamental for the reconstruction of the joint geometry, which is the basic prerequisite for the biomechanical rebalancing and correction of the limb metry in case of any pathological shortening.
Depending on whether or not it is necessary to correct the heterometry previously measured in the planning, it will be necessary to vary the length of the prosthetic neck (by modifying the head length) and in some cases also the level of stem sinking, with consequent variation of the level and orientation of the cervical osteotomy.

7) Reconstruction of joint geometry

To complete the planning it must be checked whether the stem position and the selected neck length results in a satisfactory joint geometry. In particular, the extent of the femoral offset and the lever arm of the abductors are observed. It is also evaluated whether there is a risk of impingement between the prosthetic components and the bone.
The abductor lever arm and offset measurements are extremely important parameters and must be calibrated very precisely to ensure muscular and ligamentous rebalance. This is biomechanically necessary to achieve static and dynamic joint stability, correct load transmission and physiological kinematics.

8) Reproducibility and reliability

The radiographic planning technique described above has proved to be an indispensable element in performing hip replacement surgery, both globally and in our own experience. The reliability and accuracy of the preoperative planning has been evaluated by cross-checking the planned size of the components against the actual implanted size in a sample of 80 hip replacements. A complete match was found in 94.2% of cases.

However, the method of comparing the planned position of the components with the position actually achieved has not been perfected yet. This is due to the objective difficulty of obtaining perfectly comparable pre- and post-operative radiographs. Minor changes, usually because of a different angle of rotation, can affect measurements and invalidate comparisons.

Some orthopaedic surgeons perform an additional intraoperative check of the positioning of the prosthetic components. The drawing sheet is overlayed on the image obtained with an image intensifier in order to assess during surgery if the desired geometry has been achieved. In these cases, however, great attention must be given to the resulting magnification level.

Our experience has shown that with a good pre-operative planning and a meticulous intraoperative check of the plan's accuracy, through the evaluation of anatomical parameters, a substantial elimination of postoperative dysmetria and other clinically important geometric defects have been achieved.

Three-dimensional planning

The development of new technologies has led to the introduction of computerised planning techniques. These are able to develop optimised, patient-specific planning and simulate the effects of each surgical step.

Surgical planners and simulators are part of the CAS (computer aided surgery) classified as passive systems. They are only capable of performing auxiliary surgical tasks in a non-autonomous manner: they essentially provide a range of additional information which makes the surgical procedure more precise and reproducible.

A surgical planner consists of a processing unit, represented by a computer or a computer network, and specific software that runs inside the unit. This is able to process the images of a three-dimensional CT scan performed on the patient and loaded into the computer. The images are interpolated with the virtual three-dimensional model of the prosthesis, which is preset in the software, thus enabling a real step-by-step simulation of the surgery to be carried out.

Developed on a CAD/CAM system used to design prosthetic models, surgical planner-simulators were initially introduced as stand-alone tools for planning purposes only. Nowaday, they are in fact part of more complex systems, such as image-based navigation systems, robotic assistance systems and patient-matched cutting guide systems.

Current pre-operative planning systems use three-dimensional CT images (fig. 9), which allow a very detailed assessment of the joint anatomy, that can be navigated in the three planes of space. In many cases, a precise calculation of joint parameter measurements is also possible. Dynamic overlap of virtual image of the prosthetic components takes place on the anatomical images. This, too, can be studied in the three spatial planes and even modified until the optimal implant is obtained for the specific anatomy of the hip.

In most cases, the information recorded by the planner is transferred to a navigation system or a robotic assistance system or used to build patient-matched devices. All these solutions allow a precise and accurate reproduction of the surgical plan in order to guarantee the best clinical outcome.

Bibliography

1. D'Antonio JA. Preoperative templating and choosing the implant for primary THA in the young patient. Instr Course Lect. 1994;43:339-346.

2. Ranawat CS. The pants too short, the leg too long!. Orthopedics. 1999;22(9):845-846.

3. Nercessian OA, Piccoluga F, Eftekhar NS. Postoperative sciatic and femoral nerve palsy with reference to leg lengthening and medialization/lateralization of the hip joint following total hip arthroplasty. Clin Orthop Relat Res. 1994;(304):165-171.

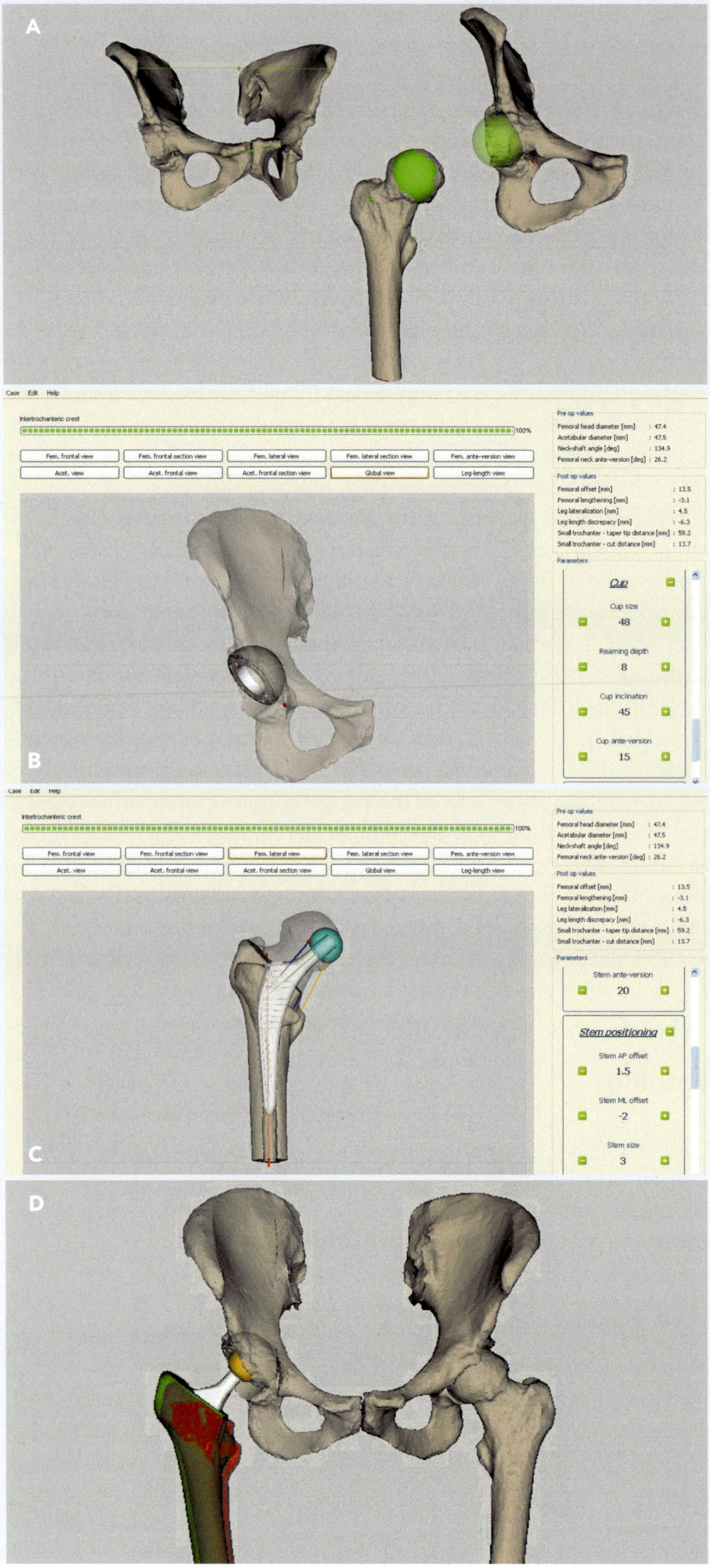

Figure 9
A) 3D study of hip joint and pelvis. B) Acetabulum with cup implantation. C) Femur with stem. D) Pelvis with planned endoprosthesis. Courtesy of Medacta International SA

4. Friberg O. Clinical symptoms and biomechanics of lumbar spine and hip joint in leg length inequality. Spine (Phila Pa 1976). 1983;8(6):643-651.
5. Gurney B, Mermier C, Robergs R, Gibson A, Rivero D. Effects of limb-length discrepancy on gait economy and lower-extremity muscle activity in older adults. J Bone Joint Surg Am. 2001;83(6):907-915.
6. McCollum DE, Gray WJ. Dislocation after total hip arthroplasty. Causes and prevention. Clin Orthop Relat Res. 1990;(261):159-170.
7. Ramaniraka NA, Rakotomanana LR, Rubin PJ, Leyvraz P. Noncemented total hip arthroplasty: influence of extramedullary parameters on initial implant stability and on bone-implant interface stresses. Rev Chir Orthop Reparatrice Appar Mot. 2000;86(6):590-597.
8. Iorio R, Healy WL, Warren PD, Appleby D. Lateral trochanteric pain following primary total hip arthroplasty. J Arthroplasty. 2006;21(2):233-236.
9. Revell PA. The combined role of wear particles, macrophages and lymphocytes in the loosening of total joint prostheses. J R Soc Interface. 2008;5(28):1263-1278.
10. Kennedy JG, Rogers WB, Soffe KE, Sullivan RJ, Griffen DG, Sheehan LJ. Effect of acetabular component orientation on recurrent dislocation, pelvic osteolysis, polyethylene wear, and component migration. J Arthroplasty. 1998;13(5):530-534.
11. Schizas CG, Parker B, Leyvraz PF. A Study of Pre-Operative Planning in CLS total Hip Arthroplasty. HIP International. 1996;6(2):75-81.
12. Eggli S, Pisan M, Müller ME. The value of preoperative planning for total hip arthroplasty. J Bone Joint Surg Br. 1998;80(3):382-390.
13. Clohisy JC, Carlisle JC, Beaulé PE, et al. A systematic approach to the plain radiographic evaluation of the young adult hip. J Bone Joint Surg Am. 2008;90 Suppl 4(Suppl 4):47-66.
14. Della Valle AG, Padgett DE, Salvati EA. Preoperative planning for primary total hip arthroplasty. J Am Acad Orthop Surg. 2005;13(7):455-462.
15. Pipino F et al. La protesi totale d'anca. Studio preoperatorio radiografico. Minerva Ortopedica e Traumatologica 1988;39-11:809-12.

The AMIS technique
Anterior Minimally Invasive Surgery

Frédéric Laude

Clinique du Sport, Paris, France

Introduction

AMIS (Anterior Minimally Invasive Surgery) is a minimally invasive anterior surgical technique for hip replacement. This follows an intramuscular and inter nerve approach that significantly reduces the risk of damage to peri-articular structures such as muscles, tendons, vessels and nerves. The anterior approach was first described by a German surgeon called Carl Hueter (1838-1882), whose work entitled 'Grundriss der Chirurgie' (The Compendium of Surgery) was published in 1881 [1].

The first anterior hip arthroplasty was performed in France in 1947 by Robert Judet, who operated on a patient in supine position on the so-called 'Judet orthopaedic table' (designed by Henry Judet, his father, in 1940) [2]. Robert Judet died in 1981 and, after this date, the anterior approach continued to be known only in Paris. In fact, in the 1990s, it was even impossible to purchase a 'Judet orthopaedic table'. The history of AMIS is closely linked to that of the anterior approach and to my personal experience with this type of surgery.

In 1987 I was an intern and my mentor was Emile Letournel, Judet brother's pupil. In his hospital, I performed a total hip arthroplasty through an anterior approach for the first time. Then, in 1996, I moved to a private hospital, where I had no access to any orthopaedic table for the anterior approach. Firmly believing in the obvious advantages of minimally invasive anterior surgery for the patient, I decided to build my own orthopaedic table in order to continue performing it. My goal is to focus on the patient's well-being, trying to preserve as much peri-articular tissue and bone stock as possible during a total hip replacement. Therefore, in 2004 I presented my project of the minimally invasive anterior approach to Medacta, asking them to support me in optimising and improving the reproducibility of this method through the development of dedicated instruments and implants. This idea matched perfectly with Medacta's vision to create the best clinical experience possible for patients in need of joint replacement. We both agreed to create a new word for this synergy: AMIS, for minimally invasive anterior surgery, which in French also means 'friends'.

The first step was to develop a leg positioner to correctly perform AMIS. In fact, a stable and replicable leg positioning is essential to allow an easier exposure and a simple and reproducible surgical procedure to restore the patient's function and biomechanics. In addition to the implants, I helped develop dedicated instruments for the AMIS

technique. These were introduced in order to protect the soft tissues, reducing the potential risk of damaging [1] nerves and muscles, facilitating both bone preparation and implantation of the prostheses.
For the past twenty years, my main activity has been hip surgery. I have performed more than 5000 total hip replacements with minimally invasive surgery through the anterior approach. In addition, I am involved in conservative hip surgery, and to date I have performed more than 300 periacetabular osteotomies and 1500 minimally invasive arthroscopies.
Over the last ten years I have organised and taken part in many courses both for beginners and experts on the anterior approach, thus having the opportunity to develop and improve the AMIS technique.

Patient selection

Basically, there are no particular contraindications for the anterior approach. In addition, more often, as the surgeon becomes an expert, it is possible to complete complex cases and revisions with a standard anterior approach or with special extensions, such as the Zarak-Nissak approach for the femoral portion. However, it is important to remember that, in the first cases a good patient selection is indispensable for a successful initial learning phase of this technique.
In principle, it is believed that the ideal patient for the first cases should be female, slim and not too muscular. This is because, in spite of the specific positioner for the operated limb, the AMIS Mobile Leg Positioner, muscular patients create the greatest difficulties, especially in femoral exposure. For the same reason, the preferred patients are the ones with a femur neck that is not too short and not too varus, with a diagnosis of arthrosis and without pelvic complications.
In fact, the longer the neck of the femur, the easier the operation becomes. The more varus the neck, with the iliac crest close to the greater trochanter, the more accuracy is required in the incision and the preparation of the joint capsule.
It is also true that in some cases the anterior approach may not be convenient. For example, in the case of previous surgery, it is reasonable to use the previous approach. This is the case of operations for an acetabular fracture or other surgeries involving the proximal femur. It is important, besides the ethical side, to bear in mind that patients who have undergone several operations sometimes have adhesions or retractions that can create difficulties in exposing the femur.
There are other cases which may cause problems or difficulties for the less experienced surgeon but can be managed once the technique has been mastered. A good example are major deformations of the proximal part of the femur (osteochondritis), with a high trochanter or a very short neck. A series of femoral fractures can lead to some errors that are not always easy to recognise using the anterior approach. Therefore, in this case, an extended femoral approach may be more suitable for the neophyte. On the other hand, it should be pointed out that a femoral neck fracture with two or three isolated screws should not create any major problems.
A coxarthrosis with acetabular protrusion is not an absolute contraindication and can be operated using the anterior approach. However, if necessary, the surgeon must be prepared to dissect the posterior capsule and short rotator muscles to obtain better exposure. Additionally, in the case of protrusions, the surgeon must apply more traction to facilitate the extraction of the femoral head and sometimes it may be necessary to remove the anterior osteophytes.
Although the normal technique is to remove the femoral head as a single piece, in some challenging cases, e.g. multiple acetabular fractures, it may be necessary to fragment the head to extract it.
In certain muscular patients, and especially when the surgeon is learning the technique, the surgical approach may be extended. Morover, do not hesitate to resect the indirect tendon of the rectus femoris in order to fully expose the acetabulum and fully release the

posterior part of the capsule to avoid malposition of the prosthesis.
Finally, it is interesting to note that, thanks to the AMIS Mobile Leg Positioner discussed below, obese patients are not a contraindication. The skin incision area is in fact among those with the thinnest adipose tissue around the hip joint. Therefore, the use of long retractors, associated in the literature with possible stress to peri-articular muscles and nerves, is not necessary to manage the surgical approach [1-3]. The only concern, given the supine position, is the risk of abdominal fat covering the surgical approach. In this case the use of patches and adhesive bandages may be sufficient to move and hold this abdominal fat tissue. Care must also be taken to sterilize the inguinal skin folds, which are often a breeding ground for bacteria that can cause complications.

Pre-operative assessment

The reparation of the patient for surgery at our clinic, an exclusively orthopaedic hospital, is based on the following protocol.
The patient is assessed one month before the admission and undergoes hematochemical tests, ECG, chest X-ray, anaesthesiological examination and dental evaluation. The latter is performed to detect the presence of caries, a dangerous gateway for bacteria, which is unfortunately becoming increasingly common. The patient then returns to the orthopaedic surgeon who must both confirm the indication for prosthetic treatment and describes the fundamental characteristics of the operation in a simplified language, trying to make the patient 'aware' of the possible sequelae of this choice.
The patient's willingness to proceed with the surgery must be confirmed by signing the informed consent form.
The low blood loss recorded in the post-operative evaluations results in a very low haemotransfusion rate, about 1-2% of patients. For this reason, we do not arrange for the collection of autologous blood bags for the operation.

Pre-operative planning

Pre-operative planning is mandatory, and neglecting it means being ready for the worst. It must be carried out rigorously, even by the most experienced surgeons.
The patient has to undergo an X-ray examination, always with a calibration marker, of: the pelvis in antero-posterior projection in both supine and standing positions; an axial projection of the femoral neck; an X-ray of the affected hip including the proximal third of the femur. These radiographic examinations are printed on film or presented on digital supports. Using the specific templates for the type of prosthesis to be implanted, the pre-operative planning is completed. The planning helps us to understand the sizes of the acetabular cup and the femoral stem. This can allow optimise the number of surgical instruments to be displayed on the instrument cart (fig. 1), making interaction with the nurse/scrub easy, fast and precise.
During planning it is possible to highlight specific measures that can help the surgeon assess the reproduction of the planning intra-operatively (fig. 2). For example, it is possible to assess the height of the femoral neck osteotomy and the cup position for the correct reproduction of the length of the operated limb.

Special features of the AMIS technique: dedicated instrumentation and leg positioner

The AMIS technique (Anterior Minimally Invasive Surgery) originates from the author's experience in hip prosthetic surgery. The author trained at the Hôpital de la Porte de Choisy with Prof. Emile Letournel, a pupil of the Judet brothers in the middle of the last century.
From the outset, the direct anterior approach was adopted as the golden standard for cup replacement surgery. It was soon clear that there were no alternatives as good as this in terms of muscle sparing and soft tissue preservation. However, it was consciously decid-

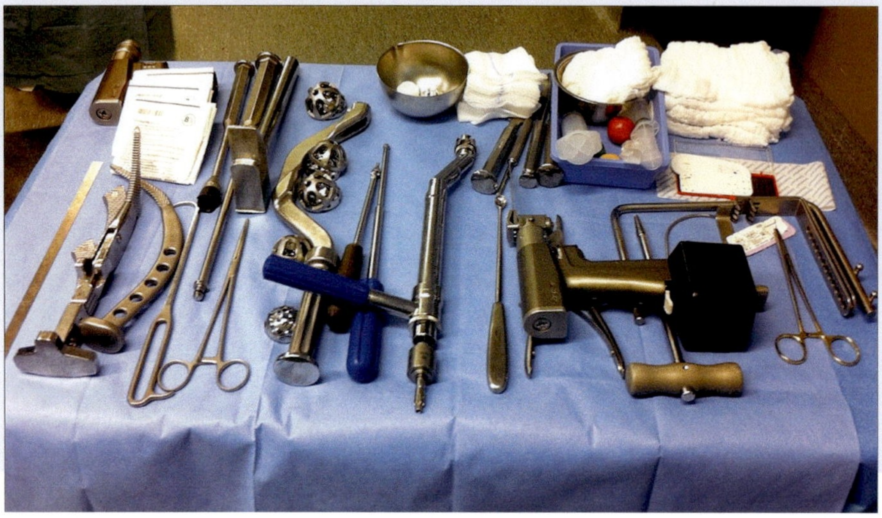

Figure 1 Surgical instrumentation on instrument table

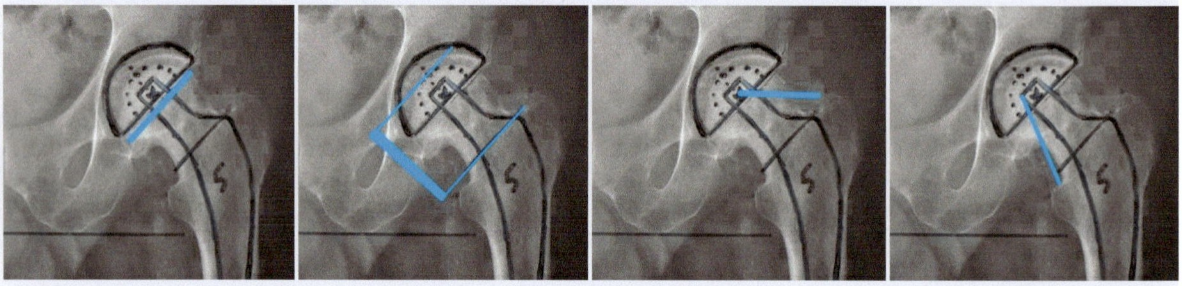

Figure 2 Measurements carried out during pre-operative planning

ed to combine this surgical approach with the use of a traction bed. This facilitated the positioning of the lower limb, thus facilitating the exposure of anatomical sites.
The Judet brothers began to develop a traction bed on the model of the one used for pelvic trauma patients. Based on the same principles, in 1994 the author began the development of a dedicated positioner. This had to maintain not only traction on the operated limb, but primarily an adequate position of the leg throughout the whole surgery (fig. 3).
In 2004 the author's increasing experience and demands led to an agreement with the Swiss company Medacta International to develop a dedicated positioner, the AMIS Mobile Leg Positioner (fig. 4). Today, this is used in many hospitals around the world that have decided to use this technique.
The main features of this device are its easy handling, its compact size and the fact that it can be connected to any surgical bed using special adapters. Every necessary position of the limb during each phase of surgery is reproduced in a stable and effective way, facilitating the surgeon's task. A special feature of this device is the automatic release of traction during the hyperextension phase for exposure of the femur. This protects the femoral nerve from being stretched.
The author's experience has led to the development of other specific tools to the AMIS technique, which owe their origin to some tools developed by H. Judet. These instruments have evolved with the idea of making the AMIS technique as elegant and conservative as possible. In the discussion of the technique we will see the use of a modified Charnley Frame that works only with the thick connective tissue of the capsule. This protects the muscle tissues encountered, to

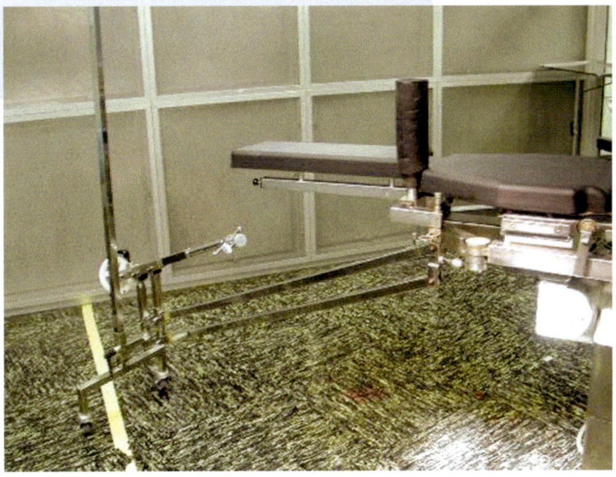

Figure 3 First leg positioner table designed by Dr. Laude

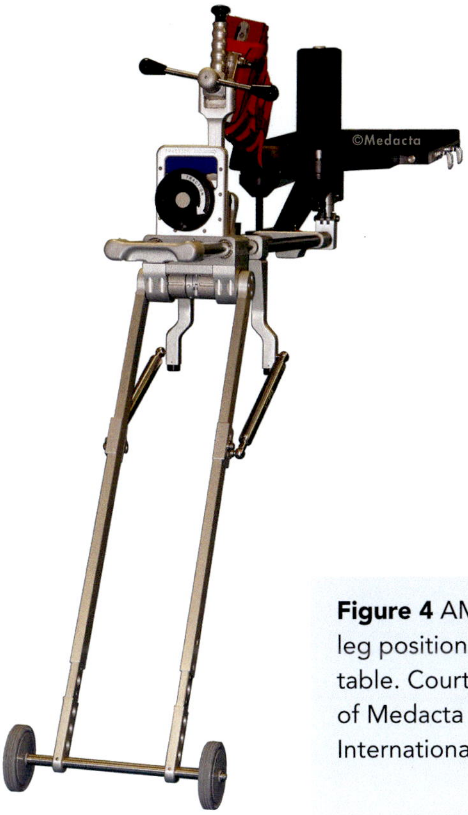

Figure 4 AMIS 2.0 leg positioning table. Courtesy of Medacta International SA

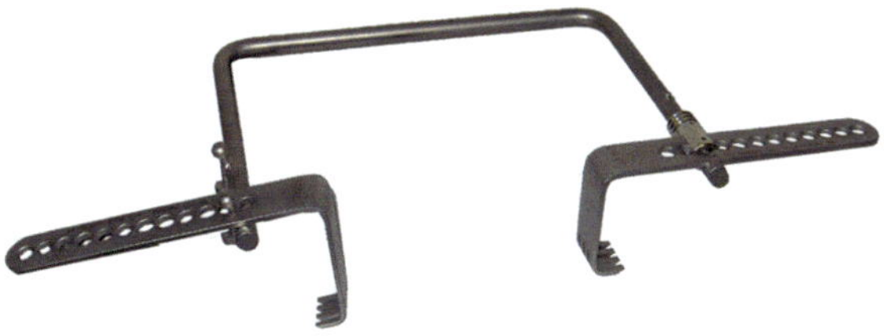

Figure 5 Charnley autostatic retractor. Courtesy of Medacta International SA

which no Hohmann applies stress.
Once the femoral head is removed, the AMIS Charnley frame (fig. 5) is positioned and is not removed again during the procedure. This avoids the constant repositioning of retractors typical of other anterior surgeries.
Cutter handles and impactors feature an offset design to work with minimal incision in the supine position.
For the same reason, a starter for the femoral canal and broaches has been developed that work at 45° to the axis of the femur. These allow the surgeon to position himself as shown in the figure (fig. 6) during the entire time of femoral implant insertion (fig. 7).
A further optimisation of the procedure has been achieved thanks to the development of the 'Gaston' (fig. 8), a pneumatic arm that is easy to manoeuvre intraoperatively and allows the positioning or stabilisation of the retractors used by the surgeon.

Patient positioning on the operating table

The patient is positioned supine on the operating table, wearing a compression stocking on the contralateral lower limb. The patient's foot is wrapped in a soft bandage to fill the shoe with which the patient's foot is tied to the leg positioner. This protects the foot and ankle of the ipsilateral limb from possible decubitus caused by the leather of the shoe. By bending the hip and knee, the heel is pushed into the support shoe, then the closing straps are tightened vigorously. This apparently trivial step is crucial, because if the grip on the ankle is lost, the tractions and rotations performed by the positioner will be less effective, if not useless. Once the patient is positioned on the operating bed, it is simultaneously checked that there is direct contact between the perineal

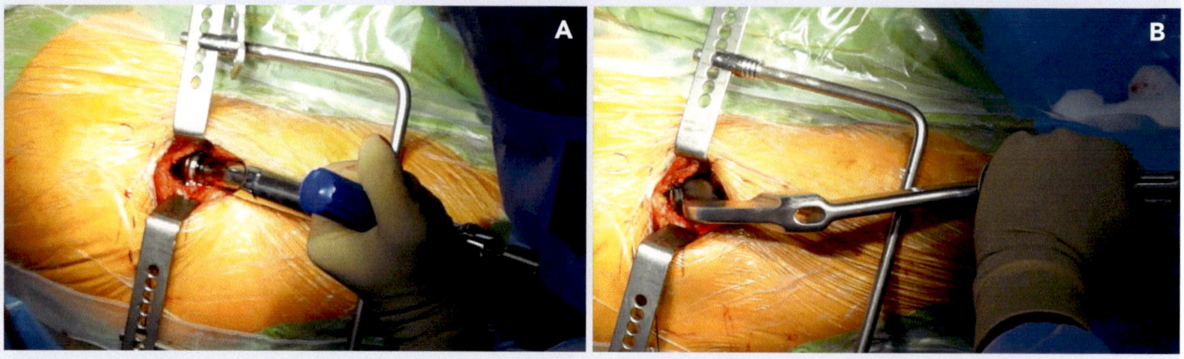

Figure 6 A) Using the reamer with off-set. B) Using the impactor with off-set

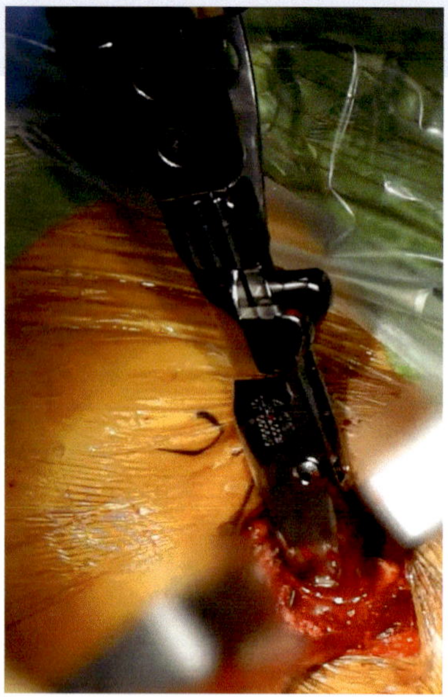

Figure 7 Using the 45° broach holder handle

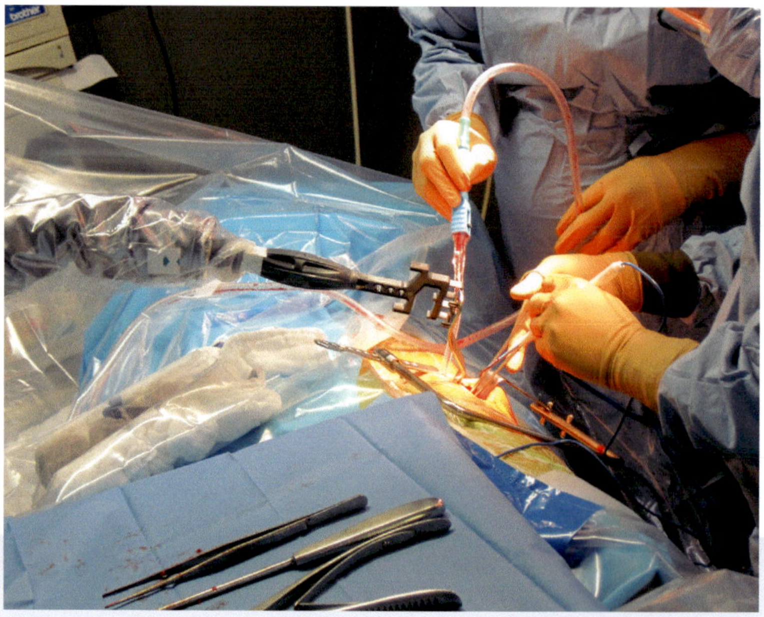

Figure 8 Using the Gaston with Hohmann retractor

support (which must be well padded) and the patient's inguinal region. At this point, thanks to the AMIS Mobile Leg Positioner (fig. 9), gentle traction is exerted, bringing the hip into flexion of approximately 10° and the knee into maximum extension with the patella at 0° (a corresponding internal rotation of the foot of 10° is not uncommon in this case).

Once the patient is correctly positioned on the bed, it is necessary to checked that the pelvis is horizontal and that the counter-thrust at the proximal part of the thigh has a space of about half a centimeter from the skin. This is to avoid any possible compressive damage to the sciatic nerve.

The patient's arm on the surgeon's side is placed on the chest and secured to it with a counter-thrust. This will also prevent the pelvis from drifting distally (obliquely) along the traction axis of the AMIS Mobile Leg Positioner.

At this point the surgical area is disinfected with Betadine alcohol solution (fig. 10). This procedure starts at least three fingers above the anterosuperior iliac spine (ASIS), reaches the umbilicus and the entire inguinal region extending distally to the knee of the operated limb. Using the AMIS Mobile Leg Positioner, only the operated leg needs to be

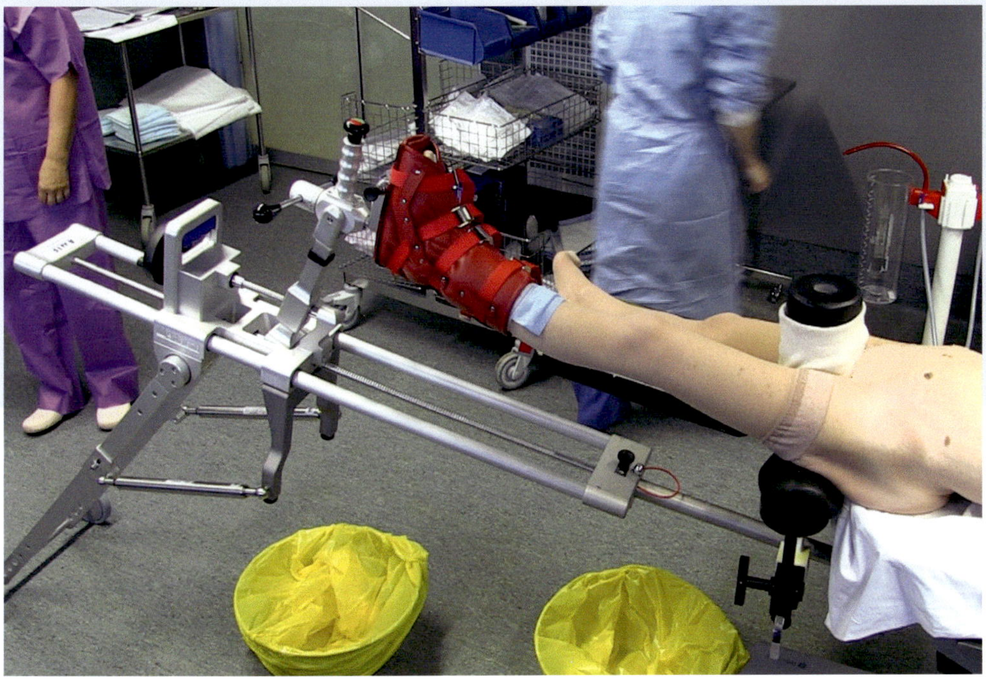

Figure 9
Starting position on AMIS leg positioner

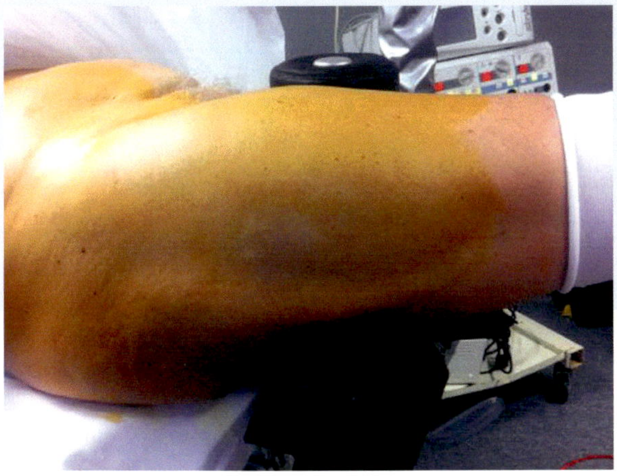

Figure 10
Area treated with alcoholic solution and Betadine

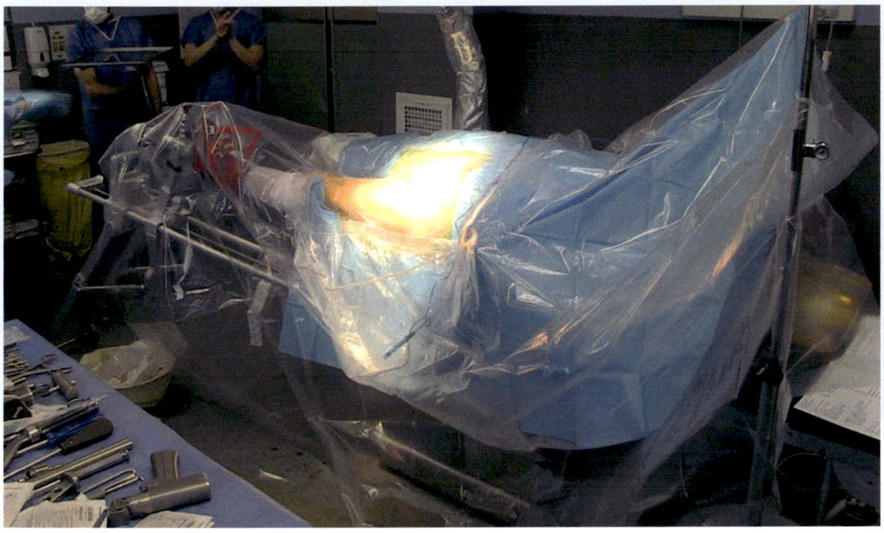

Figure 11
Sterile field completed with adhesive, transparent and classic sterile drapes

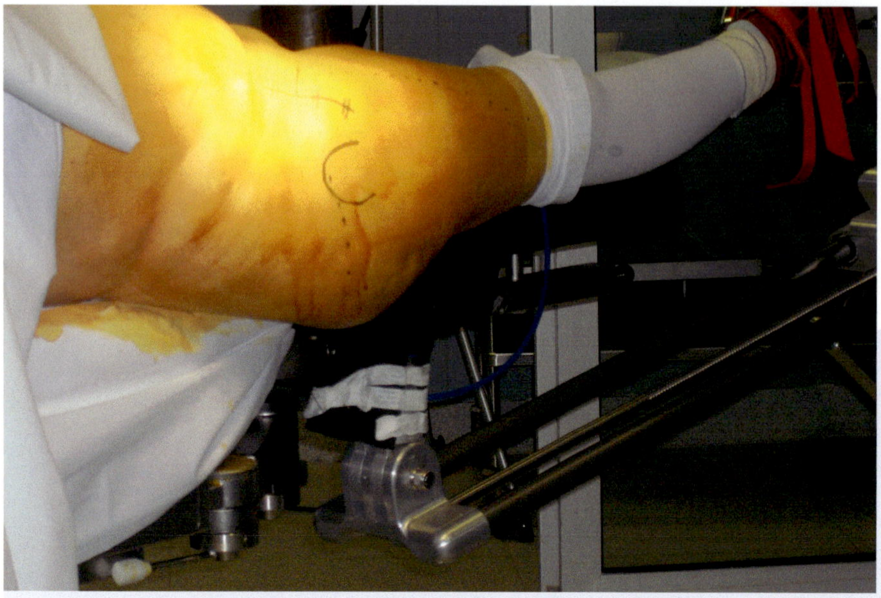

Figure 12
Incision area and anatomical landmarks outlined with sterile marker

prepared, specifically in the area described above, which saves time.
The operating field is covered with adhesive sheets, transparent if possible, allowing the surgeon (fig. 11) to constantly supervise the position of the patella, the foot and the movements of the AMIS Mobile Leg Positioner.

Surgical technique

Skin incision

Compared to the direct anterior route as described by Hueter, the skin incision is made more laterally to avoid the femoral cutaneous nerve and its branches.
The incision (fig. 12) starts 2 cm lateral and distal to the anterosuperior iliac spine (ASIS) and normally ends slightly below the vertical that passes through the apex of the greater trochanter, running parallel to the line between the ASIS and Gerdy's tubercle (fig. 13).
In the case of thin patients, it is also possible to identify the space between the tensor tensor fascia latae and sartorius muscles, starting the incision two centimeters lateral to this and two centimeters distal to the ASIS.
An alternative for patients with particularly globular abdomens is an incision along the inguinal folds ideally centered on the femoral neck but transverse to it.
In this case, however, there is a real risk of intercepting and injuring the branches of the lateral cutaneous femur nerve. It is therefore an incision that is recommended only when the learning curve has been significantly overcome and only in cases of obvious necessity.
Careful haemostasis is then carried out and the plane of the fascia lata is carefully reached.

Muscle plane

The incision extends to the aponeurosis of the tensor fascia latae. The aponeurosis is incised to expose tensor fibres which are oriented proximal to distal and directed outwards. If the muscle fibres are directed medially, there is a good chance that they are from the sartorius muscle (fig. 14).
The fascia is incised, its medial flap is lifted and the underlying tensor is detached with a finger or pliers, slipping easily between it and the sartorius muscle. The medial part of the muscle is retracted laterally, splitting the sartorius aponeurosis so as not to injure the lateral femoral cutaneous nerve. Manual mobilisation is simple and allows the tensor fascia lata muscle to be moved laterally. It is very important to have performed a good release of the aponeurosis of this muscle proximally and distally under the skin, so that the retractors do not damage the muscle. A Beckmann retractor is inserted to hold

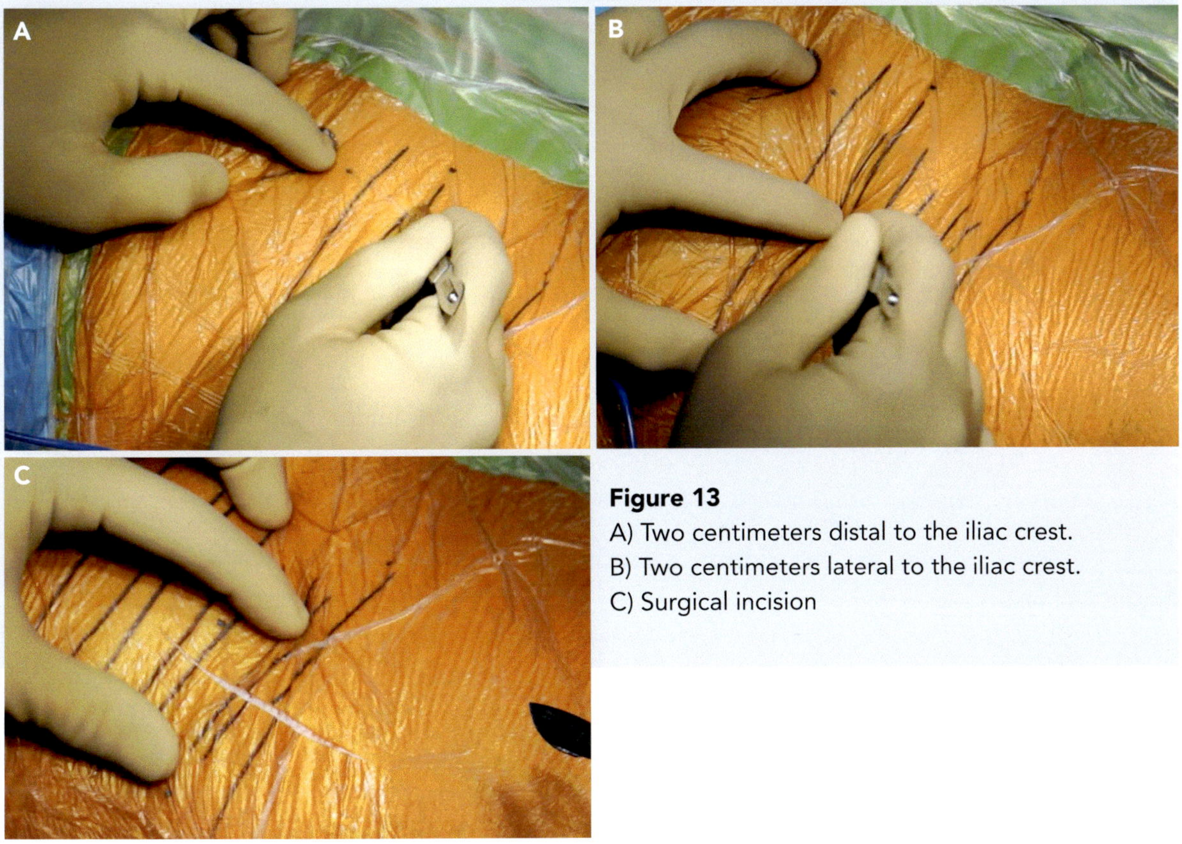

Figure 13
A) Two centimeters distal to the iliac crest.
B) Two centimeters lateral to the iliac crest.
C) Surgical incision

the tensor, then the aponeurosis of the rectus femoris is visualized.
The rectus femoris is covered with a very thin aponeurosis, which allows the muscular structure to be clearly seen. Distally and proximally you can clearly distinguish the muscle mass and its tendinous fibres which are prolonged with the direct and indirect tendons. The aponeurosis covering the red muscle mass is then incised. Here, a slight haemostasis is required almost systematically. The muscle can now be retracted medially using the Beckmann retractor.
Care must be taken not to move proximally at this level. There are venous vessels in the adipose tissue that may bleed at the slightest contact and haemostasis is often difficult. In addition, in some cases, a secondary branch of the crural nerve, which innervates the most medial part of the tensor fascia lata, may be injured.
With the Beckmann retractor positioned between the lateral part of the rectus femoris and the medial part of the tensor fascia lata, a nacreous aponeurosis or innominate fascia can be observed. This aponeurosis is the last structure that separates us from the capsule. Below this aponeurosis and a little further distally, the anterior circumflex arteriovenous bundle can be seen. The aponeurosis is thinner in the distal part of the access, and should be incised with great caution so as not to injure the circumflex vessels. (fig. 15)
After the aponeurosis has been opened, the circumflex vessels can be easily isolated with a detacher, tied with two ligatures and cut. These relatively large vessels are directly connected to the femoral artery, and a simple coagulation may not be safe enough.
The indirect rectus femoris tendon is isolated with a Lambotte. For the first operations or in cases of dysplastic acetabular cups, it is useful to resect the indirect rectus tendon. In this case, the tendon is taken with pliers and cut with an electrosurgical scalpel.
In the most medial part and underneath the rectus femoris we find the ileocapsularis muscle and, more distally, the ileopsoas tendon. This muscle is generally covered by a

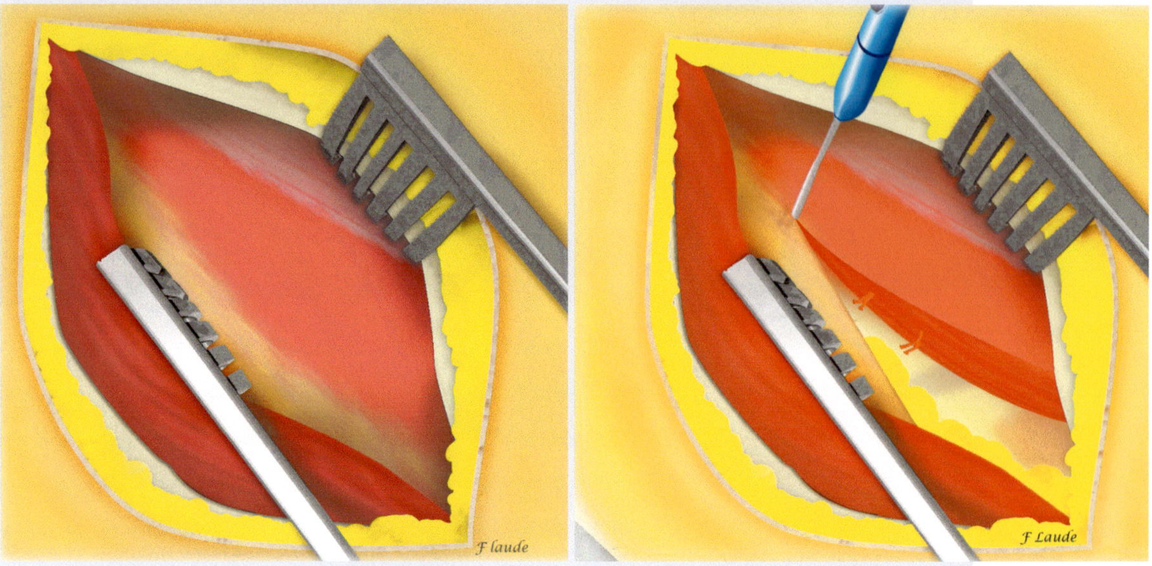

Figure 14 Muscle approach: from skin incision to the anterior circumflex vessels

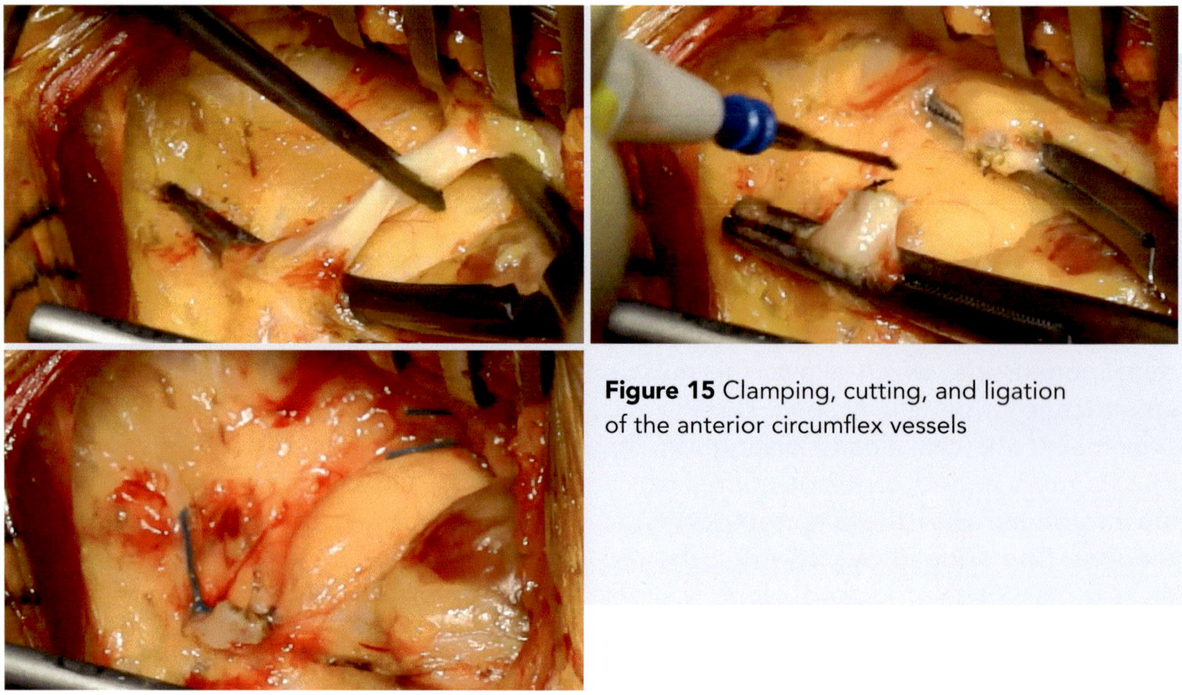

Figure 15 Clamping, cutting, and ligation of the anterior circumflex vessels

very thin aponeurosis that joins the capsule. This is especially true proximally. It does not seem useful to detach this muscle from the capsule, even if this would allow a better capsular exposure. In fact, post-operative pain may occur later, as well as some difficulty in flexing the hip.

As detailed above, it should be noted that no gluteal muscles were considered, not even for the use of retractors. As the gluteal muscles are important for transverse joint balance and gait stability, the AMIS approach therefore has a very important mini-invasive characteristic. This is one of the reasons for the excellent results expected, both in the short and long term, as described in other chapters of this book.

Access to joint space

After removing the fatty tissue overlying the capsule, the muscles around the capsule are exposed. These must not be touched. Some gluteus minimus fibres can be visualised proximally and laterally, while the ileo-capsular fibres are present on the medial side. The tensor fascia latae muscle, retracted by the Beckmann retractor, is seen on the lateral side. More distally, the vastus lateralis fibres are also visible and follow the inferior insertion of the capsule at the anterior intertrochanteric line.

The joint capsule is incised following the edge of the ileocapsularis muscle. Proximally the incision ends at the anterior edge of the acetabulum, but may slightly follow the edge of the acetabulum laterally. Distally the incision follows the medial insertion of the capsule on the femur trying to release as much medially and distally as possible. Once a good medial-distal release has been achieved, the femoral neck is exposed and a first Hohmann can be inserted. Then proceed laterally and slightly distal to the intertrochanteric line, along the fibres of the vastus lateralis (fig. 16).

A triangular flap is obtained and its medial vertex must be hooked with a traction wire. This is lifted to facilitate dissection of the capsule from the femoral neck towards the gluteus minimus fibres in the direction of the tensor fascia latae. Once the space between the gluteus minimus, the capsular insertion on the great trochanter and the femoral neck has been identified, a second Hohmann is placed. A counter-clockwise rotation of this instrument will facilitate the completion of the capsular dissection from the femoral neck.

Osteotomy of the femoral neck

The capsule release technique described above allows better visualisation of the anterior part of the neck. On the upper part of the neck, it is possible to visualised the retinaculum carrying the vessels that supply the femoral head. It is recommendable to coagulate the vessels before cutting the femoral neck. This releases the superior part of the neck.

Thanks to the AMIS Mobile Leg Positioner, the neck osteotomy is performed with the head in place without any dislocation required. This avoids possible muscle trauma or femur fractures during hip dislocation manoeuvres.

Before resecting the femur neck, traction can be increased by approximately 1 cm with the AMIS Mobile Leg Positioner, thus facilitating the opening of the osteotomy.

The osteotomy cut level is essentially identified on the basis of the cervico-diaphyseal angle and the pre-operative plan. It starts from the most lateral part of the neck, right at the union with the great trochanter, towards the femoral neck. The best anatomical landmark is the pre-trochanteric tubercle, which is located at the superior insertion of the vastus lateralis very close to the fold of the femoral neck (fig. 17).

The cut is generally made at 45° angle to

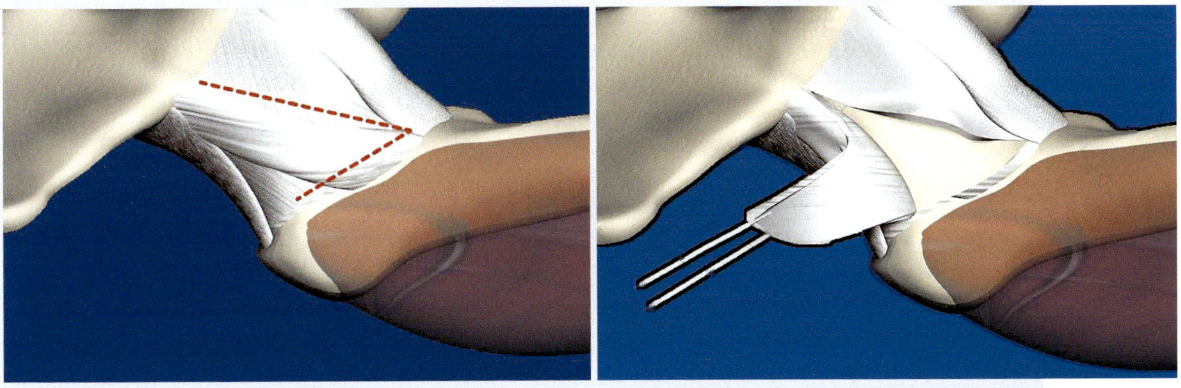

Figure 16 Triangular incision on the joint capsule. Courtesy of Medacta International SA

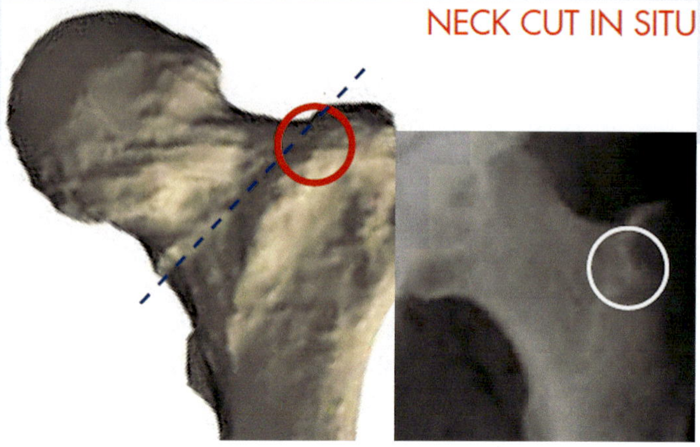

Figure 17 Pre-trochanteric tubercle and cutting line. Courtesy of Medacta International SA

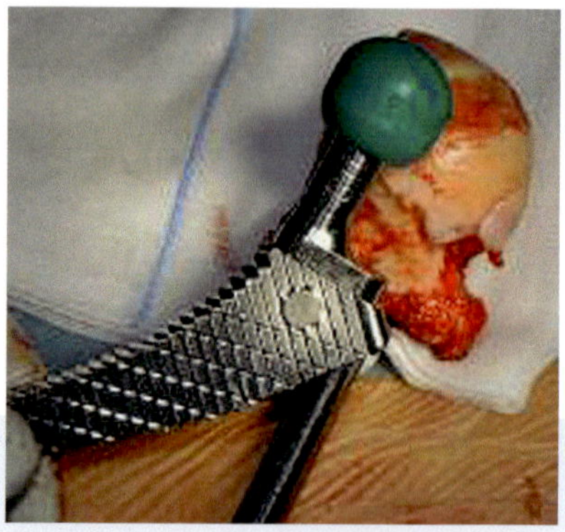

Figure 18 Intra-operative evaluation of trial broach, neck, and femoral head with anatomic neck and femoral head

the horizontal plane, just proximal to the superior fibres of the vastus lateralis. The saw must be perpendicular to the femoral neck. Before resecting the neck, the position of the lower limb should be checked by palpating the patella. The saw should preferably be narrow and long. It is important to proceed with care and caution so as not to go too far posteriorly, avoiding any injury to the posterior circumflex artery. The two Hohmanns protect the posterior vascular supply of the capsule from the action of the oscillating saw. At this point the osteotomy is opened by the gentle traction of the AMIS Mobile Leg Positioner.

It is advisable not to completely complete the osteotomy with the oscillating saw, to reduce the risk of damaging important arteries located posteriorly. An easy way to complete the osteotomy is to apply a 45° external rotation to the limb with the AMIS Mobile Leg Positioner: this rotation is usually sufficient to complete the osteotomy.

The extraction of the femoral head is completed using a 'corkscrew', screwing it as centrally as possible to the femoral neck and rotating the head consensually with the corkscrew. Caution is required as the presence of osteophytes or an irregular osteotomy may damage the surrounding musculature. Usually the posterior part of the capsule remains attached to the femoral neck and should be incised before head extraction. The retractors can be removed before completing the head extraction.

The single cut of the femoral neck makes it possible to obtain a single block which will make it easier and more accurate to determine the length of the leg. This verification (fig. 18) is carried out by overlaying the trial head and neck (chosen pre-operatively) on the patient's femoral head, trying to reproduce the physiological centre of rotation.

Acetabular preparation

Following the resection of the femoral head, any residual traction applied previously is released to facilitate the cutting of the femoral neck. The limb is already externally rotated by 45° following the previous femoral head extraction phase. This position allows the iliopsoas to be relaxed and the AMIS Charnley frame to be properly positioned.

The wire attached to the capsular flap is retrieved and lifted using it as a support. Thus, the first blade of the AMIS Charnley frame can be placed in the medial flap of the capsule, just touching the anterosuperior acetabular rim. While holding the medial blade of the retractor firmly in the anterior capsule with one hand, the adjustable lateral blade is positioned over the capsular flap that has been lifted laterally using the suture. The retractor blades are thus positioned in the capsule. As the capsule is thick in this area the grip of the blade will presumably be good. The surgeon should position the blade as laterally as possible on the flap. If the blade is positioned too deeply within the capsule, problems may occur during femoral preparation. The retractor blades are specially designed for this access. It is important to check during the operation that the retractor remains firmly in place, only gripping the capsule. Being on the ligamentous structure, the retractor will protect the muscular tissues and facilitate the post-operative recovery.

If the retractor is positioned correctly, the surgeon can leave it in place until the femoral preparation is complete. With this specific AMIS Charnley frame retractor, the capsule itself acts as a retractor. If the AMIS Charnley retractor is properly positioned, the acetabular rim is visible or palpable around its entire circumference. If it is still difficult to visualize the anterior wall of the acetabulum, a small Hohmann retractor can be placed anterolaterally to the iliac spine. The entire semi-circular joint should be visible.

The acetabular labrum is always removed to avoid impingement during cup placement. Electrocoagulation of the ligamentum teres and the residual retinacular vessels is then performed, identifying the acetabular fossa and the transverse ligament. Drilling can then begin by inserting a hemispherical drill into the acetabulum.

An offsetted bur handle is used to avoid conflict with the distal end of the incision. Impingement of the instrument at the distal edge of the incision must be avoided at this stage. This could damage the skin and produce a 'leverage effect ' leading to excessive reaming of the anterior wall of the acetabulum. If the incision is small, the burr can be placed separately in the acetabulum by hand and then locked by inserting the handle. Using the same procedure, the surgeon can remove the two components separately. The hemispherical bur may be removed with a Kocher. Drilling should preserve the subchondral bone and, if any area appears to be insufficiently drilled, it is preferable to make it bleed using a curette rather than drilling again. This avoids the risk of implanting the cup in weaker cancellous bone. After the acetabular preparation, a trial cup is inserted.

With this surgical approach, and in general with all minimally invasive procedures, care must be taken to avoid verticalization of the implant or an excessive anteversion. A useful indicator, to understand the orientation of the cup, can be the floor and obviously the axis of the lower limb. The implant should be positioned under the anterior rim of the acetabulum to avoid contact with the iliopsoas. The final cup is implanted and its stability is checked.

Preparation of the acetabular cup is completed with multiple infiltrations of local anaesthetic to control post-operative pain. Finally, it should be noted that pulsed surgical site washes are performed at each surgical stage as a preventive antiseptic measure.

Femoral exposure

Once the acetabulum has been prepared and the cup positioned, the femur is exposed. This can be easily achieved with the use of the AMIS Mobile Leg Positioner which allows to apply the necessary rotation, hyperextension and adduction of the operated limb.

This phase begins by applying slight traction and externally rotating the operated limb until the patella is rotated 90° from its initial position. This can correspond to a rotation of the foot of up to 180°, which often impresses the neophyte. It is important to emphasise that the surgeon should always accompany the rotation movements at knee level to reduce the stress on the operated leg and facilitate the movement itself. If there is difficulty in obtaining a 90° external rotation, it is advisable to release the pubofemoral ligament near the calcar. This is followed by the release of the iliofemoral ligament which can be extended proximally until a small fat pad appears. This first ma-

noeuvre is indispensable to avoid a possible bone impingment between the great trochanter and the acetabulum (fig. 19).
At this point it is necessary to release all traction to avoid an excessive stretching of the crural nerve during hyperextension. The final stage of the femoral positioning involves the full extension of the femur. Before this, it is necessary to act with a hook placed in the intramedullary canal and 'pull' the greater trochanter from the posterior profile of the cup. Failure to observe this precaution may result in rupture of the greater trochanter due to the incarceration of the greater trochanter against the cup in the final phase of femoral positioning. The AMIS Mobile Leg Positioner has a unique mechanism that automatically removes any residual traction during hyperextension. Ensure the complete absence of traction by moving the knee slightly up and down. The AMIS Mobile Leg Positioner can be lowered to the floor or locked at whatever height to allow the surgeon adequate exposure and visualization of the femoral canal. Moving the AMIS Mobile Leg Positioner under the contralateral lower limb applies adduction which exposes the femur even better (fig. 20).
If good femoral exposure has not been achieved, it is easy with the AMIS Mobile Leg Positioner to return to the starting position and repeat the movements. Repetition makes the tissues around the joint more likely to facilitate femoral exposure.
In the final position, the plane of section of the femoral neck should be horizontal. A Hohmann retractor can be inserted on the posteromedial side of the femoral neck to lateralise the proximal femur.

Femur preparation

Once the lower limb is well positioned, the surgeon should position himself with his back to the patient's feet, leaning against the patient's thigh to push it into further adduction. Depending on the type of stem used it may be necessary to clean the inside of the greater trochanter with a curette. Otherwise the surgeon may perform a compaction of the intramedullary bone of the proximal epiphysis

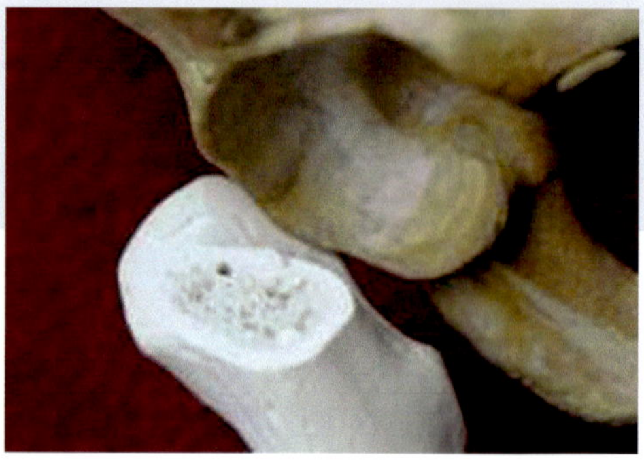

Figure 19
Bony impingement between great trochanter and acetabulum

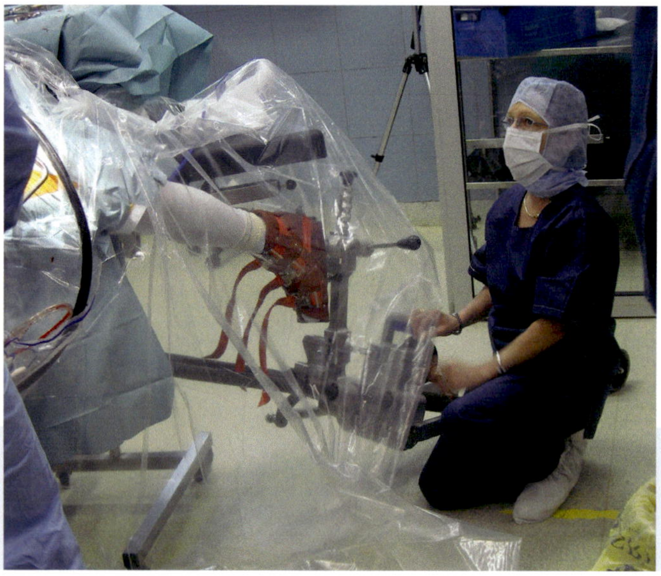

Figure 20 Hyperextension of the operated leg with AMIS positioning table

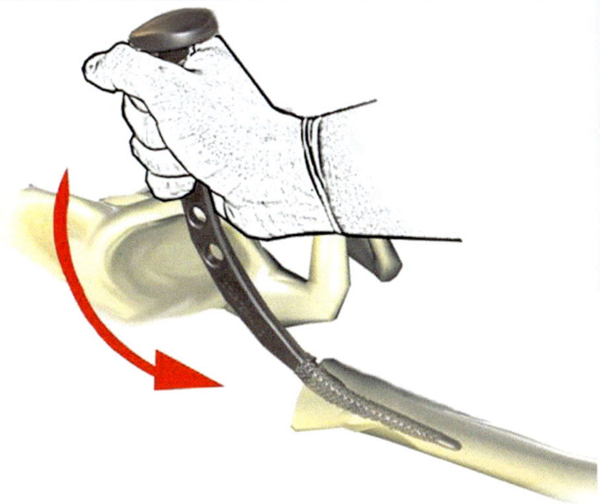

Figure 21
Femoral canal opening with AMIS starter rasp. Courtesy of Medacta International SA

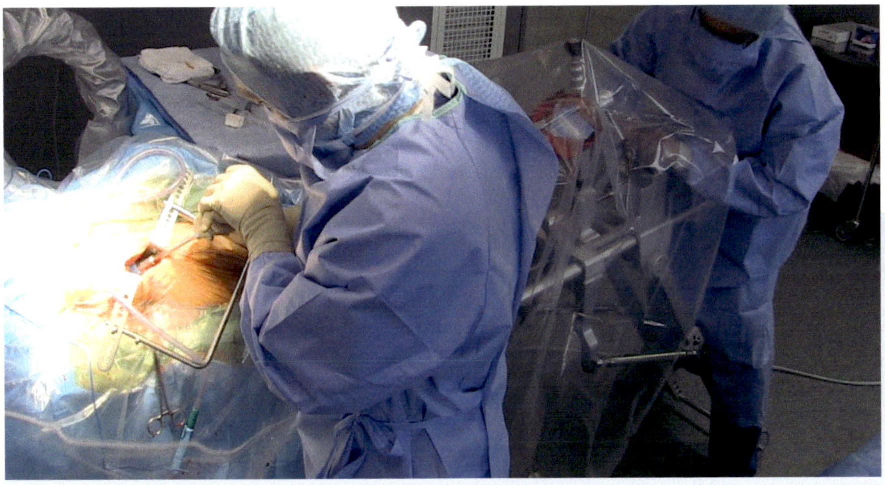

Figure 22
Reduction with AMIS leg positioner

to allow the AMIS Starter to open the femoral canal. (fig. 21).
To avoid creating an incorrect path in the canal, the hammer should never be used with the starter rasp. However, if it is necessary to 'force' the rasp into the femoral canal, the use of the hammer is recommended only after the rasp has entered at least halfway.
A flexible aspirator is used to palpate the inner cortical of the femur. The femoral preparation is continued by removing the cortical bone along the medial part of the greater trochanter.
Suitable broaches are sequentially inserted into the femur up to the chosen implant. A 45° handle is used to continue the preparation of the femoral canal in the position described above. This also avoids damage to the tensor fascia lata muscles. Each broach should be inserted as deep as possible and at the level of the femoral resection. It is advisable to push the broach down as far as possible to move it away from the calcar and thus reduce the risk of fractures. During the extraction phase it is advisable to pull the handle to reduce the risk of fractures of the greater trochanter.
This preparation is considered completed when the last inserted broach reaches the preoperatively planned level. Usually an essential landmark is palpation of the lesser trochanter.
The surgeon should not modify the physiological anteversion of the femur to reduce the risk of posterior dislocation as this risk is already significantly reduced with the AMIS approach.
Stability tests are performed with the trial components. After validating the measure-

ments in relation to the pre-operative plan, the stem is inserted and the femoral head is chosen. The length of the neck will depend on the position of the implant in relation to the planned one. It is also possible to improve accuracy by comparing the length of the neck and the final head with the natural femoral head.

To improve stability and articulation tests, the traction shoe may be disconnected from the AMIS Leg Positioner. In this case, caution must be taken to keep the surgical field sterile.

Please note that pulsed lavages on the surgical site are performed at each surgical step as a preventive antiseptic measure.

Reduction

After positioning the prosthetic components, the reduction manoeuvre is facilitated by the AMIS Mobile Leg Positioner. This system makes it possible to return to the initial position by consecutively releasing adduction, extension and rotation in a safe and reproducible manner. Traction can also be easily added during the manoeuvre if difficulties are encountered in reducing the femoral head in the cup (fig. 22). With the AMIS Mobile Leg Positioner, it is also possible to perform a quick stability test of the implanted prosthetic system by bringing the leg into 90° external rotation and applying light traction.

Closure

Surgery is completed with the application of a drainage, which will be maintained for approximately 24 hours. And at the end, sutures of the joint capsule (optional), aponeurosis of the fascia lata, subcutis and skin are performed.

Bibliography

1. Rachbauer F, Kain MS, Leunig M. The history of the anterior approach to the hip. Orthop Clin North Am. 2009;40(3):311-320.
2. Kreuzer S, Matta JM, Single-incision anterior approach for total hip arthroplasty: Smith-Petersen approach, O'Connor MI, Griffin LY, eds, Limited Incisions for Total Hip Arthroplasty, AAOS, Rosemont, 2007, 1-14.
3. HUG - Hôpitaux universitaires Genève Internal report.
4. T Stähelin et al. Tensor denervation and little abductor damage from hip replacement with the Röttinger technique. Schweiz Med Forum 2006, 6:(Suppl.32).
5. Matta JM. Anterior approach for total hip replacement: background and operative technique, in Scuderi GR, Tria AJ, Berger RA (eds), MIS Techniques in Orthopedics. Springer Science Business Media, Inc, 2005, 121-140.
6. Bhargava T, Goytia RN, et al. Lateral femoral cutaneous nerve impairment after direct anterior approach for total hip arthroplasty. Orthopedics. 2010;33(7):472.

CHAPTER 8

Minimally invasive anterior approach in hip prosthetic surgery using the AMIS Mobile Leg Positioner

Sergio Candiotto*, Vittore Costa**, Stefano Concheri***, Antonio Camporese*, Jacopo Tagliapietra*, Nelson Ojeda*, Giulio Edoardo Vigni***

*Hip and Shoulder Surgery Unit, Abano Terme General Hospital, Padua, Italy
**Hip and Prosthetic Surgery Unit, Humanitas Gavazzeni Hospital, Bergamo, Italy
***Department of Orthopaedics and Traumatology, S. Antonio Hospital, Padua, Italy
***Department of Orthopaedics and Traumatology, University of Palermo, Italy

Pre-operative clinical assessment of the patient

Before the patient enters the operating theatre, the orthopaedic examination is repeated. The previously performed examination is strictly recorded in the medical record. The assessment is carried out supine, in orthostasis and while walking.
Careful measurement of the degrees of active and passive articulation is the first phase of this examination.
Measurement of the distances between the umbilicus and medial malleoli and the distances between the spina iliaca and lateral malleoli is essential. This is both to know whether or not a dysmetria exists and to detect a pseudo-dysmetria produced by a structured or functional pelvic obliquity.
The knowledge of the actual length of the limb to be operated on will be the fundamental element in the choice of lengths when assembling the prosthesis. This will avoid unpleasant and unwanted lengthening or the risk of implant instability due to shortening.
The assessment of lumbar lordosis, whether or not associated with scoliosis (homologous or heterologous), must be done with care and precision. Assessment of pelvic tilt in the sagittal plane may reveal anteversion or, on the contrary, retroversion. These conditions must be carefully considered during the subsequent placement of the prosthetic cup.
Pelvic tilt in the frontal plane, produced by a concomitant scoliosis, or rotation in the transverse plane are two other fundamental factors that must be recognized and considered in the following steps.

Choice of instrumentation

Our habit of having two surgeons has allowed us to adopt a rapid surgical technique using Hohmann levers, without using special retractors proposed by other authors. These levers are characterised by their width, blunt tip and pronounced curvature.
The instrument set for minimally invasive anterior access necessarily also includes a set of other dedicated instruments. These include bayonet-shaped acetabular reamers and impactors, broach holders that allow the operator to position himself with his back to the patient's feet.
The relatively greater difficulty in approaching the femur compared with other surgical accesses leads us to prefer short prosthetic stems that are easier to introduce. These also tend to spare the bone tissue of the greater trochanter.

Pre-operative planning

This is an important step that must be carried out rigorously, even by the most experienced surgeons. It should be conducted with great accuracy on X-rays of the pelvis and the two hip projections, using the specific templates of the prosthesis to be implanted. The outline of the prosthesis should be drawn on a sheet of glossy paper to be overlaid on the X-ray image, identifying the key landmarks.
The recent introduction of computerisation with the digitalisation of X-rays and the use of some special software facilitate this step. It is now possible to plan directly on the screen of the most modern operating theatres. Pre-operative planning is thus accurate and easy to use.
Another advantage of the correct execution of the planning is that it allows us to limit the number of surgical instruments to be displayed on the scrub table, making interaction with the scrub nurse easy, fast and precise.

Patient preparation

The patient arrives in the operating theatre from the hospital ward. A thorough trichotomy has already been performed, proximal to the transverse umbilical line and distal to the middle third of the leg.
The scrupulous anaesthetic procedures then began, with the application of a peripheral venous catheter, administration of the established drugs and hydration. Following precise instructions from the anaesthetist, the patient is placed in lateral decubitus on the side to be operated on. Preparation of the sterile field precedes anaesthesia, which is performed by spinal injection. The patient is then returned to the supine position for the necessary time. The urinary bladder catheter is applied in accordance with known procedures.
In addition, during this waiting phase, the foot and leg of the side to be operated on are wrapped with some cotton and bandage. This will provide protection to the skeletal structures that will be subjected to traction. Therefore, it is possible to safely use the special 'shoe' to be assembled to the positioning device (AMIS Mobile Leg Positioner) which is then fixed to the operating table (fig. 1).
When authorised by the anaesthetist, the patient is transferred to the operating theatre.

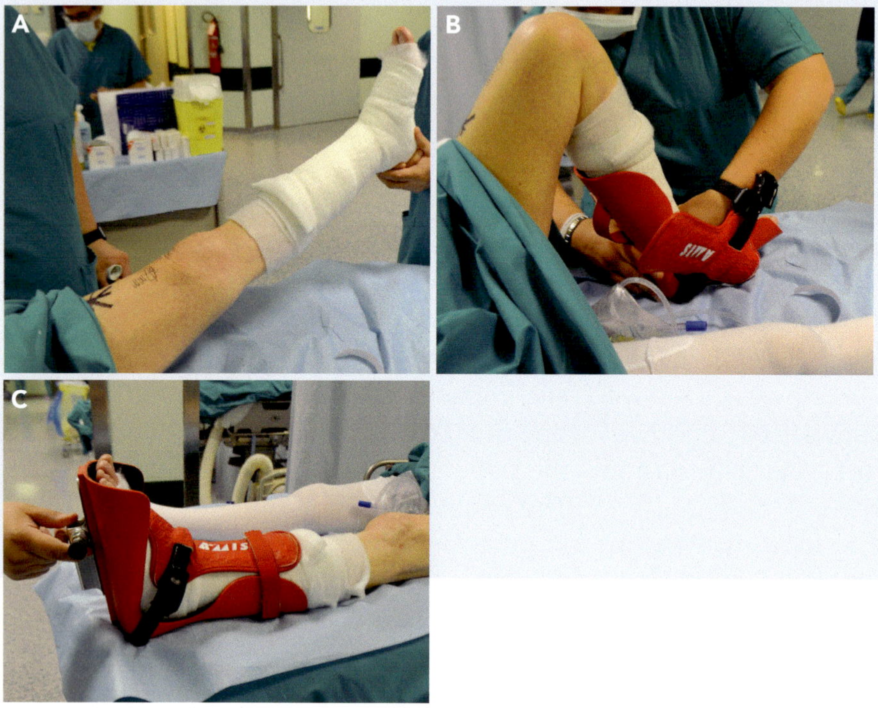

Figure 1 Leg and foot preparation in order to safely apply the 'shoe' that will be attached to the AMIS Mobile Leg Positioner

Positioning on the operating table with the AMIS Mobile Leg Positioner

In our experience, the OPT 80/OPT 100 surgical bed or the Trumpf Jupiter is used.
The patient lies supine on the orthopaedic table with the limb to be prosthetised tied to the leg positioner with the leg positioner shoe. The contralateral limb lies free on a horizontal board, without traction. The ipsilateral upper limb lies adducted and anteriorly placed with the elbow flexed and the forearm placed transversely on the thorax (fig. 2).
The situation of the pelvic-torso segment should be checked. The degree of lumbar lordosis and the inclination of the pelvis must be comparable to those normally maintained in an erect position: this must be taken into account when choosing the inclination and anteversion of the prosthetic cup.
If there is stiffness or flexion contracture of hips or knees, pads and wedges should be applied to bring the pelvis as close as possible to a 'neutral' position. Similarly, and especially in case of spinal deformities or adduction-abduction contractures of the hips, it is necessary to check that the pelvis is in the neutral position in the other planes as well. If necessary, wedges can be used under the gluteus, abducting the contralateral limb and accepting the consensual inclination-rotation of the torso.
The AMIS technique may not facilitate control of the pelvic position during surgery compared to other approaches, such as the lateral approach. In addition, traction of the limb can sometimes change the position of the pelvis, with excessive tilt towards the side to be operated on. This can produce a 'pelvic embalance' (fig. 3), which can lead to pseudo-hypermetria. In other centres, in order to limit these occurrences, it is preferred to immobilize the contralateral limb as well.
The vertical padded cylinder acting as a perineal counterthrust is carefully positioned to

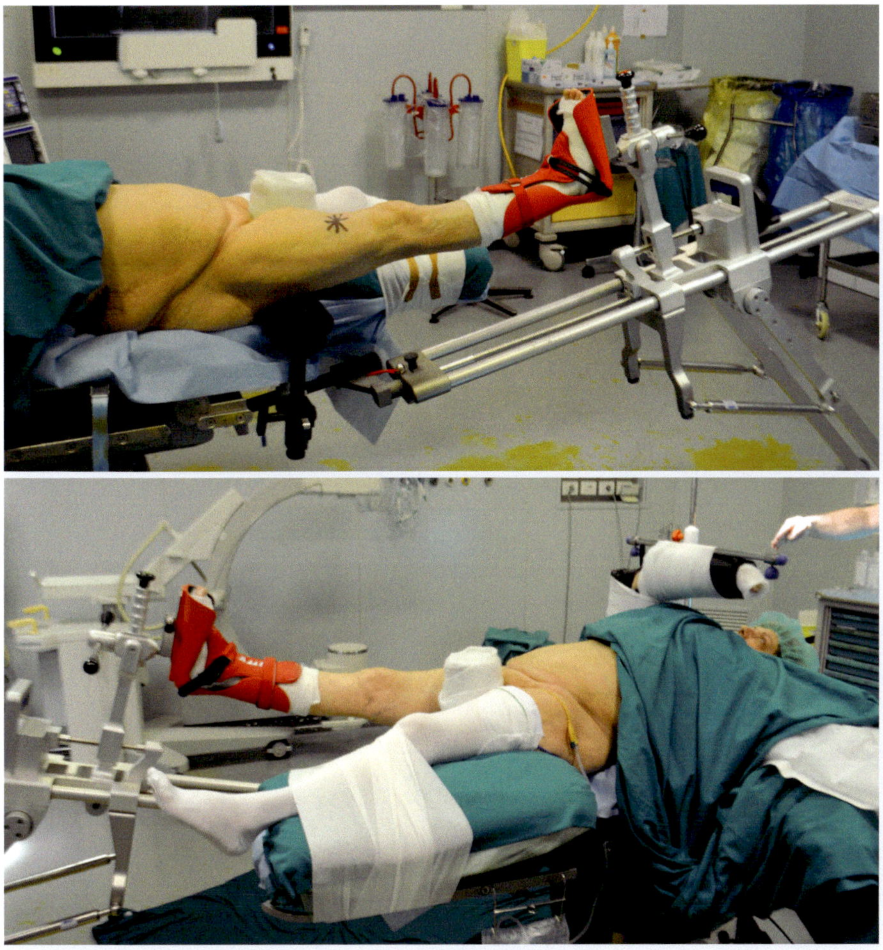

Figure 2
Panoramic photos with AMIS Mobile Leg Positioner

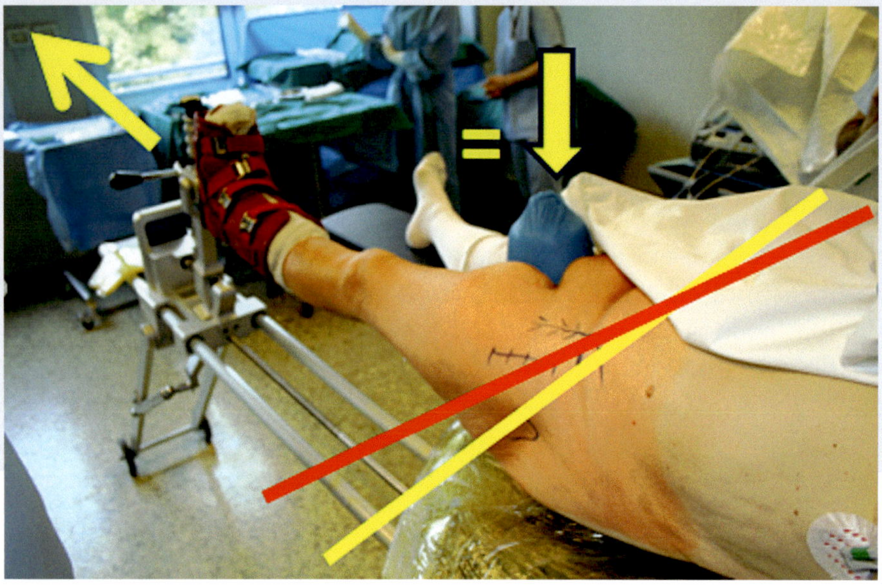

Figure 3 Traction mechanism of the limb to be operated on, which may cause pelvic obliquity in the post-surgical period

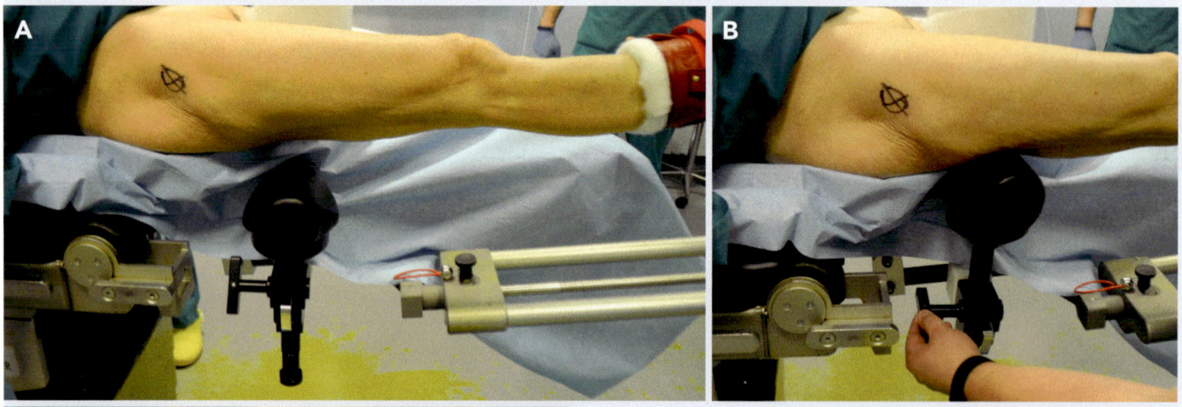

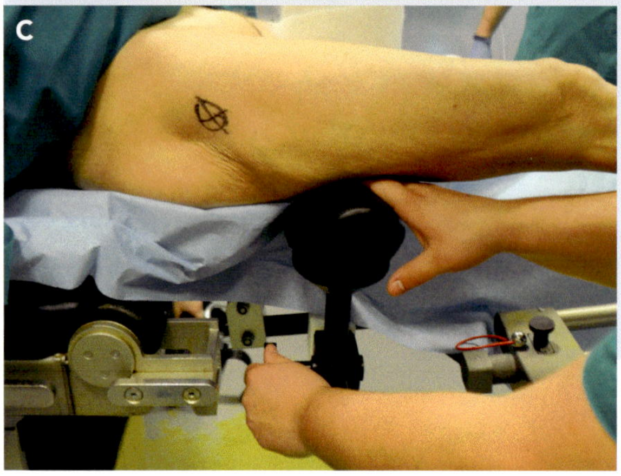

Figure 4 How to apply and check the support, to be placed under the proximal part of the femur. This guarantees a thrust that favours the 'presentation' of the proximal part of the femur in the subsequent phase of the diaphyseal canal preparation and prosthetic implantation

stabilise the pelvis without exerting excessive compression on the genitals.

An appropriately sized support is carefully prepared with cotton and gauze. This is placed posterior to the thigh, close to the femur subtrochanteric section. A sheet of anti-decubitus gel will help to make the femoral fulcrum area more comfortable and secure. A space corresponding to the thickness of a hand's palm must be kept between it and the skin in order to avoid excessive compression when extending the limb. However, a special pad is now available and is capable of exerting an upward push on the femur, without excessive pressure.

During the subsequent extension of the

limb, by lowering it using the leg positioner, this device acts as a fulcrum. It pushes the proximal femur up, making it easily accessible for surgical manoeuvres (fig. 4).
The extension of the limb must necessarily be combined with the longitudinal release of the limb, removing the traction, in order to avoid dangerous traction-compression of the femoral and sciatic nerves.
In our experience we find it useful that the contact area between the thigh and the pressor should not exceed about 10 cm^2. This makes it possible to act only on the femur without raising the lateral soft tissues during the surgery, which would make the surgical approach more difficult.
It is found unsuitable or even dangerous pressors/fulcrums consisting of a long padded cylinder mounted on a metal rod transverse to the thigh.
The surgical phase begins with careful disinfection of the skin and rigorous preparation of the operating field. TNT drapes are applied, with a window for the transparent adhesive film, which well insulates and protects the sterility of the small surgical incision and its possible extensions.
The surgical field must include proximally the area proximal to the iliac crest (at least 5 fingers from the ASIS) and distally reach at least 3 fingers past the tibial tuberosity.
The surgery begins with the limb held by the leg positioner slightly intra-rotated and flexed. This position allows the anterior tissues to be loosened and the femoral neck to be kept in an almost horizontal plane.

Surgical incision

The minimally invasive anterior approach is in fact a modification of the classic approach described by Carl Heuter in 1881.
The interstitium between the sartorius and tensor fascia lata muscles is palpated just distal to the ASIS.
It is useful for this purpose to keep the fingertips perpendicular to the skin plane and exert sufficient pressure to perceive the slight depression between the two muscles. With practice, this depression is almost always perceptible, even in asthenic or obese patients (figs. 5-7).
We make the incision on a line parallel to this

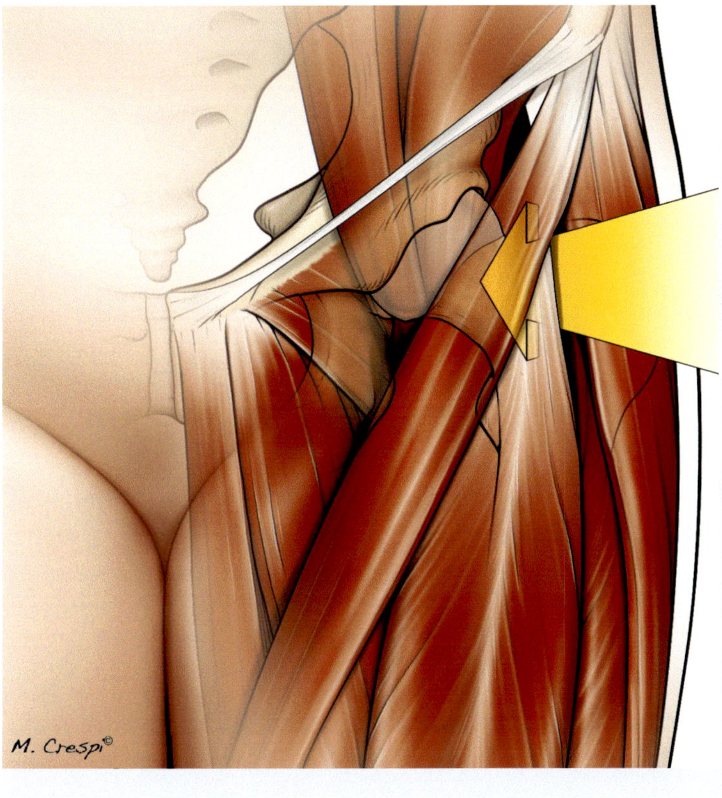

Figure 5 Anatomical and surgical illustration of the direct anterior minimally invasive approach. The space between the sartorius muscle and the tensor fascia lata muscle is shown

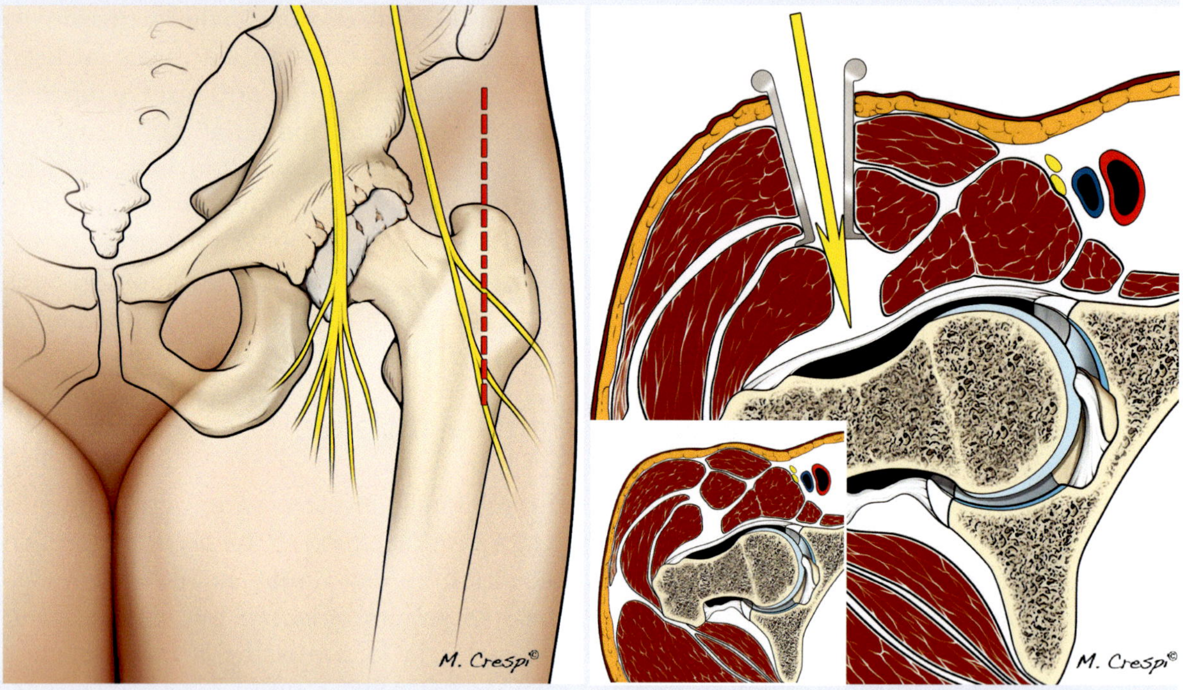

Figure 6 A) Skin incision line (dotted line) and main nerves of the area of interest.
B) Anatomical planes of surgical dissection

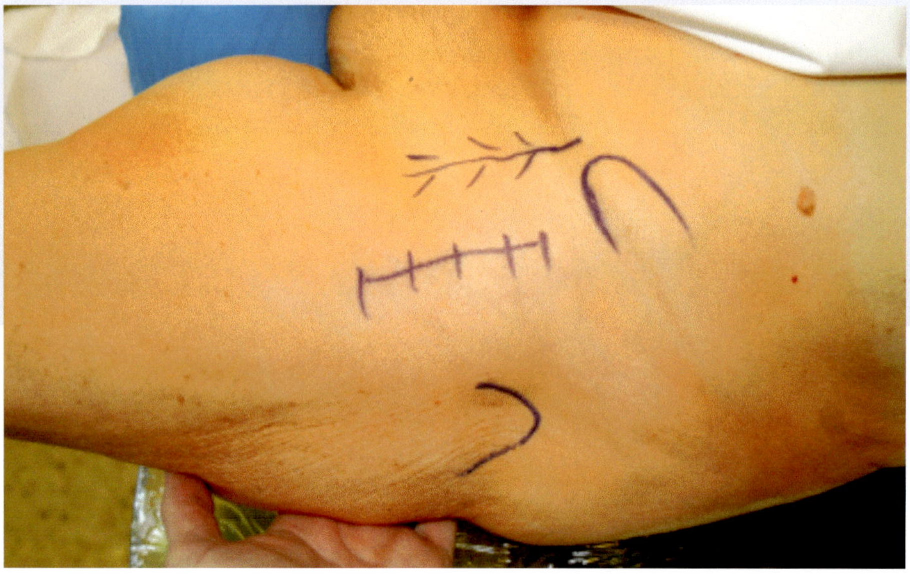

Figure 7
Drawing of landmarks, useful for identifying the exact line of the skin incision

palpable depression, staying about 3-4 cm lateral to it and pointing towards the outer margin of the patella. In practice, this corresponds in depth to the most medial portion of the tensor fascia lata. This avoids injury to the main trunk of the lateral femoral cutaneous nerve of the thigh or its lateral branches. The incision starts at approximately 2 transverse fingers inferior and lateral to the ASIS and extends distally for a variable length of 5-8 cm, depending on the experience of the surgeon and the size of the patient (figs. 8-9).

Particular caution must be taken at this stage to avoid injury to the lateral femoral cutaneous nerve (figs. 10-11).

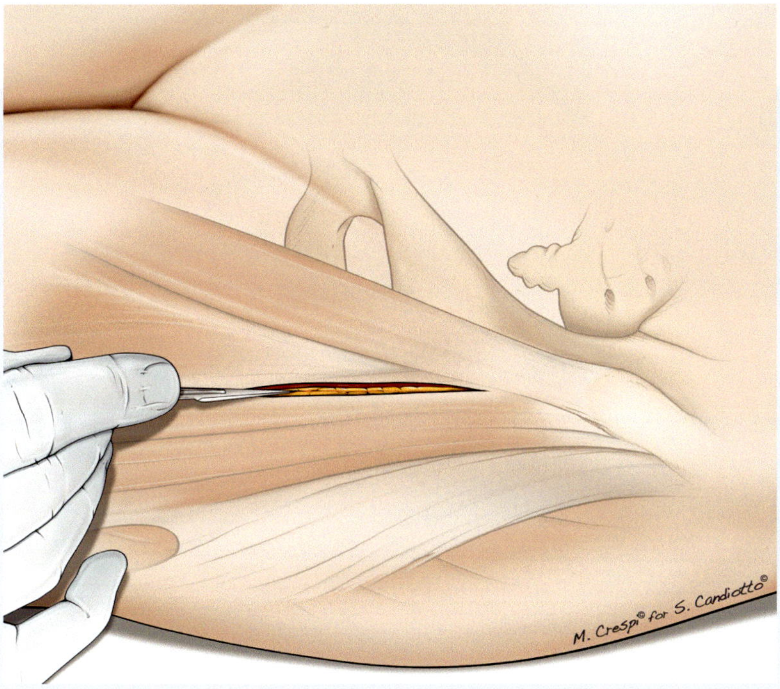

Figure 8
Skin incision

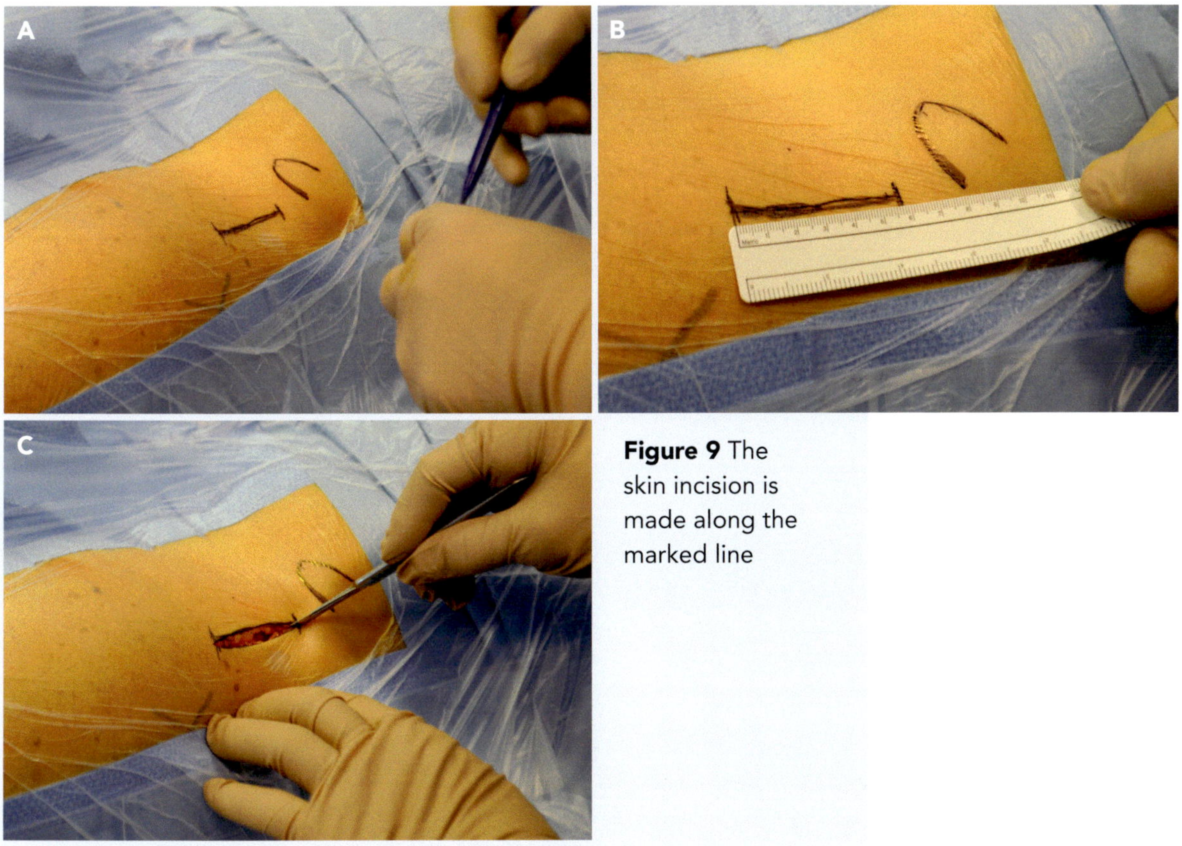

Figure 9 The skin incision is made along the marked line

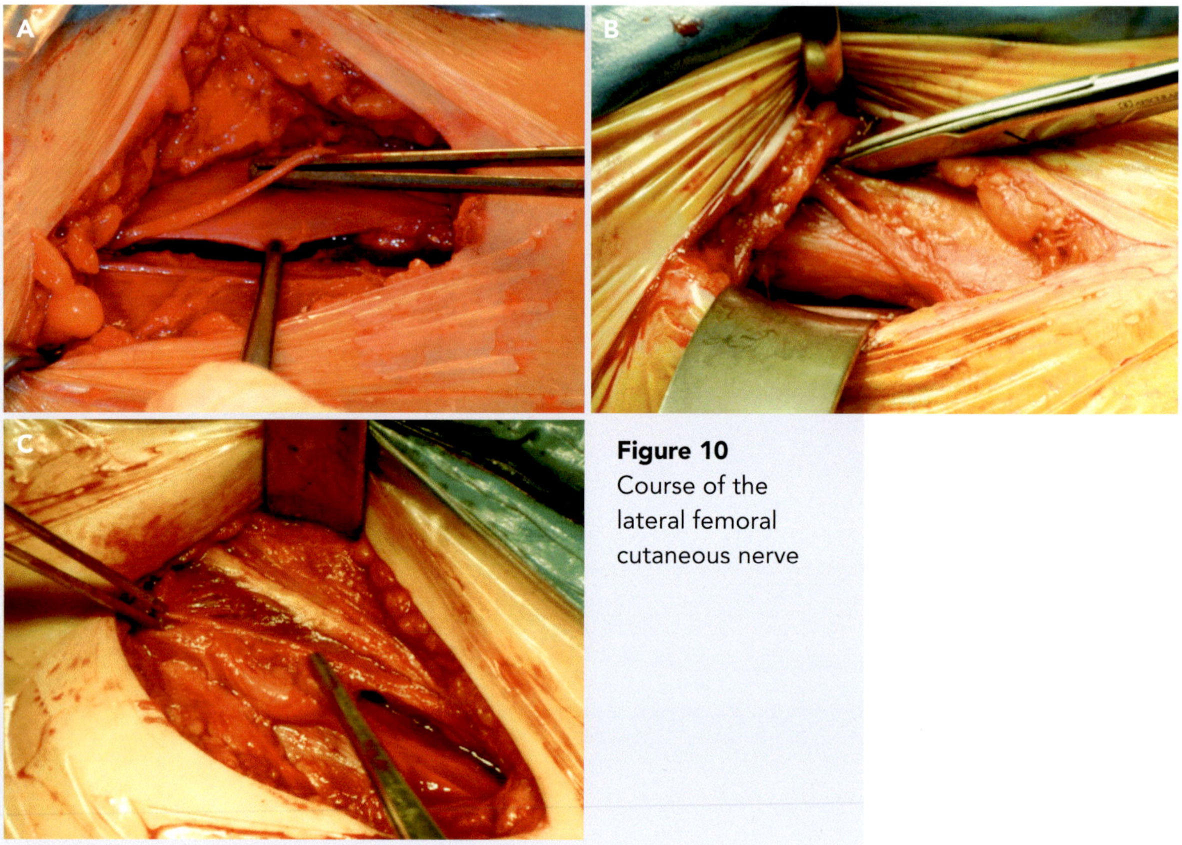

Figure 10
Course of the lateral femoral cutaneous nerve

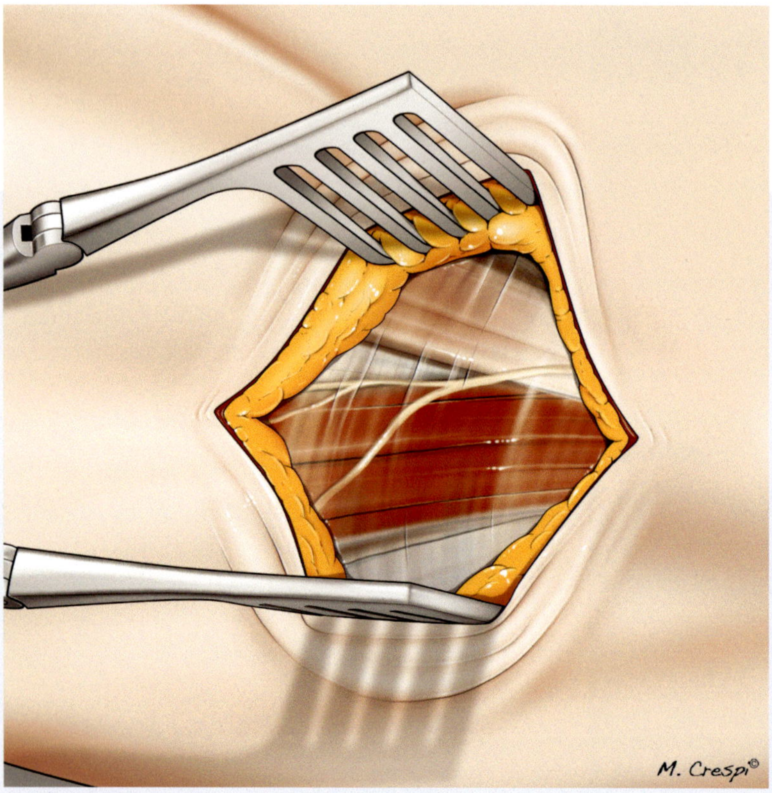

Figure 11
Subfascial layer of the lateral femoral-cutaneous nerve

Deep dissection

After the dissection of the subcutis, with an electric scalpel or blade, while performing an accurate haemostasis, the fascial plane is reached. Immediate identification in transparency of the muscular belly of the tensor fascia lata (TFL). Its fibres characteristically have a distal and lateral direction, unlike those of the sartorius muscle belly, which has instead direct distal and medial fibres.
To access the muscular plane, a small perforation of the fascia must be made with a scalpel. This should then be extended one centimetre beyond the skin incision proximally and distally to avoid compression of the TFL muscle and its ischaemia during hip hyperextension manoeuvres for femoral preparation.
The TFL muscle is then gently detached from its fascia. After identifying the interval between the TFL and the sartorius, this space is accessed directly or by incision of the thin aponeurotic fascia covering the medial margin of the TFL muscle belly. This avoids penetrating the sartorius fascia and prevents injury to the lateral cutaneous femoral nerve (fig. 12).
Spreading the two muscles with retractors, a plane appears at the bottom covered by the homonymous fascia of the rectus femoris. This, if described from medial to lateral according to a colour code, identifies a white, a red and a yellow zone. These respectively represent the aponeurosis of the rectus femoris, its muscular belly and the fat covering the joint capsule. Incising this band on the muscular margin at the border of the yellow area exposes this muscle which is then displaced medially.
The bottom of the surgical field is now covered by the underlying deep fascia ('innominate'). This is then carefully incised longitudinally so as not to injure the underlying circumflex vessels. Then the pericapsular fat is exposed, and this hides the circumflex vascular bundle.
Moving into the most proximal part of the approach, the depression between the insertion of the gluteus minimus and the lat-

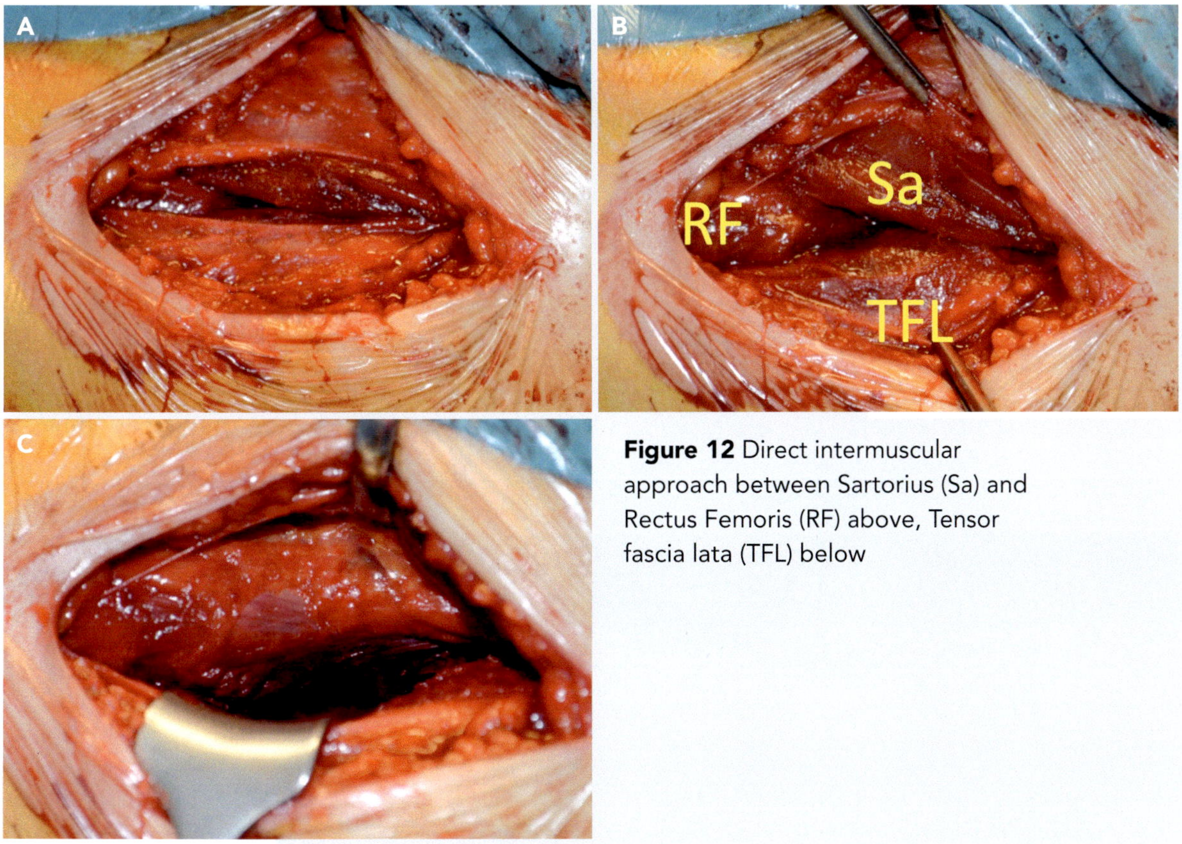

Figure 12 Direct intermuscular approach between Sartorius (Sa) and Rectus Femoris (RF) above, Tensor fascia lata (TFL) below

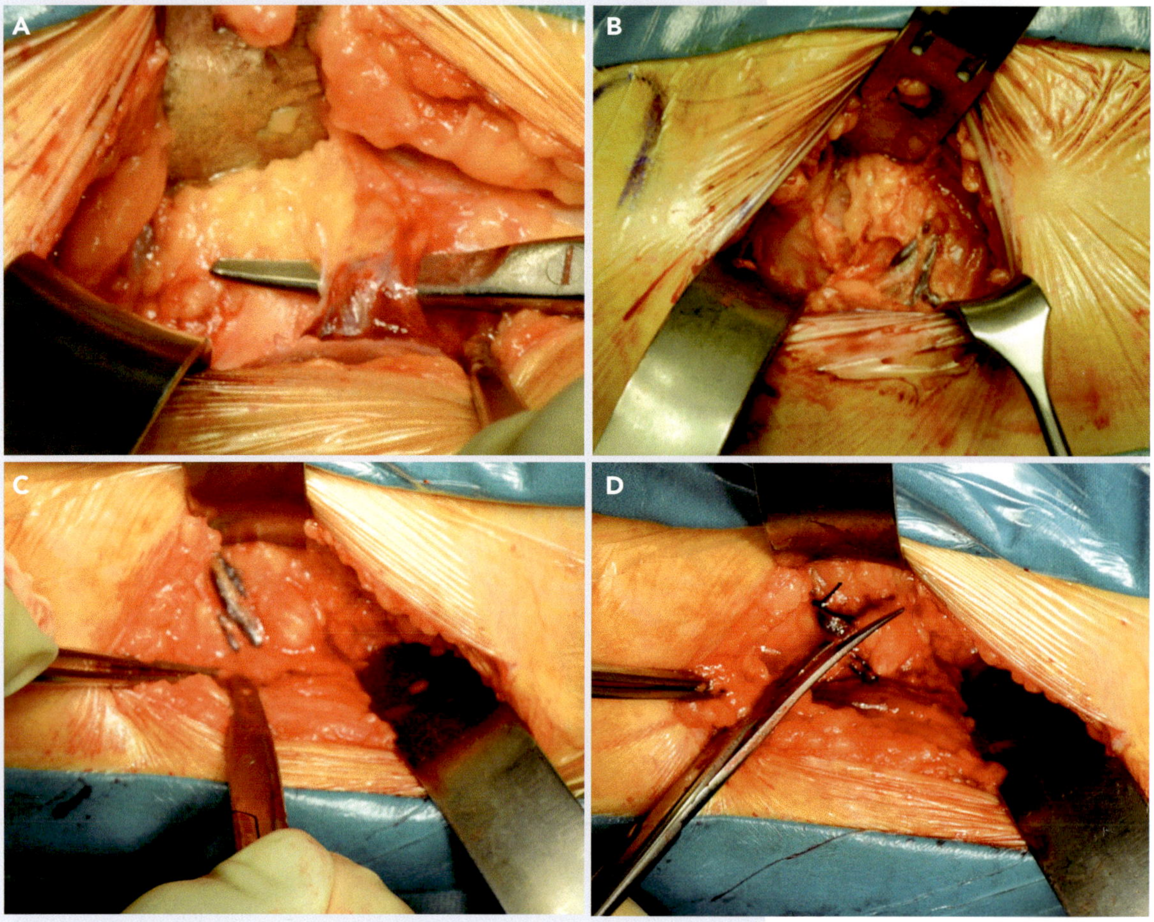

Figure 13 Identification and ligation of vessels (ascending anterior circumflex artery)

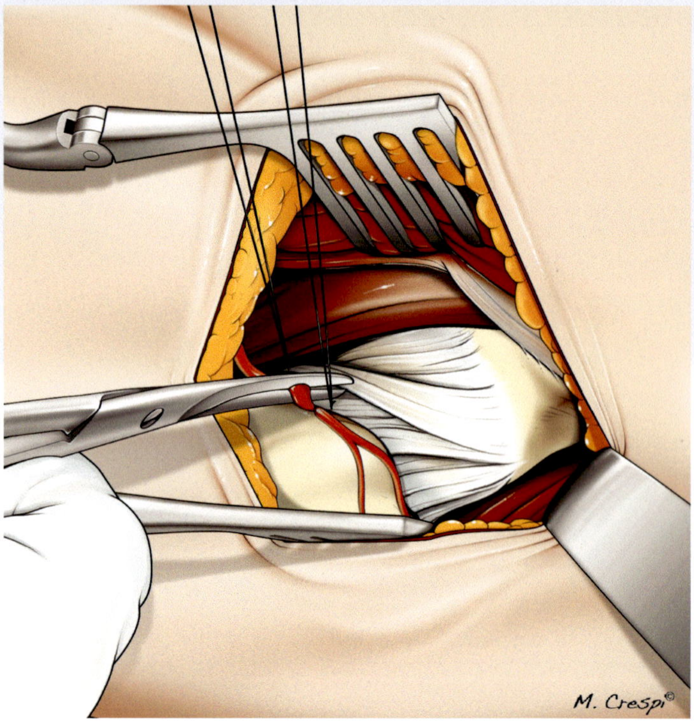

Figure 14 Ligation of vessels

eral portion of the capsule is identified by palpation. This corresponds to the lateral margin of the femoral neck where it joins the greater trochanter. A first Hohmann lever with a narrow tip is introduced there.

At this stage with a periosteal elevator or with the cautious use of another blunt instrument the surgeon tries to reach the medial margin of the joint capsule, proximally to the lesser trochanter. At this point a second Hohmann with blunt tip is gently placed and held by the assistant on the opposite side of the patient, facing the surgeon.

In order to locate the ascending branches of the lateral circumflex artery, the vascular bundle crossing the femur anteriorly in the distal half of our surgical field, it is useful to place the Hohmann lever under the tensor, just lateral to the great trochanter. By gently stretching this lever, the circumflex vessels become easily recognisable. They are carefully isolated and ligated with a suture and then dissected. Careful ligation of these vessels is absolutely necessary because post-operative bleeding at this level can produce large haematomas (figs. 13-14).

Capsulotomy

The Hohmann on the outside of the greater trochanter can now be removed and repositioned lateral to the femoral neck. Then the capsulotomy is performed along the axis of the femoral neck, delimited by the two Hohmann retractors.

This phase must always be associated with careful haemostasis of the blood vessels. We believe it is more advantageous and quicker to perform a wide excision of the anterior capsule from the cup margin to the intertrochanteric line, instead of operating with capsule sparing and performing the capsular flap (fig. 15).

After the partial section of the indirect bundle of the rectus femoris tendon and the eventual detachment of the iliopsoas muscle from the anteromedial capsule, a third Hohmann lever with a thin tip can be inserted. This can be inserted below the ASIS on the antero-superior border of the cup (at '11 o'clock' for the right hip, at '13 o'clock' for the left). This must be handled delicately due to the reduced bone strength in this area. Malpositioning or exces-

Figure 15 Exposure of the neck and femoral head after capsulotomy

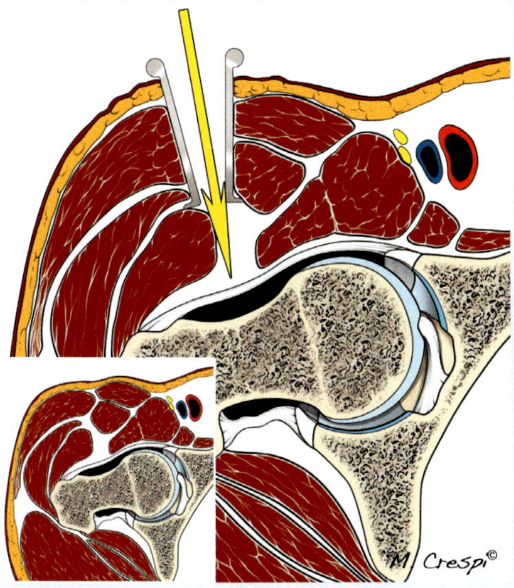

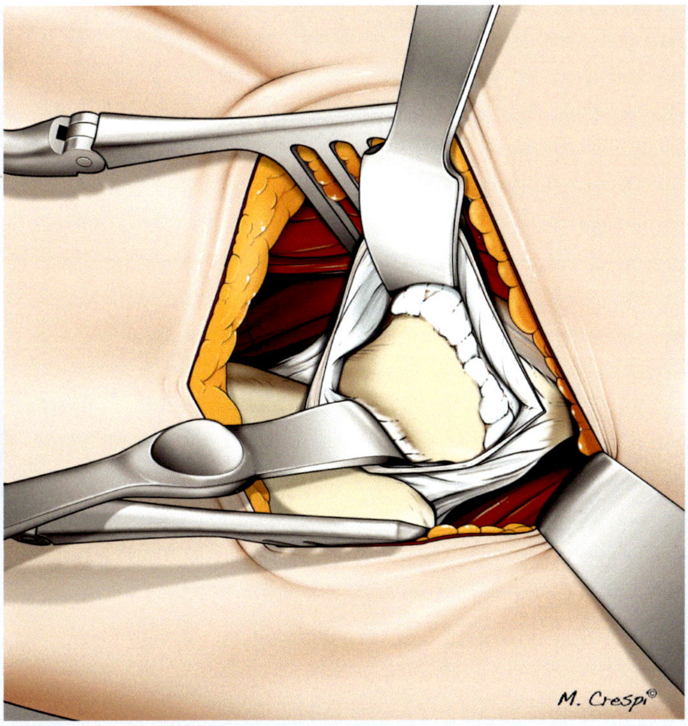

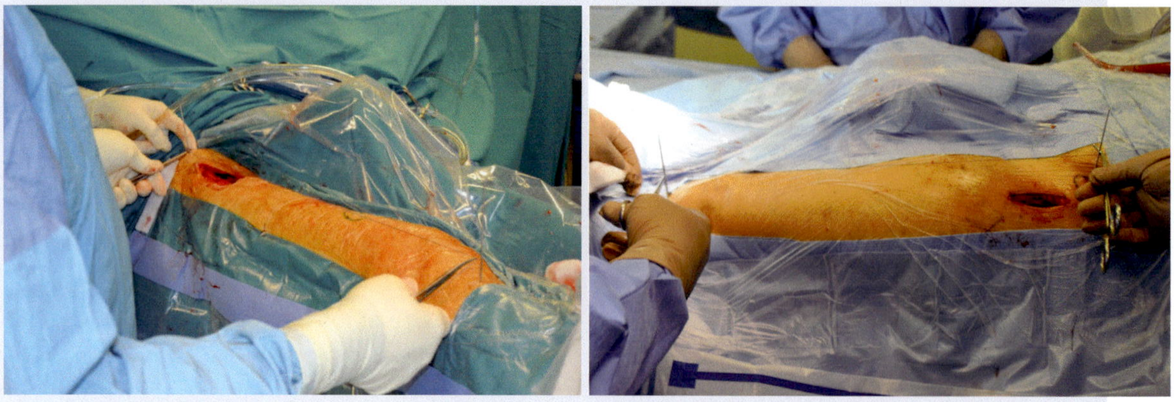

Figure 16 Checking the distance between the Kirschner wires implanted on the iliac crest and tibial tuberosity, before resecting the femoral neck. The same distance measured after implantation of the trial components will provide useful indications of limb metrics

sive traction on this retractor can damage the femur neurovascular bundle.
The visualisation of the capsule now appears optimal. After the anterior capsulectomy, the femoral neck is clearly visible. The most medial Hohmann is repositioned inside the capsule, between it and the medial side of the femoral neck. The Hohmann lever on the anterior margin of the cup is left in place. A third Hohmann with a thin tip can be placed behind the femoral neck to protect the gluteal muscles and the branches of the posterior circumflex artery. We can then proceed with the osteotomy of the femoral neck. Prior to this, however, we try to assess the existing length of the limb, which should be related to the length to be achieved at the end of the procedure (fig. 16).
It has been adopted a method for intraoperative limb length control. This involves the insertion, prior to the femoral neck osteotomy, of two fixed grips: a Kirschner wire is introduced into the ASIS and one into the anterior tibial tuberosity. A large diameter suture is placed between the two landmarks and the length is recorded by applying two Kochers. This will allow monitoring of limb length changes during surgery. Measurement of limb length is carried out before femoral neck resection and head removal. The measurement obtained will then be compared with the final measurement taken with the trial prosthesis in place.
It is also necessary for the AMIS Mobile Leg Positioner operator to accurately note the initial position of the system and then return the limb to the same position during subsequent measurements. This is because it is clear that even a small increase or decrease in hip flexion can change the distance between the landmarks.

Femoral neck osteotomy

To facilitate the osteotomy the limb can be placed in slight internal rotation so that the femoral neck lies in a horizontal plane. The Hohmann levers are positioned as described above. The correct osteotomy site is identified. This corresponds laterally to the junction between the neck and trochanter and medially is conducted with the inclination relative to the diaphyseal axis established in the planning phase.
The osteotomy is carried out with an oscillating saw in a vertical position (or in any case perpendicular to the major axis of the neck). A slight traction and extrotation of the limb open the osteotomy gap, which can be completed with an osteotome if necessary. To facilitate the extraction of the head, we usually perform a second osteotomy proximal to the first one. In this way it is possible to remove a bone cylinder of a thickness of approximately 6-10 mm ('Wafer technique') (figs. 17-18).
The femoral head thus appears more easily

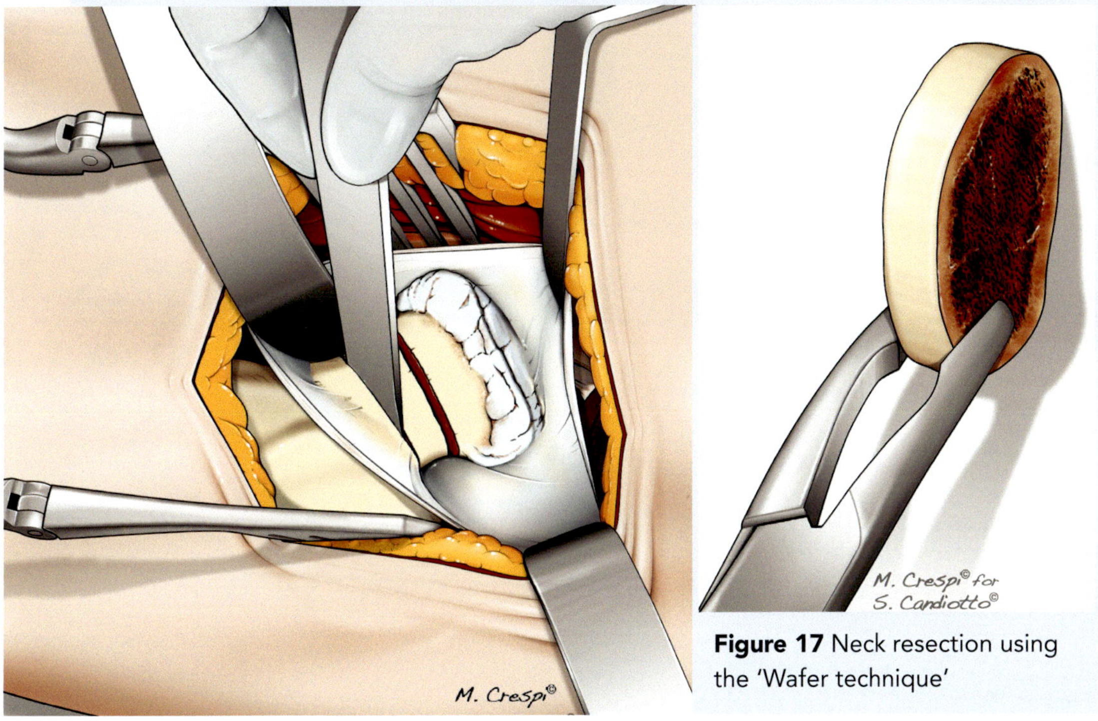

Figure 17 Neck resection using the 'Wafer technique'

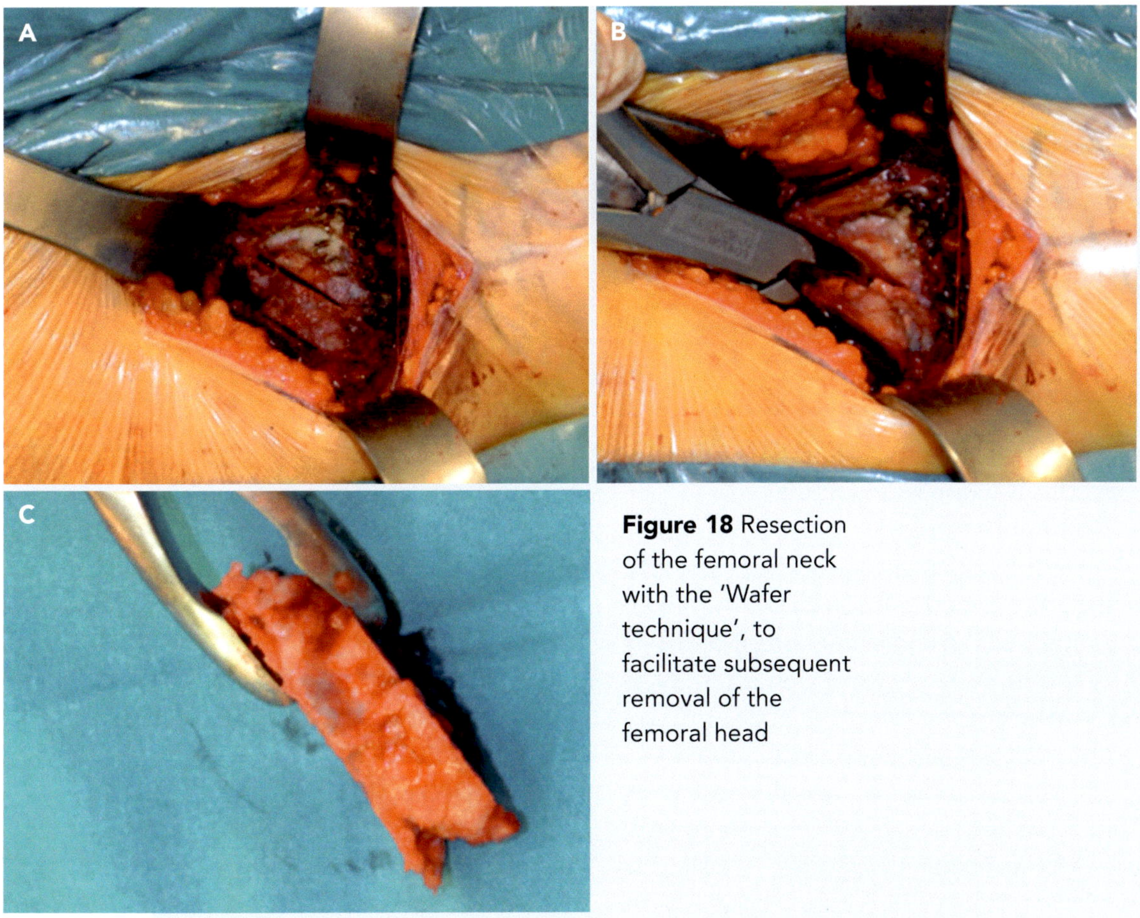

Figure 18 Resection of the femoral neck with the 'Wafer technique', to facilitate subsequent removal of the femoral head

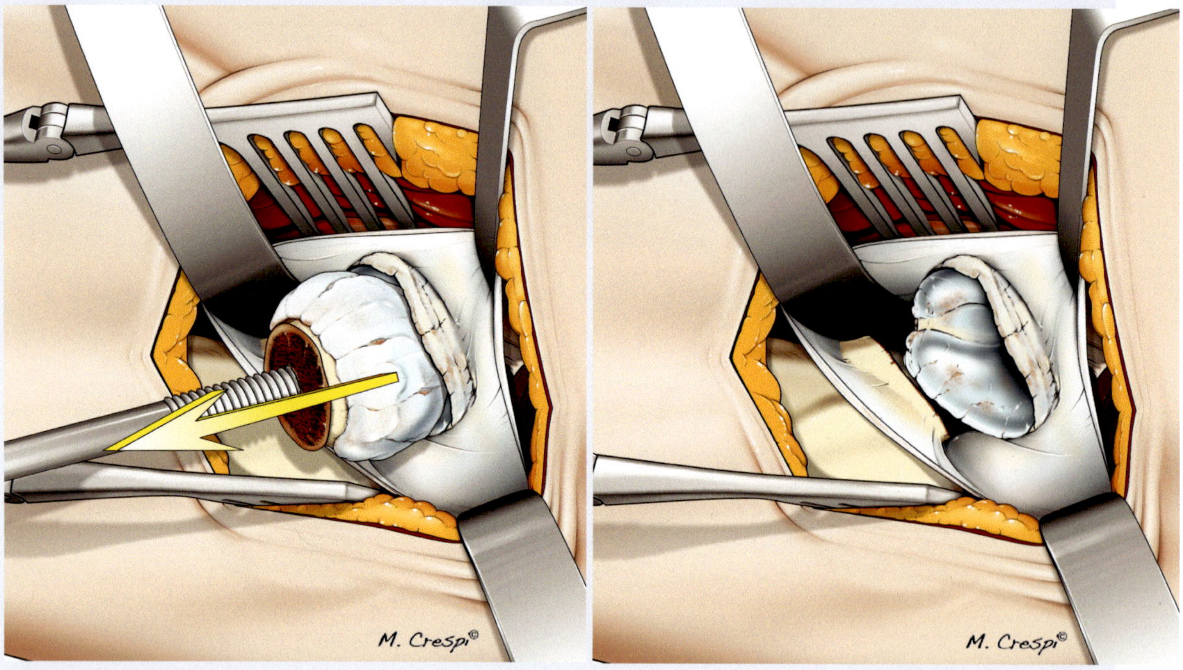

Figure 19 Excision of the femoral head

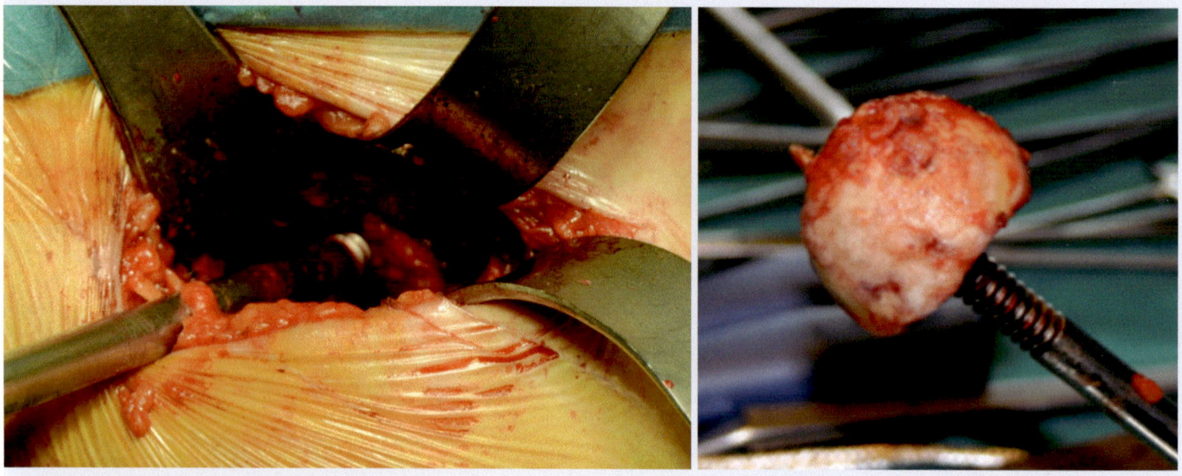

Figure 20 Excision of the femoral head

removable with the appropriate device (figs. 19-20). The traction is now released.

The Hohmann retractor, placed medial to the femoral neck, is extracted from the capsule and introduced cautiously by blunt force into contact with the medial cortex of the femur just distal to the lesser trochanter. By externally rotating the femur at approximately 90°, the capsule is placed under tension in its pubofemoral portion, which can be detached from the calcar with the electrocautery until the lesser trochanter is palpable. This is an important landmark to verify the correct plane of the osteotomy. If it is necessary to perform the osteotomy again it is advisable to put back the femur to the neutral position and then reposition the Hohmann retractors accordingly.

Preparation of the acetabular cup and application of the prosthetic cup

The femur is externally rotated at 45° and the hip slightly flexed by just lifting the leg

positioner. Slight traction to pull the femur more distally may also be useful. This leaves perfectly clear access to the acetabular cavity, and aligns the plane of the femoral osteotomy with the distal edge of the cup.
Other methods, which involve keeping the hip in greater flexion during cup preparation, can be used with neck-sparing femoral prosthesis. This would place the neck posterior to the cup margin.
A blunt Hohmann retractor is now placed on the posteroinferior edge of the cup (at '8 o'clock' for the right hip). A second Hohmann is placed on the anteroinferior edge of the cup, near the fossa and outside the transverse ligament (at '5 o'clock' for the right hip). The third, thin-tipped Hohmann remains cautiously positioned on the anterosuperior acetabular rim. With surgical experience, however, this third retractor can be omitted.
The position of the Hohmann retractors allows ideal exposure of the acetabular cavity. This makes it easy to remove the fibrous labrum and possible osteophytes and to prepare the cup with the dedicated hemispherical burs with increasing diameter. These are mounted on a special 'bayonet' handpiece with offset.
The shape of the acetabular reamer helps to avoid contact with the femur which, acting as a fulcrum, could alter reaming and cause ovalisation or unwanted changes in cup inclination. It is recommended to go appropriately deep with reaming. We mention this because in the early stages of the learning curve excessive caution is often observed. It is also recommended to be very careful not to exceed the anteversion and verticalization of the prosthetic cup. To avoid this error, the floor of the operating theatre should be taken as a reference plane and our degree of version can be measured using it. While orientation in the frontal plane and therefore the horizontal/vertical position is always calculated with the axis of the lower limb. However, the transverse ligament of the acetabulum must always be taken into account. This will serve as a guide to check the orientation of the prosthetic cup (figs. 21-22).

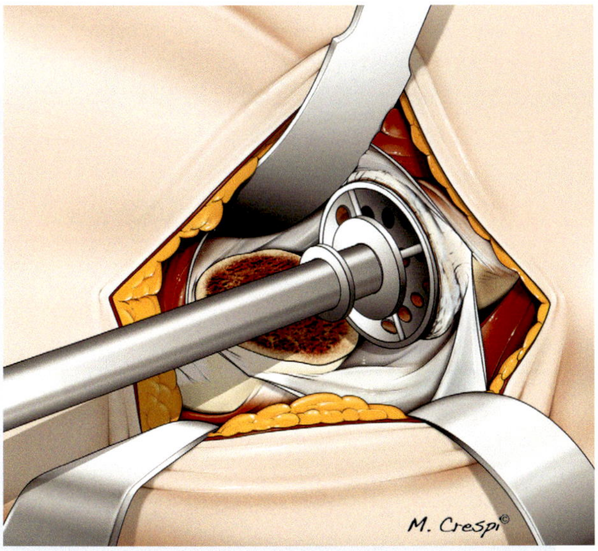

Figure 21 Drilling of the acetabular floor to prepare for the prosthetic cup

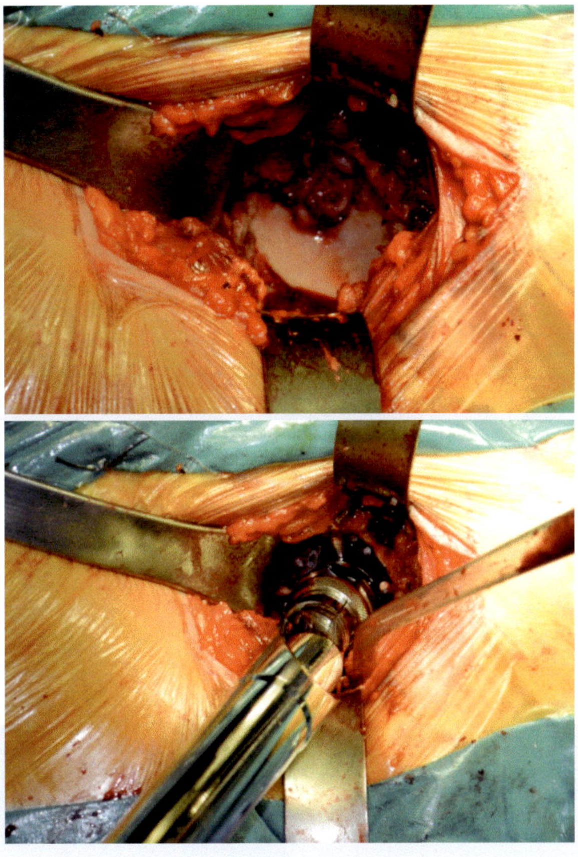

Figure 22 Adequate exposure of the cup and preparation of the acetabular floor with the acetabular burs

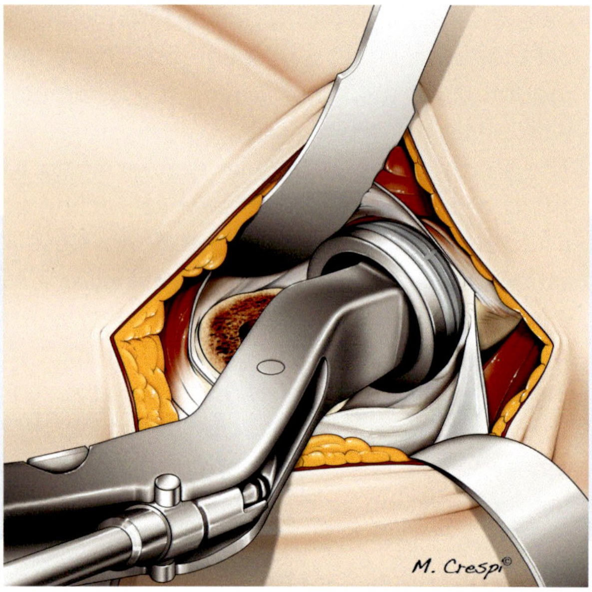

Figure 23
Application of press-fit prosthetic cup

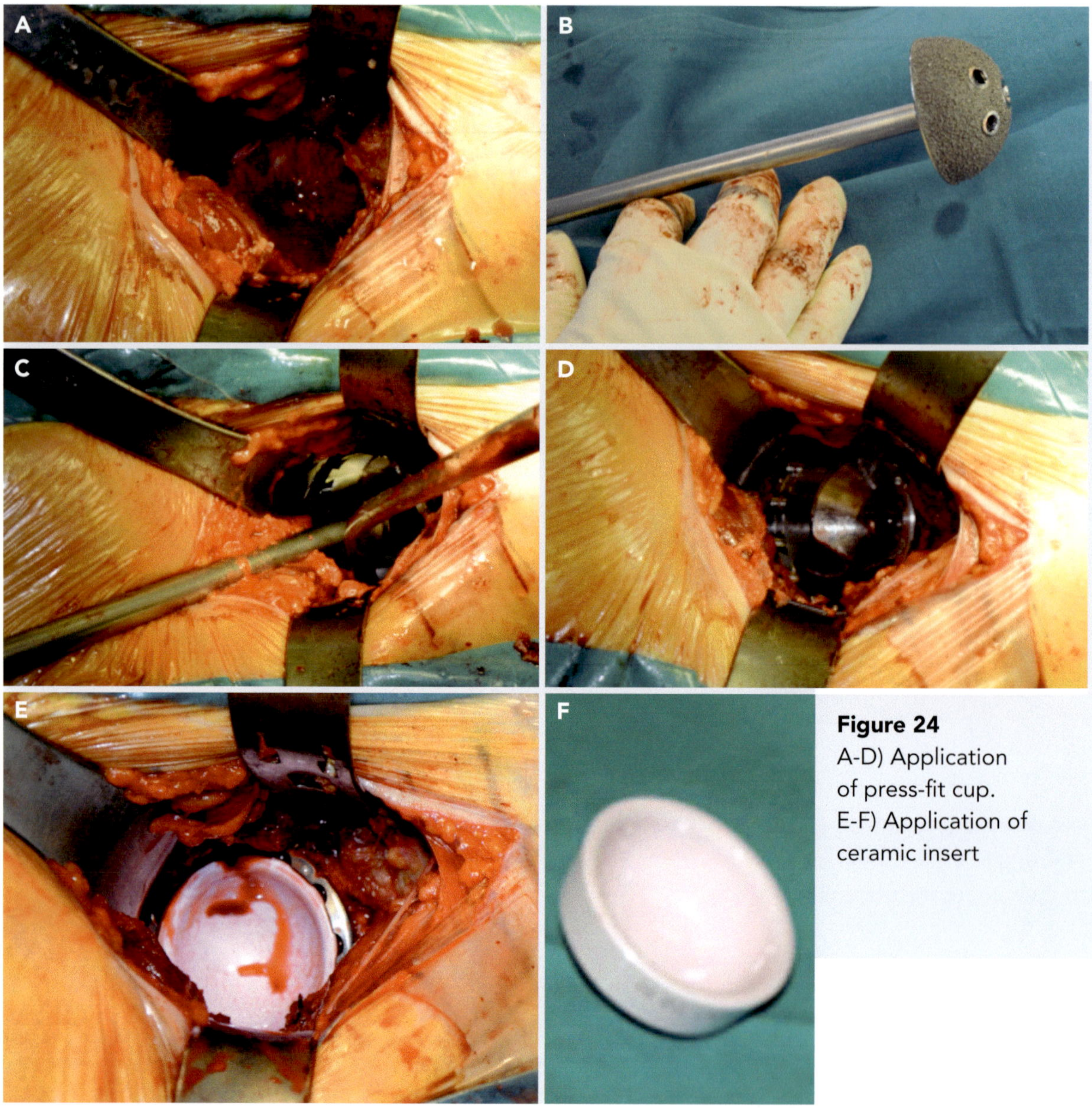

Figure 24
A-D) Application of press-fit cup.
E-F) Application of ceramic insert

It is preferred to use a traditionally shaped hemispherical cup with a very wrinkled bone anchoring surface. We usually use ceramic-ceramic bearings (figs. 23-24).

Capsular release and 'presentation' of the femur

Our experience with minimally invasive anterior access began before the availability of limb extension aids such as the AMIS Mobile Leg Positioner. The femoral surgical phase has always represented the most difficult step of the operation, especially in patients with pronounced femoral varus and great muscle mass.
The AMIS Mobile Leg Positioner therefore seemed to us to be able to simplify accessibility to the femur, with a considerable decrease in the risks of iatrogenic fracture, malpositioning of the stem in varus and nerve damage to the femoral nerve.
In fact, this device allows to align the femur with the small surgical incision, by lowering and externally rotating the limb. Furthermore, thanks to the action of the posterior fulcrum, constituted by the presser described above and adequately set up under the thigh, a variable degree of upward thrust of the proximal femur is obtained ('push up' effect).
However, this effect on the femur requires a release of the capsule. Without this release, the extra-rotation of the femur tightens it posteriorly on the cup, where the greater trochanter tends to lock during extension.
The difficulty of this 'presentation' of the femur, which is especially required when using longer stems, has been considerably reduced since we gave preference to shorter stems. With these it was possible to significantly reduce the degree of lowering of the limb and anteposition of the proximal femur required during femoral time.
At this point the moderate traction on the limb is removed. The Hohmann retractors are removed from the cup. The limb is placed in an external rotation of approximately 90° and the Hohmann is placed medial to the femur, immediately distal to the small trochanter. This retractor is used to assess that the detachment of the capsule at the level of the calcar is adequate (interruption of the pubofemoral ligamentous component).
The limb is now placed in neutral rotation and the femur is pulled laterally with a hook. This makes it easier to highlight the iliofemoral and ischiofemoral capsular components, which often counteract this trans-

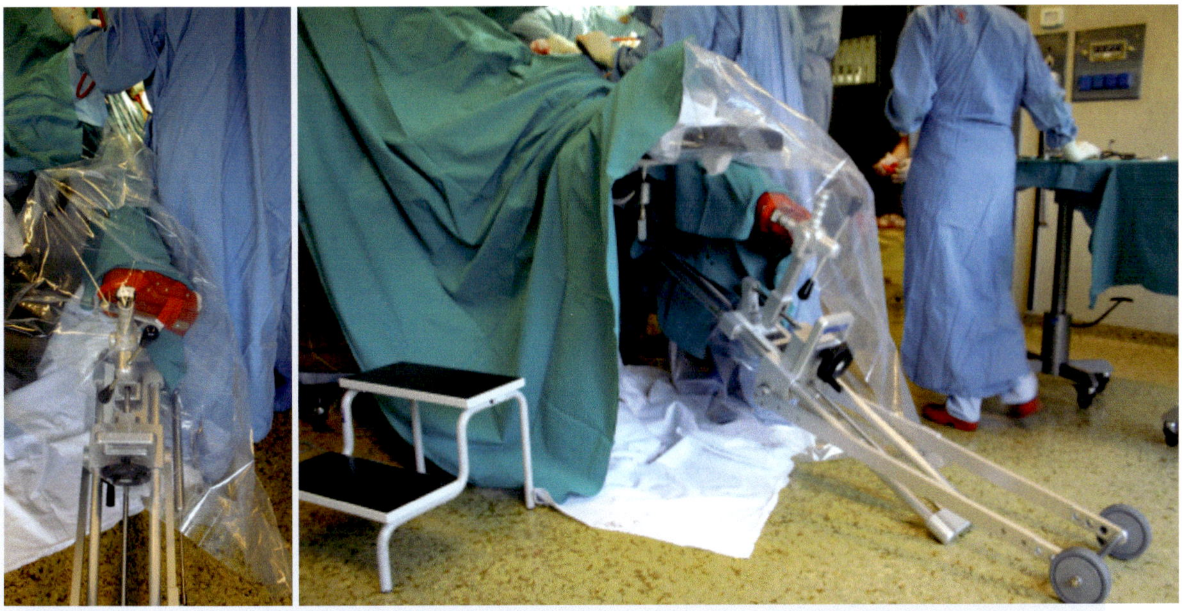

Figure 25 Position in full extension and external rotation of the limb during diaphyseal canal preparation and subsequent implantation of the prosthetic stem

lation. They should cautiously be dissected close to the femur and superficial use of the electrocauter, following the supero-medial profile of the great trochanter for 1-2 cm.
If the release is considered adequate, the external rotation and extension manoeuvre of the limb is now tried. The limb is forced into external rotation with the toes pointing towards the floor (fig. 25).
This rotation must be carried out by the surgeon or an assistant, acting on the knee and avoiding sole rotation of the foot through the boot. This is to minimise the risk of fractures or capsuloligamentous injury to the knee. The limb is now lowered to an intermediate level. At the same time, acting with a hook on the calcar, the surgeon tries to pull the femur laterally and anteriorly with gentle movements.
It should be possible to bring the greater trochanter over the posterior margin of the cup and anteriorly.
In case of some difficulties during this manoeuvre, the capsular release procedure should be repeated from the beginning before extending the hip to its maximum. With the almost complete lowering of the limb, necessary in relation to the type of femoral stem chosen, the anteposition of the femur is observed. This emerges more superficially in the surgical field, with the osteotomy plane tending to lie in the horizontal plane.
It should be noted, however, that in patients with particular morpho-functional conditions (marked joint stiffness, cervical-diaphyseal varus, short femoral neck, deep coxa, etc.), it may not always be possible to achieve the desired capsular release and consequently a lesser degree of femoral anteposition and 'presentation' may occur. It should be noted that the AMIS Mobile Leg Positioner incorporates a device that automatically and instantaneously releases traction during lowering (extension) of the limb to prevent stretching of the femoral and sciatic nerves.
In cases of particular stiffness, the anaesthetist may be asked to convert spinal anaesthesia to general anaesthesia to achieve the appropriate level of muscle relaxation and allow the procedure to proceed smoothly.

Femoral preparation and stem application

A Hohmann retractor with blunt tip is placed medially to the calcar and is held by the assistant on the opposite side of the patient. It should be used with caution and alternately released to avoid prolonged tension on the femoral vascular nerve bundle. A second fine-tipped Hohmann is placed supero-laterally to the apex of the greater trochanter to retract the tissues that are obstructing the introduction of the rasps. It also avoids contact of the rasps and the prosthesis with the skin. It can also help anterior translation of the femur. In order to optimise the central position of the femur in the operating field, it may be necessary to increase or decrease the degree of rotation of the limb and abduct it using the AMIS Mobile Leg Positioner. The surgeon is now facing the head of the patient and will perform the whole femoral step in this position trying also to push the limb in forced adduction. First, a 'banana' (or 'channel finder') rasp is used and introduced into the femur close to the calcar (figs. 26-27). Proceeding with a gentle oscillatory action of the rasp handle to find the canal. In this way the tip of the rasp remains in contact with the medial femoral cortex, which is now, given the extra-rotation of the limb in an anterior position. If necessary, careful percussion of the rasp handle can be applied, but only if at least half of it has entered the femoral canal.
We then proceed with broaches of increasing size, taking care to avoid excessive anteversion: it is useful to keep them parallel to the posterior margin of the osteotomy of the femoral neck (which in the surgical field now is located medially) (figs. 28-29).
The preparation of the femoral canal exposes the patient to the risk of fracture of the calcar in the insertion phase or of the greater trochanter in the extraction phase. To avoid this, it is recommended to push the handle of the broach posteriorly during insertion, so as to move it away from the calcar. On the other hand, during the extraction phase, it is recommended to pull the handle towards

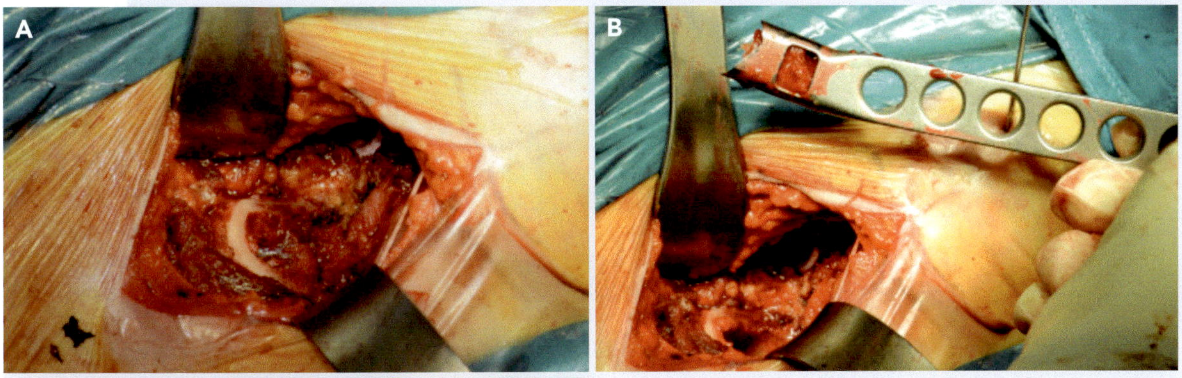

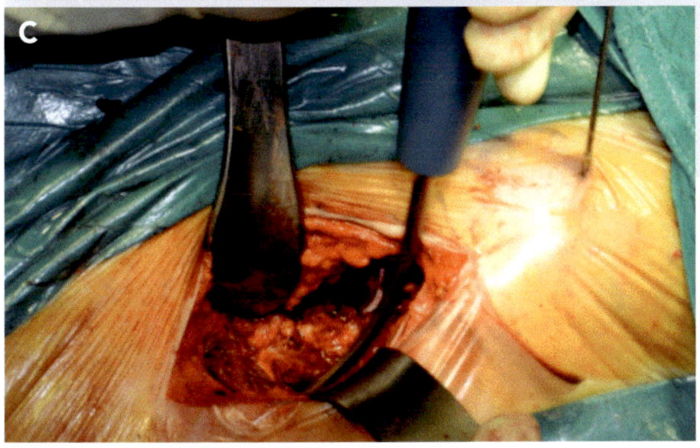

Figure 26 Exposure of the femoral neck, which is opened with the specific 'box' osteotome and curved spoon

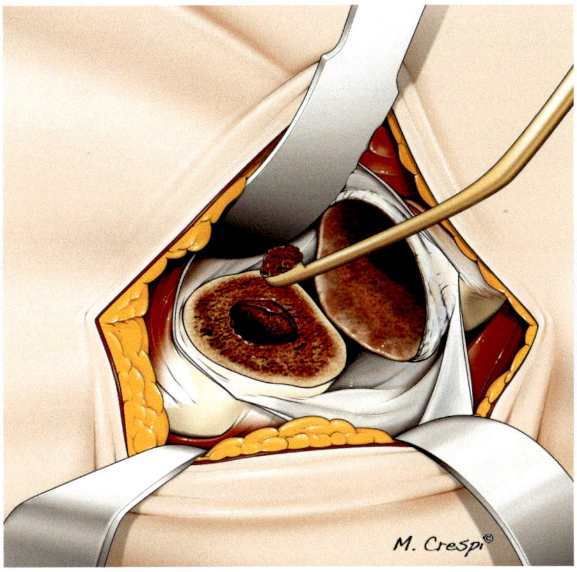

Figure 27
The diaphyseal canal is explored with the curved spoon

yourself to move the broach away from the greater trochanter. The broach should drop down until the thread/signal disappears into the channel trying to align the end of the thread with the calcar.

The sensation of correct 'fit and fill' occurs when the noise from the percussive action on the broach changes. At this point the stability, especially rotational stability, of the broach is checked.

In the presence of femoral varus it is found useful to remove a small amount of bone tissue with a spoon or Luer from the inside of the greater trochanter to prevent varus positioning of the stem.

With the last rasp used and the insertion of a temporary head we then perform the reduction. This is achieved by raising the limb to its initial level, releasing the external rotation, applying moderate traction to the limb and rotating it internally. At the same time the head is pushed into the cup with a presser. The sensation of an easy or difficult reduction is assessed, remembering that difficulty is always an indication of probable lengthening.

Checking that the limb is in the same position as noted before the osteotomy, the distance between the two previously applied Kirschner wires is checked. In our experience it is usually considered adding about 2-3 mm to this measurement to approximate the real change in length of the limb. This is because the distance between the landmarks can eas-

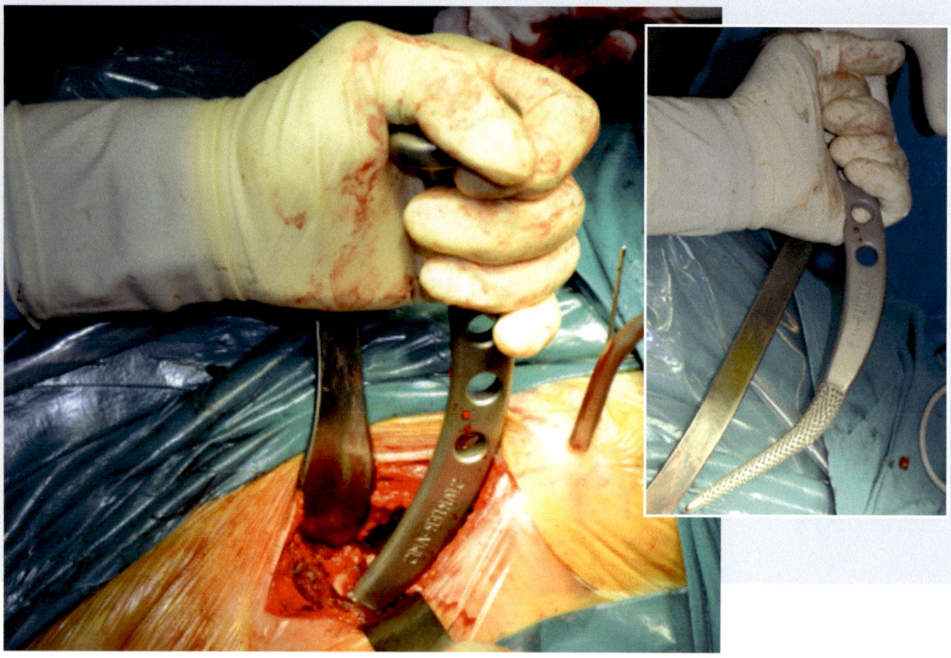

Figure 28 Further preparation of the diaphyseal canal with the curved 'banana' rasp

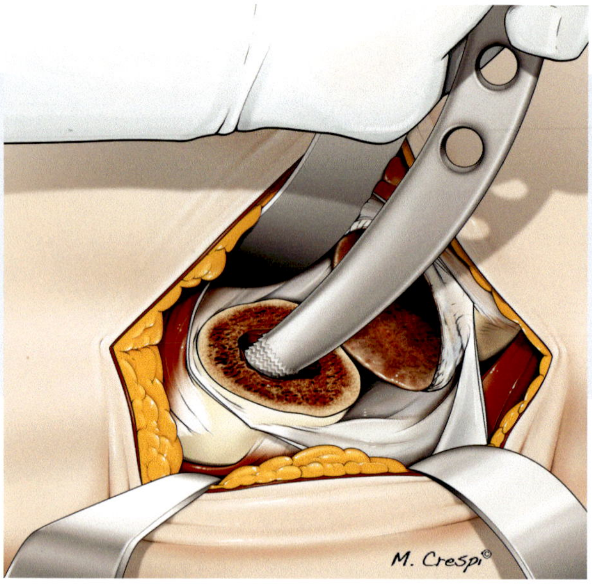

Figure 29 The access to the diaphyseal canal is widened with the curved 'banana' rasp

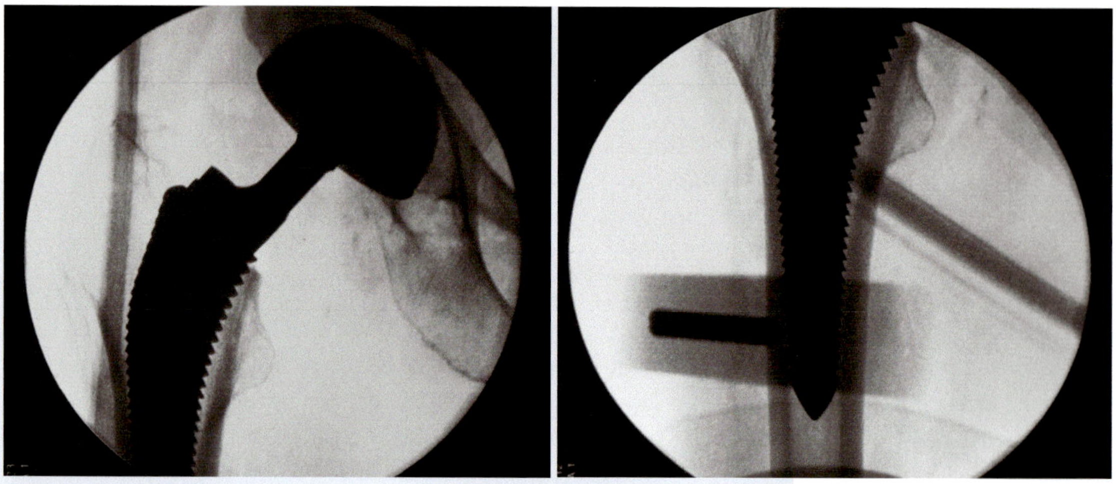

Figure 30 Fluoroscopic examination of the position, orientation and size of prosthetic components

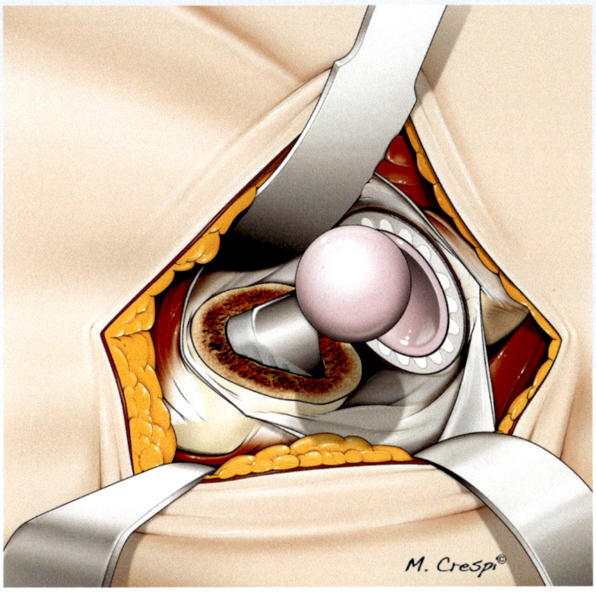

Figure 31
Final position of stem and head

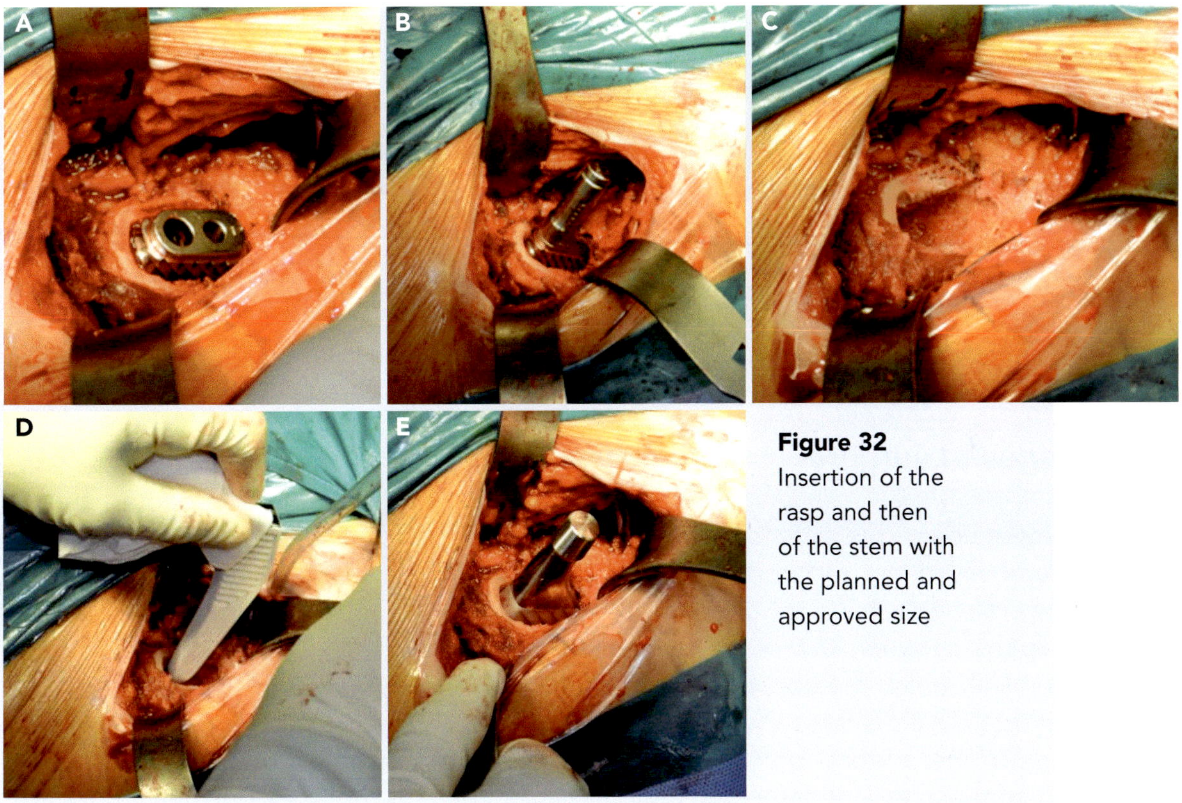

Figure 32
Insertion of the rasp and then of the stem with the planned and approved size

ily be affected by a minor displacement of the pelvis or an imperfect position of the limb.
Since the anterior hip approach using the leg positioner offers the possibility to easily perform a fluoroscopic check, it is our habit to regularly perform one to verify the correct positioning of the implant and in particular of the stem (fig. 30).
A gauze left around the trial neck now facilitates the dislocation manoeuvre, which is performed by combining gentle traction and external rotation. By holding the femur with the same gauze, while the thigh is externally rotated and the femur lowered, the femur is easily returned to the 'presentation' position: it is sufficient to reposition the two Hohmann retractors to complete the operation by applying the definitive stem and head (figs. 31-33) or continue the preparation with another broach.

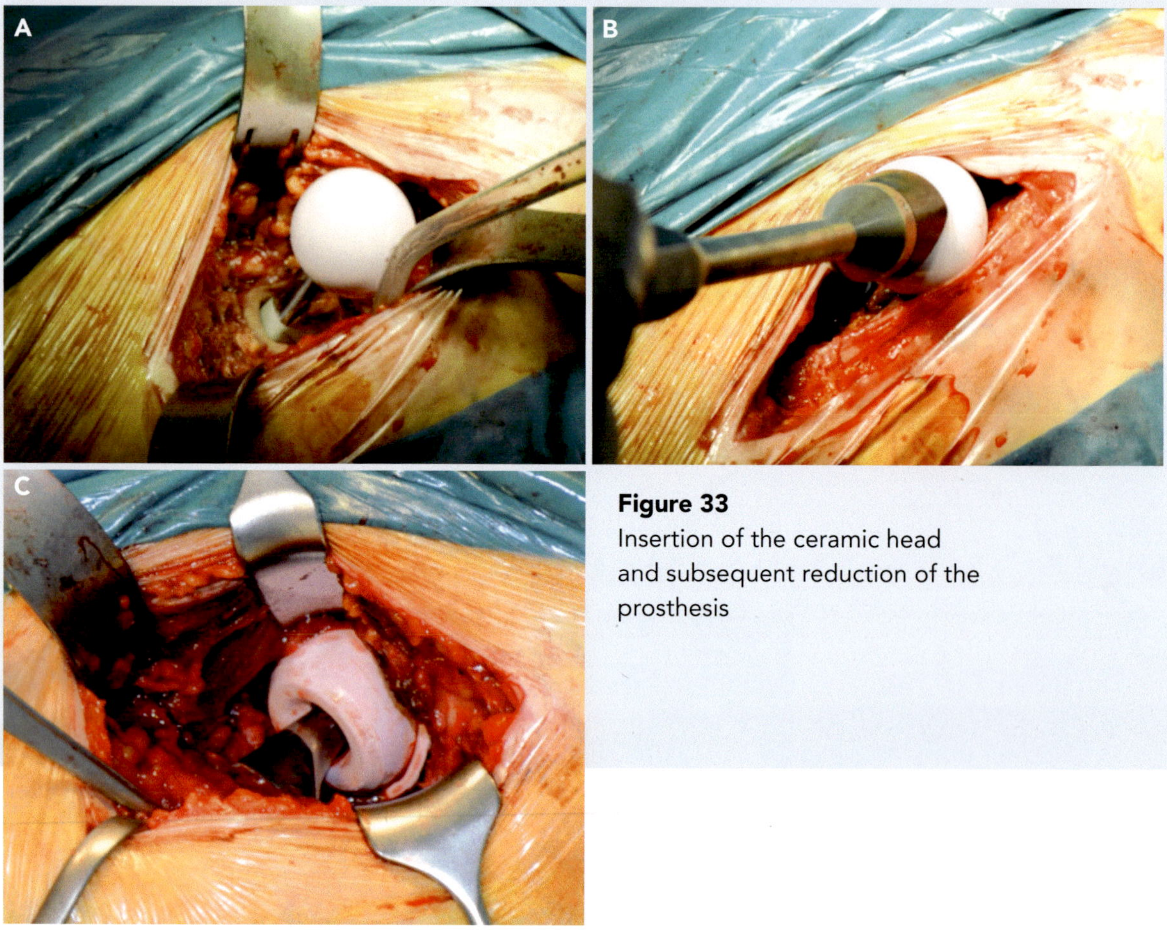

Figure 33
Insertion of the ceramic head and subsequent reduction of the prosthesis

Final stages of surgery

After the reduction of the definitive implant and the removal of the retractors, we observe the spontaneous 'closing' of the intermuscular space between the sartorius and the TFL, through which the approach to the joint was made. This confirms the real mini-invasiveness of the surgical procedure and the respect of the muscular tissue.
Simple tests will be performed on the limb free to rotate without traction, which will allow us to assess the stability of the implant. Some of these are the moderate and cautious forced external rotation of the femur and, with the patella positioned at Zenith, the traction of the prosthetic neck with a hook, testing the difficulty to pull the femur laterally.
A final check of the haemostasis is advisable after restoration of the normal pressure regime (we normally operate under spinal anaesthesia with controlled hypotension). The vessels most prone to bleeding are the posterior branches of medial circumflex. In addition to these, there are the ascending branches of the lateral circumflex, which have already been ligated and cauterised during surgery. Bleeding from the posterior circumflex branches post-operatively can have significant consequences. This is because there is no inextensible anatomical compartment which, under pressure, would counteract the bleeding.
Even when haemostasis appears perfect, it is always applied a drain in the joint. Before the closure of the layers we proceed with a thorough pulse wash, which has already been carried out before the placement of the cup and the definitive stem.
Given the sacrifice of the joint capsule, the suture is limited to the superficial fascia (where care must be taken to avoid the lateral femoral cutaneous nerve) and the sub-

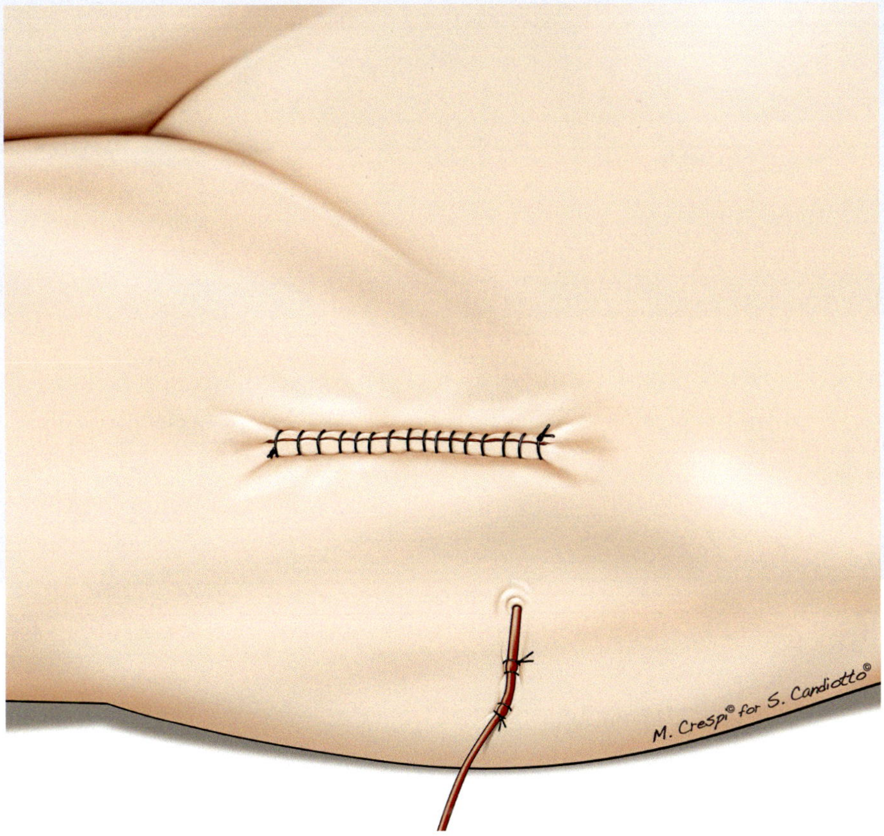

Figure 34
Application of suction drainage and suture of the skin

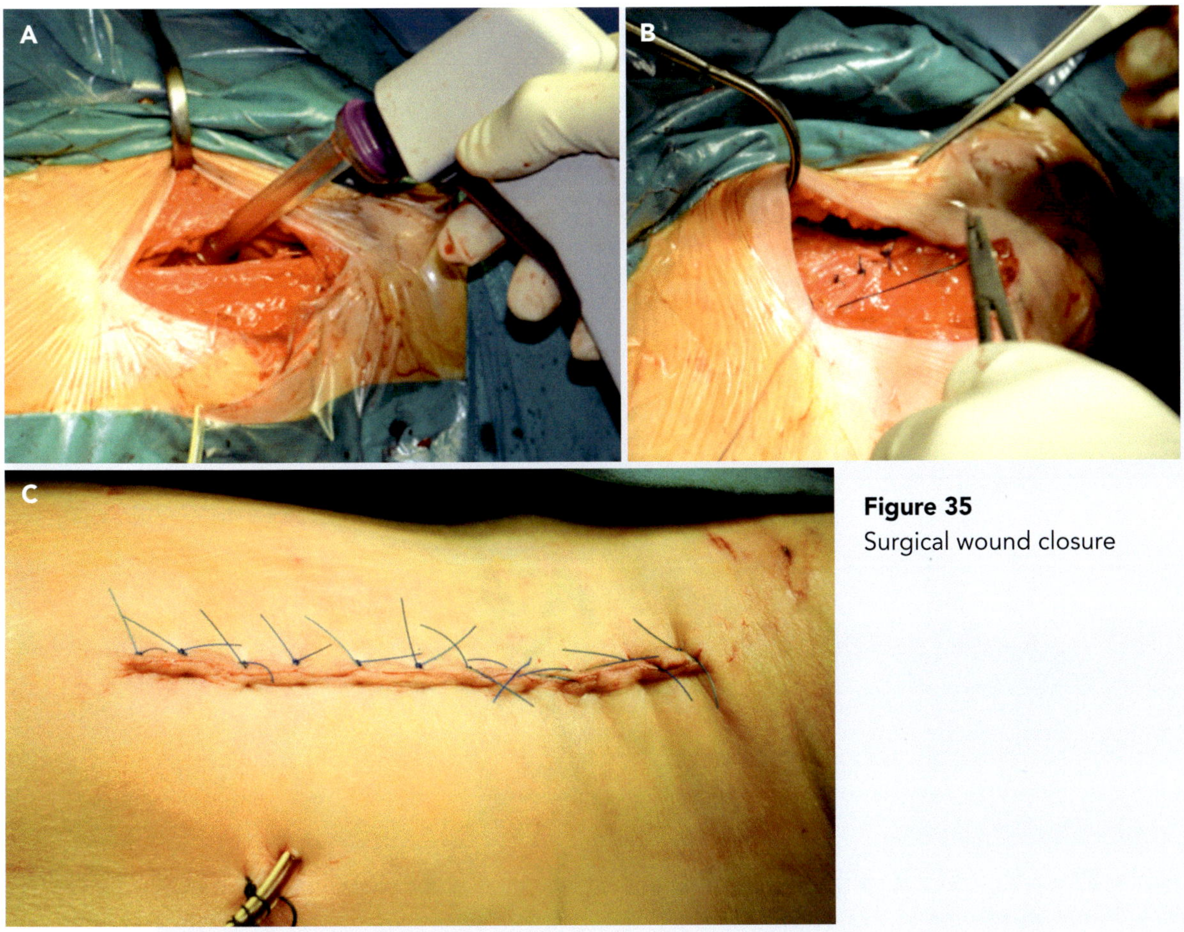

Figure 35
Surgical wound closure

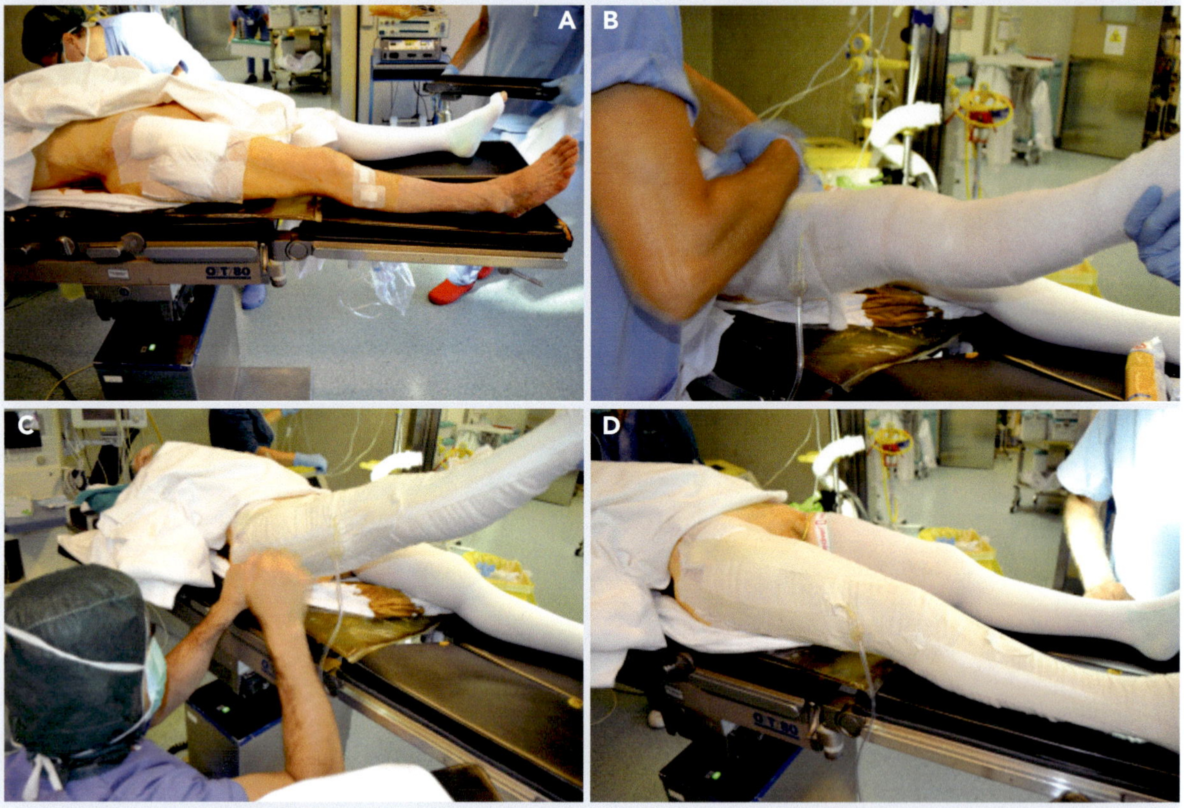

Figure 36 Dressing and bandaging of the operated limb

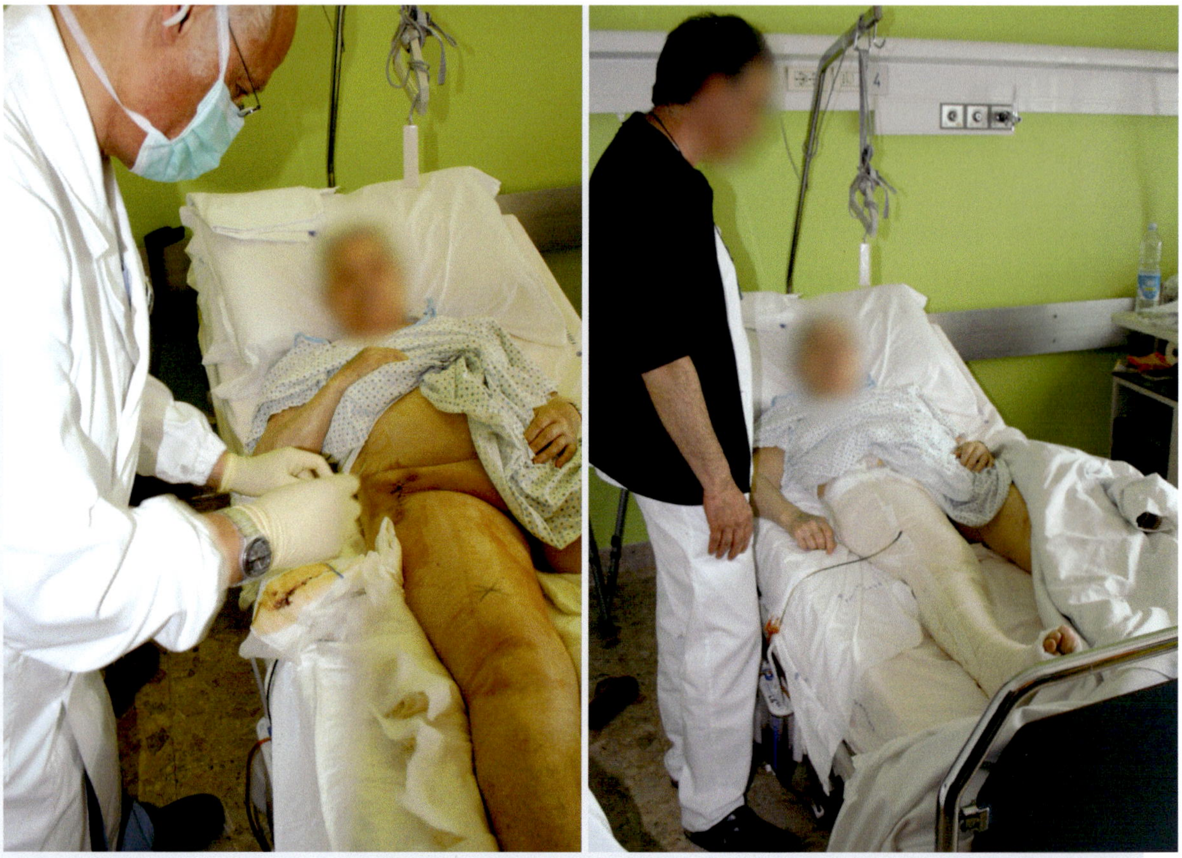

Figure 37 Patient management in the immediate post-operative period and drain removal at 36-48 hours after surgery

cutaneous and cutaneous plane (figs. 34-35). The dressing is always completed by the application of an elastic bandage starting from the foot and ending at the inguinal area (where it is fixed to the skin with some short longitudinal strips of tape so that it does not loose) and that constitutes a further barrier to possible bleeding (fig. 36).
Obviously final confirmation of limb length is only possible after removal of the leg positioner's shoe and a comparison of the malleoli. The patient is placed in bed with a spreader cushion between the lower limbs which is kept in place for at least 12 hours. The drain is removed after approximately 24-36 hours (fig. 37).
Weight bearing is permitted in the immediate post-operative period, in accordance with the patient's general condition. Antibiotic prophylaxis begins at induction of anaesthesia. Thromboembolic prophylaxis with low molecular weight heparin or the most modern oral anticoagulant drugs is prolonged according to common protocols (5 weeks).

Strategy to avoid limb dysmetria

A method proposed by other authors involves capsular sparing with assessment of any limb length variations at the time of suturing the capsular flaps. Another method is to overlap the rasps on the resected femoral head in order to have visual confirmation of the correct osteotomy level and offset. In our hands these two methods are not feasible, the anterior capsule is removed and a double osteotomy of the femoral neck is performed. The importance of preoperative planning is therefore maximal along with intraoperative confirmation of the level of the osteotomy, through the measurement of the distance between it and the lesser trochanter. We have also adopted the method of placing a Kirschner wire on the ASIS and one on the anterior tibial tuberosity to monitor limb length. However, we believe that no single method, if used alone, is effective in ensuring correct limb length. A good practice must involve the use of multiple methods at the same time. It should also be remembered that if there is any difficulty, even moderate, in reducing the implant, a limb lengthening should always be suspected.

CHAPTER 9

The bikini incision anterior approach in minimally invasive arthroplasty of the hip

Florian Fischer, Agostino De Felice, Andrea Fossali, Elia Creta, Vanni Benito Petrachi

Scientific Institute Auxologico Capitanio Hospital, Milan, Italy

Introduction

Total hip arthroplasty has become one of the most successful orthopedic treatments over the last decades. Due to continue research for progress and efforts to improve patients' satisfaction, even the surgical approach has become an important issue within minimally invasive techniques and tissue sparing surgery. Better knowledge of structural and functional anatomy has raised huge interest – not just among surgeons, but also among well informed patients (internet) - for the renaissance of the anterior approach to the hip. Historically, the first description of the 'modern' anterior approach to the hip was published in 1881 by Carl Hueter [1], a german surgeon. Over the years its application was continued and further modified for the treatment of the septic and dysplastic hip and trauma surgery of the proximal femur and the acetabulum by well-known authors as Smith-Petersen (1917) [2] and Judet (1947) [3] and has found its first mini-invasive version by Matta in 2005 [4].
In the last decade every existing hip approach has been modified in terms of muscle sparing surgery. The direct anterior hip approach for THA allows the implantation through an inter-nervous and intermuscular plane without muscle detachment from bone. The potential advantage over other surgical approaches is mainly given by not damaging the abductor function of the lateral hip structures, which results in fast functional recovery and in fewer Trendelenburg-positive patients when compared to lateral or in a lower dislocation rate when compared to posterior approaches [5].

Definition

Originally, the longitudinal incision of the anterior approach to the hip was placed over the TFL (tensor fasciae latae) muscle belly, starting at 2 fingerbreadths distal and lateral from the ASIS (anterior superior iliac spine) heading toward the fibular head. As the longitudinal incision did not follow the anatomic skin crease, scar widening, and hypertrophic wound healing could be observed. For this reason, Leunig et al. [6] started to perform the anterior hip approach with a short oblique incision in the inguinal crease, following the main folding lines (Langer's lines) of the skin, reducing thus poor cosmetic results while maintaining the potential benefits of the anterior approach (fig. 1).

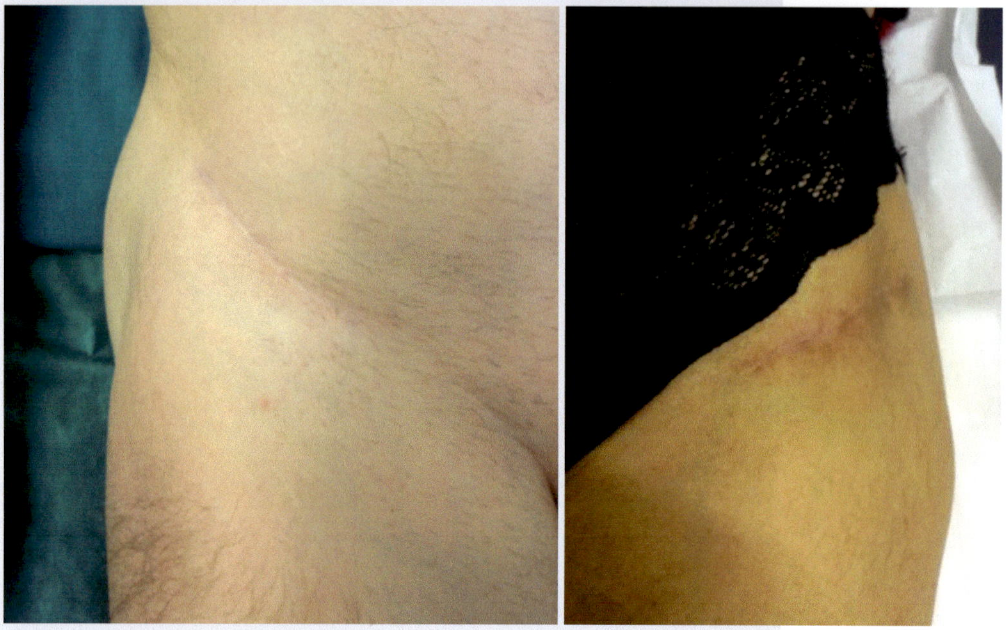

Figure 1 Good cosmetic results with the bikini incision

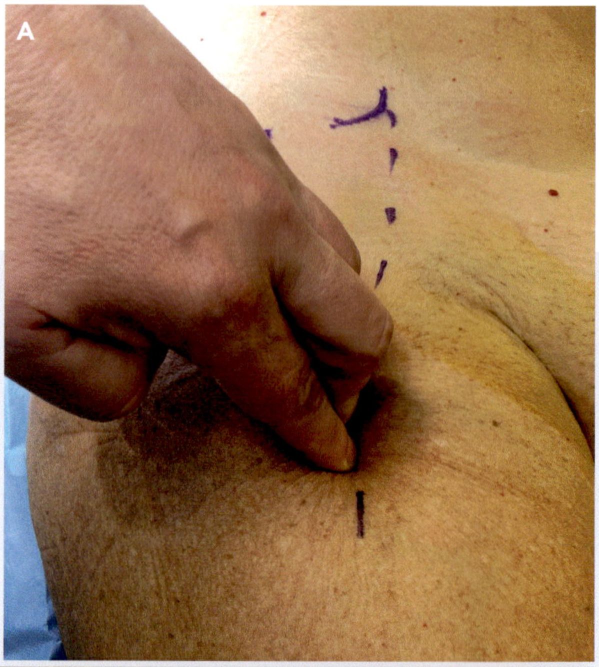

Figure 2
A) When the interval between TFL and sartorius is palpable, the bikini incision anterior approach can be easily performed. B) Standard setup with conventional dressing, the C-arm is ready for the later intra-operative controls

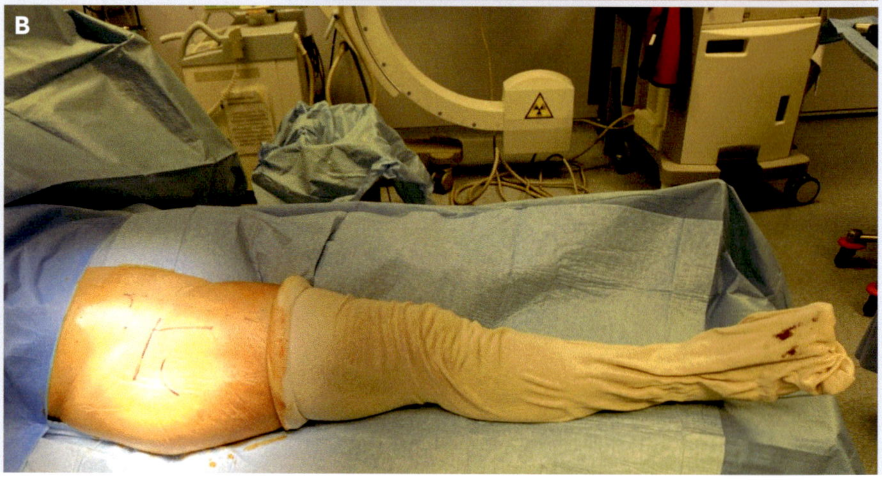

Indication

At the beginning of our experience, the bikini incision was reserved for the 'average' patient with primary osteoarthritis of the hip. To avoid difficult cases as too small or too tall and muscular patients with a short or varus femoral neck, we performed the bikini incision only in patients where the interval between the TFL and the sartorius was easily palpable from the outside (fig. 2A). During our learning process, we gradually extended the indication on almost every type of patient and pathology, such as necrosis, dysplastic hips and femoral neck fractures, even in obese patients, in case of revision of a former done bikini approach or in femoro-acetabular impingement as a mini-open treatment.

Contraindications

Contraindications for the anterior bikini approach to the hip regard general medical status and risk profile, high grade dysplasia, very muscular males (interval between TFL and sartorius not palpable) and local skin lesions or infections. Some of the very first papers about the anterior hip approach, especially the inguinal, raised concerns about higher infection rates for incisions in proximity to the genitalia, but have not been confirmed [7,8].

Preparation

The patient's pre-operative preparation for THA with bikini incision does not differ for other surgical accesses regarding antibiotic and antithrombotic prevention. On the contrary to the direct lateral approach, we do not perform any pharmacological prevention of heterotopic ossifications.
The intra-operative setup requires a standard operating table (we do not use extension devices), standard sterile patient's dressing (fig. 2B). (we considered preparation with the initially used special drape and scrubbing of both extremities too time-wasting), instrumentation for anterior access and a C-arm.
The patient is placed in a supine position on a standard operating table, with his hip over the hinge of the bendable stilts (this position can be very useful for the later preparation of the femoral canal). Be careful to shift the table distally, until You get easy access with the C-arm for the intraoperative radiological control.
The entire extremity up to the umbilicus gets scrubbed and draped, on the other side we just prepare the leg with a sterile stockinette for the rare use of the figure-4 position and the final control of leg length.

Surgical technique

The main surgical landmarks (tip of greater trochanter, ASIS) are found, and the inguinal crease is identified by putting the hip into flexion (fig. 3).
In our first cases we placed the skin incision two thirds laterally and one third medially of the ASIS, nowadays we incise the inguinal fold completely lateral, keeping the LFCN (lateral femoral cutaneous nerve) at secure distance. A stich at the medial extremity of the incision may be useful to prevent from accidental skin rupture and medial extension.
With the use of two retractors, the superficial (electrocautery) and deep (bluntly with gauze pad) layer of the subcutaneous fat is dissected and the TFL fascia exposed (fig. 4). It is mandatory to clearly identify the muscle with the following three references:

1. touch the ASIS with Your fingers – the TFL originates from its lateral part;
2. the muscle belly has a blue discoloration under the fascia, while the gluteus medius has a whiter more appearance (fig. 5);
3. identify the TFL perforator vessel (fig. 6) (from the ascending branch of the lateral circumflex femoral artery) and incise the fascia just medially to it (fig. 7). Even for experienced surgeons, this part can be challenging due to the restricted operative space in mini-invasive surgery and can complicate the further procedure a lot.

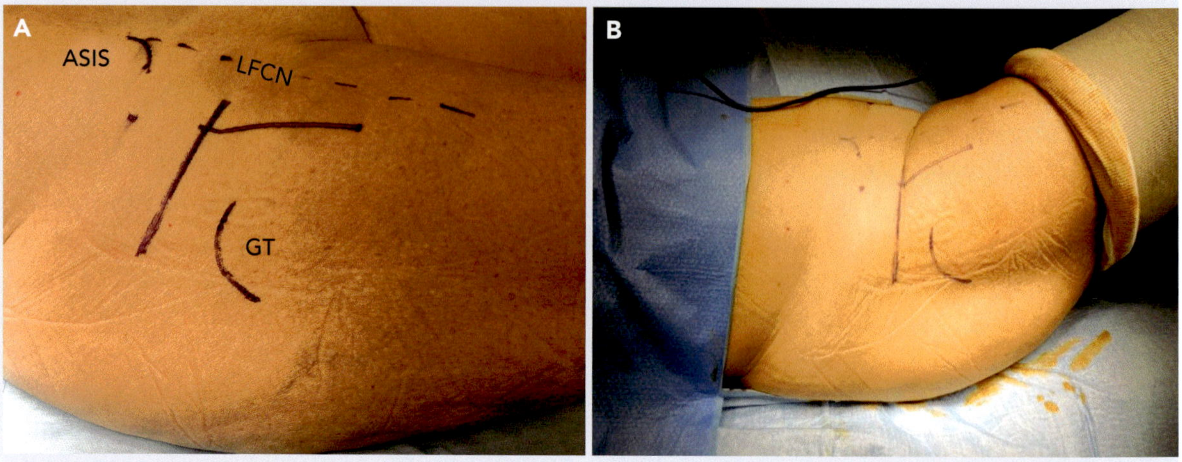

Figure 3 A) The signed landmarks are ASIS, great trocanter GT and the lateral femoral cutaneous nerve LFCN. B) Finding of the inguinal crease putting the hip into flexion. The incision is entirely lateral to the ASIS

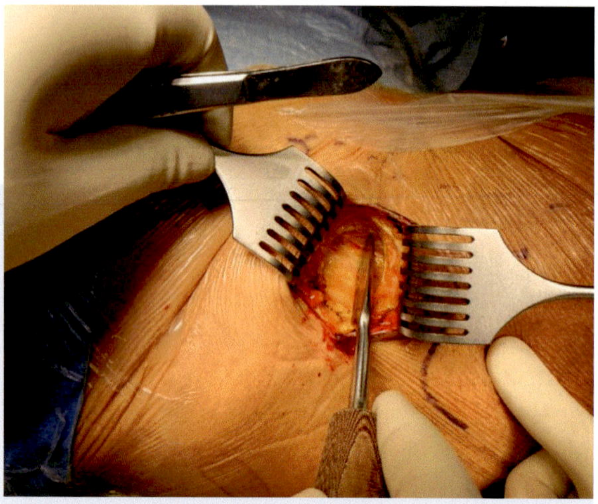

Figure 4 Using two retractors the TFL fascia is exposed by blunt dissecting of the subctaneous fat

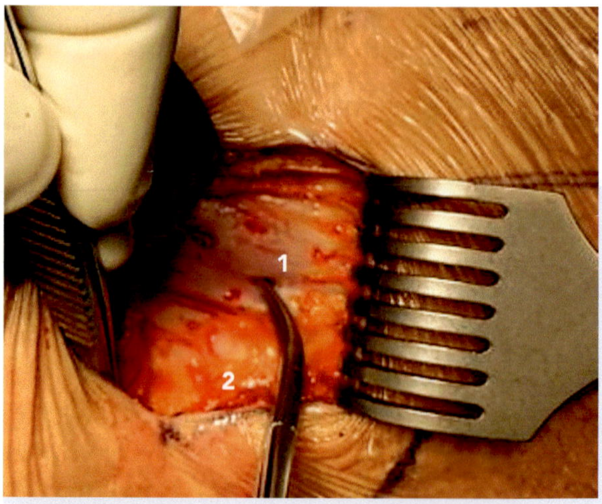

Figure 5 Notice the different colorations of the TFL (blue 1) and the gluteus medius fascia (white 2)

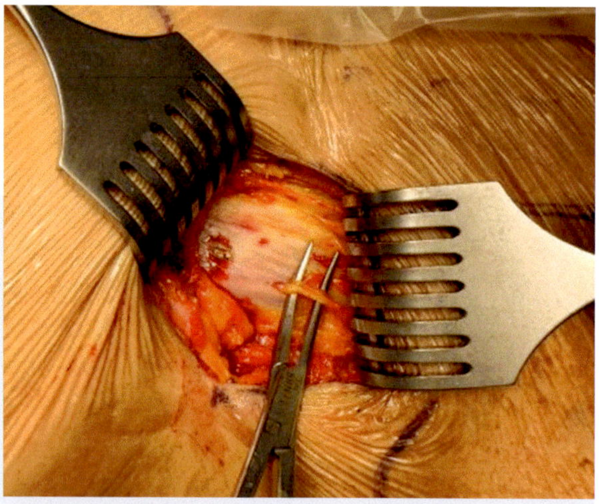

Figure 6 The TFL perforator vessel is an important landmark

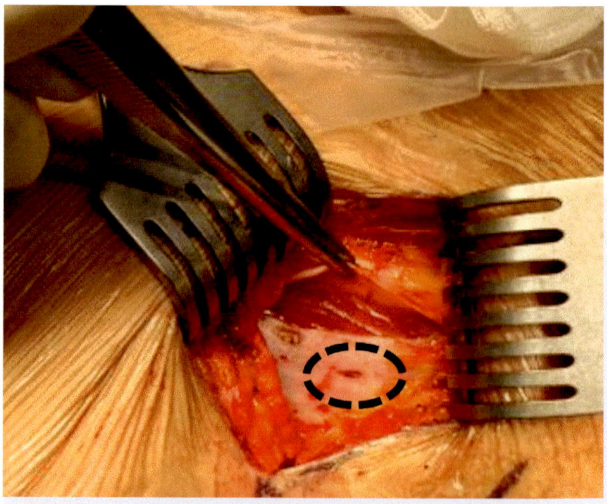

Figure 7 The TFL fascia is incised just medially to the vessel perforation

Now the medial layer of the opened fascia can be elevated with a pincette and the blunt dissection of the Smith-Petersen interval performed with the index finger (fig. 8). Hereafter two deep Hohmann retractors are placed laterally, behind and over the great trochanter and a Langenbeck medially to widen the interval (fig. 9). The deep branches of the lateral circumflex vessels can now be identified and coagulated/ligated (fig. 10) and the remaining fascial sheet is incised until the precapsular fat pad is visible and can be removed.

At this time the articular capsule is exposed by 3 or 4 Hohmann retractors: one medially to the neck into the soft-spot, the second laterally to the shoulder of the greater trochanter, the third on the acetabular roof under the rectus femoris tendon (always perpendicular to the inguinal ligament to avoid damage to the femoral nerve and vessels) and eventually the fourth around the great trochanter (fig. 11).

At this point the anterolateral capsulotomy is performed (fig. 12) and two blunt Hohmann retractors (medial and lateral) are repositioned intracapsularly around the neck preventing from injury to the posterior soft

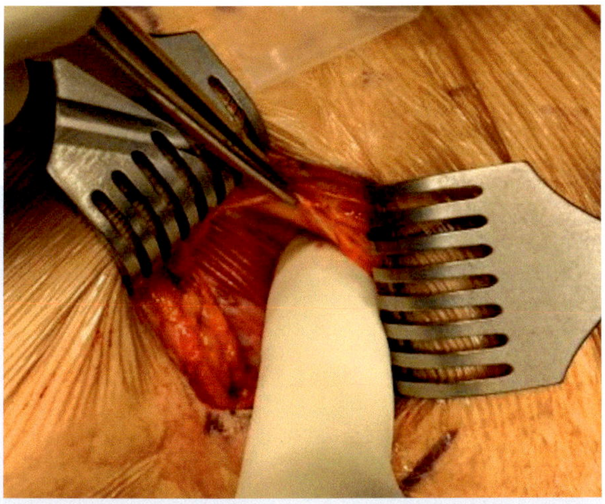

Figure 8 Exploring the Smith-Petersen interval with the index finger

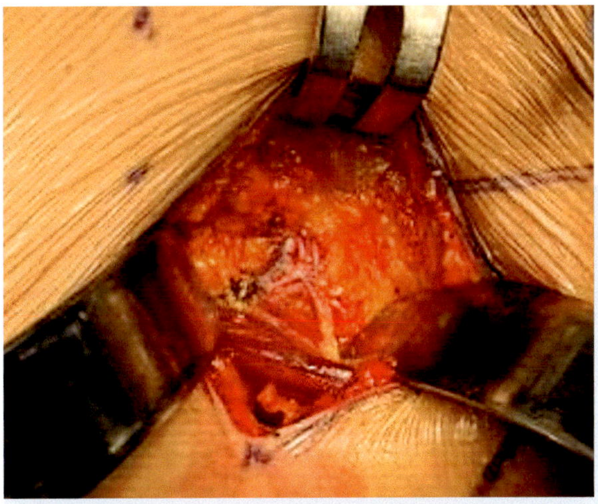

Figure 9 Opening of the interval by two lateral Hohmann retractors around the great trochanter and a medial Langenbeck

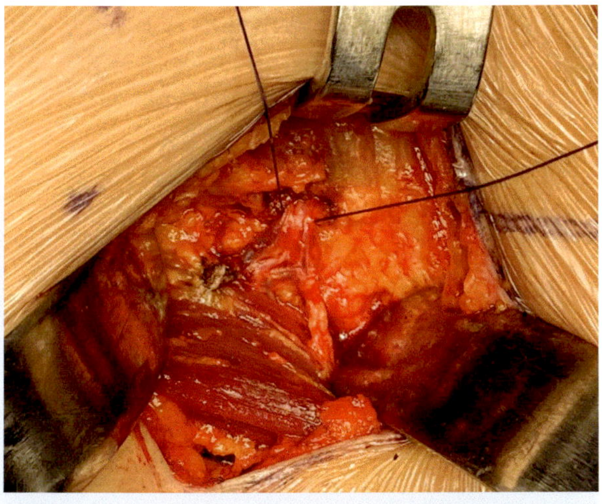

Figure 10 The deep vessels are coagulated or ligated

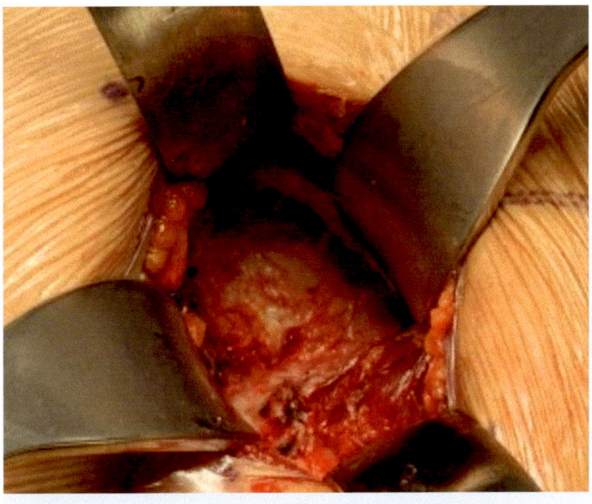

Figure 11 Exposition of the articolar capsule by four Hohmann retractors

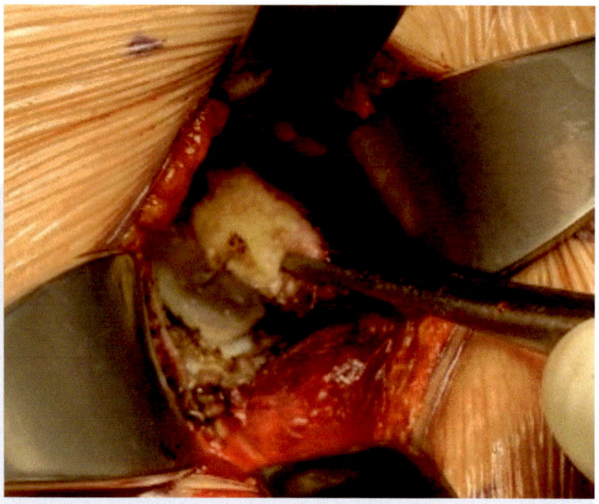

Figure 12 Anterolateral capsulectomy

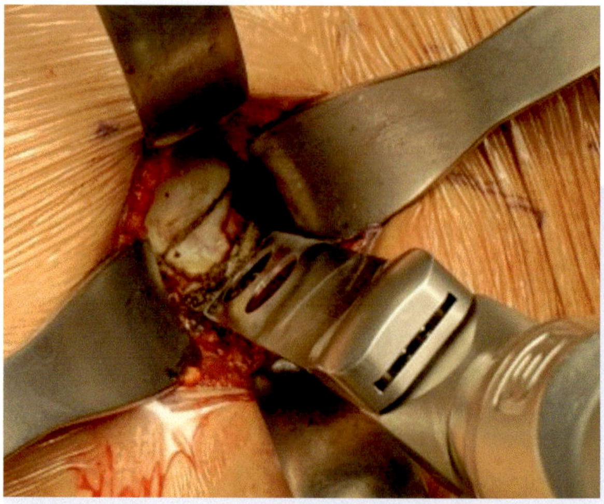

Figure 13 Exposition of the articolar capsule by four Hohmann retractors

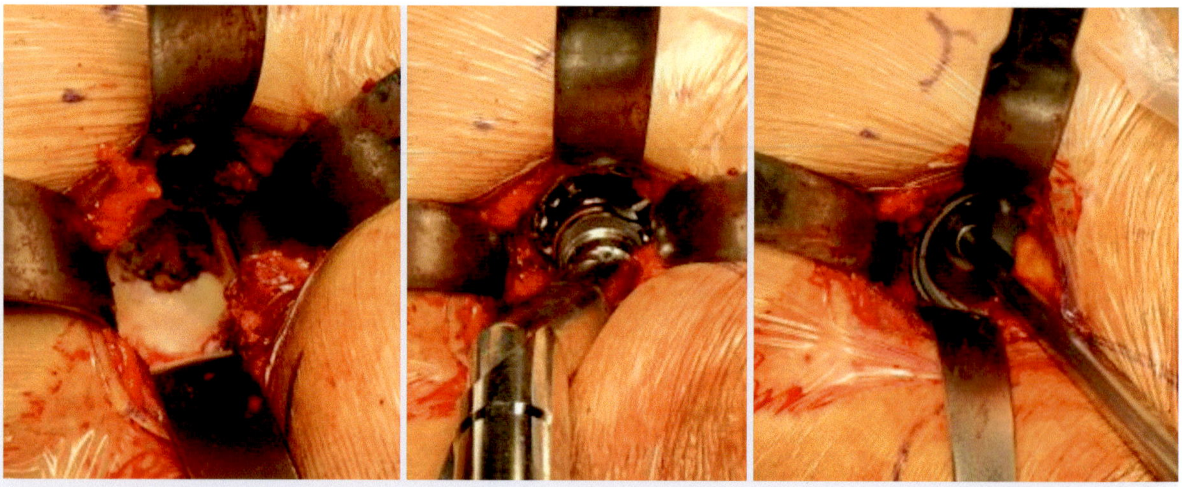

Figure 14 Good exposition, reaming and implant of the cup

tissues by the oscillating saw. A double osteotomy is completed (fig. 13), the neck section removed and eventually corrected and the femoral head extracted.

Now the acetabulum can be prepared with straight or curved (soft tissue impingement is not to underestimate and may increase antiversion of the cup) instruments in the standard fashion (fig. 14).

The femoral preparation is more challenging and depends mostly on the type of the chosen implant. While a calcar guided short stem does not necessarily require any further soft tissue release or special instrumentation, the use of a standard straight stem with a bikini incision anterior approach has to be carefully evaluated and facilitated:

1. bend the operating table to hyperextend the hip (fig. 15);
2. lever the femur with a bone hook in the calcar area of the neck (fig. 16);
3. perform some additional posterolateral release (fig. 17) until the femur rises;
4. put a retractor between trochanter and gluteus medius to elevate the femur.

At this stage, a second Hohmann retractor is put in place on the medial neck and femoral broaching can be done even in a lazy 4 position (figs. 18-19).

We normally check the correct size and posi-

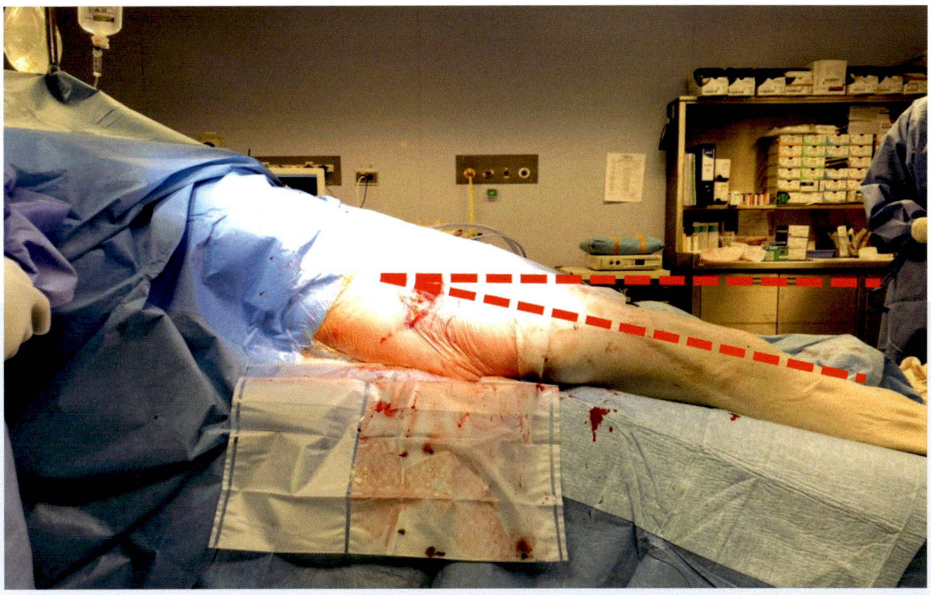

Figure 15 Breaking the table over the hinge facilitates the entry in the femoral canal

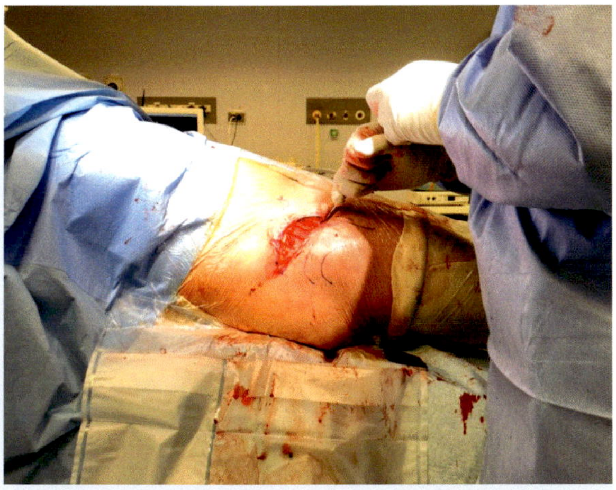

Figure 16 A bone hook in the calcar region helps to bring the femur up

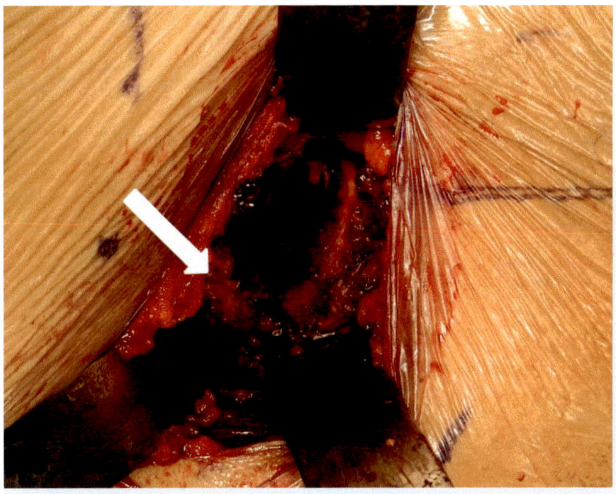

Figure 17 The posterolateral capsule waiting to be released

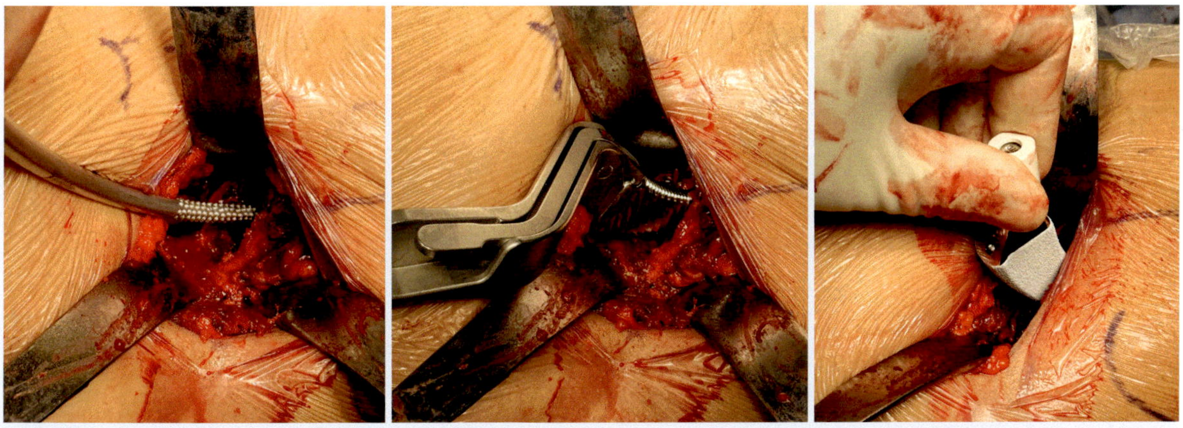

Figure 18 Preparing and broaching of the femoral canal

tion of the implant with the C-arm intraoperatively. At the end of surgery, the wound is debrided, a redon drain can be placed and the TFL fascia is closed with few stiches to avoid damaging the lateral femoral cutaneous nerve (fig. 20).

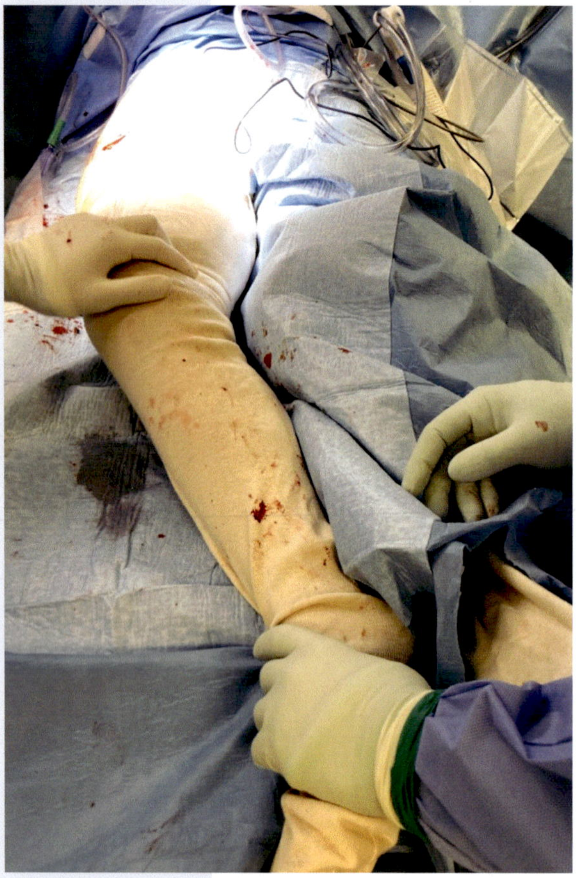

Figure 19 The lazy 4 position

Difficulties and complications

Especially during the learning curve the implantation of a THA via the anterior hip approach can be a technically challenging procedure. Due to neck-preserving technique and the oblique bikini incision the 'working space' is even more reduced, with limited visibility of the surgical site. Therefore, surgeons should first be familiar with the longitudinal incision before performing the bikini approach.

The most frequent specific complications are:

1. accidental opening and preparation of the wrong muscle-interval, mostly medial to the sartorius, rarely into Watson-Jones. Those errors make the exposition of the articular capsule quite difficult and may influence the positioning of the whole implant. Always check the anatomic landmarks before incising the fascia;
2. incorrect cup positioning with to high antiversion by impingement of the soft tissue can be avoided using curved instrumentation;

Figure 20 At the end of surgery, the TFL fascia gets closed by a few stiches and a redon can be placed

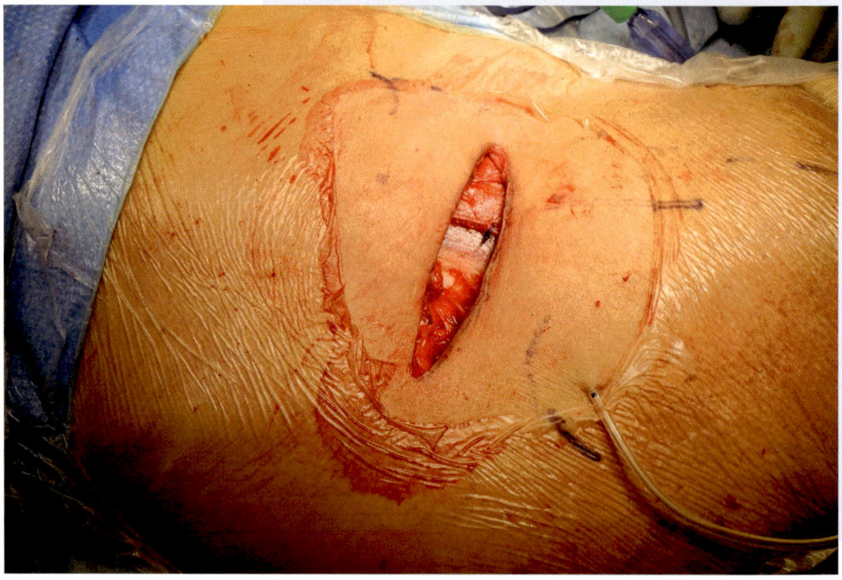

3. insufficient preparation of the proximal femur can lead to either damage of the TFL by a too strong lever of the femoral elevator or to trochanter fractures and a canal perforation due to incorrect entry-point to the femoral canal: based on the surgeon's choice of the implant, the femur is to release, elevate and bring up by table breaking in case of a straight conventional stem. None of those facilitations are required in case of a calcar-guided short stem, that can be implanted on a normal operating table without the risk of malposition;
4. due to the proximity of the LFCN to both surgical incisions for the anterior hip approach (longitudinal and oblique), injury is to avoid, especially at the beginning of the learning curve. The sensory nerve can be cut and torn or compressed by the final suture. Its symptomatology is described as meralgia paresthetica – a very painful condition in the patient's lateral thigh with a severe impact on patient's life. While a slightly higher incidence of LFCN dysaesthesia could be observed when the bikini incision was initially placed for one third medially to the ASIS crossing the LFCN, nerve complications, performing the approach completely lateral to the ASIS, were comparable to the longitudinal anterior approach [9]. However, recent anatomic studies have shown that due to a large number and variability, 20,5% of the LFCN branches enter the thigh lateral to the ASIS and that both approaches (direct and oblique) cross the main branch in 100% of the cases anyway [10].

Old patients

Over the last years short stems have gained popularity even in older patients, because fewer complications were reported due to their less invasive operating technique by less broaching-demanding implants. Less surgical trauma, shorter operative times, a lower transfusion rate and fewer periprosthetic infections compared to a standard-length stem, while maintaining good axial and rotational stability, removed the initial doubts about the secure use of short stems in even octogenarian patients [5,11]. Moreover, the use of calcar-guided implants avoids the need of further soft-tissue release and more extensile femur preparation and for us, combined to the bikini incision anterior hip approach, has become the best solution for a short hospital stay and fast recover, even for the elderly patient (fig. 21).

Obese patients

The direct anterior hip approach has been associated with increased wound healing problems and lesser cosmetic results, especially in the obese patients. The poor skin in

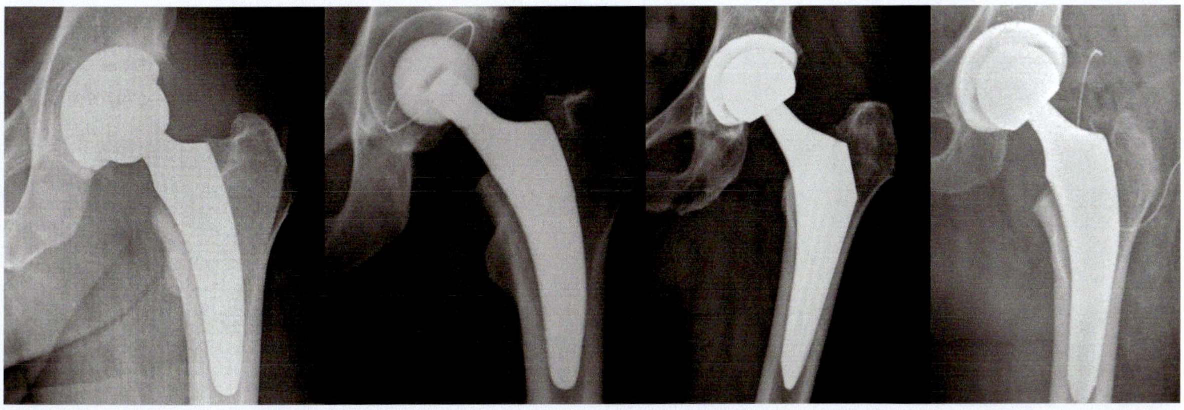

Figure 21 Very good results of short stems even in elderly patients

the proximal part of the incision, the overhanging panniculus and the adjacent genitalia increase the risk of superficial infection [12]. The horizontal bikini incision, along Langer's lines, does not show any delay in wound healing and therefore does not compromise the natural skin barrier avoiding bacterial penetration of the perilesional soft tissues. Instead, acute skin infections or frequent local dehiscences in the skin folds are contraindications to surgery.

Tips and tricks

Tips and tricks for an easy-going bikini incision anterior approach to the hip are:

- get experience with the longitudinal incision before trying the bikini incision anterior approach;
- clearly identify the TFL fascia with the described landmarks;
- use special instruments (double offset broaches, etc.);
- be careful of too much cup – antiversion;
- avoid too much stress to the femoral canal;
- identify the LFCN before the closure of the wound.

Bibliography

1. Hueter C. Grundriss der Chirurgie 2. Leipzig: FCW Vogel; 1883. Fünfte Abtheilung: Die Verletzung und Krankheiten des Hüftgelenks; pp. 129–200.

2. Smith-Peterson MN. A new supra-articular subperiosteal approach to the hip joint. J Bone Joint Surg Am. 1917;s2-15:592–5.

3. Judet J, Judet R. The use of an artificial femoral head for arthroplasty of the hip joint. J Bone Joint Surg Br Vol. 1950;32-B(2):166–73.

4. Matta JM, Shahrdar C, Ferguson T. Single-incision anterior approach for total hip arthroplasty on an orthopaedic table. Clin Orthop Relat Res. 2005;441:115–24.

5. Holzapfel BM, Rak D, Kreuzer S, Arnholdt J, Thaler M, Rudert M. Short stem hip arthroplasty via the minimally invasive direct anterior approach. Oper Orthop Traumatol 2021;33:288-303.

6. Leunig M, Faas, M, von Knoch F, Naal FD. Skin Crease "Bikini" Incision for Anterior Approach Total Hip Arthroplasty: Surgical Technique and Preliminary Results. Clin Orthop Relat Res 2013;471:2245-2252.

7. O'Connor CM, et al. Direct Anterior Approach Total Hip Arthroplasty Is Not Associated with Increased Infection Rates. JBJS Reviews 2021;9(1):e20.00047.

8. Nizam I, Dabirrahmani D, Alva A, Choudary D. Bikini Anterior Hip Replacements In Obese Patients Are Not Associated With An Increased Risk Of Complication. Arch Orthop Trauma Surg 2021 Sep 12.

9. Wang Q, Yue Y, Yang Z, Chen L, Li Q, Kang P. Comparison of Postoperative Outcomes Between Traditional Longitudinal Incision and Bikini Incision in Total Hip Arthroplasty via Direct Anterior Approach: A Randomized Controlled Trial. J Arthroplasty. 2021;36:222-230.

10. Thaler M, Damerer D, Hechenberger F, Hoermann R, Van Beeck A, Stofferin H. The Anatomical Course of the Lateral Femoral Cutaneous Nerve in Relation to Various Skin Incisions Used or Primary and Revision Total Hip Arthroplasty With the Direct Anterior Approach. J Arthroplasty. 2021;36:368-373.

11. Gkagkalis G, Goetti P, Mai S, Meinecke I, Helmy N, Bosson D, Kutzner KP. Cementless short-stem total hip arthroplasty in the elderly patient – is it a safe option?: a prospective multicenter observational study. BMC Geriatr 2019;19:112.

12. Manrique J, Paskey T, Tarabichi M, Restrepo C, Foltz C, Hozack WJ. Total Hip Arthroplasty Through the Direct Anterior Approach Using a Bikini Incision Can Be Safely Performed in Obese Patients. J Arthroplasty. 2019;34(8):1723-1730.

CHAPTER 10

Robotic assistance in minimally invasive hip prosthetic surgery

Silvia Pierantoni*, Marco Zamperetti*, Jacopo Tagliapietra*, Alberto Procura*, Salvatore Gravinese*, Giulio Edoardo Vigni**, Antonio Camporese*

*Hip and Shoulder Surgery Unit, Abano Terme General Hospital, Padua, Italy
**Department of Orthopaedics and Traumatology, University of Palermo, Italy

Introduction

Prosthetic hip replacement surgery can be considered one of the most successful surgical procedures, with a survival rate of 95% after 10 years and 80% after 25 years [1]. Progress in this field often encounters the limitation of achieving insignificant differences in clinical benefit in the short term, having to turn its efforts more to the reduction of complications in the long term.
The main cause of failure in hip prosthesis surgery within the first year after surgery remains dislocation. The rate of dislocation, from an average of 1% after first prosthesis implantation, rises to 25%, according to some case reports, in revision prostheses [2,3], occupying the top ranks among the reasons for surgical revision [4].
While an acute episode has a better prognosis in terms of risk of recurrence [5], dislocations in chronic cases are often accompanied by a higher risk of recurrence and multifactorial causes. They also require high costs for the patient and the healthcare system and despite this lower success rates than primary implant prosthetics.
Estimates of the impact of 'unstable prostheses' report a 300% increase in hospital management costs [6,7]. Without forgetting the role of the patient's subjective factors, scientific interest in recent years has focused on investigating the role played by implant alignment. This parameter influences not only the risk of dislocation, but also that of impingement, premature wear, mechanical stress and periprosthetic fractures. These factors are being addressed not only in the interest of longer-term patient care, but also in the interest of saving economic resources.
The goal of implant durability has been pursued over the years and continues to this day. Its study has delved into tribology, which investigates the wear relationships between materials, since John Charnley introduced the concept of 'low-friction arthroplasty' in 1965 [8,9] and in the research of perfecting the positioning of prosthetic components and its reproducibility.
In the latter area, it will come as no surprise that the positive correlation between surgical experience and implant accuracy is widely evidenced [10-12]. Rather, it may be interesting how studies on the reproducibility of the results have revealed a non-negligible variability even in experienced hands and reference centres [13-16]. This is the margin of human error, which, without any strange digressions, has always fuelled the drive towards automation, representing its main rationale in all fields, including medicine and surgery.

Historical notes

The application of robotic assistance in orthopaedic prosthetic surgery took its first steps in the early 1990s. Today, one must first distinguish between three different types: passive, active and semi-active [17].

In the first type, the passive type, the robotic assistance always remains under the control of the surgeon. In the active type, the robot performs pre-operative planning and, based on this, carries out the procedure under the surgeon's supervision. In the semi-active type, on the other hand, the surgery is carried out by the surgeon with real-time robotic assistance, using (visual/tactile) sensors.

Over time, the semi-active type of surgical assistance has become the preferred one. A further distinction must be made between assistance systems based on pre-operative image acquisition and others that do not include it, therefore called 'imageless'.

A recent literature review [17], identified four main robotic assist systems in hip surgery worldwide: the ROBODOC system (THINK surgical, Inc., Fremont, CA, USA) in its new generation TSolution One [18), the CASPAR system (Universal Robot Systems Ortho, Germany), the ACROBOT system (COMPANY), and the Rio MAKO ROBOT system (Stryker, FL, USA). The ROBODOC and Rio MAKO ROBOT systems represent the most widely used systems worldwide today.

The main 'imageless' systems include the Intellijoint system (Intellijoint Surgical Inc., Waterloo, Canada), the Brainlab Hip system (Brainlab, Munich, Germany) and the Stryker Orthomap system (Stryker Corporatio, Kalamazoo, MI, USA). All are based on the acquisition of intraoperative retrievals only. These are identified before and after implant preparation to provide the surgeon with real-time three-dimensional guidance on component positioning and the possibility of verifying parameters like version, offset and length.

As its use has become more widespread, robotic assistance has adapted its applicability to the main surgical approaches used in prosthetic surgery.

The advantages that have emerged in favour of the minimally invasive anterior technique (such as the reduction of tissue damage and intraoperative bleeding, the reduction of post-operative pain and hospitalisation time, as well as the faster functional recovery in the immediate post-operative period) [19-21] make it particularly promising in combination with robotic assistance despite the technical and economic limitations that still accompany it.

'Safety zones' in hip prosthetic surgery

The first proposal to identify a 'safety zone' in the placement of prosthetic implants was made by Lewinnek and his colleagues in 1978. It concerned the acetabular component and was defined in terms of abduction/inclination in the range of 40° ± 10° and anteversion in the range of 15° ± 10° [22].

For the femoral component, the range of anteversion considered 'safe' was between 10° and 15° from the posterior intercondylar line [23,24]. These ranges represented the standard for the next forty years, during which their limitations were noted and modifications proposed.

Several studies have shown, for example, that dislocation can occur even when the acetabular component is correctly seated in the safety zone [25,26].

The popularity of cementless implants, meanwhile, has highlighted the great inter-individual variety in the geometry of the proximal metaphyseal femoral region. This has motivated the push towards resurfacing surgery, modularity, and the 'customisation' of stems. These are all strategies finalised to the maximum respect of the native morphology [27].

The next conceptual step was to consider not only the version of the individual implant components, but their reciprocal relationship. Thus the 'combined anteversion' in prosthetics began to be discussed in the 1990s [28-30]. It is defined as the sum of femoral anteversion and cup anteversion.

The normal range commonly considered

'safe' for maximising range of motion in relation to the risk of conflict or dislocation is between 30° and 60° [30]. A 6.9 higher dislocation risk is reported in the literature for combined anteversions outside the safe range [31].

The objective of respecting this parameter, together with the widespread use of cementless implants that are more dependent on metaphyseal geometry than cemented ones, has also led to the definition of a dedicated surgical technique, the so-called 'Combined Anteversion Technique'. This technique consists of preparing the femoral implant before the acetabular one. It therefore allows the limits related to the geometry of the proximal femur to be compensated with the cup placement [32]. The most current debate has ultimately focused on the analysis of the dynamic relationships between pelvis and hip, in the postural transition between sitting and standing [33]. When standing, the lumbar lordosis increases and the pelvis tilts forward. This increases the anterior coverage of the acetabulum over the femoral head, thus reducing the relative acetabular anteversion. In contrast, when sitting, lordosis reduces, the pelvis tilts posteriorly and the acetabulum increases its relative anteversion.

These variations influence the range of motion in flexion-extension of the hip: in a sitting position, flexion is facilitated due to less anterior coverage [34].

The variation of the pelvic tilt is globally estimated at an average value of 20° (sacral slope of about 40° standing to about 20° sitting).

The correlation between this variation and the 'relative' anteversion of the acetabulum has been quantified as approximately 0.8° for each degree of pelvic tilt variation (15° total for 20° pelvic variation) [35,33].

However, there is considerable interpersonal variability. In particular, stiffnesses of the lumbar spine (fusions or deformities of the vertebral bodies, scoliosis or arthritic degenerative discopathy] will reflect negatively on the adaptation to the postural transition, increasing the risk of femoral-acetabular conflict and/or dislocation.

Based on these considerations, some authors have proposed the introduction of the sacral slope calculation in the pre-operative planning. This has been proposed using x-rays in latero-lateral projection performed in sitting and standing position [34). Other authors, are experimenting the use of EOS scans for this purpose [36).

What is most important is how deeper knowledge of spino-pelvic-femoral relationships has transformed the concept of the safety zone from 'static' to 'functional' [33).

Linked to this change, it is plausible that the focus on the radiographic aspect of implants should also change in favour of functional considerations [37).

Therefore, it will be clear how technological progress in robotic assistance has been enriched each time with the conceptual achievements mentioned above, offering conventional surgery the result of the elaboration of all these parameters.

Pre-operative planning

In semi-active robotic assistance, the robot is equipped with the following: a data processing station, the so-called 'mind', a screen for displaying the 3D model and a motorised 'arm'.

The operating system requires the calibration of some anatomical landmarks on the patient for data processing [17). Initially, in the ROBODOC system (THINK surgical, Inc., Fremont, CA, USA], the application of the landmarks required an additional surgical procedure prior to the CT scan, which was not without risk of morbidity [38-39].

Motivated to reduce this critical issue, calibration based on optical sensors and probes placed intraoperatively on specific skeletal landmarks was introduced in 1999. This was the so-called DigiMatch technique, which proved to be safer and still effective, despite an increase in surgical time [40].

The Rio MAKO ROBOT system (Stryker, Fort Lauderdale, FL, USA) is based on the use of optical (infrared) sensors. The use of this system began in 2008 with knee surgery and in 2010 with hip surgery [17].

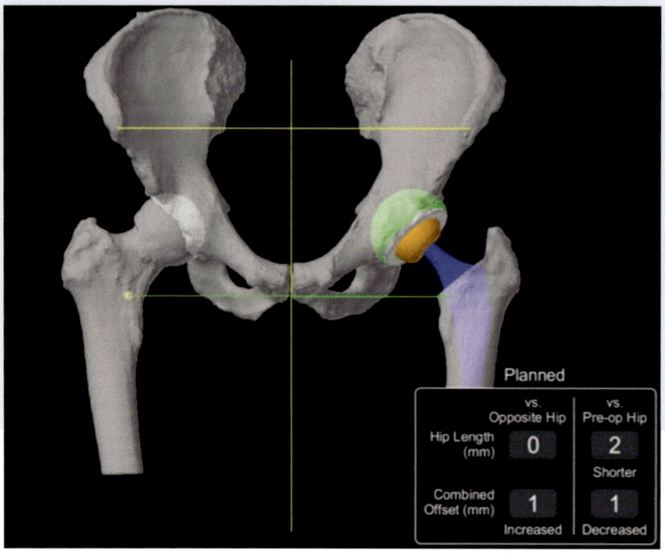

Figure 1
3D model of the pre-operative implant at the end of the planning. Courtesy of Stryker

The Italian experience started with this system in 2012 thanks to Dr Perazzini's team at the San Francesco Clinic in Verona. The initial application used anterolateral surgical approach and since 2016 also the minimally invasive anterior approach [41]. We will therefore report the main features of this system, which then gradually spread throughout our country.

This system requires a pre-operative CT scan of the pelvis and the proximal and distal femur. Thus, the orientation of the condyles is assessed for cervical-diaphyseal anteversion analysis (dedicated CT scan protocol).

Data processing is carried out by the Stryker Team, which creates a virtual 3D model of the pelvis and femur. Implant planning is performed in collaboration with the surgeon [42]. The software allows control of multiple parameters, including length, hip offset and native centre of rotation (COR), compared to the contralateral. Pelvic tilt can also be calculated, but it must be remembered that the CT scan is obtained in the supine position.

Clinical assessment remains particularly important for the integration of the lower limb metrics. This measurement is calculated by the software as the distance between the line joining the anterosuperior iliac spines and the line joining the lesser trochanters. Therefore, this cannot take into account heterometries distal to the lesser trochanter.

The offset is calculated as the 'combined offset', defined as the distance between the line passing through the pubic symphysis and the anatomical axis of the femurs (which is verticalised in the pre-operative CT planning).

The native center of rotation (COR) is the landmark during component selection. This is in order to best respect the characteristics of the native hip and consequently the related subjective comfort with the implant [43].

Having a choice of various implant models, planning usually begins with the choice of cup size and orientation and continues with that of the femoral component [42]. The CT data allow the maximum depth of the acetabular reaming to be accurately determined, protecting the medial wall thickness. It also allows the inclination and version of the acetabular cup to be modified according to the depth of the cotyloid walls. When preparing the femoral implant, the height and inclination of the cervical osteotomy are calculated, always based on the COR. Through the choice of the femoral implant it will be possible to compensate for the variations made by the acetabular implant on the native COR. This will be possible by relying on the concept of 'combined offset' and the availability of modular heads and different types of prosthetic stems. In the choice of the femoral implant, it has already been anticipated how the morphology of the proximal femur influences the final version of the stem, especially if uncemented.

Therefore, once the femoral planning is complete, planning will focus on analysing the 'combined anteversion'. This will allow subsequent adjustments on the cup version. Alternatively, it will be possible to use polyethylene liners with constraints, for minor corrections, or to use cemented stems or modular collars, in case of major corrective needs [42]. At the end of the planning, the software will provide the surgeon with a 3D model of the preliminary implant (fig. 1) [44]. Usually the planning is carried out within 2 months prior to the planned surgery.

Intraoperative robotic assistance

The surgeon can choose between two different modes of intraoperative assistance: the Enhanced Femoral Workflow and the Express Femoral Workflow. The first modality implies that robotic assistance follows all stages of implant preparation. It therefore requires the intraoperative acquisition of acetabular and femoral landmarks in order to be able to compare and guide all the parameters analysed in the pre-operative planning in real time (length, combined offset, combined anteversion, COR). This requires the implantation of optical sensors on the pelvis and femur and, in addition, a pelvic landmark.

The second modality reduces the intraoperative verification parameters, renouncing femoral osteotomy guidance and concentrating mainly on length verification and combined offset. It involves the implantation of optical sensors only on the pelvis, in addition to a landmark on the pelvis, one on the greater trochanter and one distal. The latter can be at the level of the anterior tibial tuberosity or the patella, if the surgical technique respectively involves the traction bed or not.

The acetabular and femoral landmarks are acquired intraoperatively using a pointer or probe. The acquired data are compared with the CT scan of the pre-operative planning to verify their correspondence, with a margin of error of 1 mm as tolerance.

Once data acquisition is complete, depending on the selected mode, the software assists with the preparation of both the femoral osteotomy and acetabular reaming (Enhanced Femoral Workflow). Alternatively, it assists in the preparation of the acetabular component only (Express Femoral Workflow), which therefore follows the cervical osteotomy performed manually by the surgeon. The 'motor arm' of the system guides the preparation phase, allowing minimal intraoperative correction by the surgeon and providing a 'virtual protective barrier'. In the preparation of acetabular reaming, for example, the reamer is positioned in the acetabulum manually by the surgeon who then sees it visualised on the 3D CT model. Based on this model, the surgeon orients its inclination and version until it matches the values established pre-operatively. The intraoperative variation margin is about 15°. At this point, the system allows the desired position to be 'locked'. The motor arm then holds the position obtained, allowing the surgeon to control only the push along the axis of the reamer.

Once the reaming has been performed, the 3D CT model will provide a chromatic and metric guide of the reaming depth, up to the limit defined pre-operatively so as not to affect the medial wall. If the reaming exceeds the limits of the pre-operative planning, the robotic arm will increase its resistance to the surgeon's action and the system will emit an acoustic warning signal, eventually blocking the motor arm [45]. Once the positioning of the components is complete, the pre-operative and post-operative parameters can be checked.

Surgical procedure

The anterior minimally invasive surgical approach to the hip allows excellent visualisation of the acetabulum. It can also be extended proximally up to the iliac crest in the case of acetabular problems. However, this approach allows a less optimal view of the femur. In the event of complications on the femur, it can only be extended distally by passing to the lateral side of the thigh or, more often, by making a second lateral approach [46].

With these premises, this approach seems particularly suitable for the application of

robotic assistance with the Express Femoral Workflow, which will be described below.
The surgical team includes two operating surgeons, the surgical scrub nurse and the Stryker Specialist. Preparation begins with the OR set-up.
The Mako Robot system, i.e. the 'motor arm', is positioned on the same side as the surgery. The infrared optical detector, on the other hand, is placed on the opposite side together with the monitor displaying the 3D model and the Stryker Team Specialist's workstation (fig. 2) [44].
The procedure is conducted under spinal anaesthesia and sedation or under general anaesthesia, in supine decubitus on the operating bed. The use of a traction system is not essential; the choice is based on the surgeon's preference. Preparation of the surgical field requires an additional sterile field on the region of the iliac crest contralateral to that of the prosthetic implant. The preliminary fixation of the optical sensor is achieved with the application of two or three pins on the iliac crest. Once the transmitter is attached to these pins, it communicates with the software through the infrared camera. It is essential that the fixation is stable and that there is smooth communication between the transmitter and the infrared sensor before starting the surgical procedure. Usually before proceeding with the incision, the landmark at the level of the patella or the anterior tibial tuberosity (monocortical pin) is also applied.
Some authors [41] suggest the usefulness of slightly modifying the classic anterior approach to facilitate the trochanteric exposure where one of the landmarks will be applied. The approach is directed more obliquely, towards the thigh. Following the intermuscular plane between the tensor fascia lata and the

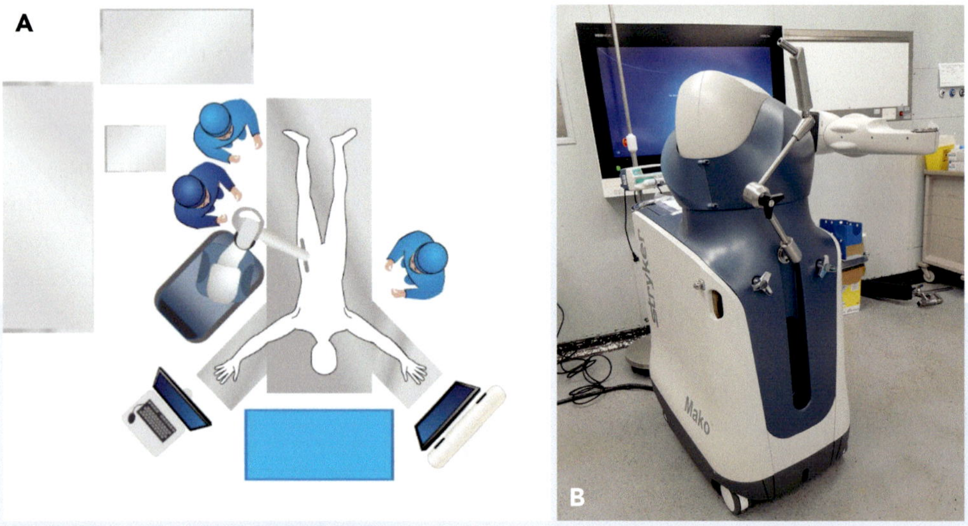

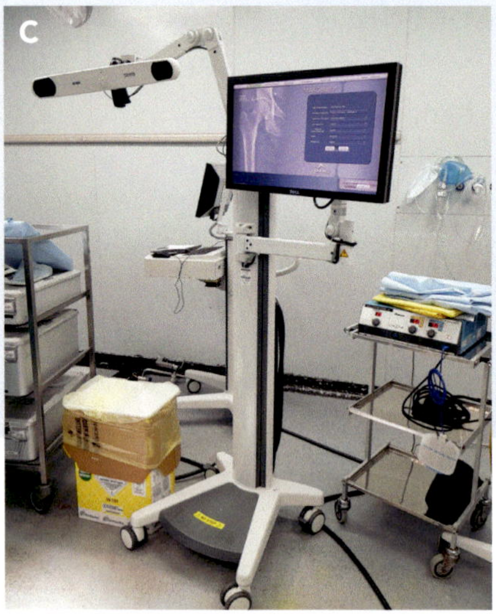

Figure 2 A) Setting suggested by Stryker. B) The MAKO Robot system or 'motor arm', positioned on the side of the hip to be operated.
C) Infrared sensor and monitor placed on the side opposite the limb to be operated on.
Courtesy of Stryker

sartorius, the branches of the lateral circumflex artery are ligated and the rectus femoris and its reflex tendon are detached in a disto-proximal direction. This is done in order to obtain a wide exposure of the joint capsule up to its insertion on the anterosuperior acetabular rim. Having performed the capsulotomy along the fibres of the iliofemoral ligament, the anterosuperior margin of the acetabulum is exposed. Here, the first landmark is to be applied. Distally, the greater trochanter must be exposed for the implantation of a second landmark, possibly laterally and distally where the trochanter cortical thickness guarantees a more stable fixation. The three landmarks applied so far will be acquired by the sensor through a pointer or probe, in order to establish a real-time correspondence between the patient's anatomy and the 3D model, before starting the preparation of the articular surfaces.
The femoral component is approached first. The Enhanced Femoral Workflow modality requires the dislocation of the hip and the acquisition of the cervicocephalic landmarks for the identification of the osteotomy line. The femoral stem is implanted in order to take advantage of the assistance in verifying the final version of the stem. All this while maintaining a margin of correction in the version of the subsequent acetabular implant in order to respect the desired values of combined anteversion. In the anterior approach, sacrificing these verification parameters, the saving of technical time and femoral exposure may justify the preference of a manual cervical osteotomy, as provided in the Express Femoral Workflow. After the osteotomy and removal of the femoral head, the exposure of the femur is completed by partial release of the femoral insertions of the pubofemoral and ischiofemoral ligaments. This facilitates the anterior translation of the greater trochanter in the extension and external rotation manoeuvres required for the preparation of the femoral canal.
When preparing the acetabulum, the cotyloid rim and the round ligament of the femur must be removed. On the other hand, removal of any osteophytes is not performed before mapping the acetabular cup with the probe or pointer. This will eventually be done after the acetabular cup implantation. After verifying the correspondence between the intraoperative acquisitions and the pre-operative CT data, with a maximum margin of error of 1 mm, the software will reproduce the 3D model of the acetabulum on the monitor (fig. 3). The surgeon will then apply the chosen ream-

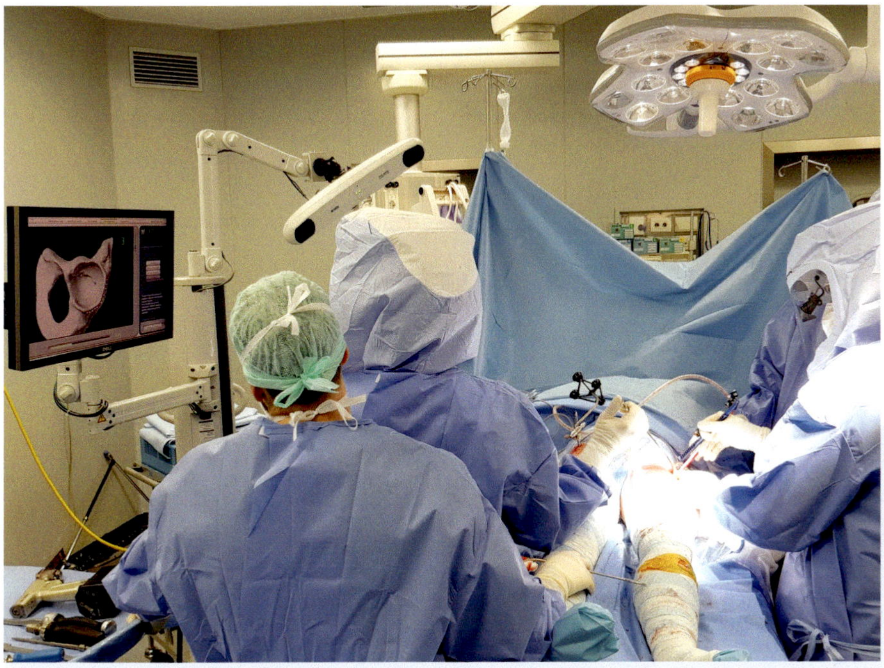

Figure 3
The acquisition of the acetabular landmarks with the pointer or probe

er to the MAKO Robot system by manually introducing it into the acetabular cavity. This will then be displayed on the monitor. The surgeon will have the option to adjust the tilt and version according to the parameters defined in the planning, shown on the monitor, or according to corrections deemed necessary (fig. 4). Having found the desired orientation, the surgeon will instruct the Stryker Specialist to 'lock' the chosen position.

The surgeon will be allowed at this point to proceed with the preparation of the cotyloid surface without variation on any vector other than the axial thrust vector to the reamer. A chromatic and metric guide will be reproduced on the monitor during reaming to provide the surgeon with constant feedback on the acquired depth (fig. 5). As already mentioned, an acoustic system will provide an alarm if the desired value is exceeded, blocking the action of the motor arm to protect the acetabular wall. It will be possible to proceed with the preparation with progressive drills or directly with the one selected pre-operatively for the cup seating. The implantation operation will retrace the same steps in terms of positioning and 'locking' as described for the reaming (fig. 6). Finally, the operation will be completed with the preparation of the femoral canal, the implantation of the chosen prosthetic stem and the final verification of conformity with the combined length and offset parameters defined by the pre-operative planning (figs. 7-8).

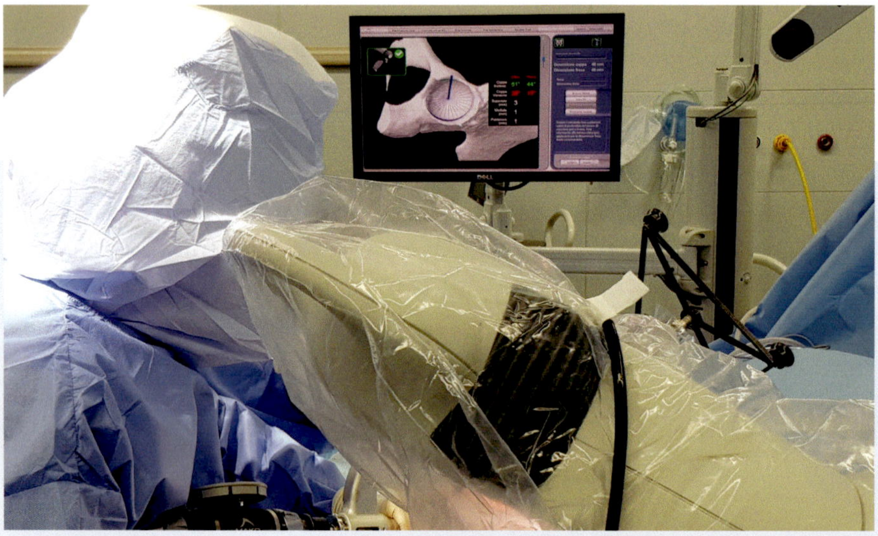

Figure 4 The surgeon sees the reamer reproduced on the screen as a ridged dome and looks for its correct orientation prior to engagement

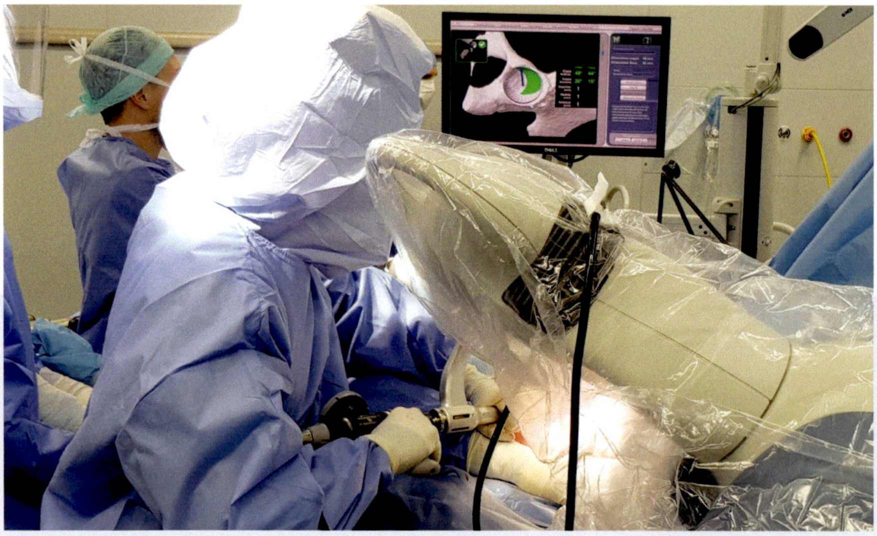

Figure 5 The coloured guide indicates the surface to be reamed

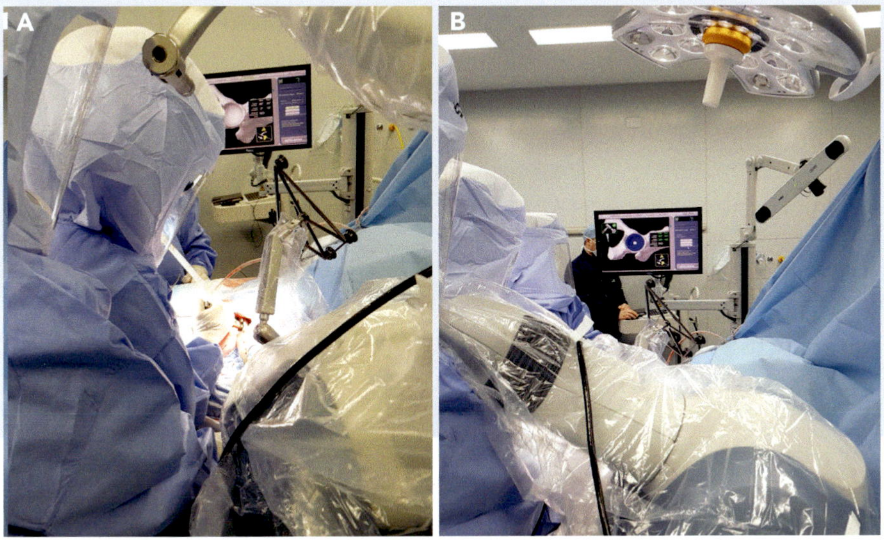

Figure 6
A) Manual seating of the prosthetic cup in the acetabulum.
B) 3D model representation in order to achieve the correct inclination and version

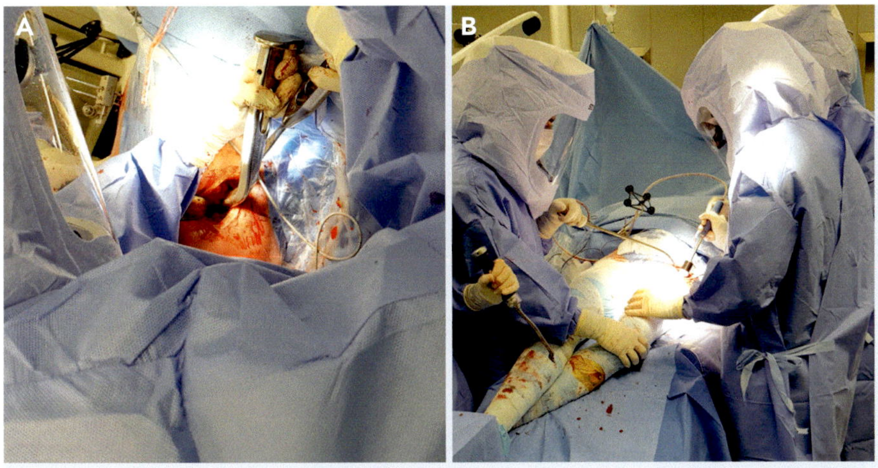

Figure 7
A) Preparation of the femoral canal.
B) Implantation of the head after performing the appropriate checks with the trial components and the stability manoeuvres

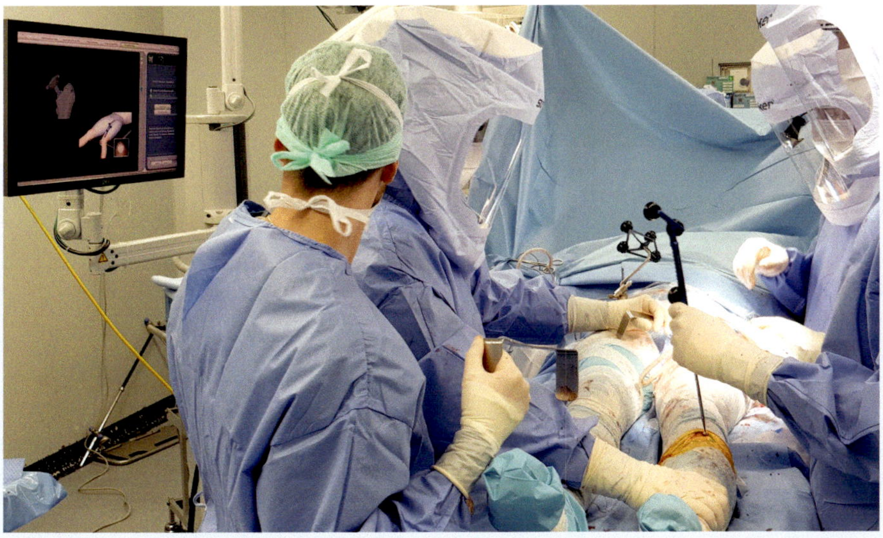

Figure 8
Final assisted checks

Authors' experience and clinical cases

The experience of using robotic assistance with the Rio MAKO ROBOT system (Stryker, FL, USA) at the hip surgery unit of the Policlinico di Abano Terme, Padua, began thanks to the efforts of Dr Camporese and his collaborators in 2017. The case history now reaches 200 implants with the minimally invasive anterior approach. The clinical cases shown as examples in the following pages are taken from this case history.

CASE REPORT 1

50-year-old female patient. Severe arthrosis due to aseptic necrosis of the left femoral head (X-rays and MRI). -7 mm heterometry on the left, resolved post-operatively. Pre and post-operative X-ray evaluations and surgical timing. The patient was not transfused during her hospital stay, and was discharged to an external rehabilitation centre during the second post-operative day.

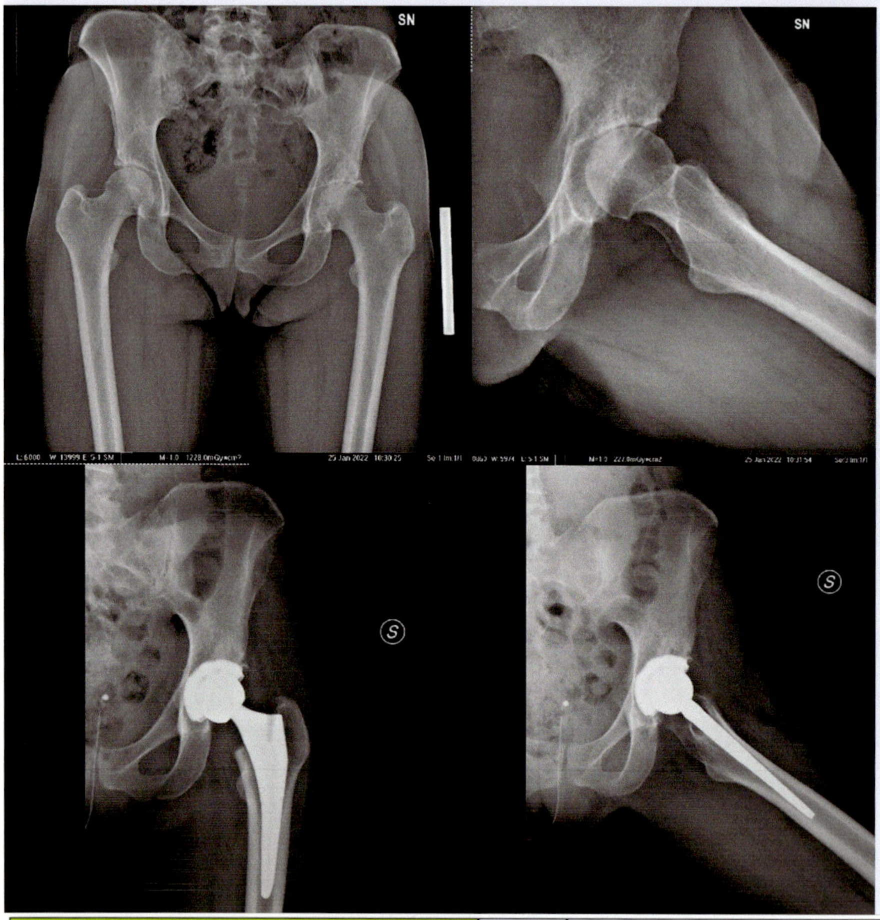

Validato	✓ VALIDA - DETTAGLI VALIDAZIONE	Registrato	Operato

Tempi operatori

Tempo	Data registrata	Ora registrata	Data	Ora
ARRIVO NEL BLOCCO			17/02/2022	13.40
PREPARAZIONE PAZIENTE			17/02/2022	13.45
INDUZIONE ANESTESIA			17/02/2022	13.50
ENTRATA IN SALA			17/02/2022	14.15
INIZIO INTERVENTO - INCISIONE			17/02/2022	14.40
FINE INTERVENTO - SUTURA			17/02/2022	15.38
FINE MEDICAZIONE			17/02/2022	15.45
RISVEGLIO			17/02/2022	00.00
USCITA DALLA SALA			17/02/2022	15.50
INIZIO PULIZIA			17/02/2022	
FINE PULIZIA			17/02/2022	
USCITA DAL BLOCCO			17/02/2022	

CASE REPORT 2

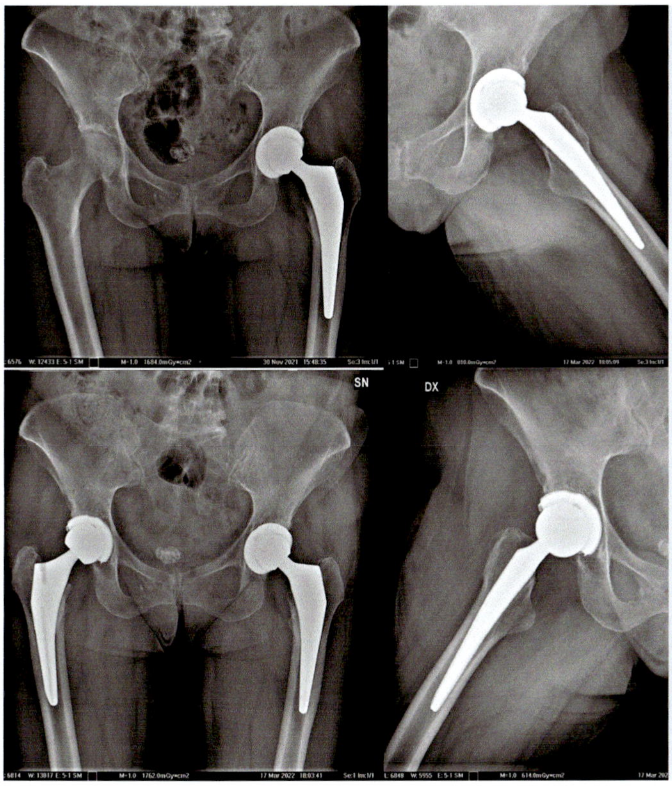

78-year-old female patient. Bilateral coxarthrosis. On the left the patient had already been treated elsewhere with an outcome of +2.5 cm dysmetria on the left. Pre- and post-operative X-rays. The patient was admitted to the rehabilitation ward on the first post-operative day, and was not transfused during her stay. The dysmetria was resolved.

10

CASE REPORT 3

Patient 37 years old, male. Severe right arthrosis with CAM deformity; no heterometry; pre and post-operative X-ray and surgical timing. Discharged home on post-operative day 4.

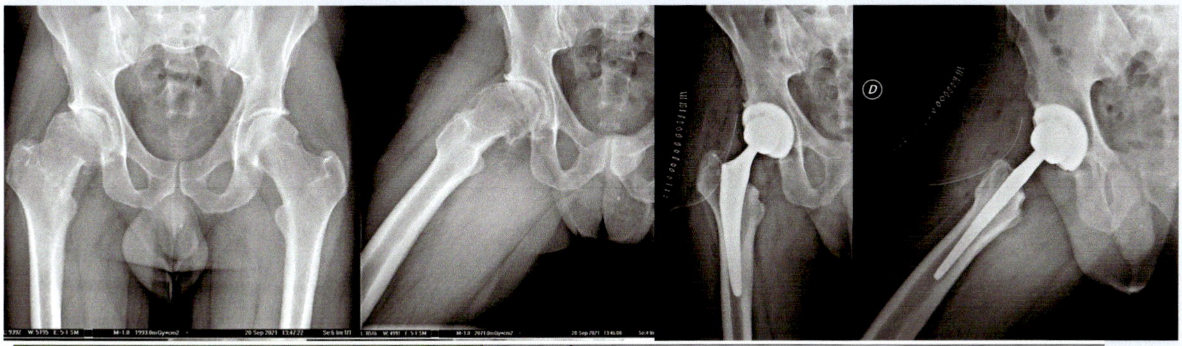

Validato | VALIDA - DETTAGLI VALIDAZIONE | Registrato | Operato

Tempi operatori

Tempo	Data registrata	Ora registrata	Data	Ora
ARRIVO NEL BLOCCO			05/11/2021	09.50
PREPARAZIONE PAZIENTE			05/11/2021	10.00
INDUZIONE ANESTESIA			05/11/2021	10.30
ENTRATA IN SALA			05/11/2021	10.55
INIZIO INTERVENTO - INCISIONE			05/11/2021	11.25
FINE INTERVENTO - SUTURA			05/11/2021	12.35
FINE MEDICAZIONE			05/11/2021	12.40
RISVEGLIO			05/11/2021	00.00
USCITA DALLA SALA			05/11/2021	12.45
INIZIO PULIZIA			05/11/2021	
FINE PULIZIA			05/11/2021	
USCITA DAL BLOCCO			05/11/2021	

CASE REPORT 4

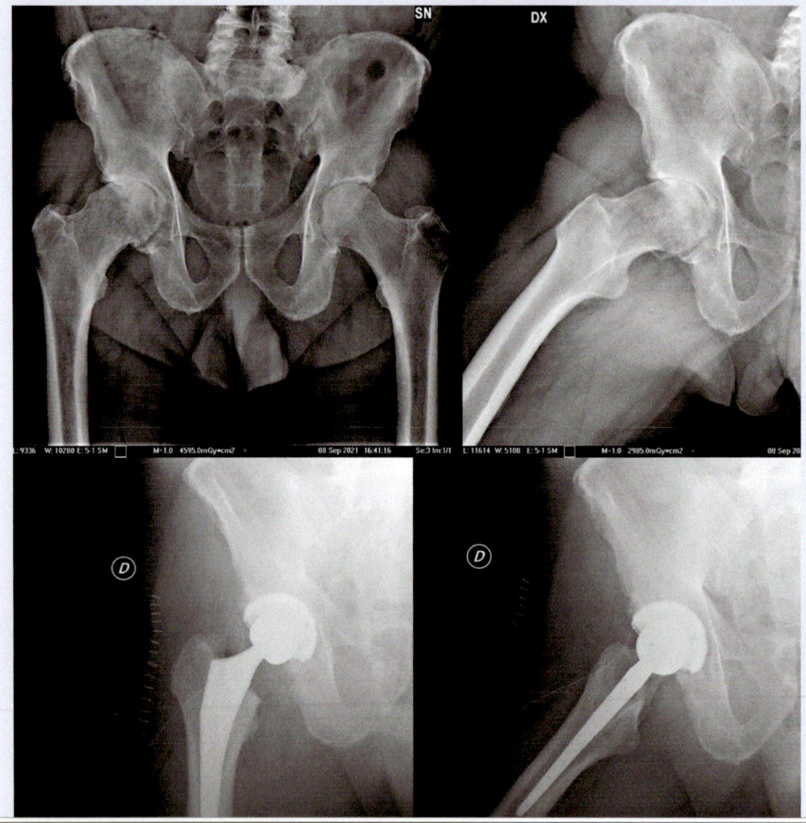

Patient 65 years old, male. Severe right cox-arthrosis. No heterometry. Pre- and post-operative X-ray and surgical timing. Discharged home on post-operative day 4.

Validato | VALIDA - DETTAGLI VALIDAZIONE | Registrato | Operato

Tempi operatori

Tempo	Data registrata	Ora registrata	Data	Ora
ARRIVO NEL BLOCCO			05/11/2021	07.10
PREPARAZIONE PAZIENTE			05/11/2021	07.20
INDUZIONE ANESTESIA			05/11/2021	07.45
ENTRATA IN SALA			05/11/2021	08.15
INIZIO INTERVENTO - INCISIONE			05/11/2021	08.40
FINE INTERVENTO - SUTURA			05/11/2021	10.00
FINE MEDICAZIONE			05/11/2021	10.05
RISVEGLIO			05/11/2021	00.00
USCITA DALLA SALA			05/11/2021	10.30
INIZIO PULIZIA			05/11/2021	
FINE PULIZIA			05/11/2021	
USCITA DAL BLOCCO			05/11/2021	

Limitations of robotic surgery

The current main limitations of robotic care are cost, surgical time and potential complications related to it. The economic aspect can be considered as the main factor limiting its diffusion. To get an idea, costs of $793,000 are reported for the MAKO system, a sum not including maintenance costs [47]. The economic budget, in fact, includes not only the equipment and the software, but also preparatory and intra-operative assistance, additional material compared to the conventional implant (pins and disposable items), maintenance and updating costs. To these must also be added the expenses related to higher average surgical and operating room times. Finally, the need for CT scanning represents not only an economic but also a biological cost for the patient. Patient exposure is only partly mitigated by eliminating the need for intraoperative radioscopic control. Rather, the operators' exposure is reduced.

The main antithesis to these considerations is the prospect of cost amortisation in the long term due to the benefits arising from its

use. Moreover, it is to be expected that the expansion of its use will produce a gradual reduction in costs, also due to the effect of increased demand on supply [48-49].
In terms of surgical times, a progressive reduction in the difference between conventional and robotic prosthetic surgery can be traced over time. In 2013, a study reported that robotic surgery took an average of 27 minutes longer [50]. When considering the time required for the assisted procedure, the influence of the surgical learning curve and possible intraoperative technical difficulties must be taken into account. Considering the latter, estimates reveal a declining trend over time (from 18% in cases in 2003 [51] to 10% in 2011 [52]).
As for the surgical learning curve, a 2015 study showed that increasing experience correlated with a reduction in time, from an average of 80 minutes for the first 35 cases, to an average of 69 minutes after 70 cases [53]. Perazzini and colleagues suggest an average of 30 procedures in quick succession for the acquisition of a good proficiency [42]. The reduction in surgical time also reduces possible related complications, i.e. anaesthesiological and infectious risks [39]. In addition, greater surgical experience and skill leads to a reduction in tissue damage. This is also a factor in the placement of the landmarks, over time there is an advantage in the rate of heterotopic ossifications, which is higher in the beginning [54-55].

Advantages of robotic surgery

Regarding estimates of the benefits of robotic assistance in hip prosthetic surgery, the limitations of the recent introduction and the slow spread of its use related to costs should be noted.
However, the trend of results in the literature is increasingly in favour of its use. The comparison in terms of clinical outcome has not changed the first findings of substantial equivalence of the two methods, although to date there is evidence of a superiority of robotic surgery also in this parameter [55,56]. On the other hand, the advantages in terms of reduced intra- and perioperative complications, accuracy of implant positioning and compliance with lower limb metrics were consolidated. In terms of the accuracy of the femoral implant, superiority was evaluated in terms of fit, varus-valgus orientation, alignment, as well as reduction of intraoperative fracture complications [51,57]. Studies on cadavers have documented an increase in bone-implant contact from 60.1% to 93.2% when comparing manual and robotic techniques [58]. Given this finding, a better preservation of the bone-stock is also documented, which is maximised by the use of short stems [50]. Better bone-stock preservation is also present at pelvis level. This is suggested by the identification of a significant correlation between robotic assistance and the use of smaller acetabular cups [59]. In the context of acetabular alignment, there are many evidences of cup seating in the 'safety zones' as defined by Lewinnek [60,61]. The relevance of these findings has certainly decreased with the evolution of the concept of implant stability as a function of spino-pelvic dynamics. In this field, the new frontiers of technological development involve systems that also include these considerations, such as the 'optimised positioning system' produced by the Corin Group, UK (OPS, Corin, Cirencester, UK), which has already published encouraging results [62]. Due to its direct clinical implication, accuracy in the preservation of lower limb metrics must also be valued. Differences in these correlate not only with possible patient dissatisfaction [63], but also with trochanteric pain [64], limping [65], lumbar pain [66], and even possible nerve suffering from stretching [67,42]. Estimates of the mean length discrepancy following conventional hip replacement surgery have been reported in the literature to range from 1 to 15.9 mm [68]. Analysing this parameter, the superiority of robotic assistance over conventional surgery emerged from the very first studies [51,62], with statistical mean error of length discrepancy in the order of 1 mm in robotic surgery [69]. Certainly, the benefit is attributable to the possibility of planning the implant

with great precision thanks to technological elaboration. It must be remembered that to date the role of clinical findings remains irreplaceable: the dysmetria, in fact, may be true (structural), or apparent (functional), and the two types may variously combine in some patients. Also, it should be pointed out that the robotic system analyses the length parameter only on the hip, not on the entire lower limb, and in a static position. Therefore, medical collaboration from planning to implementation remains essential, comforting the more traditionalists.

Conclusions

Although hip prosthetic surgery is considered a successful procedure, some challenges remain, motivating continued refinement of the technique [27]. Recent literature reports that the need for revision after primary surgery varies between 3% and 8% at 14 years [70]. The main causes identified are in order of frequency: aseptic loosening (48%), dislocations (15%), periprosthetic fractures (10%) and infectious issues (9%) [70-71]. The risk of having to undergo revision surgery understandably correlates not only with the characteristics of the implant but also with the age of the patient. For implants performed before the age of 50, a 30% risk of possible future revision has been estimated [71].

We must then consider that, regardless of gender and race, many other variables influence the anatomical features of the hip, some constitutive others pathological [27]. It is estimated that up to 6% of the healthy population, for example, has acetabular retroversion [72]. This percentage increases to 20% in subjects with coxarthrosis and up to 42% in subjects with Legg-Calvé-Perthes disease [72-73]. The prevalence of hip dysplasia varies between 3.6% and 4.3% in the adult population (2017 data, on Chinese population) [74], while that of coxa profunda varies between 5% and 20% in the literature [75].

Further complexity to the subjective anatomical variability is added by spino-pelvic dynamics [76]. With these premises, each hip seems to be defined by an enormous combination of anatomical and functional parameters. The use of robotic assistance appears to be a valid strategy towards the 'customisation' of implants. These customised implants are intended to be more anatomically and biomechanically appropriate to the single patient and therefore also more durable over time [27]. The most recent results are confirming this potential. This is in addition to the fact that technology is proving effective in reducing the margin of human error, supporting surgical skill in optimising and reproducing the result.

In a final balance between advantages and limitations of robotic assistance, minimally invasive surgery appears to have a synergistic effect on the former and a compensatory effect on the latter [77].

The main advantages of minimally invasive surgery, which are increasingly recognised and appreciated, are as follows. This surgery leads to a decrease in muscle-tendon and vascular tissue damage with a consequent reduction in blood loss and transfusions [78]. Further benefit of this approach comes from the impact on the immunohistochemical response produced by the surgical procedure. A favourable change in the chemical factors of inflammation, evidenced by a decrease in the values of pro-inflammatory cytokines (IL6, IL8 and TNF-alpha) [79]. Furthermore, the volumetric reduction of 'surgical dead space', shorter surgical times and easier post-surgical pain control must be considered. These factors are associated with a reduction in hospitalisation time and a faster functional recovery, which also reaches high levels of activity [80]. Finally, this surgery has the advantage of a reduced complication coefficient (infections, DVT, instability). These benefits make the combination of robotic assistance and minimally invasive anterior approach desirable at scale, as it is promisingly effective and sustainable.

Bibliography

1. Deep K, Shankar S, Mahendra A. Computer assisted navigation in total knee and hip arthroplasty.

Sicot J. 2017; 3:50.
2. Patel PD, Potts A, Froimson MI. The Dislocating Hip Arthroplasty. Prevention and Treatment. J Arthroplasty 2007;22(4 Suppl 1):86-90.
3. Australian Orthopaedic Association National Joint Replacement Registry (AOANJRR). Hip, knee and shoulder arthroplasty 2018. www.aoa.org.au.
4. Bozic KJ, Kurtz SM, Lau E, et al. The epidemiology of revision total hip arthroplasty in the United States. J Bone Joint Surg Am 2009 91(1):128-33.
5. Woo RY, Morrey BF. Dislocation after total hip arthroplasty. J Bone Joint Surg Am 1982;64(9):1295-306.
6. Sanchez-Sotelo J, Haidukewych GJ, Boberg CJ Hospital cost of dislocation after primary total hip arthroplasty J Bone Surg Am 2006;88(2):290-4.
7. Abdel MP, Cross MB, Yasen AT, Haddad FS. The functional and financial impact of isolated and recurrent dislocation after total hip arthroplasty Bone Joint J 2015;97-B(8):1046-49.
8. Charnley J. A biomechanical analysis of the use of cement to anchor the femoral head prosthesis J Bone Joint Surg Br 1965; 47:354-63.
9. Charnley J. An artificial bearing in the hip joint: implications in biological lubrification. Fed Proc 1966;25(3):1079-81.
10. Manley M, Ong K, Lau E, Kurtz SM. Effect of volume on total hip arthroplasty revision rates in the United States Medicare population. J Bone Joint Surg Am 2008;90(11)2446–51.
11. Solomon DH, Losina E, Baron JA, et al. Contribution of hospital characteristics to the volume-outcome relationship: dislocation and infection following total hip replacement surgery. Arthritis Rheum 2002;46(9):2436–44.
12. Shervin N, et al. Orthopaedic procedure volume and patient outcomes: a systematic literature review. Clin Orthop Relat Res 2007;457: 35–41.
13. Padgett DE, Hendrix SL, et al. Effectiveness of an acetabular positioning device in primary total hip arthroplasty. HSS J 2005;1(1): 64–67.
14. Dorr LD, Wan Z, Malik A, et al. A comparison of surgeon estimation and computed tomographic measurement of femoral component anteversion in cementless total hip arthroplasty. J Bone Joint Surg Am 2009;91(11):2598–604.
15. Callanan MC, Jarrett B, Bragdon CR, et al. The John Charnley Award: risk factors for cup malpositioning: quality improvement through a joint registry at a tertiary hospital. Clin Orthop Relat Res 2011;469(2):319-29.
16. Barrack RL, Krempec JA, Clohisy JC, et al. Accuracy of acetabular component position in hip arthroplasty. J Bone Joint Surg Am 2013;95(19):1760–768.
17. Subramanian P, Wainwright TW, Bahadori S and Middleton RG. A review of the evolution of robotic-assisted total hip arthroplasty HIP International 2019;29(3):232–38.
18. Wasterlain AS, Buza JA, 3rd, Thakkar SC, et al. Navigation and robotics in total hip arthroplasty. JBJS Rev 2017;5(3):e2.
19. Higgins BT, Barlow DR, Heagerty NE, Lin TJ. Anterior vs. posterior approach for total hip arthroplasty, a systematic review and meta-analysis. J Arthroplasty. 2015;30(3):419–34.
20. Martin CT, Pugely AJ, Gao Y, Clark CR. A Comparison of Hospital Length of Stay and Short-Term Morbidity Between the Anterior and the Posterior Approaches to Total Hip Arthroplasty. J Arthroplasty. 2013;28(5):849-54.
21. Galakatos GR. Direct Anterior Total Hip Arthroplasty. Review Mo Med. 2018;115(6):537–41.
22. Lewinnek GE, Lewis JL, Tarr R, Compere CL, Zimmerman JR. Dislocations after total hip-replacement arthroplasties. J Bone Joint Surg Am. 1978;60(2):217–20.
23. Lazennec JY, Thauront F, Robbins CB, Pour AE. Acetabular and femoral anteversions in standing position are outside the proposed safe zone after total hip arthroplasty. J Arthroplast. 2017; 32(11):3550–556.
24. Rivière C, Lazic S, Villet L, Wiart Y, Allwood SM, Cobb J. Kinematic alignment technique for total hip and knee arthroplasty: the personalized implant positioning surgery. EFORT Open Rev. 2018;3(3):98–105.
25. Seagrave KG, Troelsen A, Malchau H, Husted H, Gromov K. Acetabular cup position and risk of dislocation in primary total hip arthroplasty. Acta Orthop. 2017; 88(1):10-17.
26. Abdel MP, von Roth P, Jennings MT, Hanssen AD, Pagnano MW. What safezone? The vast majority of dislocated THAs are within the Lewinnek safe zone for acetabular component position. Clin Orthop Relat Res. 2016;474(2):386-91.
27. Rivière C, Vendittoli PA. Personalized Hip and Knee Joint Replacement. Springer Ed. 2020.
28. Ranawac CS, Chitranjan S, Maynard MJ. Modern techniques of cemented total hip arthroplasty.

Tech Orthop 1991; 6:17–25.
29. Widmer KH, Zurfluh B. Compliant positioning of total hip components for optimal range of motion. J Orthop Res. 2004;22(4):815-21.
30. Nakashima Y, Hirata M, Akiyama M, et al. Combined anteversion technique reduced the dislocation in cementless total hip arthroplasty. Int Orthop. 2014;38(1):27-32.
31. Jolles BM, Zangger P, Leyvraz PF. Factors predisposing to dislocation after primary total hip arthroplasty: a multivariate analysis. J Arthroplasty 2002;17(3):282–88.
32. Dorr LD, Malik A, Dastane M, Wan Z. Combined anteversion technique for total hip arthroplasty. Clin Orthop Relat Res 2009; 467(1):119–127.
33. Tezuka T, Heckmann ND Bodner RJ Functional Safe Zone for Total Hip Arthroplasty: Why the Lewinnek Safe Zone is not always predictive of Stability. The Journal of Arthroplasty 2019;34(1):3-8.
34. Kawanade V, Dorr LD, Wan Z. Predictability of acetabular component angular change with postural shift from standing to sitting position. J Bone Jt Surg Am 2014;96(12):978-86.
35. Lembeck B, Mueller O, Reize P, Wuelker N. Pelvic tilt makes acetabular cup navigation inaccurate. Acta Orthop 2005;76(4):517-23.
36. Esposito CI, Carrol KM, Sculco PK, et al. Total hip arthoplasty patients with fixed spinopelvic alignement are at higher risk of hip dislocation. J Arthroplasty 2018;33(5):1449-454.
37. Jacofsky DJ, Allen M. Robotics in arthroplasty: a comprehensive review. J Arthroplasty 2016;31(10):2353-363.
38. Nogler M, Maurer H, Wimmer C, et al. Knee pain caused by a fiducial marker in the medial femoral condyle: a clinical and anatomic study of 20 cases. Acta Orthop Scand 2001;72(5):477–480.
39. Schulz AP, Seide K, Queitsch C, et al. Results of total hip replacement using the ROBODOC surgical assistant system: clinical outcome and evaluation of complications for 97 procedures. Int J Med Robot 2007;3(4):301–306.
40. Nakamura N, Sugano N, Nishii T, et al. Robot-assisted primary cementless total hip arthroplasty using surface registration techniques: a short-term clinical report. Int J Comput Assist Radiol Surg 2009;4(2)157–162.
41. Perazzini P, Trevisan M, Sembenini P, Alberton F et al. The MakoTM robotic arm-assisted total hip arthroplasty using direct anterior approach: surgical technique, skills and pitfalls. Acta Biomed 2020;91(4-S): 21-30.
42. Catani F. Robotic surgery for total hip and knee replacement. Ed Minerva Medica S.p.a. 2021.
43. Dungy DS, Netravali NA. Active robotics for total hip arthroplasty. Am J Orthop 2016;45(4):256-59.
44. Stryker, Mako Total Hip Direct Anterior Approach Surgical Reference Guide.
45. Perets I, Mu BH, Mont MA, Rivkin G, Kandel L e Domb BG. Current topics in robotic-assisted total hip arthroplasty: a review. Hip International 2020;30(2):118-124.
46. Perazzini P, Marangon A, Montanari M, Trevisan M Robotically-assisted Total Hip Arthroplasty using the Direct Anterior Approach (DAA) in "Robotic surgery for total hip and knee replacement". Catani F, Minerva Medica Ed. 2021.
47. Lang JE, Mannava S, Floyd AJ, et al. Robotic systems in orthopaedic surgery. J Bone Joint Surg Br 2011;93(10):1296-299.
48. Solow RM. A contribution to the theory of economic growth. Q J Econ 1956;70:65–94.
49. Swan TW. Economic growth and capital accumulation. Econ Rec 1956;32:334–361.
50. Lim SJ, Ko KR, Park CW, et al. Robot-assisted primary cementless THA with a short femoral stem: a prospective randomized short-term outcome study. Comput Aided Surg 2015;20(1):41–46.
51. Honl M, Dierk O, Gauck C, et al Comparison of robotic-assisted and manual implantation of a primary total hip replacement. A prospective study. J Bone Joint Surg Am 2003;85(8):1470-478.
52. Chun YS, Kim KI, Cho YJ et al. Causes and patterns of aborting a robot-assisted arthroplasty. J Arthroplasty 2011;26(4):621-625.
53. Redmond JM, Gupta A, Hammarstedt JE, et al. The learning curve associated with robotic-assisted total hip arthroplasty. J Arthroplasty 2015;30(1):50–54.
54. Siebel T and Käfer W. Clinical outcome following robotic assisted versus conventional THA: a controlled and prospective study of seventy-one patients. Z Orthop Ihre Grenzgeb 2005;143(4):391–398.
55. Nakamura N, Sugano N, Nishii T, et al. A comparison between robotic-assisted and manual implantation of cementless THA. Clin Orthop Relat Res 2010; 468(4):1072-1081.
56. Bargar WL, Parise CA, Hankins A, et al. Fourteen year follow-up of randomized clinical trials of

active robotic-assisted total hip arthroplasty. J Arthroplasty 2018;33(3) 810–814.
57. Nishihara S, Sugano N, Nishii T, et al. Comparison between hand rasping and robotic milling for stem implantation in cementless THA. J Arthroplasty 2006;21(7:)957–966.
58. Wu L, Hahne HJ, Hassenpflug J. The dimensional accuracy of preparation of femoral cavity in cementless THA. J Zhejiang Univ Sci 2004;5(10):1270–1278.
59. Suarez-Ahedo C, Gui C, Martin TJ, et al. Robotic-arm assisted THA results in smaller acetabular cup size in relation to the femoral head size: a matched-pair controlled study. Hip Int 2017;27(2)147–152.
60. Domb BG, El Bitar YF, Sadik AY, et al. Comparison of robotic-assisted and conventional acetabular cup placement in THA: a matched-pair controlled study. Clin Orthop Relat Res 2014;472(1):329–336.
61. Domb BG, Redmond JM, Louis SS, et al. Accuracy of component positioning in 1980 total hip arthroplasties: a comparative analysis by surgical technique and mode of guidance. J Arthroplasty 2015;30(12):2208–218.
62. Jerabek SA, Carroll K, Maratt JD, et al. Accuracy of cup positioning and achieving desired hip length and offset following robotic THA. In: Poster S18 presented at 14th annual CAOS meeting, Milan, Italy, 18–21 June 2014.
63. Wylde V, Whitehouse SL, Taylor AH, et al. Prevalence and functional impact of patient-perceived leg lenght discrepancy after hip replacement. Int Orthop 2009;33(4):905-909.
64. Sayed-Noor AS, Sjodén GO. Greater trochanteric pain after total hip arthroplasty: the incidence, clinical outcome and associated factors. HIP Int 2006;16(3):202-206.
65. Tanaka r, Shigematsu M, Motooka T, et al. Factors influencing the improvement of gait ability after total hip arthroplasty. J Arthroplasty 2010;25(6):982-985.
66. Clarck CR, Huddleston HD, Schoch EP, et al. Leg-lenght discrepancy after total hip arthroplasty. J Am Acad Orthop Surg 2006;14(1):38-45.
67. Hofmann AA, Skrzynski MC. Leg-length Inequality and Nerve Palsy in total hip arthroplasty: a Lawer awaits! Orthopedics 2000;23(9):943-944.
68. Konyves A, Bannister GC. The importance of leg lenght discrepancy after total hip arthroplasty. J Bone Joint Surg Br 2005;87(2):155-157.
69. Nawabi DH, Conditt MA, Ranawat AS, et al. Haptically guided robotic technology in THA: a cadaveric investigation. Proc Inst Mech Eng H 2013;227(3):302–309.
70. Ferguson RJ, Palmer AJ, Taylor A, Porter ML, Malchau H, Glyn-Jones S. Hip replacement. Lancet. 2018;392(10158):1662–671.
71. Commitee NS. National Joint Registry for England, Wales, Northern Ireland and the Isle of Man: 15th annual report 2017. National Joint Registry Centre. 2018.
72. Wassilew GI, Heller MO, Janz V, Perka C, Müller M, Renner L. High prevalence of acetabular retroversion in asymptomatic adults: a 3D CT-based study. Bone Jt J. 2017;99-B(12):1584–589.
73. Krebs V, Incavo SJ, Shields WH. The anatomy of the acetabulum: what is normal? Clin Orthop. 2009;467(4):868-875.
74. Tian FD, et al. Prevalence of developmental dysplasia of the hip in Chinese adults: a cross-sectional survey. Chin Med J. 2017;130(11):1261–268.
75. Diesel CV, Ribeiro TA, Coussirat C, Scheidt RB, Macedo CA, Galia CR. Coxa profunda in the diagnosis of pincer-type femoroacetabular impingement and its prevalence in asymptomatic subjects. Bone Joint J. 2015;97-B(4):478–483.
76. Endo K, Suzuki H, Nishimura H, Tanaka H, Shishido T, Yamamoto K. Characteristics of sagittal spino-pelvic alignment in Japanese young adults. Asian Spine J. 2014;8(5):599-604.
77. Reininga IH, Zijlstra W, Wagenmakers R, Stevens M. et al. Minimally invasive and computer-navigated total hip arthroplasty: a qualitative and systematic review of the literature. BMC Musculoskelet Disord. 2010;11:92.
78. Chimento GF, Pavone V, Sharrock N, Kahn B, Cahill J, Sculco TP: Minimally invasive total hip arthroplasty: a prospective randomized study. J Arthroplasty 2005;20(2):139-144.
79. Bergin PF, Doppelt JD, Kephart CJ, et al. Comparison of minimally invasive direct anterior versus posterior total hip arthroplasty based on inflammation and muscle damage markers. J Bone Joint Surg Am. 2011;93(15):1392-398.
80. Lloyd JM, Wainwright T, Middleton RG. What is the role of minimally invasive surgery in a fast track hip and knee replacement pathway? Ann R Coll Surg Engl. 2012 Apr;94(3):148-51.

CHAPTER 11

The anterior lateral decubitus intermuscolar approach in hip arthroplasty

Serafino Carta, Mattia Fortina

Department of Orthopaedics and Traumatology, Siena University Hospital, Italy

Introduction

For any surgical procedure the main priority is to obtain the resolution of the existing pathology, minimizing the anatomical damages unavoidably correlated to the surgical act.
In general, the dimension of the surgical access can directly quantify the extent of tissue damage caused by surgical procedure itself; hence, the attempt to limit the biological impact has led to the need of limiting the size of the incision. However, over time experience has shown that obsessive research of its dimensioning paradoxically exposes skin and underlying anatomical layers to worst damages, as well as to an increase in the risk of prosthetic components malpositioning and intraoperative complications.
Considering 'tissue sparing surgery', every surgical access must represent the best possible compromise between the attempt to minimize biological damage and the need to obtain optimal results, reproducible in terms of implant positioning within a reasonable duration of the surgical procedure.
Consequently, every single surgical access is strongly influenced by the personal skills and experience of the lead surgeon.
Therefore, specialists inevitably adapt the surgical procedure to their own experience, personalizing it in the small details but still maintaining a codified basic algorithm.
In addition to dimensions, a second fundamental aspect of the surgical access to be considered in the field of tissue sparing surgery regards its anatomical characteristics.
Concerning surgical approaches for hip replacement, the anterior approach (performed between sartorius and tensor fasciae latae muscles) appears to be the only anatomic route that allows the reaching of the hip joint without compromising structural, vascular and neural integrity of coxofemoral musculotendinous units.
Undoubtedly these features made this method the gold standard in hip surgery, representing the end-point of tissue sparing approach – which results in blood loss, post-operative pain and functional impotence reduction in the immediate – and in full and complete recovery of the prosthetic joint in the long-term, a key point in the forgotten prosthesis.
Practical application of the aforementioned features of anterior approach encountered many obstacles that conditioned its broad transmission.
The critical points proved to be related not so much to difficulties in performing the surgical access as such, but rather to the optimal exposure of the cup and the femur for their adequate preparation and the subsequent positioning of prosthetic components.

Consequences translated in a higher risk of intraoperative complications than traditional access routes, in terms of musculotendinous and neurovascular damage due to excessive tension during retraction, intraoperative fractures and implant malposition.

Prerequisites for ALDI approach (Anterior Lateral Decubitus Intermuscular Approach)

Criticalities described and reported in literature, as well as experiences gained in outpatient setting of specialized centers where anterior approach was regularly used, led us to consider supine positioning as the first and key reason of our reluctance to use this access. This was due to two main aspects, i.e. the preparation of the surgical field and the vision of both the acetabulum and the femoral metaphysis, in addition to the numerous difficulties related to their exposures in terms of excessive tension during retraction and consequent muscular lesions. This had us facing a paradox in which an access route that represents the gold standard of atraumaticity translates in a more damaging technique than the traditional access in terms of tissues integrity and preservation.

As mentioned above, the common experience in using the anterior access consists in positioning the patient in supine decubitus on the operating table, in contrast with the consolidated practice of traditional and most commonly used surgical accesses such as the posterolateral, the direct lateral and the antero-lateral as well.

Looking back, direct lateral and antero-lateral surgical accesses were initially described and performed with the patient positioned in supine decubitus, whilst, the postero-lateral entry was the only one to require a lateral decubitus related to the placement of the surgical window for obvious reasons.

Presumably the reasons why supine decubitus was commonly used at the beginning are related to the general surgical tradition and to its key role in the facilitation of the management of the anesthesia: possibly, the evolution in time of anesthesiologic techniques has allowed the use of different positions including the lateral one, in the attempt to optimize and facilitate the surgical procedure. In fact, in the field of orthopedic surgery it is now extremely common to place patients in various positions, thanks to the extremely versatile operating tables that allow to facilitate the surgery and to reduce intra-operative complications: this further underlines how significant the patient decubitus is.

For these reasons, coming from a consolidated experience of direct lateral access in lateral decubitus, we considered crucial to evaluate the possibility to perform anterior access while maintaining lateral decubitus with the aim of conserving the highest number of structures.

The need for valid and constant reference points in prosthetic surgery (for correct implant positioning) is now an established and indispensable element and has a fundamental relevance for shortening the learning curve, for optimal results and less complications when using a surgical access other than the usual one.

The assumptions made for the use of lateral decubitus were the following:

- the possibility to prepare the surgical field in the traditional way;
- the reduction of blood loss with respect to supine decubitus due to gravitational blood shift;
- a better joint and bone exposure with consequent reduction in the tension exerted on retractors because of the higher degree of movement of the lower limb in both extension and abduction, which result limited in supine decubitus even with the help of specific beds;
- an unchanged visual on the acetabulum that allows a preparation similar to the one performed with traditional accesses and, in particular in our own experience, with the direct lateral approach.

Once the chance to associate anterior access with lateral decubitus was contemplated, in 2007 we performed the first surgery. The case was of a female patient with normal BMI

and ideal cervical-diaphyseal parameters suffering from femoral neck fracture eligible for partial hip replacement. While selecting the first patient, we therefore relied on criteria that are unanimously considered valid in the use of the anterior access.
The first operation confirmed our theoretical assumptions to be correct and demonstrated that the surgery would be carried out without excessive difficulties, showing that the wider mobility of the lower limb permitted by lateral decubitus allowed for better access to the femoral meta-diaphysis in behalf of its preparation compared to that observed in procedures performed in supine decubitus.
Noticeably, the learning process has allowed us to refine the capsular release step and to determine a precise algorithm in its intraoperative timing.
The first case was followed by a second intervention of total hip replacement for femur fracture, as we considered this type of patients to be ideal as they did not have retractions or deformities typical of arthritis.
Over time, experience has enabled us to extend the indications to more complicated cases in terms of arthritic features, coxofemoral morphology and patient's morphometry.
At the end of this learning process, we were able to extend the use of this approach to all cases, regardless of patient's characteristics and joint pathology, while amplifying the use of ALDI approach also in severe dysplasia and acetabular and femoral revisions, as well as in periprosthetic fractures.
Obviously, the extension of the technique required us to conceive and adapt the possibility to extend the anterior access both proximally and distally: also, in this case we appreciated the advantages of lateral decubitus that appears to be essential to achieve this goal.
Ultimately, the path we took with the introduction of lateral decubitus allowed us to obtain a safe, tissue-sparing and versatile surgical access with the addition of proximal and distal extension. Since 2008 we have performed more than 2000 THA via ALDI Approach and approximately 200 THA revisions.

Surgical technique

The first step in a surgical procedure is to position the patient on the operating bed. As stated in the introduction, the ALDI approach involves direct anterior access to the hip with the patient positioned in lateral decubitus. Therefore, there are no substantial differences compared to the lateral decubitus positioning generally used in direct lateral access. In fact, compared to our previous experience with the latter nothing has changed except for a greater attention to the positioning of the patient on the edge of the operating bed on the posterior side of the patient; the use of sacral and pubic supports remains exactly the same. As shown in the picture (fig. 1), the draping and the preparation of the limb are the same as in the direct lateral access, whilst the landmarks for the skin incision are specific for the anterior access, i.e. a line that, starting one centimeter posterior to the anterior superior iliac spine, runs distally for a length of about 12 centimeters along the course of the fibers of the tensor fasciae latae muscle. The ideal extension of this line would reach the Gerdy's tubercle when keeping the limb aligned with the trunk.
Regarding the length of the skin incision in traditional surgical approaches, it is appropriate to perform a minimally invasive cut by reducing the length of the incision in the attempt to limit the musculotendinous damage as much as possible.
The length of the incision per se is not important in the anterior access, if not for cosmetic purposes only, because it exploits an intra-vascular and intra-nervous gap in the anatomical space between the tensor fasciae latae and the sartorius. This area has different dimensions depending on the height of the patient, so that a longer skin incision in a taller patient is not an indication of greater invasiveness, provided that the length of the anatomical interval described is respected, which in practice corresponds to the length of the tensor fasciae latae itself.
The incision of the skin and the dissection of the adipose tissue allow us to expose the tensor fasciae latae with the respective

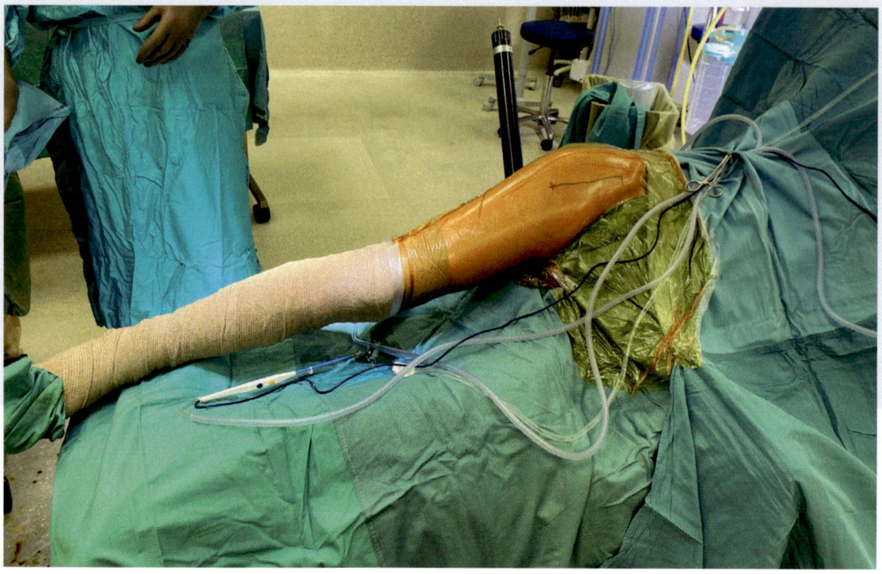

Figure 1 This image shows the positioning of the patient in lateral decubitus with the subsequent draping. The surgical incision is shown on the skin

epimysium that covers it (fig. 2). This thin fibrous sheath should be cut at the anterior third of the width of the muscle belly (fig. 3). To correctly locate this interval, the perforating arteries that cross the epimysium from the subcutis and enter the underlying muscle tissue, can be used as landmarks and should be cauterized prior to the incision of the thin fibrous sheath. The dissection and incision of the epimysium is performed by using thin scissors which exploit the point where the perforating artery crosses the fascia. The dissection proceeds in a cranial direction towards the anterior superior iliac spine (ASIS) (fig. 4). At this point it is possible to delicately dissect the anterior third of the tensor fasciae latae from the epimysium accessing the space that separates it from the sartorius (fig. 5). In order to facilitate this operation, it is of fundamental importance to reduce the tension of the muscle in question thanks to the abduction of the lower limb (fig. 6) that until now was in a neutral position. Already in this first step we take advantage of the freedom of movement of the lower limb permitted by the lateral decubitus. In fact, it allows to accompany the surgical phases by positioning the limb in order to minimize muscle tension and to obtain a better surgical window in terms of width and visibility.

Once the tensor is isolated and loaded posteriorly with the retractor 1, the fascia overlying the rectus femoris is exposed in the deeper layers; fibers of the rectus muscle are visible in transparency (fig. 7).

The thin fascia should be cut posteriorly to the margin of the rectus femoris, which is then loaded anteriorly with retractor 2 thus exposing a thin vascular branch that feeds the muscular belly at this level; the uncovered vessel is then cauterized (figs. 8-9).

After carefully incising the underlying fibrous septum, it is possible to expose the transverse branch of the lateral circumflex artery of the femur (CL) (fig. 10), which must be clamped and cauterized or ligated according to the operator's preference (fig. 11).

Once the transverse branch of the circumflex artery has been dissected, it is possible to expose the capsular plane (CF) bordered superiorly and posteriorly by the gluteus minimus and gluteus medius (GL), distally by the vastus lateralis (VL) and anteriorly by the rectus femoris previously displaced by retractor 2 (fig. 12).

The exposure of the capsular plane, performed to allow its incision and subsequent release, requires as a first step the section of the fibrous structures produced between the gluteus minimus and the upper portion of the capsule (fig. 13), which play a key role in the abduction of the hip by allowing the capsular lift, subtracting it from the conflict between the neck and the acetabular margin (fig. 14). The resection of these expansions

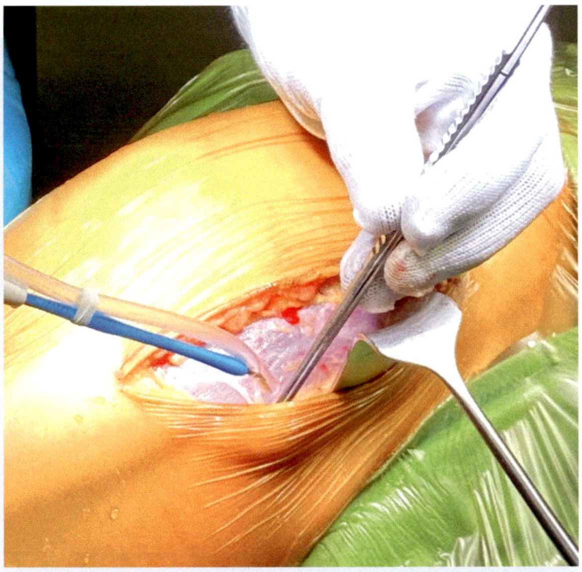

Figure 2 Exposure of the tensor fascia lata (TFL) after dissection of the subcutaneous adipose tissue

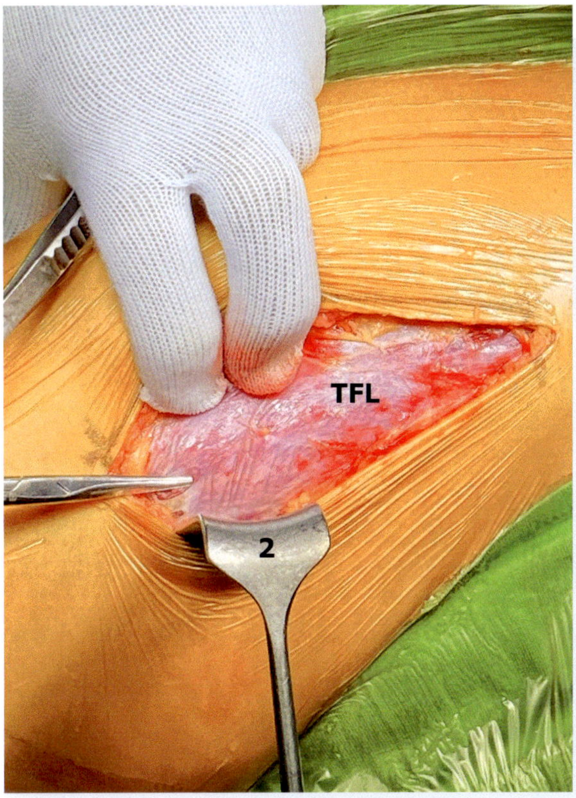

Figure 3 Epimysium incision of the TFL is made at the anterior third of the width of its muscular belly and is at the vascular lacuna through which one of the perforators of the subcutaneous tissue runs

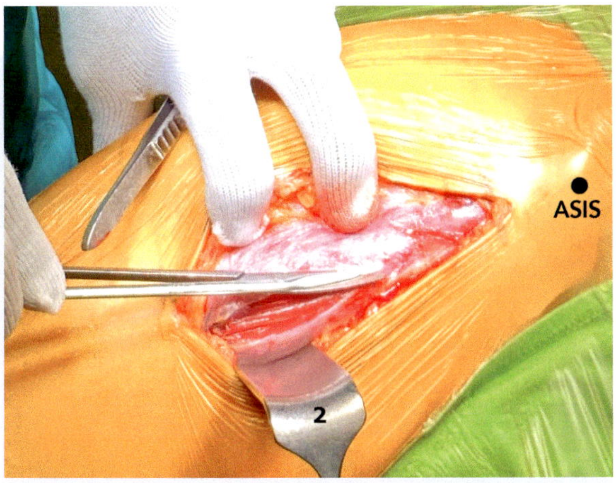

Figure 4 In this image, the course of the epimysium incision can be appreciated. This proceeds cranially towards the antero superior iliac spine (ASIS)

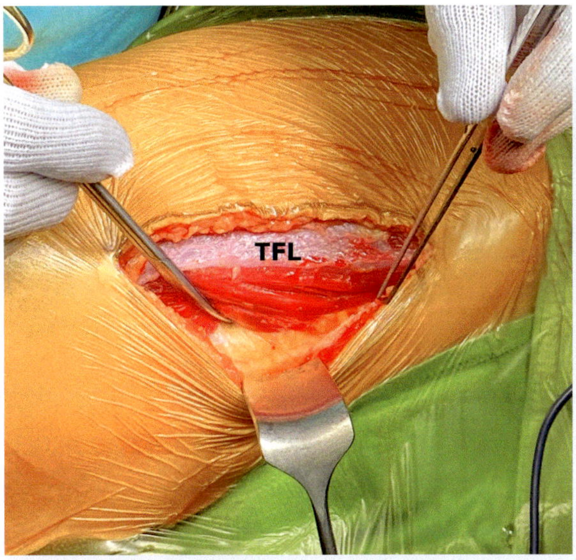

Figure 5 Posterolateral retraction of the TFL with exposure of the interval (the sartorius muscle is not visible in the image)

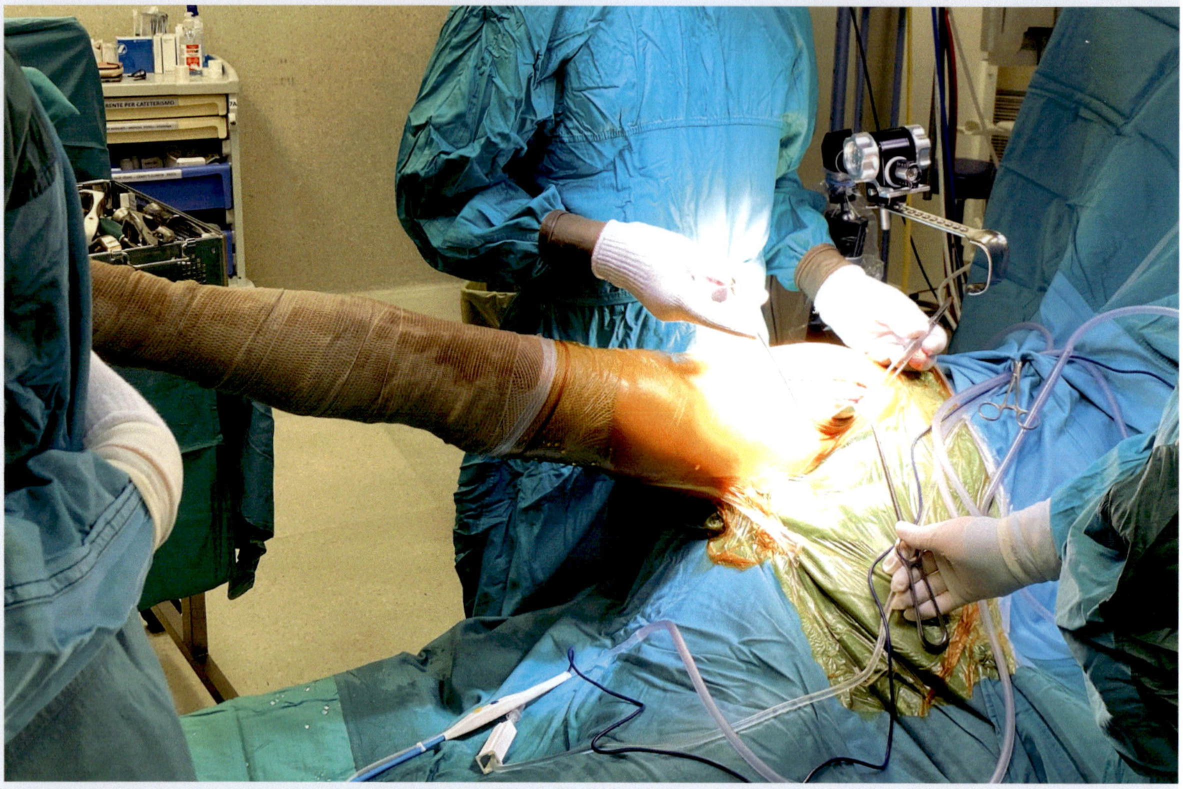

Figure 6 The abduction of the limb allows for a reduction in the tension of the TFL and abductor muscles as well as the skin. This facilitates divarication and management of the surgical area

is performed with an electrosurgical scalpel by lifting the small gluteus (GL) which gets appropriately detached by positioning the lower limb in abduction (fig. 15). The dissection of these expansions allows to create a supra-capsular interval in which a Homann (retractor 3) is placed (fig. 16).

The learning process about the anterior access has led us to notice that the capsular release is of fundamental importance as it allows an adequate mobilization of the femur minimizing the tensions, hence obtaining a better surgical window as well as lowering the risk of fractures or injuries related to the stresses that would be necessary for an adequate exposure of the segments in the absence of a complete capsular release. In addition, capsular release is of major significance in avoiding unnecessary tension on the prosthetic implant after surgery in several daily activities, as documented by Crowninshield in Pathologic ligamentous constraint of the hip [16].

In the practice, the release results on the femoral side following the base of the femoral neck, whilst at the acetabular level it is sufficient to partially disengage the capsule below the reflex tendon of the rectus femoris at the antero-inferior iliac spine (figs. 17-18). After this, the capsulotomy is performed in the proximal distal sense using as proximal reference point the reflex tendon of the rectus femoris (TR) until reaching its femoral insertion at the vastus lateralis (VL) fibers (figs. 19-20).

The capsular section allows the removal of the extracapsular retractor 3 and the positioning of retractor 5 in an intracapsular location lying on the superior margin of the femoral neck (fig. 21).

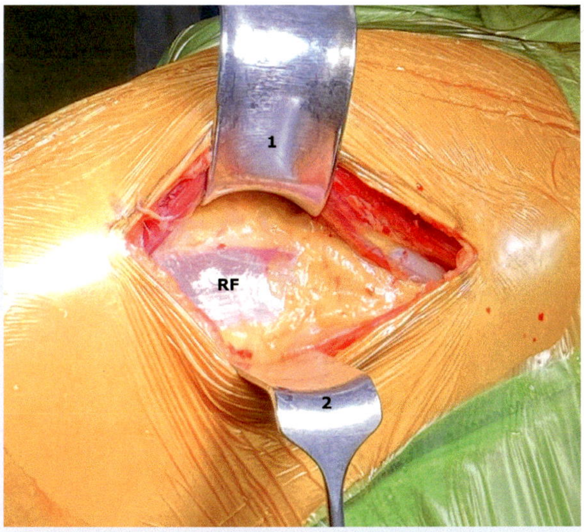

Figure 7 Retraction of the TFL and exposure of the rectus femoris (RF), whose fibres are recognisable in transparency below the thin fibrous sheath

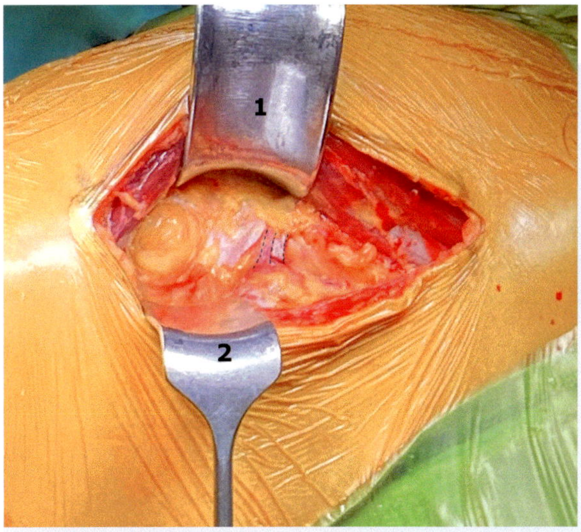

Figure 8 The muscle belly of the RF is mobilised antero-medially by retractor 2, exposing the thin vascular branch that feeds it (this is shown by the dotted line)

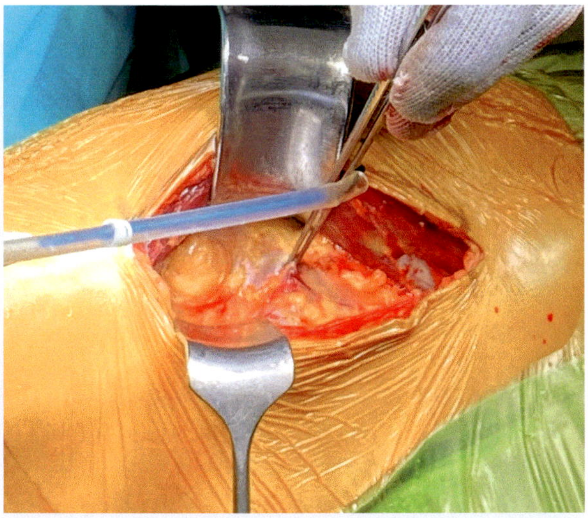

Figure 9 Cauterization of the vascular branch of the RF allows the antero-medial retraction of this muscle to be completed

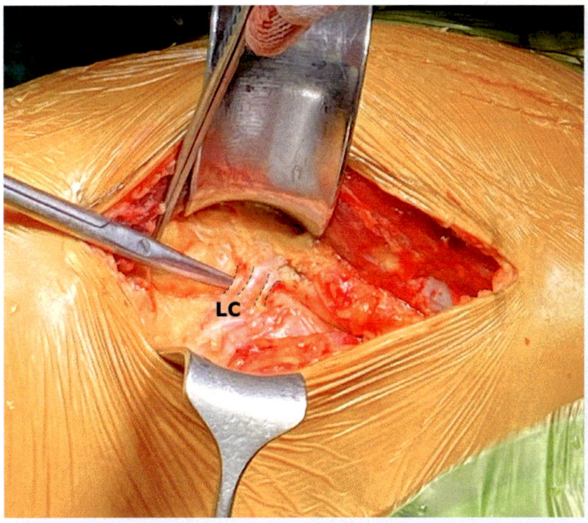

Figure 10 Exposure of the transverse branch of the lateral circumflex artery of the femur (LC)

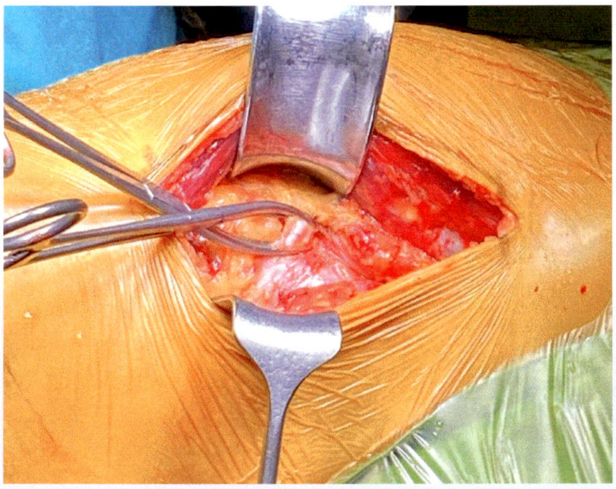

Figure 11 Clamping and cautery of the LC

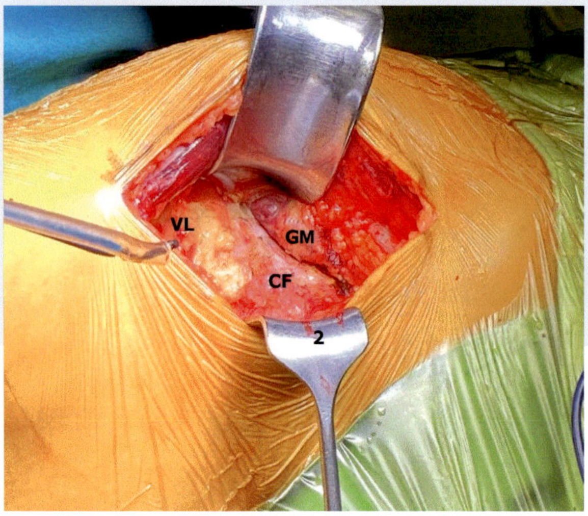

Figure 12 Exposure of the antero-medial portion of the femoral capsule. This is delimited superolaterally by the gluteus minimus (GM), medially by the rectus femoris (not visible in the image because it is displaced by the retractor) 2) and inferiorly by the vastus lateralis (VL)

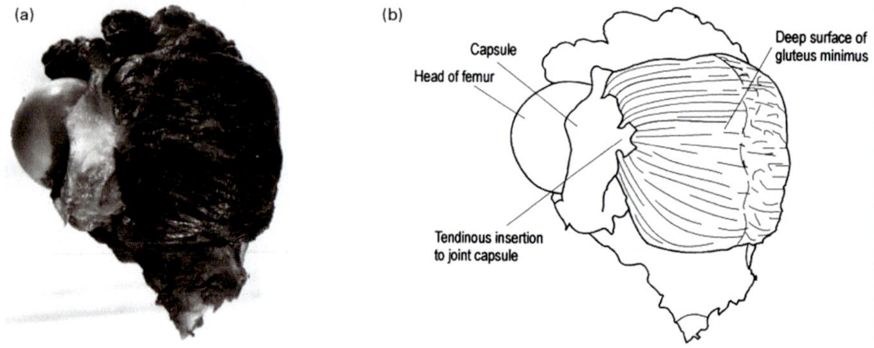

Figure 13 Anatomical representation of the fibrous expansions that unite the gluteus minimus to the upper portion of the joint capsule

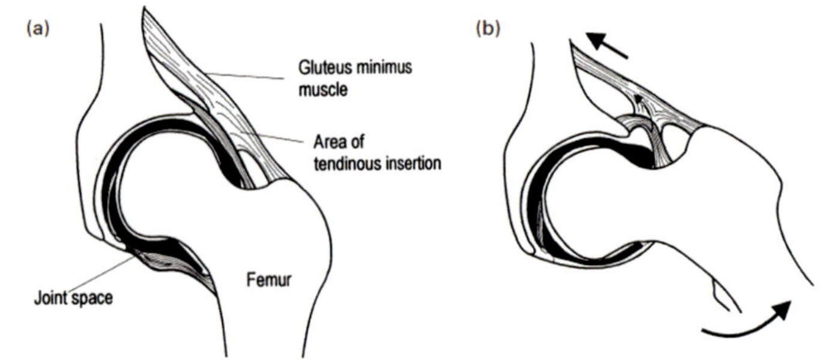

Figure 14 Graphical representation of the role of the fibrous expansions that unite the cranial side of the capsule to the gluteus minimus (GM). This allows the capsule to be plicated. Thus, the capsule is protected from entrapment between the femoral neck and the acetabular rim during hip abduction movements

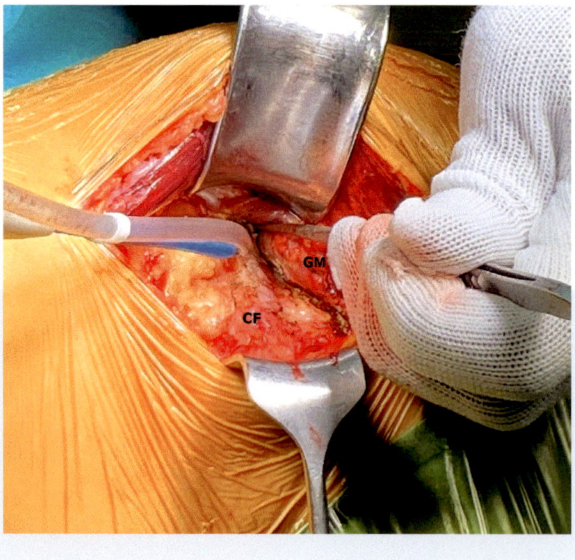

Figure 15 Resection of the fibrous expansions between the gluteus minimus (GM), retracted by the forceps, and the capsule (CF)

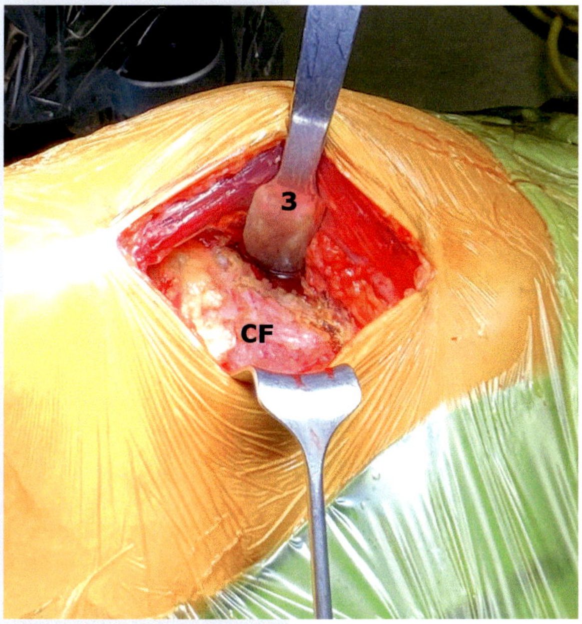

Figure 16 Complete exposure of the femoral capsule (CF). Retractor 3 is inserted in the interval between it and the gluteus minimus, which is released from the fibrous expansions between the two structures

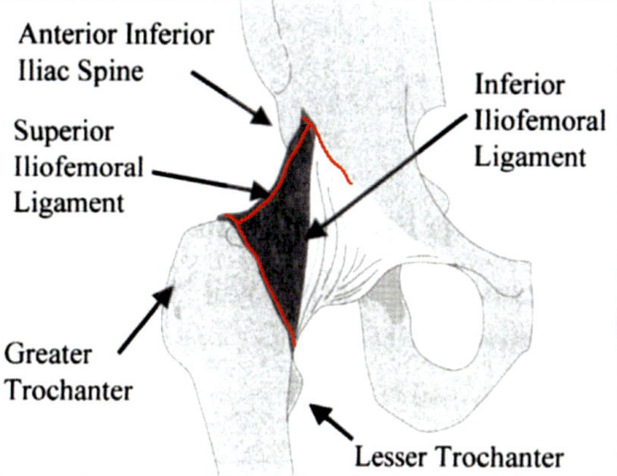

Figure 17 Graphic representation of the anterior joint capsule and its component structures. The red continuous line represents the capsular incision made during surgery

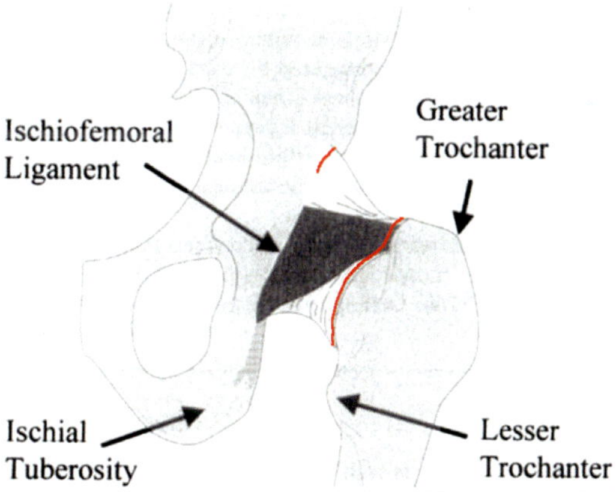

Figure 18 Graphical representation of the posterior joint capsule and its component structures. The red continuous line represents the capsular incision made during surgery

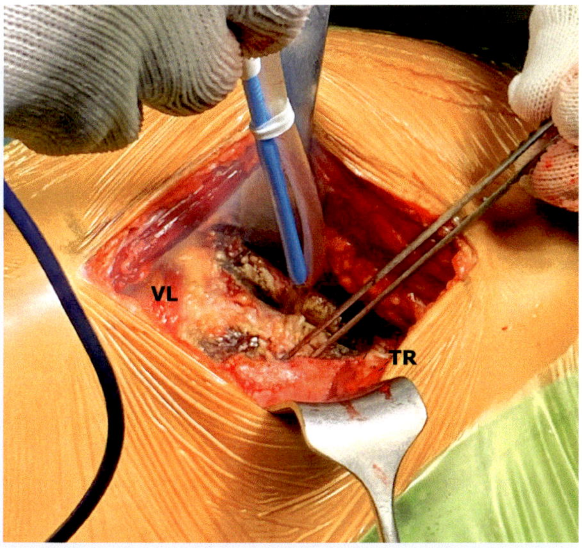

Figure 19 Capsulotomy performed with the electrocautery from proximal to distal. This runs from the reflected head of the rectus femoris (TR) to the base of the neck near the muscle belly of the vastus lateralis (VL)

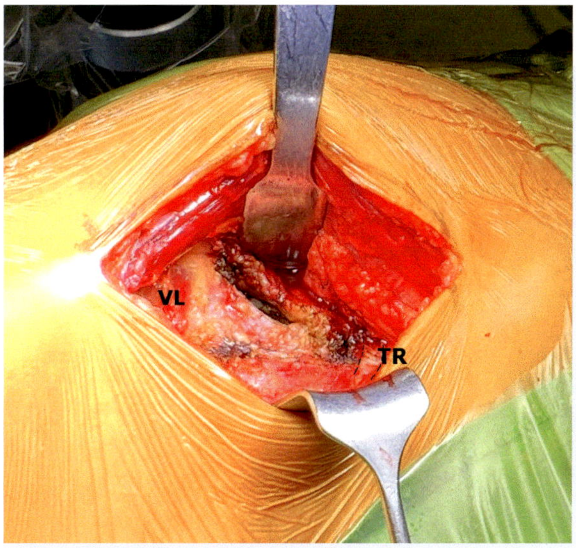

Figure 20 Capsulotomy line on the antero-superior side of the capsule, as shown in figure 17

The positioning of a suture thread to isolate and suspend the antero-distal portion of the capsule (figs. 22-23) facilitates the extension of the capsulotomy along the base of the neck; the retraction of the vastus lateralis by means of a Farabeuf allows the identification of the descending branch of the lateral circumflex artery (CLD) and of the pectineus muscle (P) that must be properly protected and spared (fig. 24).
Once the capsulotomy is completed on the anterior side of the femoral neck, the retractor 3 is positioned under the capsule, resting on the medial surface of the femoral head (fig. 25). In this way it is possible to visualize the femoral neck and, if necessary, it is possible to proceed with the removal of the osteophytes first and terminate with the resection of the femoral neck.
A corkscrew is placed on the femoral head to allow its removal (fig. 26). Then, to facilitate the extraction of the head the limb is brought into slight abduction (fig. 27) to determine a slippage of the resection (fig. 28) that generates a lever action that facilitates the removal of the head (fig. 29).
Once the head has been detached (fig. 30), the next step is the capsular release around the femoral calcar (CF) (fig. 31), which is exposed via the extra-rotation and slight flexion of the limb. In this phase the retractor 3 is positioned in front of the anterior cotyloid margin (fig. 32), thus allowing the cleaning of any osteophytes and the visualization of the base of the ileopubic branch (IP).
At this point, by intra-rotating the limb it is possible to expose the apex of the great trochanter (GT) behind which the retractor 4 is positioned, thus dislocating the small and middle gluteus and exposing the superior capsule (CF) (fig. 33).
The limb is now extra-rotated and extended in order to allow the completion of capsular disengagement and its detachment from the plane of the extra-rotators (ER) (fig. 34) and from the posterior surface of the femoral neck. With this last step, the integral release of the joint capsule is achieved, and the cup preparation can begin.
To allow an adequate exposure and visualization of the acetabulum, the retractor 4 is positioned behind the posterior acetabular rim and, to easily perform this operation, the limb is slightly abducted, intra-rotated and extended (fig. 35) in order to relax the abductor muscles. At this point the retractor 3 is positioned in front of the anterior margin of the acetabulum and the retractor 5 in correspondence of the obturator incisura radiographically identified with a drop shape (fig. 36).
For the preparation of the cup, a cutter-holder handle with double offset is used (fig. 37), which allows to correctly incline the drill avoiding an excess of verticality.
Once the preparation of the cup has been completed and the ideal size of the acetabular component has been identified (fig. 38), it is possible to proceed with the implantation by using a handle with double offset (fig. 39). However, to complete the positioning, a straight handle is preferable for a better mechanical transfer on the prosthetic cup of the percussion generated by the hammer (fig. 40). The liner housing (fig. 41), in this case made up of ceramic material, completes the acetabular phase (fig. 42).
To proceed with the preparation of the femur, the retractor 4 is brought back behind the apex of the great trochanter and the surgeon moves anteriorly to the patient while the limb is positioned in extra-rotation, adduction and extension (fig. 43). To allow adequate access to the femoral stump, a femoral elevator (retractor 6) is placed below the femoral neck (fig. 44). Next steps are the opening of the femoral canal with a specific instrument (fig. 45) and the interruption of the cortical ring of the femoral neck on the great trochanter side (fig. 46) in order to allow a correct lodging of the stem shoulder and to reduce the risk of excessive bone tensions as well, which could increase the risk of fracture. In the femoral preparation, too, double offset handle is of great help in facilitating the procedure, as well as the use of short prosthetic stems with a slender shoulder, that allows to follow a curvilinear trajectory in its introduction (fig. 47), saving the femoral bone stock as well. With this type of preparation, the risk of varus posi-

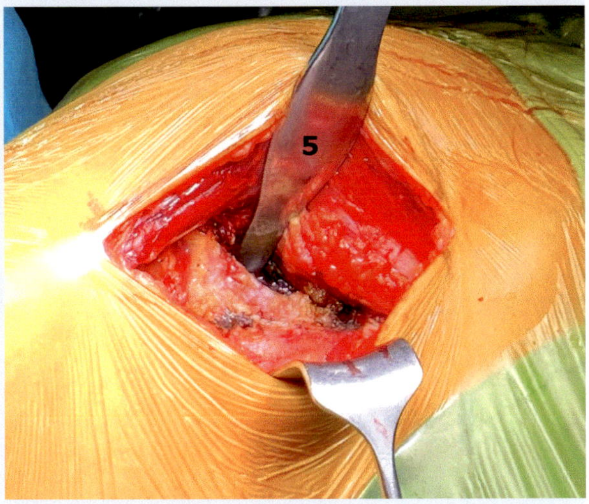

Figure 21 Retractor 5 is in an intra-articular position. This is located on the superior portion of the femoral neck and allows retraction of the capsule and muscle structures

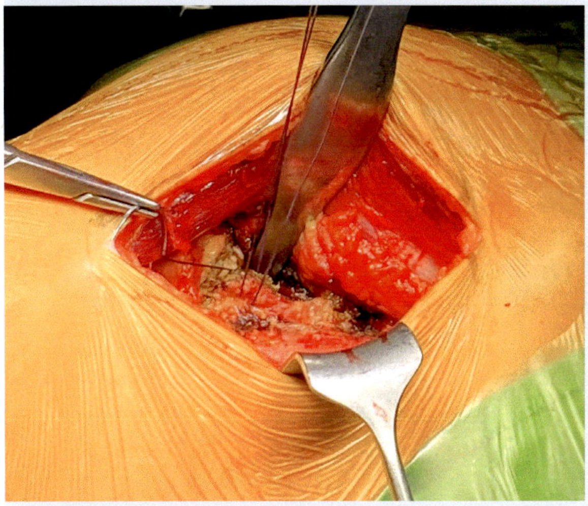

Figure 22 Placement of suspension wire on the inferomedial margin of the capsule, exposed through capsulotomy

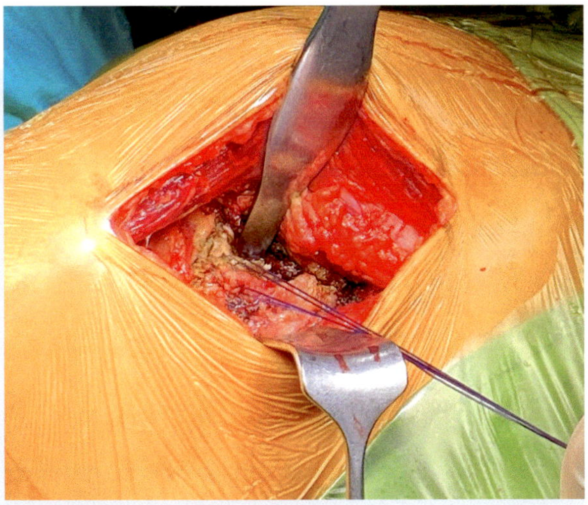

Figure 23 The wire allows retraction of the capsular flap during its detachment along the base of the femoral neck to the superomedial margin of the vastus lateralis belly as shown in figure 17

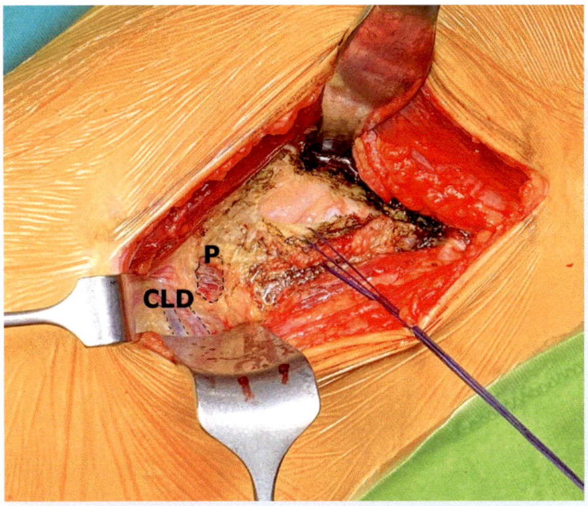

Figure 24 The extension of the capsulotomy along its inferomedial insertion will expose the fibres of the pectineus muscle (P) and the descending branch of the circumflex artery of the femur (CLD), thus allowing its sparing

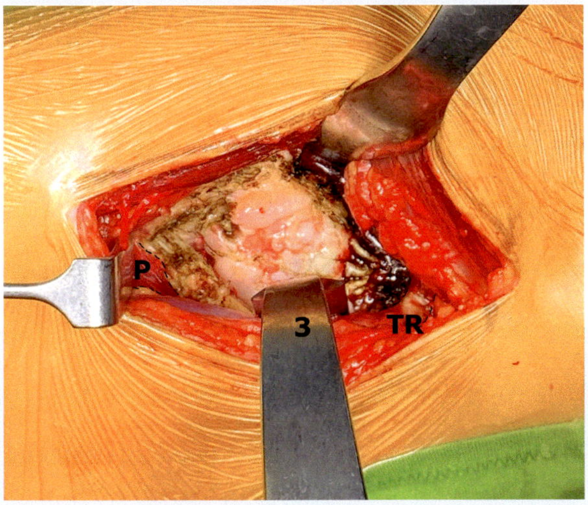

Figure 25 With the anterior capsulotomy completed and the retractors in the intra-articular position, complete exposure of the femoral neck is achieved, allowing its resection

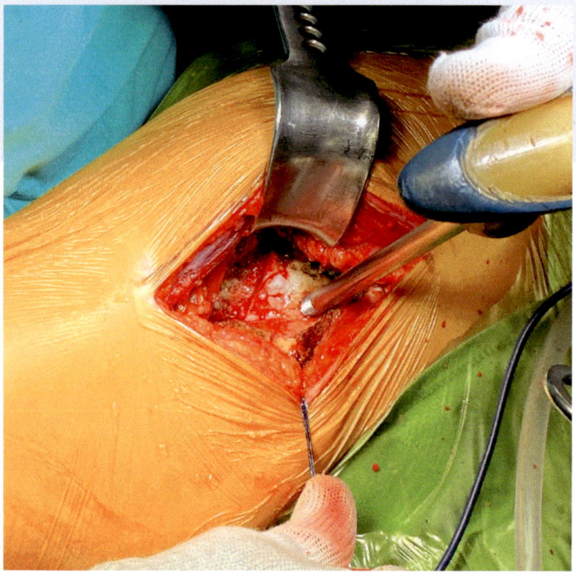

Figure 26 Once the cervical osteotomy has been completed, the corkscrew is placed on the femoral head

Figure 27 During the extraction of the femoral head, the lower limb is abducted and internally rotated

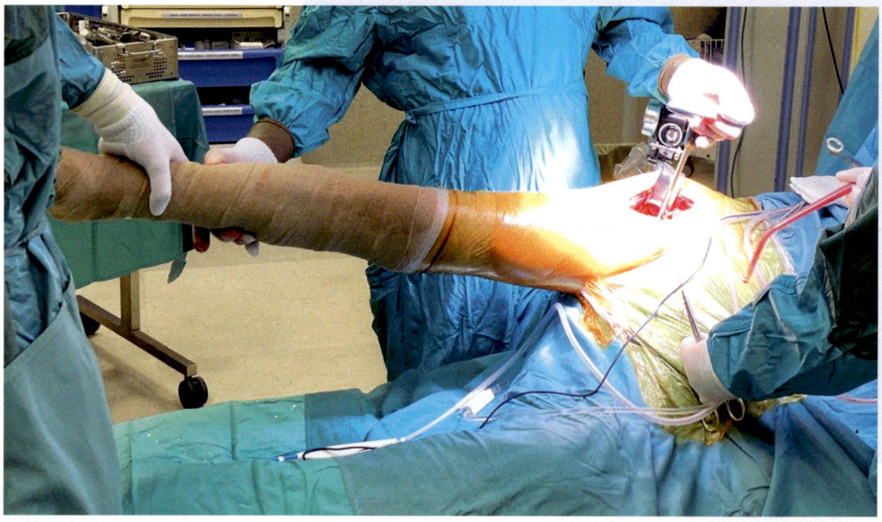

Figure 28 This image shows the posterior sliding of the distal margin of the femoral neck resection in relation to its proximal counterpart. This facilitates the extraction of the head

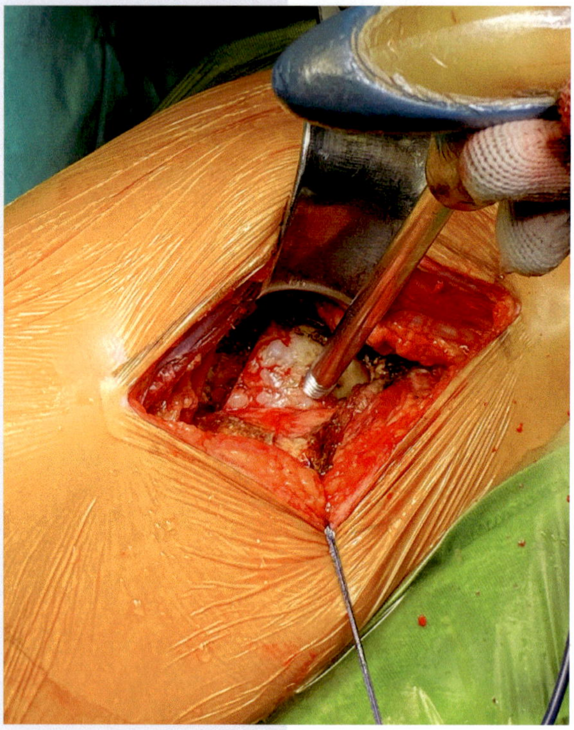

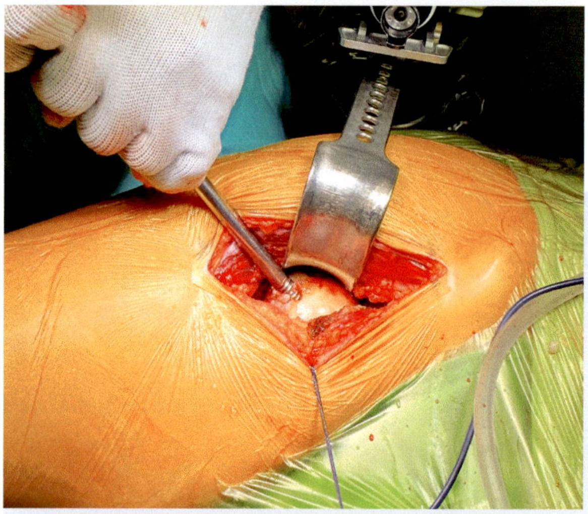

Figure 29 The inclination of the corkscrew handle towards the distal margin of the incision combined with slight traction allows the femoral head to be extracted. The process is facilitated by the sliding of the resection planes shown in figure 28

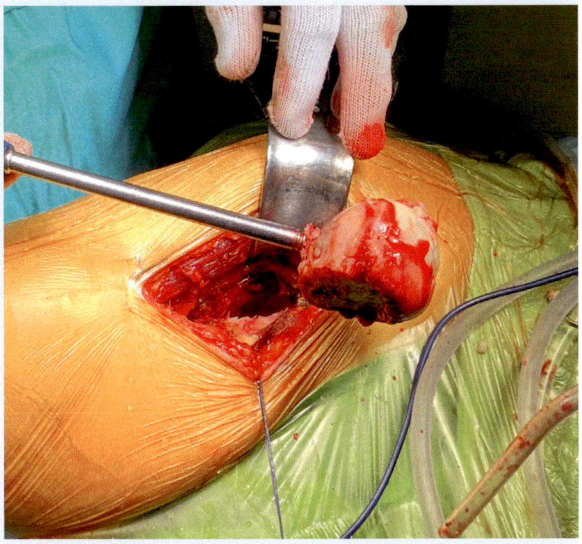

Figure 30 Image of the femoral head after its removal

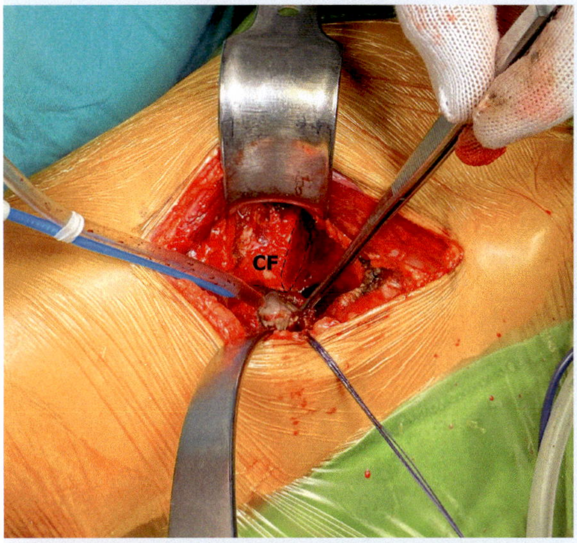

Figure 31 External rotation and abduction of the lower limb allows exposure of the inferior aspect of the resected femoral neck (CF). This allows the release of the joint capsule to proceed as depicted in figures 17 and 18

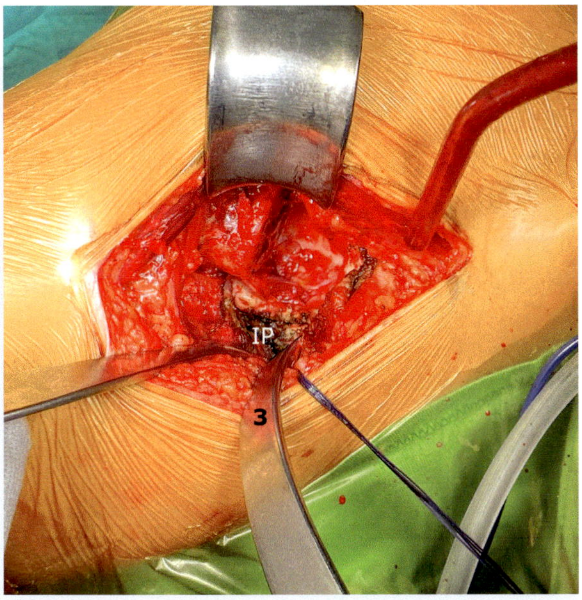

Figure 32 This image shows the exposure of the anteroinferior acetabular margin (dashed black line) at the insertion of the ileopubic branch (IP). Retractor 3 is positioned medial to the anterior cotyloid rim and below the capsule and the iliopsoas tendon

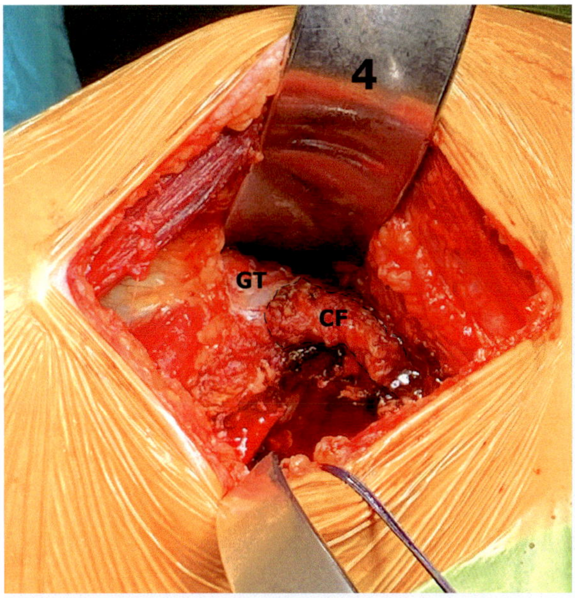

Figure 33 Retractor 4 is positioned lateral and proximal to the greater trochanter (GT) and below the tendon of the gluteus minimus. This allows the upper portion of the joint capsule (CF) (delineated by the dashed black line) to be exposed

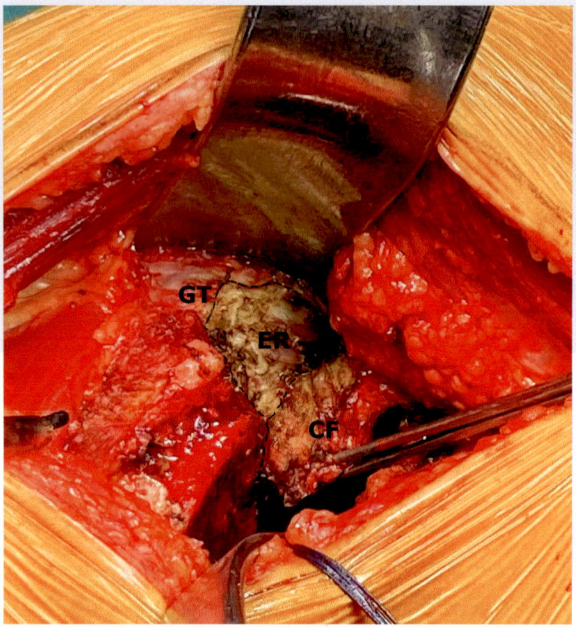

Figure 34 The capsular margin (CF), detached along the dashed black line, allows the capsular release to be completed.
In doing so, the femur is completely released from this structure and the external rotators (ER) can be exposed

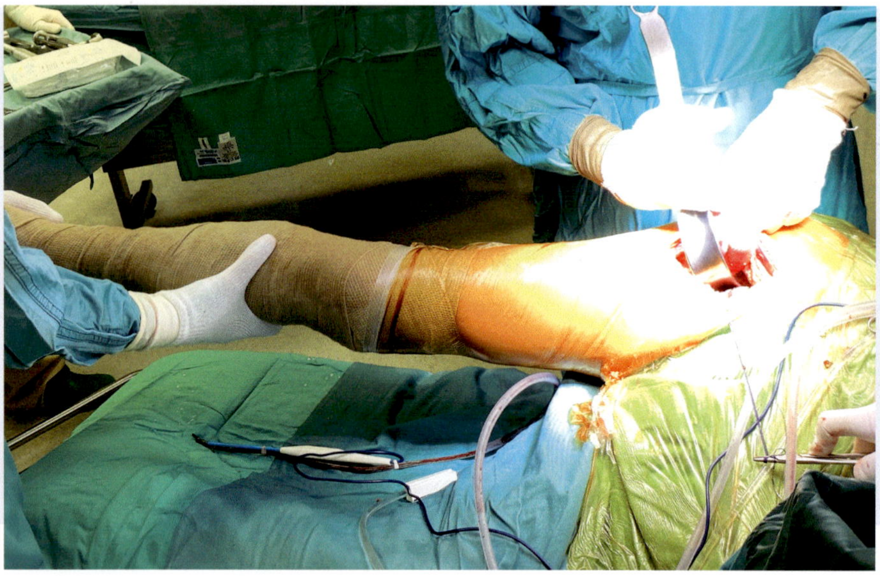

Figure 35 The abduction and extension of the limb allows the positioning of Retractor 4 behind the posterior margin of the cup

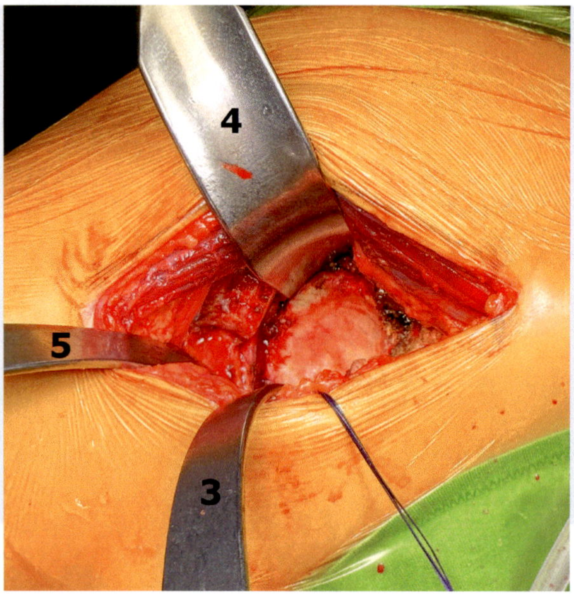

Figure 36 Retractor 4, positioned behind the posterior cotyloid margin, retracts the resected femoral neck stump and the gluteal and TFL muscles. Retractor 3 is placed behind the anterior acetabular margin. Retractor 5 is placed below the obturator incisura once the transverse acetabular ligament or osteophyte has been removed.
This allows complete exposure of the acetabular cavity

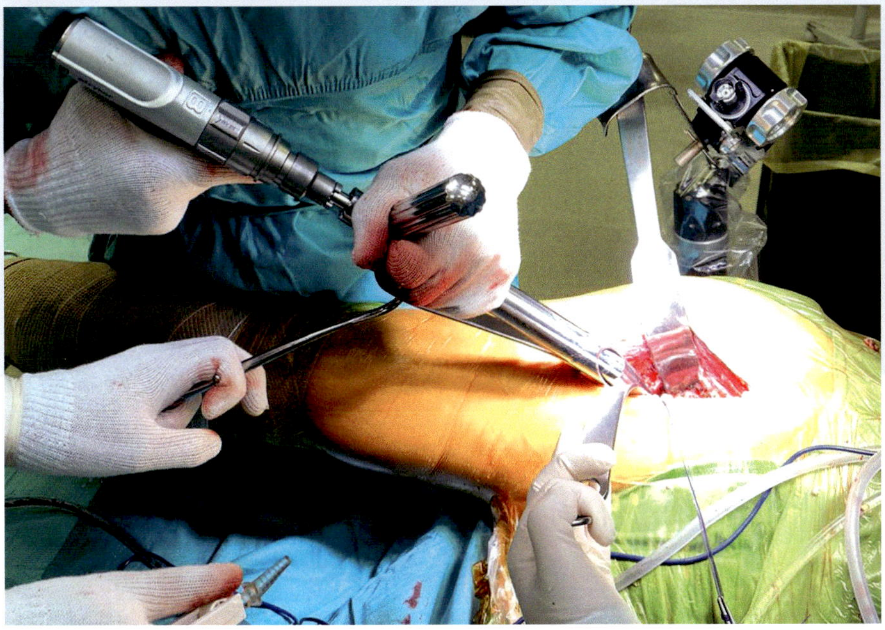

Figure 37 Shown is the acetabular preparation with double offset handle. This facilitates correct positioning, limiting conflicts with the surgical field

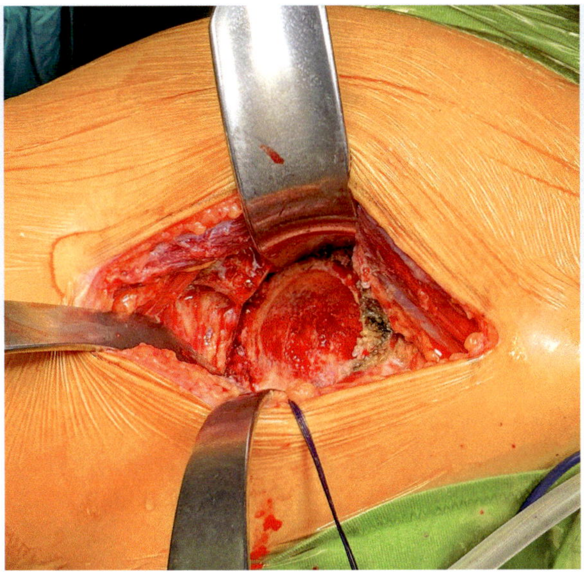

Figure 38 The figure shows the acetabular cavity at the end of the preparation and the exposure of the subchondral bone

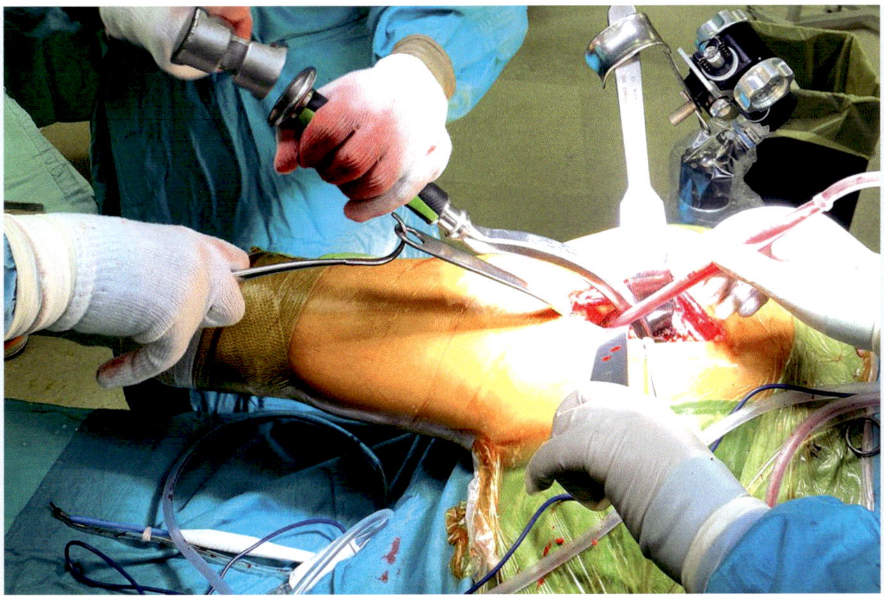

Figure 39 This image shows the positioning of the acetabular prosthetic component with the double offset handle. As seen in figure 37, this instrument allows for correct positioning without conditioning due to conflict with the surgical field margins

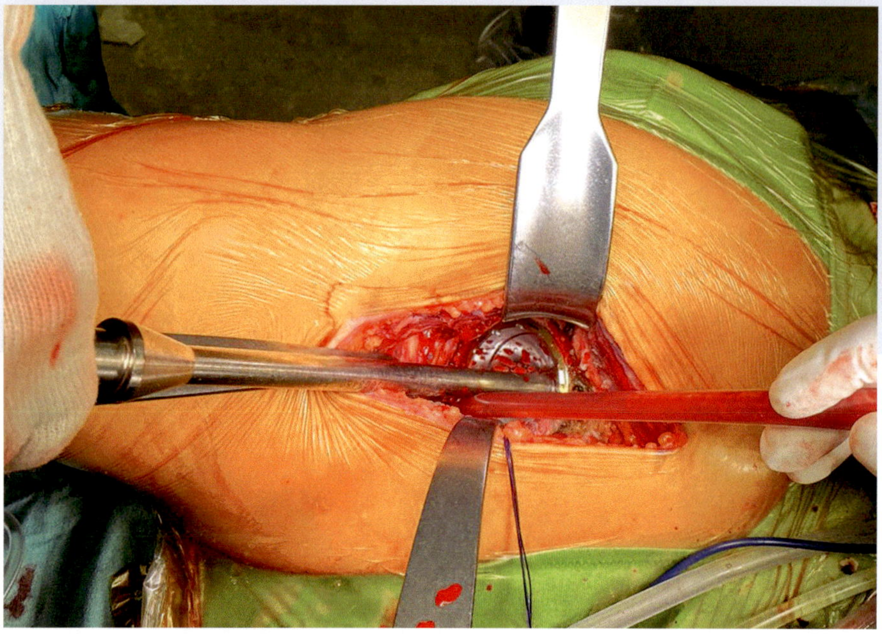

Figure 40 The use of a straight handle allows better mechanical transfer of percussion for correct implant positioning

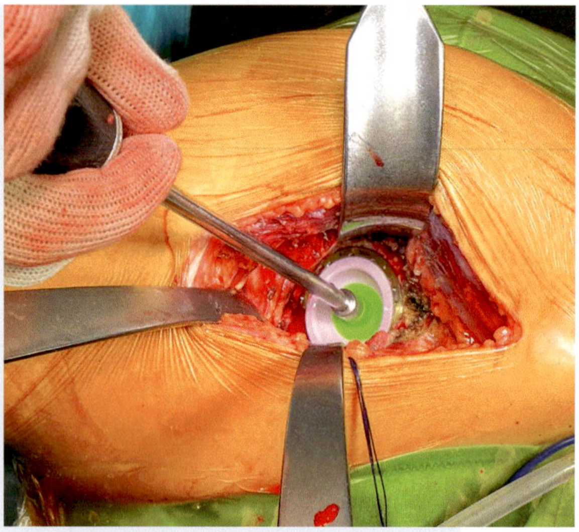

Figure 41 Placement of the ceramic prosthetic liner

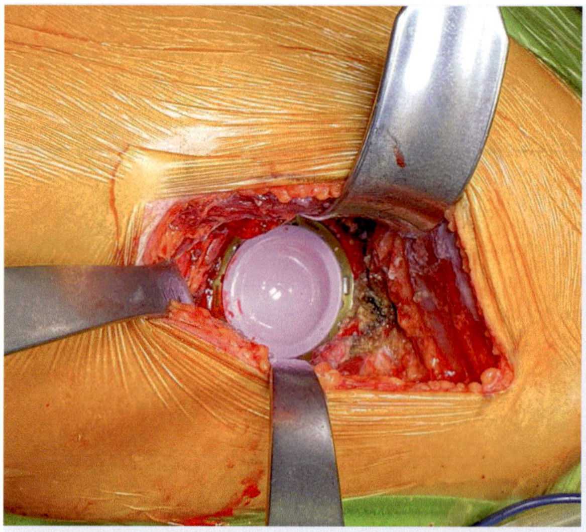

Figure 42 The image shows the complete view of the prosthesised acetabular cavity together with the placement of the retractors described earlier

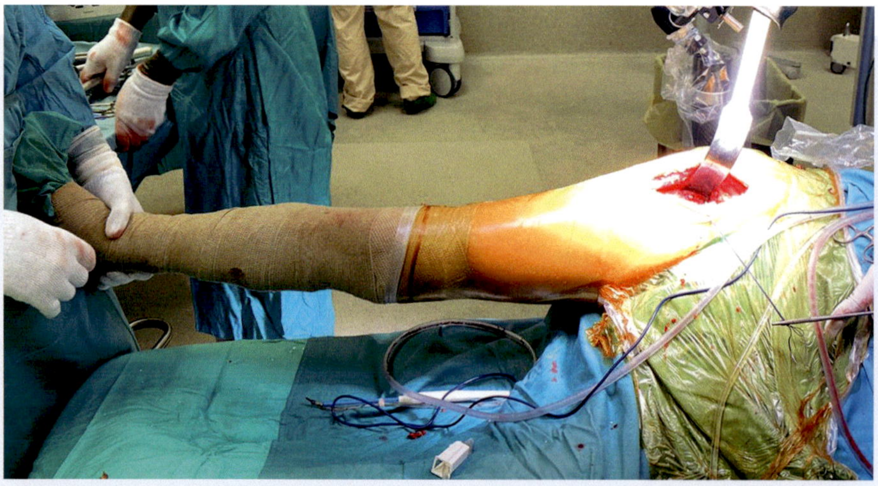

Figure 43 Proper exposure of the femur requires placement of retractor 4 behind the apex of the greater trochanter as described earlier in figure 33

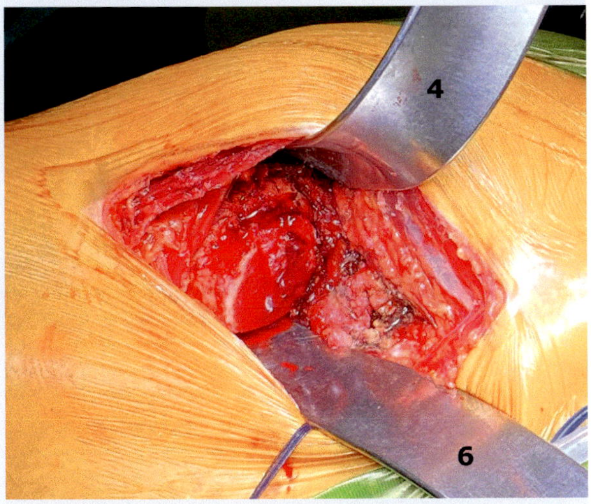

Figure 44 Correct exposure of the femur requires, in addition to the retractor 4 positioned as described in figure 43, a femoral elevator (6) placed below the posteroinferior margin of the resected femoral neck

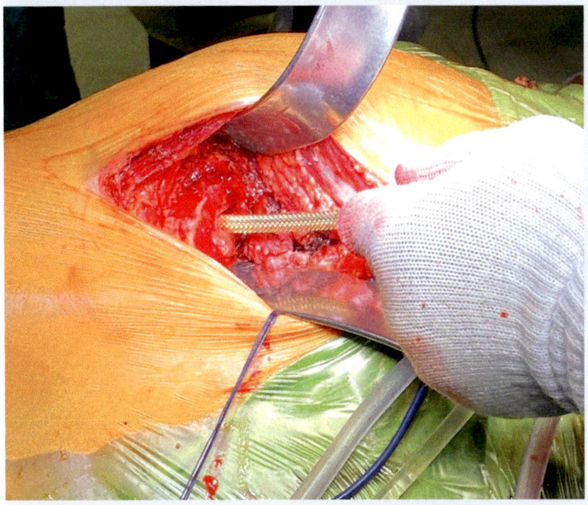

Figure 45 The image shows the opening of the femoral canal with a special instrument

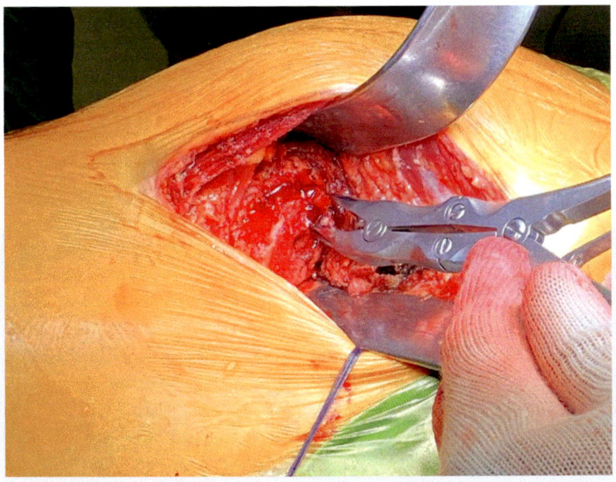

Figure 46 The cortical ring of the base of the femoral neck is interrupted towards the greater trochanter, allowing easier preparation and limiting the risk of fractures

tioning is greater than with the classic straight introduction. For this reason, the cortical interruption towards the greater trochanter reduces the risk of this type of alignment error.
Once the preparation of the femur is completed, it is possible to proceed with the introduction of the prosthetic stem, always with a curvilinear trajectory, by striking the prosthesis in a latero-distal direction (figs. 48-49).
Once the prosthetic stem is introduced, the retractors 4 and 6 are removed and, while retractor 1 loads the TFL, the head is implanted after an appropriate joint stability tests (fig. 50). At this stage, the surgeon returns to the initial position at the back of the patient.
Once the prosthetic implant is completed, the capsular margins are selected for suturing (fig. 51). The suture is first completed in the craniocaudal direction along the direction of the neck (fig. 52) and then some stitches are applied at the base of the neck below the vastus lateralis (figs. 53-54).
The capsular reconstruction (fig. 55) aims at recreating an anatomical barrier between the intra- and the extra-articular space to facilitate the re-establishment of the hip anatomy, but it does not play any role in reducing the risk of implant dislocation.
The intervention is completed by the suturing of the epimysium of the TFL with detached stitches (figs. 56-57) and by the final skin suture (fig. 58).

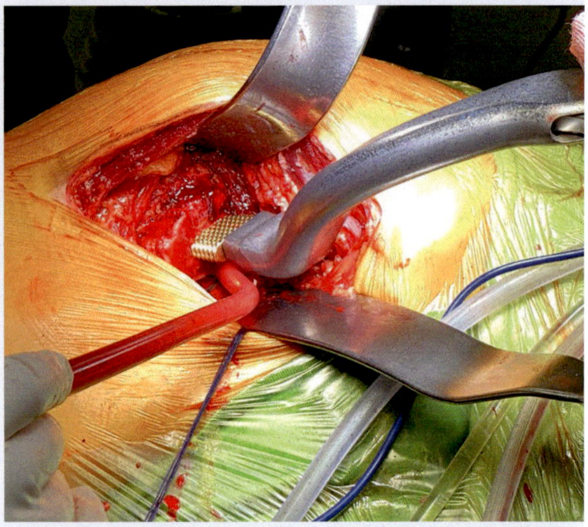

Figure 47 The preparation of the femoral canal is facilitated by the use of a double offset handle. As in the acetabular preparation, this instrument makes it possible to limit the risk of incorrect positioning due to conflict with the surgical field

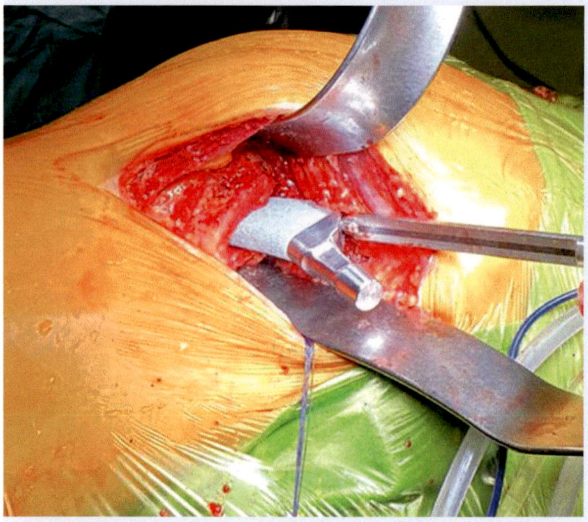

Figure 48 Once the femoral preparation has been completed, the prosthetic component is introduced following a curvilinear trajectory that requires lateral and distal percussion

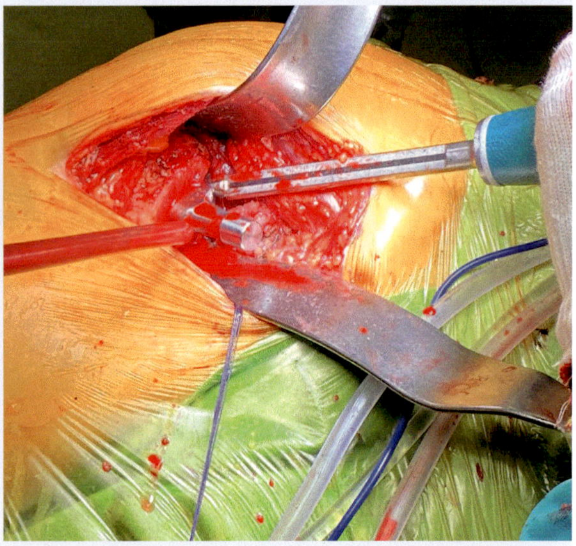

Figure 49 The final positioning of the stem allows the restoration of the anatomical cervical metaphyseal axis

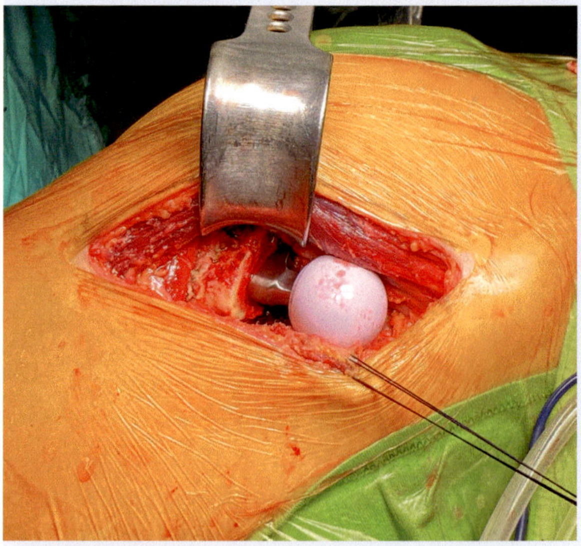

Figure 50 The image shows the positioning of the ceramic prosthetic head after the joint stability and lower limb length tests

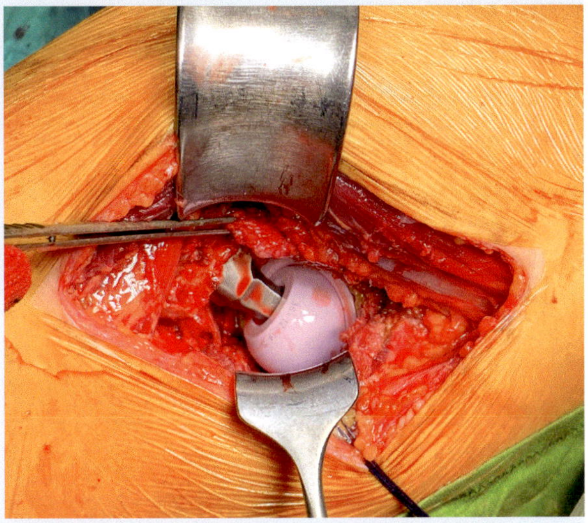

Figure 51 Prosthetic implant is reduced and the anatomical integrity of the periarticular structures is preserved

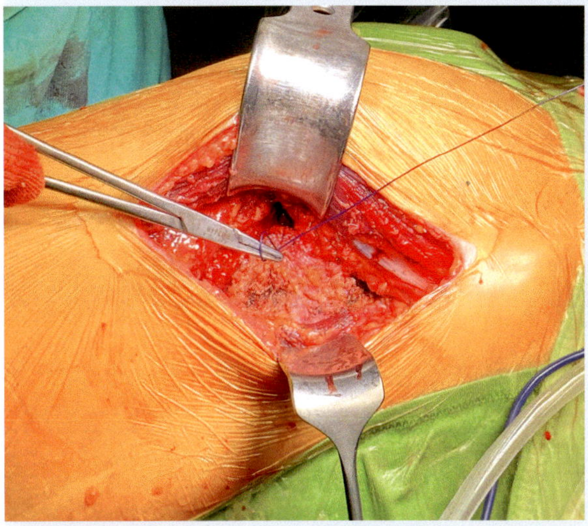

Figure 52 The image shows the suture with single interrupted stitches of the capsular margins along the capsulotomy described in figure 20

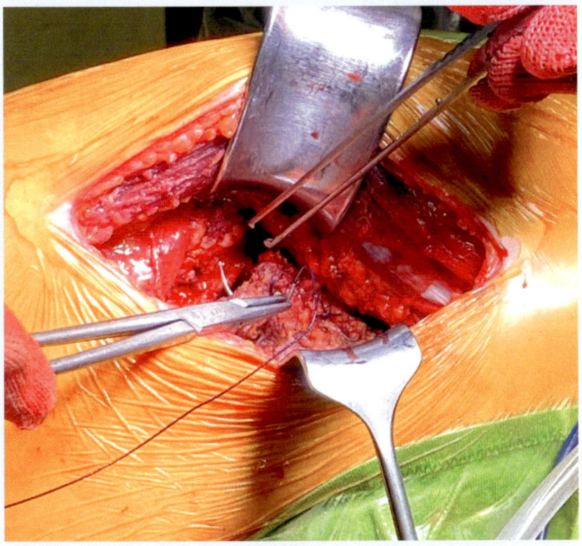

Figure 53 Reinsertion of the anteroinferior capsular margin along the base of the neck in the direction of the vastus lateralis

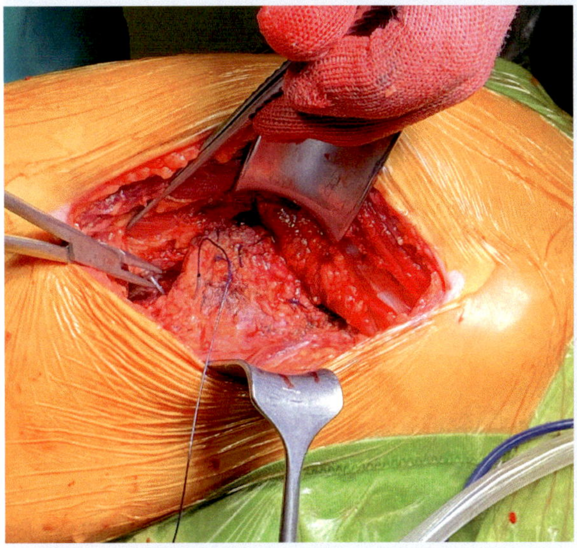

Figure 54 The image shows the complete reinsertion of the distal capsule below the muscular belly of the vastus lateralis, which, in the figure, is retracted by the surgical forceps

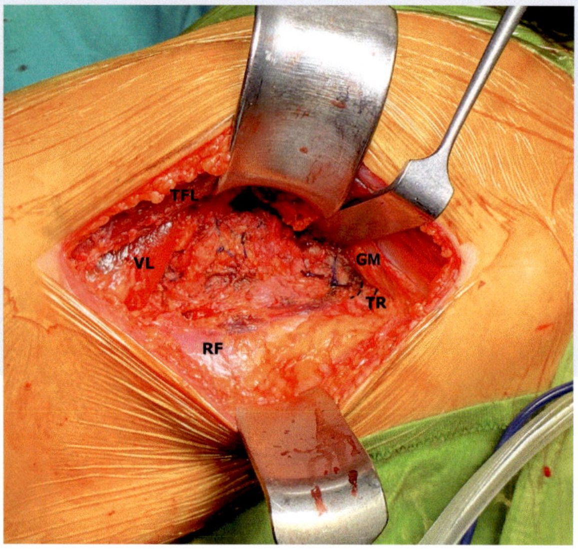

Figure 55 The capsular suture recreates the anatomical continuity of this structure, delimiting the articular space from the extraarticular space. The image displays the anatomical structures delimiting the anterior approach (the TFL and sartorius) and shows their integrity after surgery

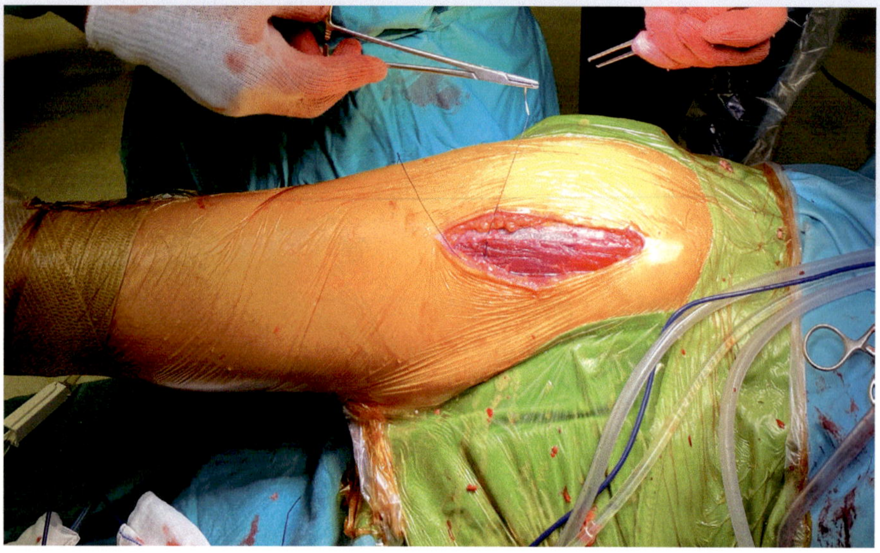

Figure 56 The tensor fascia lata recovers its anatomical position after removal of the retractors

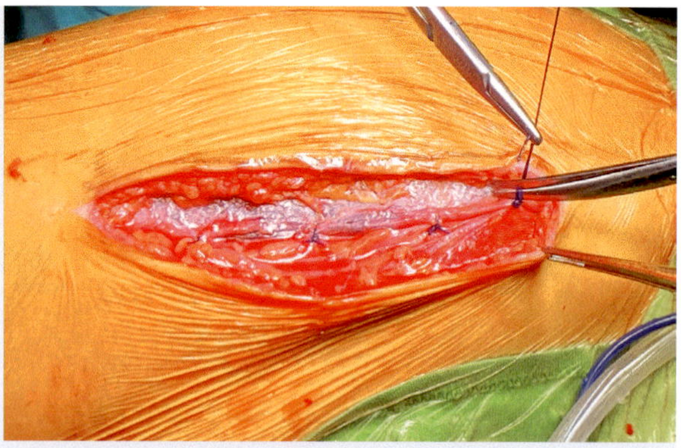

Figure 57 Reconstruction of the fascial plane that overlays the tensor fascia lata with single interrupted stitches

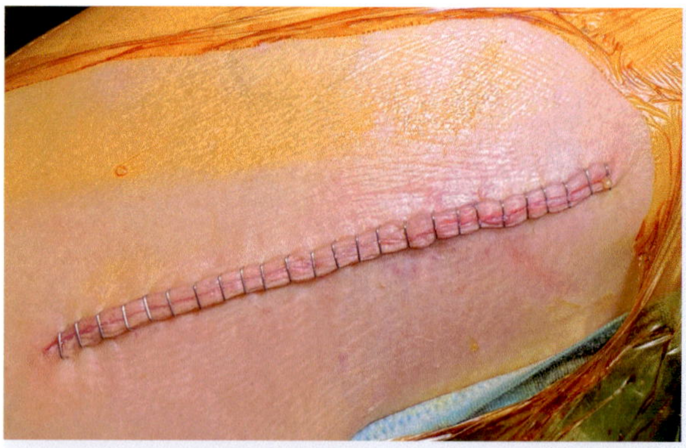

Figure 58 The completed skin suture is shown. No signs of margin distress are visible due to correct tension management during retraction

Incidents, difficulties and possible complications in the ALDI Approach

The learning curve and the more than ten-year path with the ALDI Approach ensured the progression from an initial phase where a patient selection was necessary to the current situation where this surgical technique can be used regardless of the patient's morphology, BMI or joint morphology, as well as to the possibility to treat cases of prosthetic revision – both acetabular and femoral – or periprosthetic fractures, as shown in the collected radiographic documentation about some clinical cases treated with this access.

As mentioned, the learning curve initially forced us to select patients in terms of general morphological characteristics related to adipose and muscular features and joint morphology. As already known, normal weight, limited muscular mass and standard articular morphology, e.g., coxa valga with mild degenerative features, represent the ideal choice to practice the first experiences of hip prosthesis with any surgical access – and even more with the anterior access, in order to find familiarity with the divarication, the hemostasis and the timing of the capsular release, to allow a correct exposure of both acetabular and femoral sides.

For its consolidation, the learning process of a surgical procedure requires the same features that are typical of a climb, i.e. to proceed to the next step the preceding one must be firmly established, to reduce to the minimum all the related risks of an activity that, even if carried out with all the possible precautions, still retains the possibility of unexpected events and complications. In this sense, evaluating the possible problems related to a surgical access – and in particular in the anterior one – it is easy to understand how these are the direct consequences of an incongruous management of the divarication step, which might lead to:

- muscular-tendinous and/or vascular-nerve damage;
- an inadequate acetabular and femoral exposure, leading to incorrect positioning of the components;
- intraoperative fractures.

In all these cases, the pathogenesis of the complication constantly lies in the attempt to remedy an inadequate exposure by forcing the divarication, in particular with the Homann, the hook and the femoral elevator. Analyzing the literature, the anterior approach appears to be particularly affected by these problems to the point of inducing surgeons to abandon it and to return to traditional accesses.

According to the complications reported in the literature of the anterior access, the most frequently reported ones are the fractures of the proximal metaphyseal area – both on the calcar and on the greater trochanter – caused by the hook used to lift the femur; although less frequently, other possible fractures related to the patient positioning are those involving the ankle, caused by the use of the traction bed.

Understanding the difficulties related to a surgical practice is of fundamental importance; the learning curve described can be thus considered completed only once the surgeon is effectively able to manage those difficulties, limiting the risk that they may evolve into intra-operative complications.

Taking into consideration our personal learning experience and the familiarity we obtained, we are able to indicate which are the critical issues related to each phase of surgery and their possible evolution into complications if not properly managed.

1. Surgical access

The initial difficulty in the execution of the anterior access is the correct identification of the tensor fasciae latae muscular belly, achieved by using the superior anterior iliac spine as a reference point (fig. 2). An error in this step might lead to failure to identify the space between the TFL and the sartorius. The literature describes the false path as represented by the passage anterior to the sartorius, mistakenly identified as the TFL. However, in our practice with the lateral decubitus this error has never occurred, whilst in some other circumstances the incision of the TFL is performed posterior to the tensor: in these cases, once understood the error, it is possible to suture the fascia and to proceed to move anteriorly to the muscle belly, thus correctly identifying the anatomical space between the TFL and the sartorius. This kind of error is more frequent in patients with a greater adipose layer, in which the identification of the iliac spine is less precise. In these situations the cutaneous incision is followed by the dissection of the adipose tissue and the exposure of the fascial plane, allowing the palpation of the iliac spine directly under the skin.

Once the tensor has been spread posteriorly, on the underlying anatomical space an effort should be made to correctly identify the position of the rectus femoris (fig. 7), which, if incorrect, leads to a possible passage anteriorly instead of posteriorly between this structure and the vastus lateralis and the small and medium gluteus. In our experience this eventuality did not occur, but we have verified that the abduction and the extension of the limb (fig.6) allow an adequate posterior divarication of the TFL and the correct identification of the anatomical space.

Isolation and cauterization of the lateral circumflex has never been a source of possible complications or difficulties (fig. 10).

The isolation of the capsule and its incision has never been burdened by errors or difficulties either, whilst the refinement of its complete release from the femur has been the subject of a progressive and quite long work that, once perfected, has allowed us to obtain adequate acetabular and femoral exposure, thus extending the use of the anterior access to all patients with coxo-femoral joint pathology regardless of morphological and articular characteristics.

2. Acetabular preparation and prosthetic implantation

The correct acetabular preparation and implantation of the cup necessarily require an adequate exposure that does not condition the orientation of the drills and subsequently of the implant. For this to occur, it is necessary to mobilize the femoral metaphysis beyond the posterior acetabular rim by means of retractor 4 (fig. 36) in association with limb extension. This maneuver is particularly difficult in the protruded coxa vara due to the medial, proximal position of the metaphysis and the reduced length of the periarticular musculature as a whole – in particular of the extrarotators. Inadequate acetabular exposure in the preparation and positioning of the implant leads to excessive anteversion and inclination of the prosthetic cup, a complication reported in the literature of anterior access.

In this phase, in the absence of an adequate exposure, the attempt to remedy by forcing on the retractor 4 might be responsible for a posterior acetabular wall fracture or for the anterior margin of the femoral neck collapse at the resection site.

In our experience an insufficient acetabular exposure due to inadequate mobilization of the femoral metaphysis has always forced us to return to the capsular release with the aim to obtain a better mobility and a consequent reduced tension, thus avoiding fractures as described.

Regarding the anterior margin of the resection on the femoral neck, the cortical thickness is particularly reduced and therefore subject to yielding. In our experience this problem is not uncommon, especially in implants on patients with cervical fractures and, when performed, it involves a small portion of the neck proximal to the vastus lateralis that does not compromise the femoral integrity and does not require specific treatments. Potentially also the spread on the anterior margin with the retractor 3 could be a cause of complications; however, in our experience we have never had fractures on the anterior acetabular wall, whilst we face more frequently the risk of insulting the iliopsoas tendon by inserting the retractor in its area.

The attention paid in obtaining a constant acetabular exposure, as already pointed out, allows to achieve a reduction in fracture complications and especially to avoid malpositioning in terms of anteversion and inclination.

3. Femoral preparation and prosthetic implantation

Since the beginning of our experience with the anterior access we have noticed that the femoral preparation was the real challenge and difficulty, in fact while the acetabular preparation was very close to the experience with direct lateral access, the femoral one required the development of a gesture substantially different from the one previously developed, necessitating the femur to be aligned to the surgical window, the lower limb to be positioned in extension and extra-rotation (fig. 59) and the surgeon to be placed anteriorly with respect to the patient. As previously seen, also in this phase potential complications arise first from the retraction. Specifically, the positioning of the retractor 4 behind the apex of the great trochanter (fig. 44) can lead, particularly in patients with reduced bone quality, to its introduction into the territory of the greater trochanter, creating the conditions for an apical fracture. Since we have personally experienced retractor malpositioning, we always visually check its position before proceeding to the preparation of the femur, correcting it if necessary. Consequently, we have never had trochanteric fractures that required osteosynthesis but only some infringement of the apex of the greater trochanter that has not affected in any cases the rehabilitation path and the functional recovery.

Another element determined to be fundamental to the reduced incidence of problems and complications on the greater trochanter is the type of prosthetic stem – as the absence of a pronounced shoulder allows to safeguard the trochanteric bone stock increasing its resistance.

In addition to the retractor 4 in the femoral exposure, the femoral elevator 6 (fig. 44) is crucial, placed in correspondence of the calcar and exploiting the strongest portion of the femoral neck. Also in this case, it is necessary to avoid forcing the elevation in an excessive way in order to prevent leading to support point failure or to an avulsion of the piriformis insertion, which is, once the capsular release is completed, the anatomical structure that hinders the lifting and the anteposition of the femoral metaphysis. In very few cases we found an avulsion of the trochanteric apex in correspondence of the piriformis insertion, confirming the fact that, after the postero-superior capsule, this is the main obstacle to a correct femoral exposure.

To avoid complications, once an inadequate exposure is verified and the complete postero-superior capsule is released, the detachment of the piriformis should be performed, if necessary, e.g., in case of protruded coxa vara. The correct positioning of the femoral metaphysis with respect to the surgical window is fundamental for the femoral preparation and to avoid complications like the risk of postero-lateral meta-diaphyseal cortical perforation due to an excessive inclination of the instrument in the opening of the canal (fig. 45) or a bad positioning of the stem with excessive varus deviation and extrarotation. Also, in this phase of the learning curve it was consolidated the habit of searching for an adequate metaphyseal exposure (fig. 59) before proceeding with the opening of the canal and then with the preparation of the femur, allowing to avoid false paths and malpositioning.

Thanks to these attentions, along our experience we have had only three cases of femoral fissuring that have required the removal of the prosthetic stem and the metaphyseal cerclage, due to rotational stresses during the implant reduction maneuvers and to the interruption of the cortical ring of the resected femoral neck in the direction of the great trochanter (fig. 46), which at the time of the introduction of the definitive stem has caused a failure at the level of the calcar. As mentioned, in these cases the removal of the stem allowed a closure of the fissure that, once stabilized with one or two cerclages, allowed the positioning of the stem without having to proceed to increase the size of the implant. In all the cases mentioned, complete healing was obtained and only greater caution was exercised in the granting of the load during the first month after surgery.

Acknowledgment: thanks to Dr Alice De Sensi for reviewing English translation

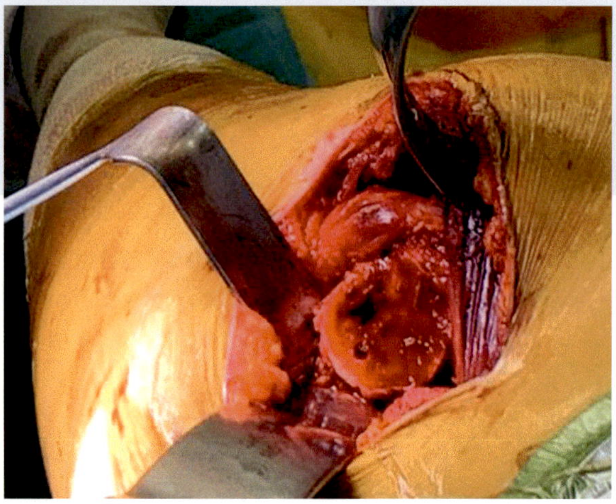

Figure 59 The image shows the correct femoral exposure. The stump obtained from the neck resection appears correctly aligned with the surgical field

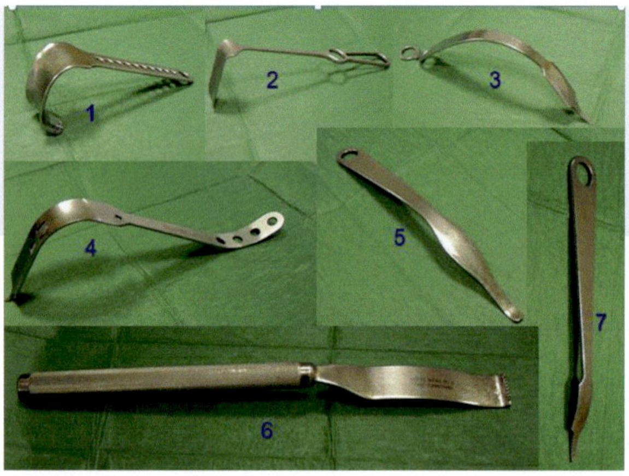

Figure 60 The image shows the retractors used in the ALDI Approach and their relative numbering

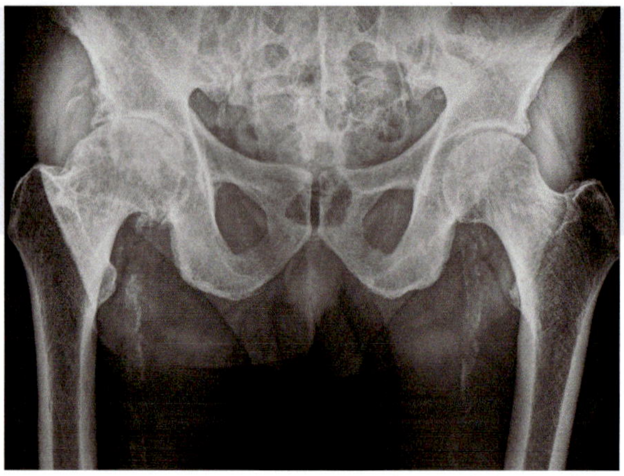

Figure 61 Pre-operative radiographic assessment

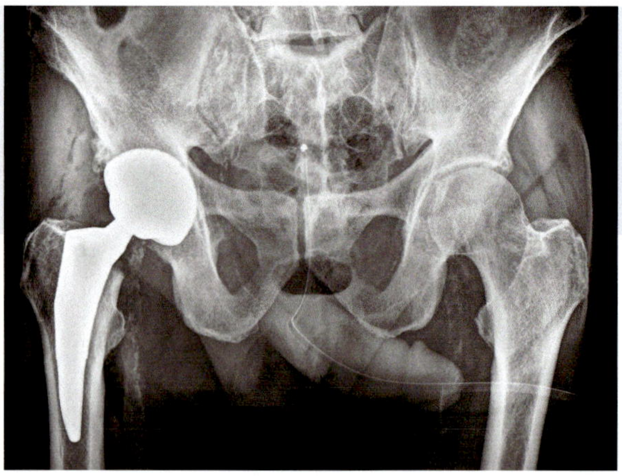

Figure 62 Post-operative radiographic examination

Bibliography

1. Carta S, Fortina M, Scipio D, Pichierri P, Riva A, Ferrata P. ALDI (Anterior Lateral Decubitus Intermuscular) approach: new developments in total hip arthroplasty with anterior approach. 94th Annual Congress of the Orthopaedics and Traumatology Italian Society. Milan, 7-11/11/09 J Orthop Traumatol, 1 (1 Suppl) (2009), p. S32.
2. Carta S, Fortina M. ALDI (Anterior Lateral Decubitus Intermuscular) approach to the hip: Comprehensive description of the surgical technique with operative video. Orthop Traumatol Surg Res. 2019;105(5):923-930.
3. Schneeberger AG, Schulz RF, Ganz R. Blood loss in total hip arthroplasty. Lateral position combined with preservation of the capsule versus supine position combined with capsulectomy. Arch Orthop Trauma Surg. 1998;117(1-2):47-49.
4. Locher S, et al. Blood loss in total hip prosthesis implantation: lateral versus supine position. Z Orthop Ihre Grenzgeb. 1999;137(2):148-152.
5. Ropars M, Morandi X, Huten D, Thomazeau H, Berton E, Darnault P. Anatomical study of the lateral femoral cutaneous nerve with special reference to minimally invasive anterior approach for total hip replacement. Surg Radiol Anat. 2009;31(3):199-204.
6. Walters J, Solomons M, Davies J. Gluteus minimus: observations on its insertion. J Anat. 2001;198(Pt 2):239-242.
7. Beck M, Sledge JB, Gautier E, Dora CF, Ganz R. The anatomy and function of the gluteus minimus muscle. J Bone Joint Surg Br. 2000;82(3):358-363.
8. Hewitt J, Guilak F, Glisson R, Vail TP. Regional material properties of the human hip joint capsule ligaments. J Orthop Res. 2001;19(3):359-364.
9. Martin HD, Savage A, Braly BA, Palmer IJ, Beall DP, Kelly B. The function of the hip capsular ligaments: a quantitative report. Arthroscopy. 2008;24(2):188-195.
10. Sotereanos NG, Miller MC, Smith B, Hube R, Sewecke JJ, Wohlrab D. Using intraoperative pelvic landmarks for acetabular component placement in total hip arthroplasty. J Arthroplasty. 2006;21(6):832-840.
11. Smith-Petersen MN. Approach to and exposure of the hip joint for mold arthroplasty. J Bone Joint Surg Am. 1949;31A(1):40-46.
12. Yoon YS, Hodgson AJ, Tonetti J, Masri BA, Duncan CP. Resolving inconsistencies in defining the target orientation for the acetabular cup angles in total hip arthroplasty. Clin Biomech (Bristol, Avon). 2008;23(3):253-259.
13. Pilot P, Kerens B, Draijer WF, et al. Is minimally invasive surgery less invasive in total hip replacement? A pilot study. Injury. 2006;37 Suppl 5:S17-S23.
14. Matsuura M, Ohashi H, Okamoto Y, Inori F, Okajima Y. Elevation of the femur in THA through a direct anterior approach: cadaver and clinical studies. Clin Orthop Relat Res. 2010;468(12):3201-3206.
15. Ogonda L, Wilson R, Archbold P, et al. A minimal-incision technique in total hip arthroplasty does not improve early postoperative outcomes. A prospective, randomized, controlled trial. J Bone Joint Surg Am. 2005;87(4):701-710.
16. Crowninshield RD, Johnston RC, Brand RA, Pedersen DR. Pathologic ligamentous constraint of the hip. Clin Orthop Relat Res. 1983;(181):291-297.

CASE REPORT 1

62-year-old male.A) Preoperative X-ray in hip arthrodesis due to articular infection 30 years before surgery. B) Post-operative X-ray THR via ALDI Approach extended distally on the femur to allow screw and plate remouvement. C) Post-operative 1-year X-ray.

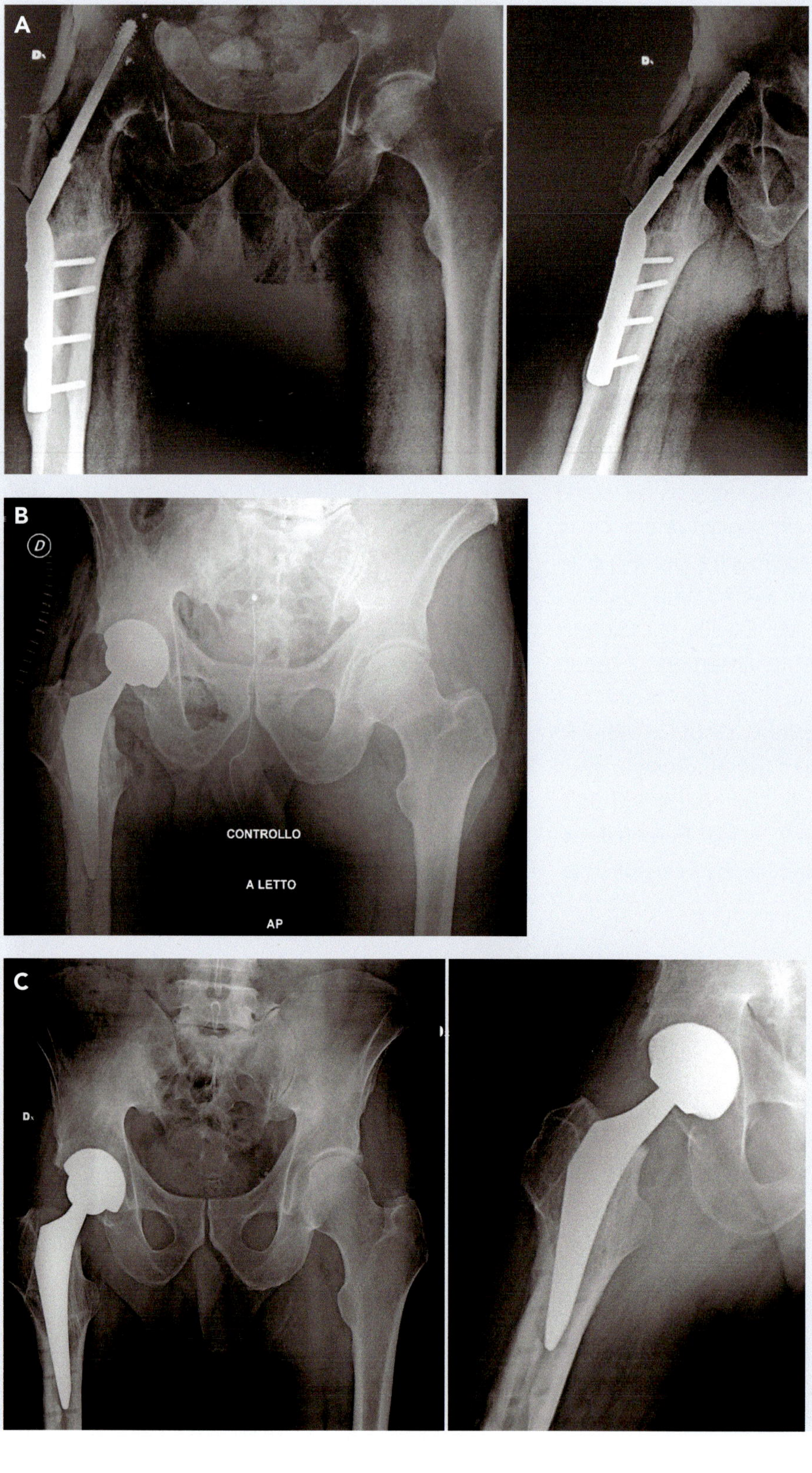

CASE REPORT 2

71-year-old female. A) Periprostetic fracture (B2) preoperative CT scan. B) Treatment: ALDI Approach extended distally in order to expose the femoral fracture, stem replacement with long modular stem and osteosynthesis with multiple cercalge wire. Post-operative X-ray. C) Xray at 1 year: complete fracture healing and stem osteointegration. D) Due to left side arthrosis at one year the patient is proposed for total hip replacement: preoperative X-ray. E) Post-operative X-ray of left THR performed with ALDI Approach. F) Post-operative X-ray at 2 years (right) and 1 year (left).

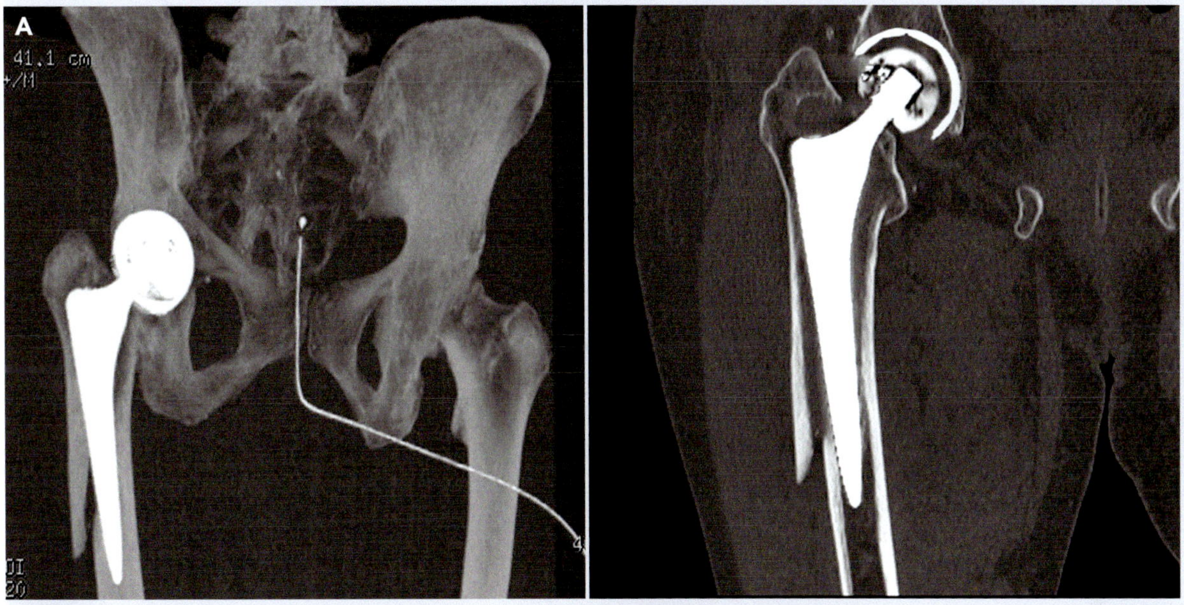

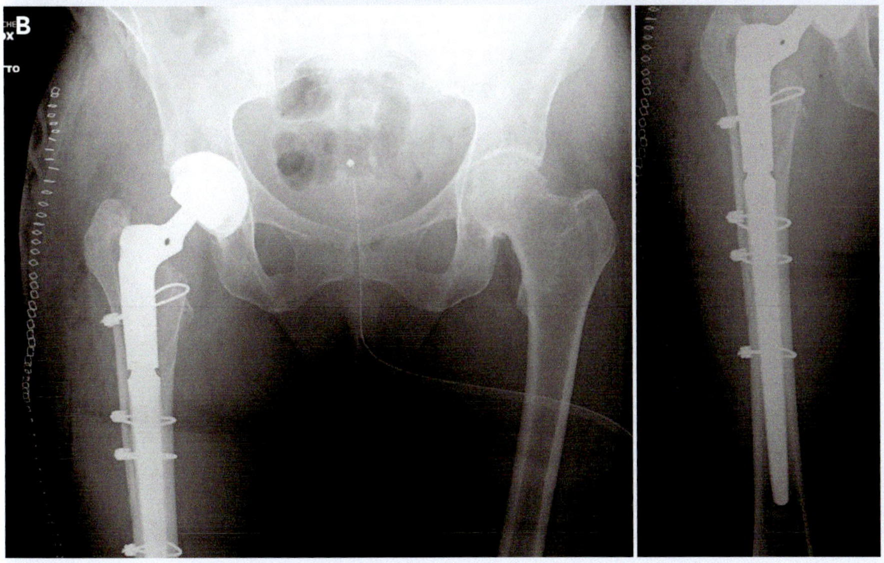

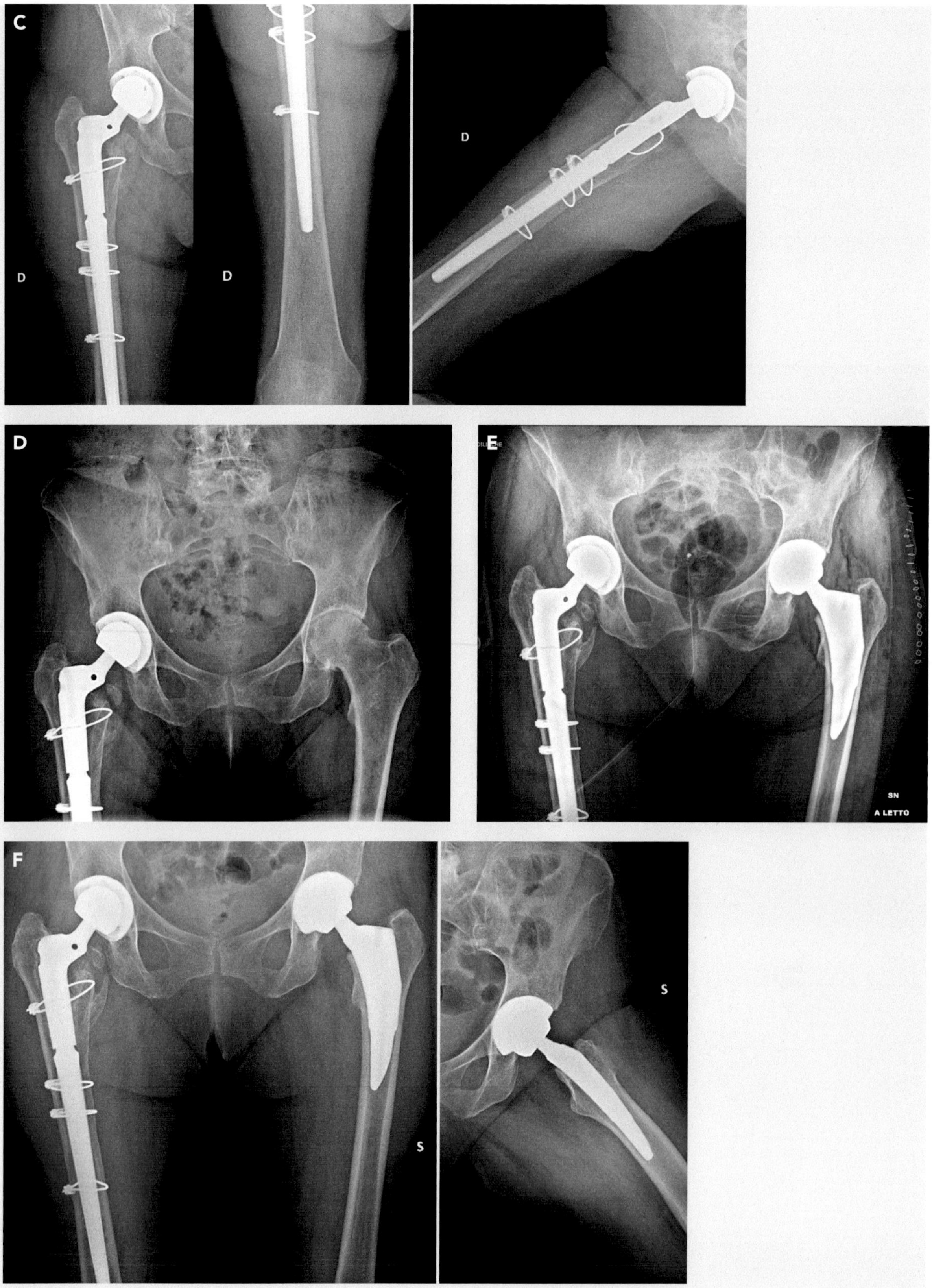
C
D
D
D
D
E
SN
A LETTO
F
S
S

CASE REPORT 3

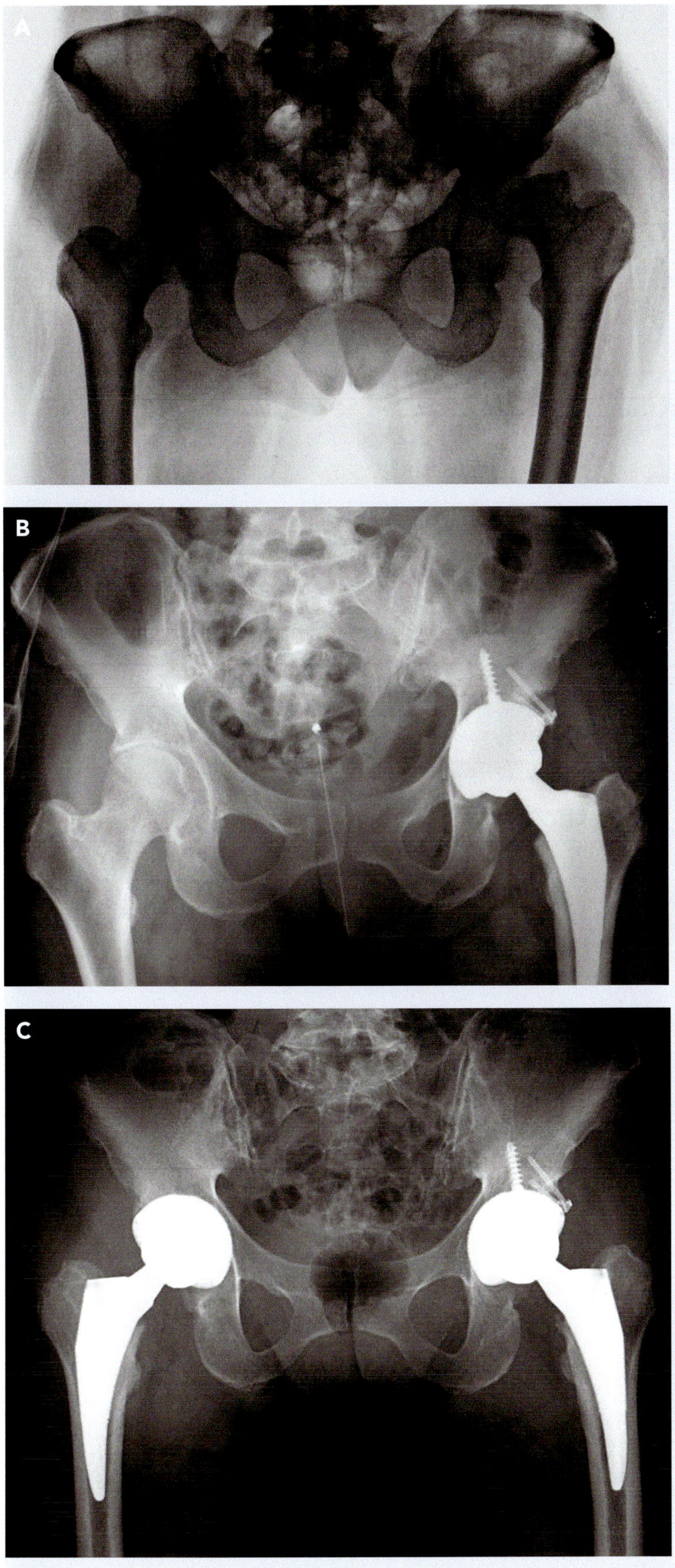

50-year-old female. A) Preoperative X-ray in left dysplastic hip and Perthes disease. B) Postoperative X-ray. Treatment: ALDI Approach with THR, restore of the anatomical hip rotation center (HCR) filling the cranial dysplastic acetabular defect with head bone fragment stabilized by two screws. C) X-ray at 2 years at the moment of the right THR performed with ALDI Approach as well.

CASE REPORT 4

65-year-old female. A) Preoperative X-ray. Bilateral partum releted hip dislocation treated with repeated surgical osteotomy. B) Post-operative X-ray. Treatment: ALDI Approach extended proximally along the iliac wing and distally exposing the femoral shaft. Restore of the acetabular anatomical position in the paleocotile. After plate remouvement, femoral osteotomy in order to restore the bone axis and to allow metaphiseal distalisation using a modular revision stem. C) Post-operative at 10 months X-ray. Complete healing of the femoral osteotomy and prosthetic ostheointegration. D) Post-operative left THR X-ray, performed with ALDI Approach partially extended proximally along the iliac wing. E) Post-operative X-ray at 4 years (right) and 3 years and 2 months (left).

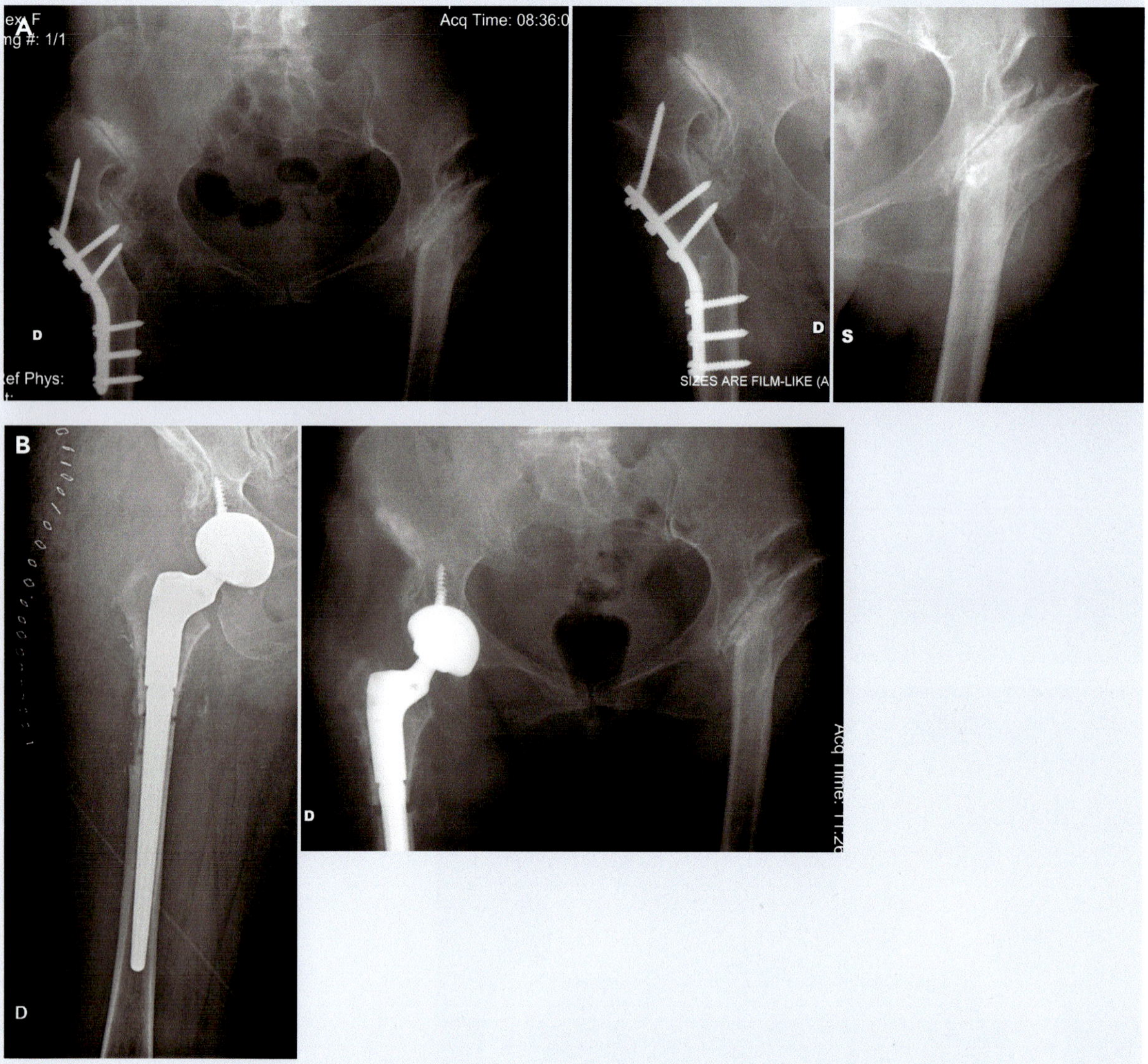

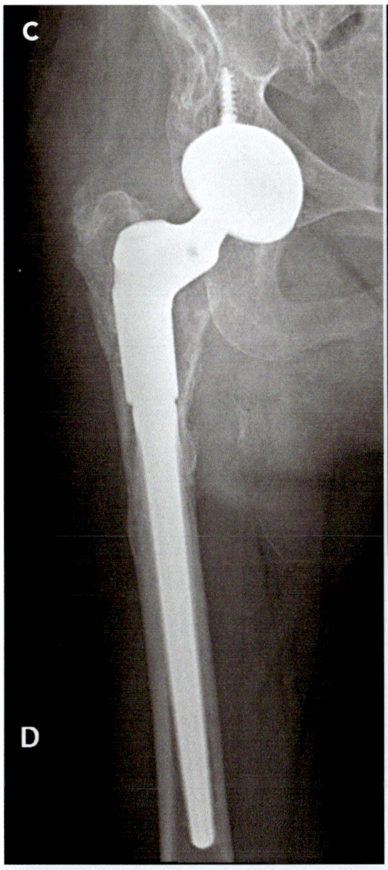
C
D

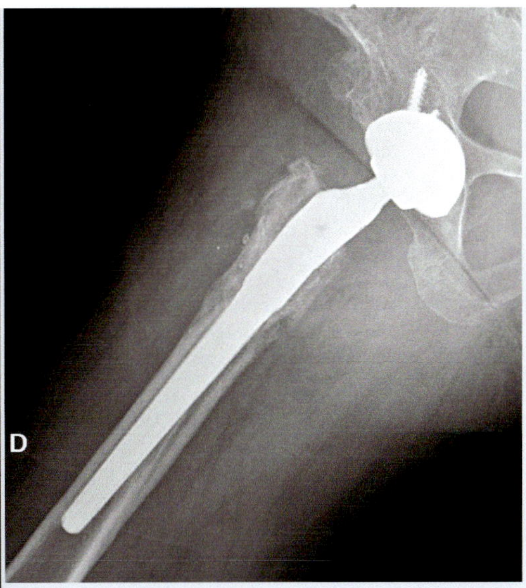
D

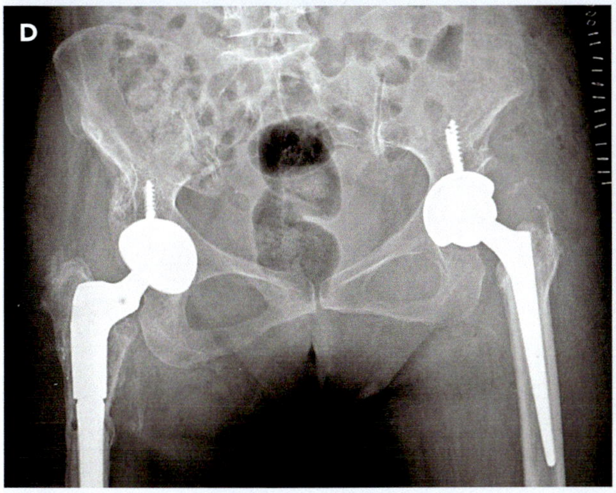
D

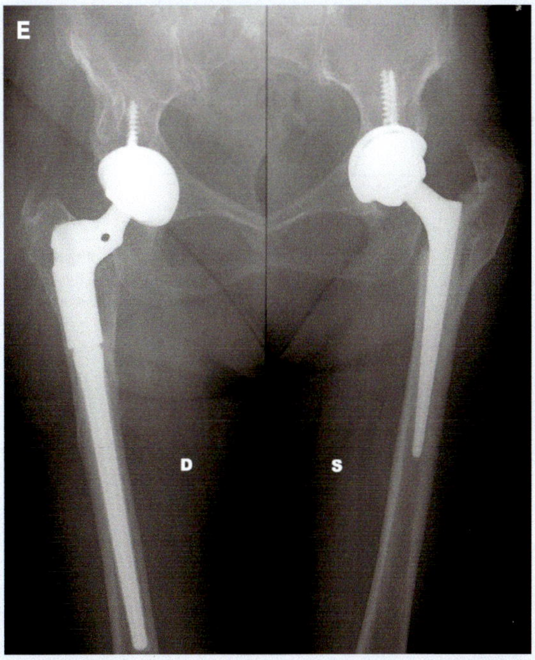
E
D
S

CASE REPORT 5

29-year-old female. A) Preoperative X-ray in right dysplastic femur with hypoplasic head due to Perthes disease. B) Post-operative X-ray. Right THR performed with ALDI Approach correcting the leg length discrepancy. C) 2 years X-ray. Complete prosthetic ostheointegration.

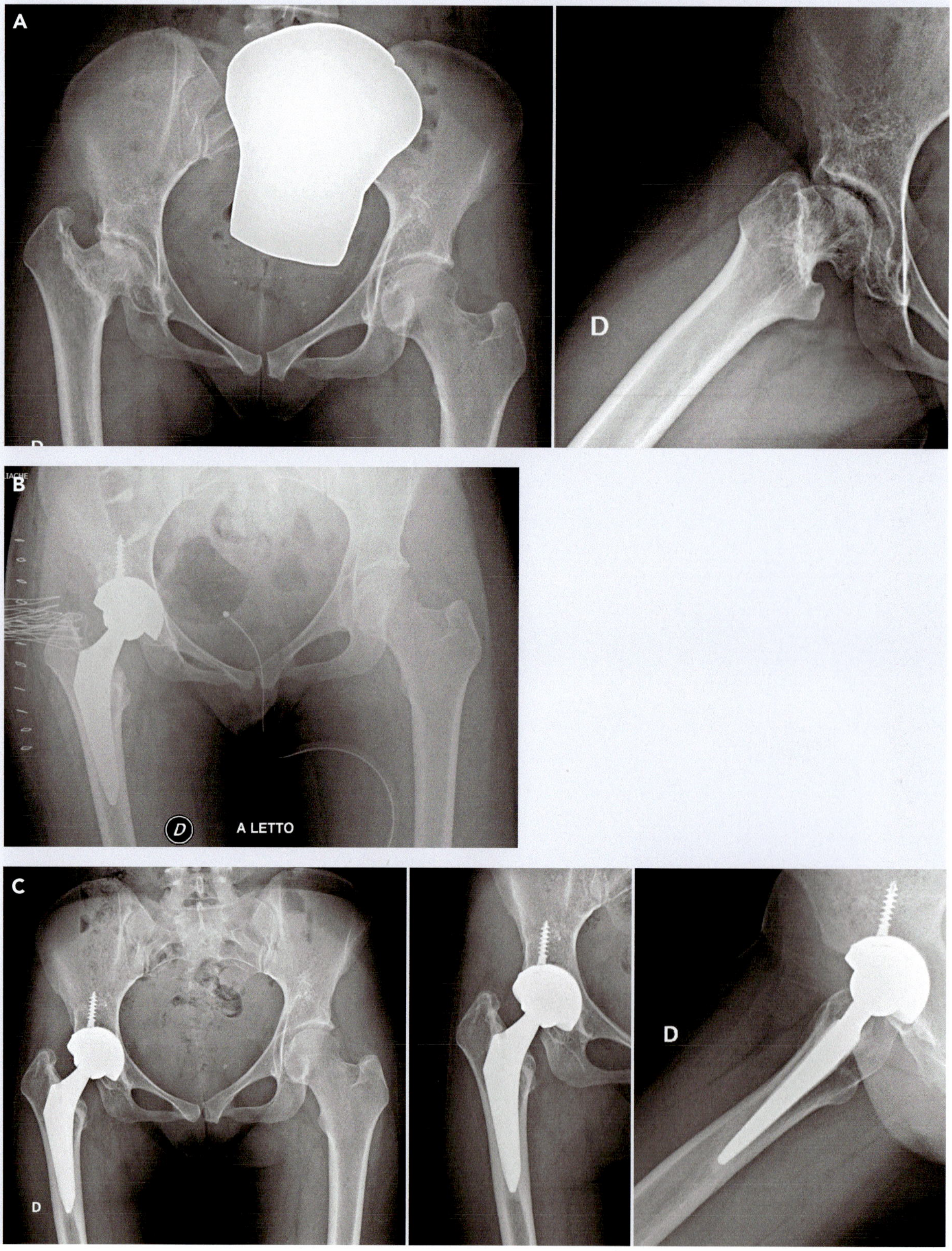

CASE REPORT 6

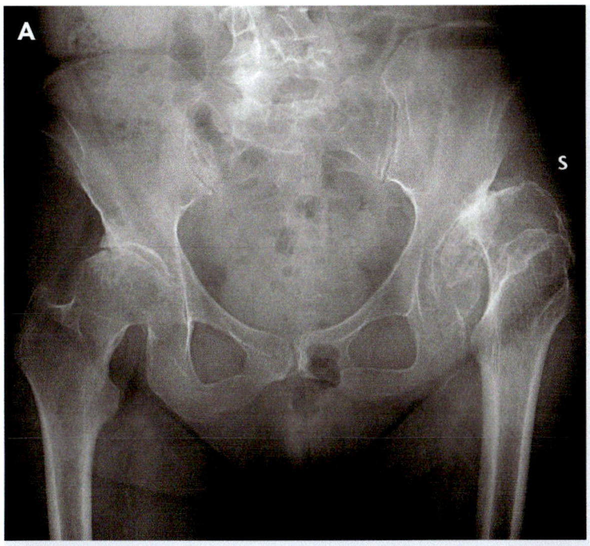

66-year-old female. A) Preoperative X-ray in patient with right hip arthrosis and left hip dysplasia. B) Post-operative X-ray right THR performed with ALDI Approach. C) Post-operative X-ray. After 15 months left THR performed with ALDI Approach restoring the HRC and correcting the leg length discrepancy. D) Post-operative X-ray at 4 years (right) and at 3 years (left).

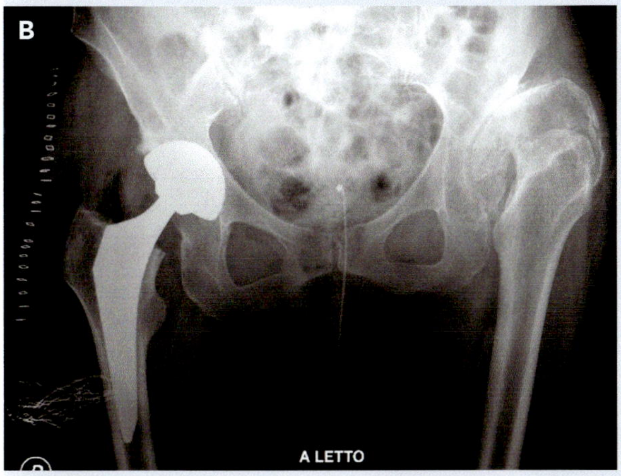

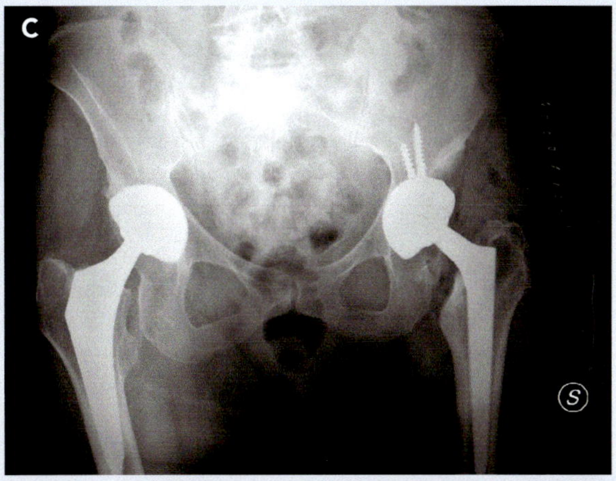

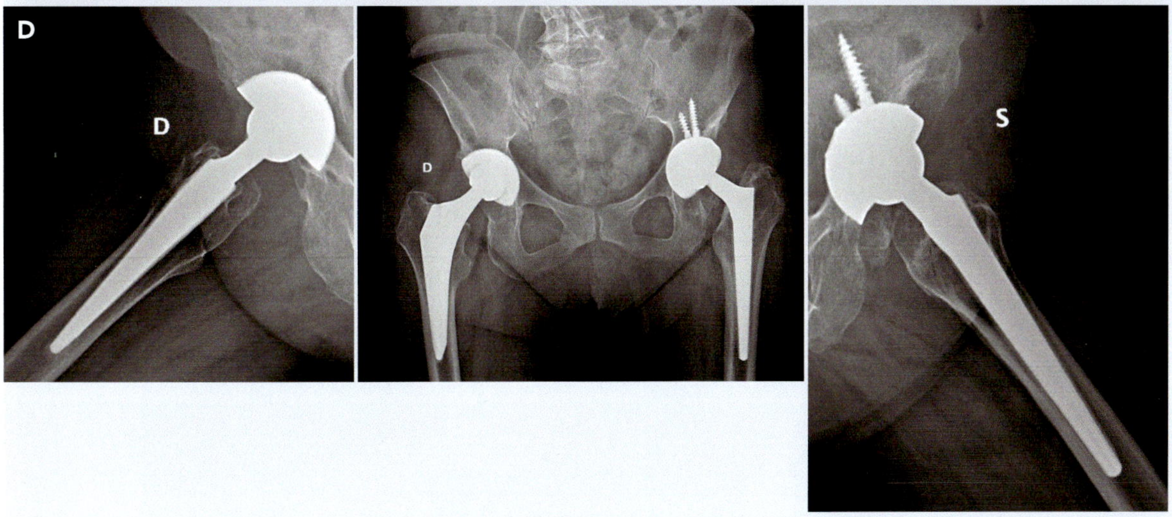

CASE REPORT 7

31-year-old female. A) Preoperative X-ray. Hip arthrosis with dismorphism due to neck fracture treated with cervical screws. B) Post-operative X-ray. THA via ALDI Approach with intraoperative complication as calcar fracture due to torsional stress during implant reduction maneuvers, treated with double wire cerclage. C) Post-operative X-ray at 11 years. Complete healing and implant osteointegration after 11 years.

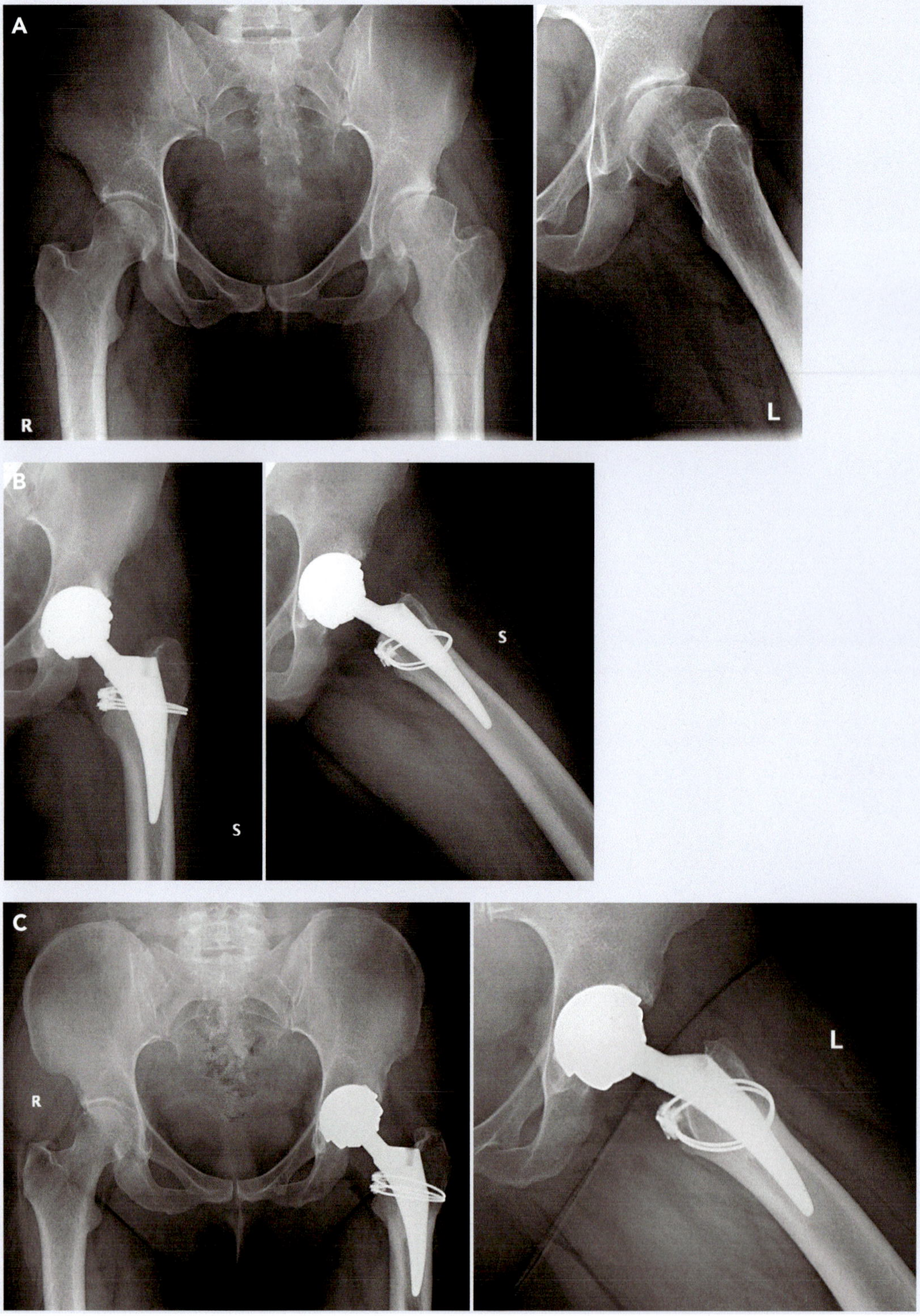

CASE REPORT 8

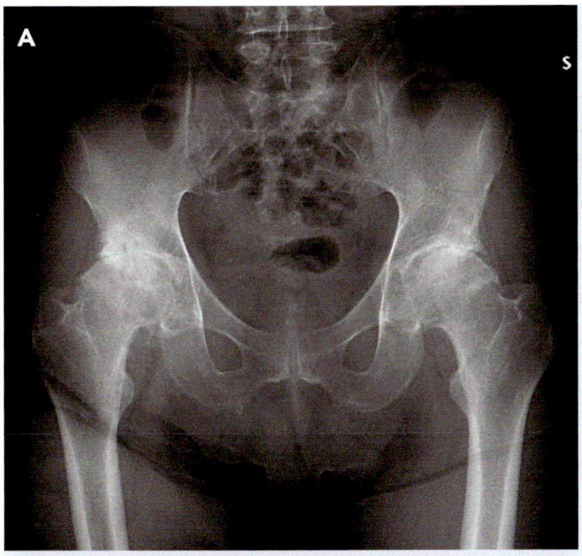

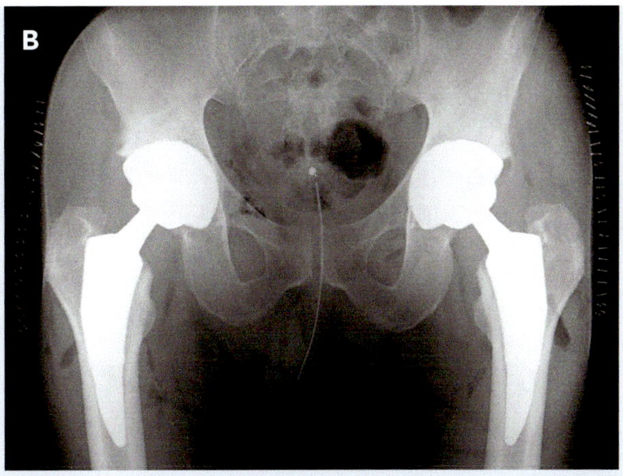

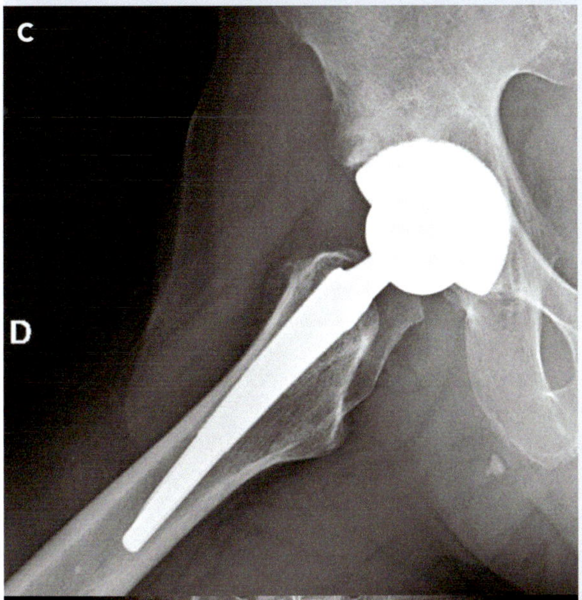

49-year-old male. A) Preoperative X-ray in bilateral hip arthrosis. B) Post-operative X-ray in bilateral simultaneous THR performed via ALDI Approach. C) Post-operative X-ray at 1 year.

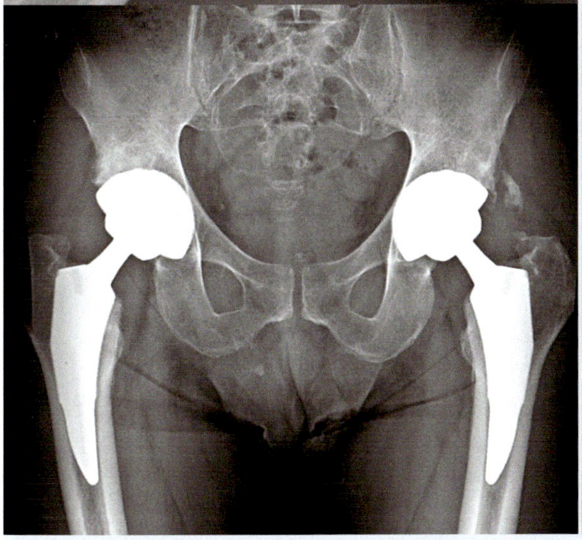

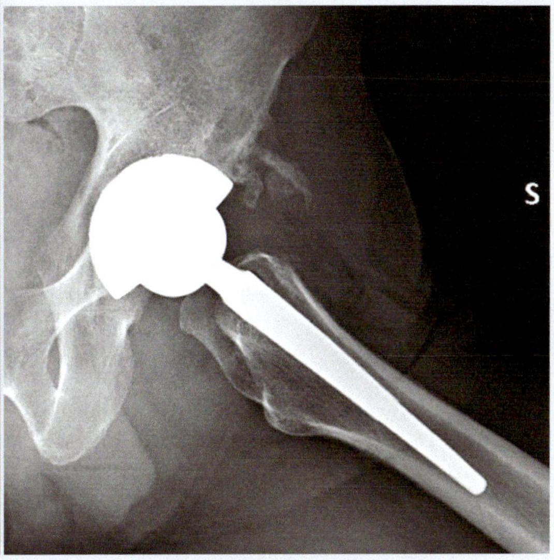

11

CASE REPORT 9

93-year-old female. A) Preoperative X-ray of bilateral hip arthrosis in varus femur and head protrusion. B) Post-operative X-ray. THR of the right hip performed with ALDI Approach. C) Post-operative X-ray left THR. After 1 year hip replacement on the left side by ALDI Approach. D) Post-operative X-ray at 2 years of the right THR. E) Post-operative X-ray at 1 year of left THR.

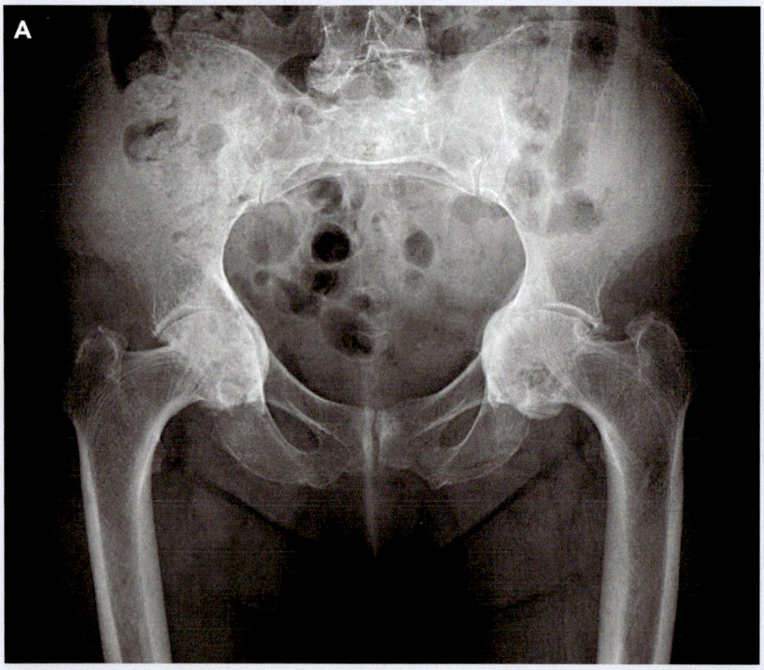

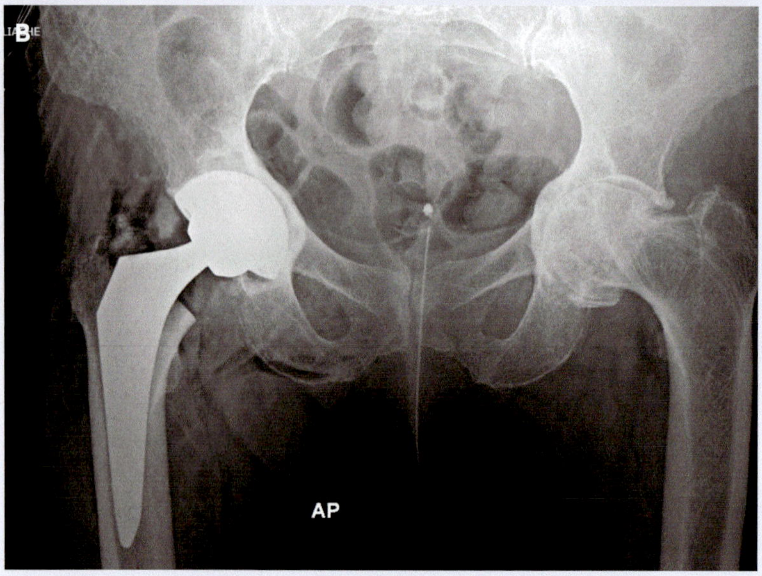

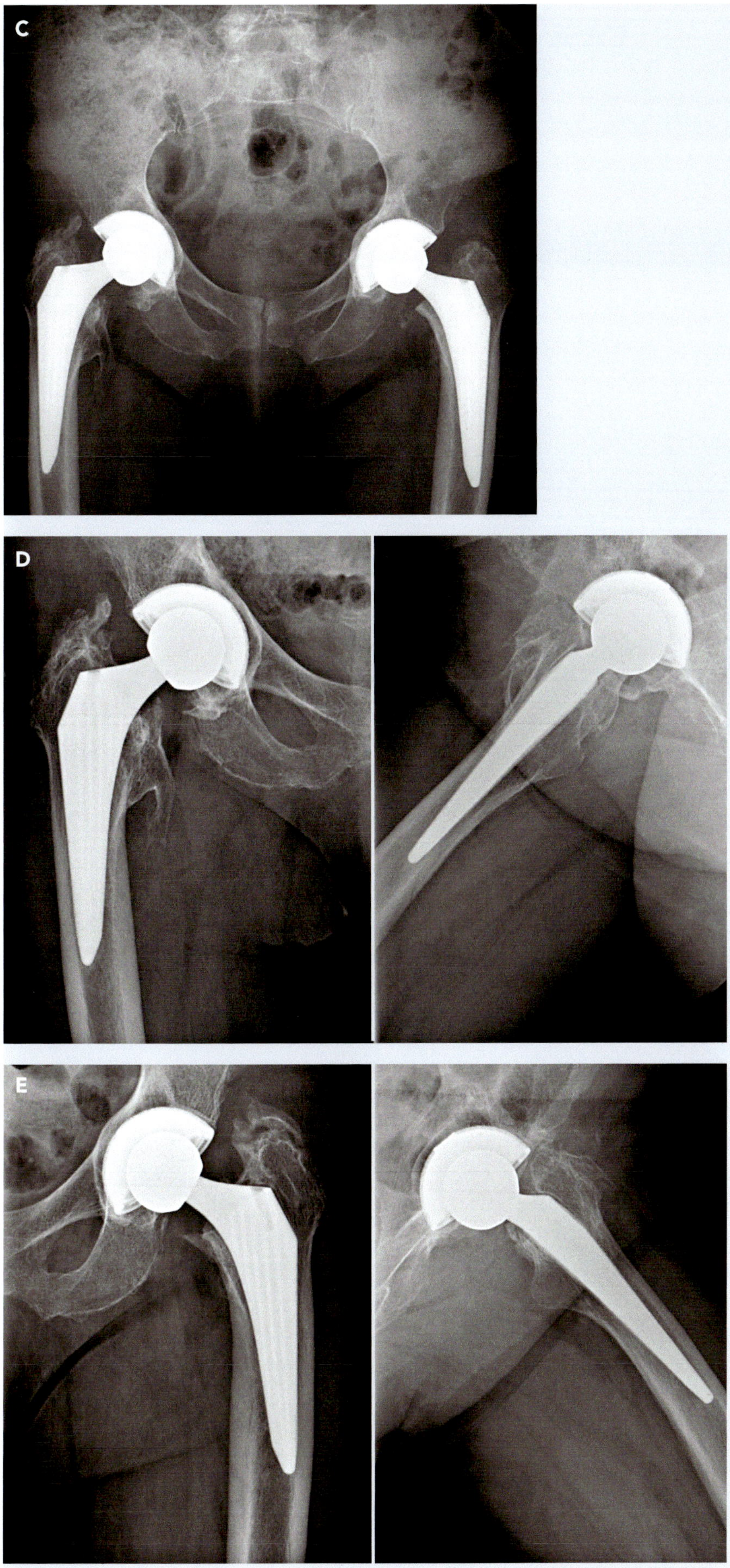
C
D
E

CASE REPORT 10

65-year-old male. A) Preoperative X-ray. Left dysplastic hip arthrosis. B) Post-operative X-ray. Left THR performed by ALDI Approach. C) Post-operative X-ray at 4 years.

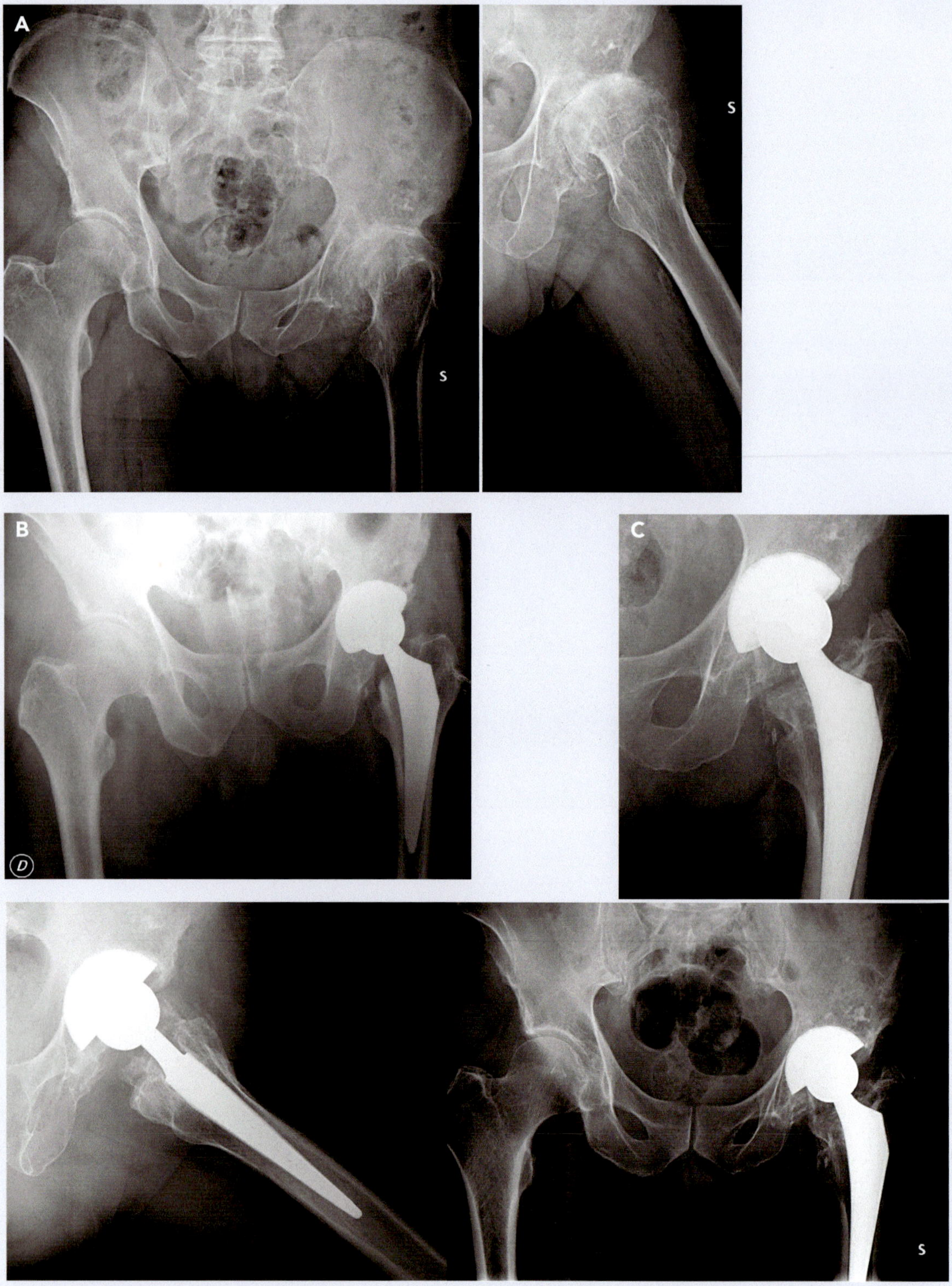

CASE REPORT 11

64-year-old female. A) Pre-operative control in coxarthrosis for existing bilateral congenital dislocation of the left hip. B) Post-operative X-ray 2 months after left hip replacement surgery performed with ALDI Approach. Positioning of the acetabular component on the paleocotyl and filling of the bone defect with autologous graft obtained from the femoral head and stabilized with screws. C) Right hip post-operative X-ray control 6 months after left hip replacement surgery performed with ALDI Approach. Also on the right side, positioning of the acetabular component on the paleocotyl and filling of the bone defect with autologous graft obtained from the femoral head and stabilized with screws. D) Post-operative X-ray at 4 years on the left side and 3 years on the right side demonstrating the osseointegration of the implants and autologous supracotyloid bone grafts.

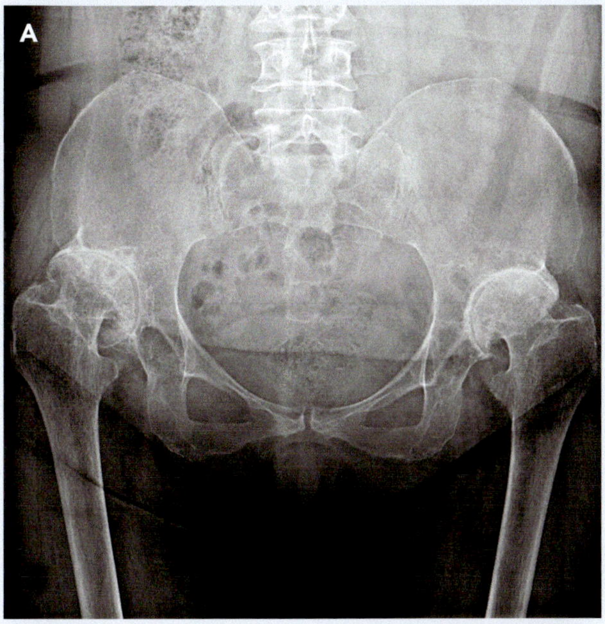

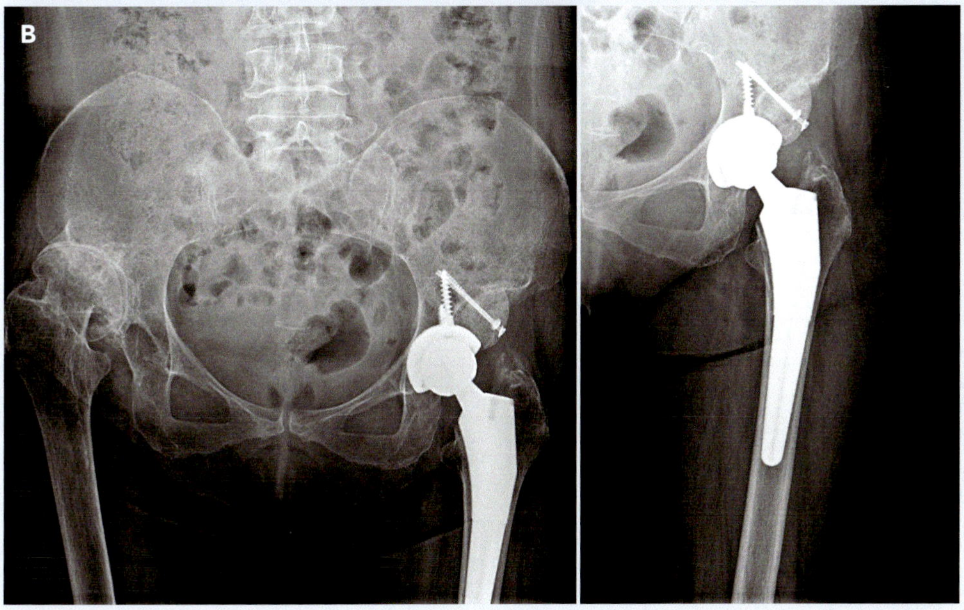

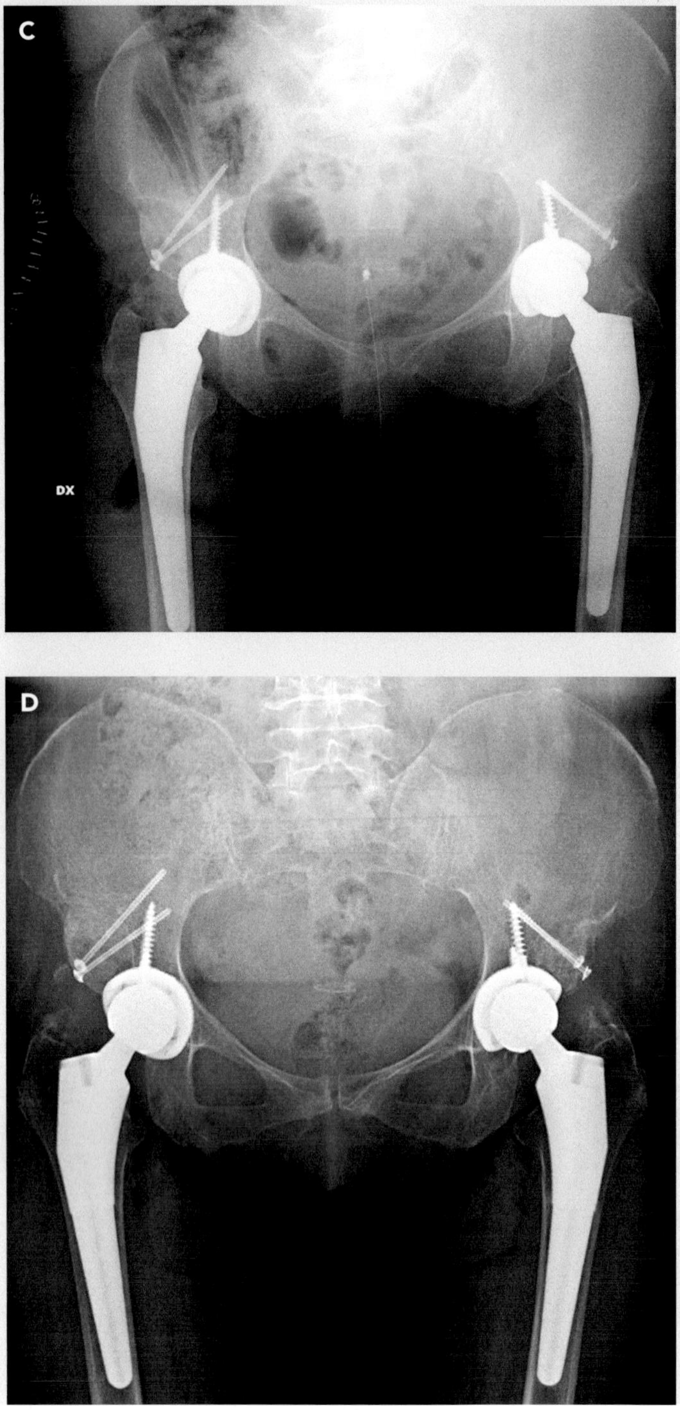
C
DX
D

The minimally invasive anterolateral approach in total hip replacement

Giovanni Francesco Grano, Maria Pavlidou

Department of Orthopaedics and Traumatology, Bassano del Grappa Hospital, Vicenza, ULSS 7 Pedemontana/Veneto, Italy

Introduction

Over the last twenty years, hip prosthetic surgery has improved its standard in prosthetic models, biomechanics, materials, anesthetic techniques, pre- and post-operative protocols and surgical approaches.

In terms of surgical technique, over the last decade, minimally invasive surgery (MIS), characterised by greater respect for all those tissues not involved in the pathology, has become popular [1].

As for the surgical approach, the concept of using intermuscular planes has now prevailed. This allows the muscles and their tendon insertions to be respected, resulting in less bleeding and less post-operative pain. In addition, there are undoubted advantages in the rehabilitation process due to the preservation of muscle strength and hip proprioception [2,3].

Starting from the classic approaches (anterior of Smith-Petersen [4], antero-lateral of Watson-Jones [5], direct lateral of Hardinge [6] and posterior of Gibson-Moore [7]) each surgeon, using the best known and most familiar approach, has tried to optimise it.

In the standard anterolateral approach of Watson-Jones, surgical damage to the abductor muscles is associated with altered proprioception and reduced muscle strength, which can result in Trendelenburg gait [8].

This chapter describes a new minimally invasive anterolateral access called 'detachment free' (DF) as it completely respects the abductor tendon and muscle structures.

Indications

In order to use minimally invasive approach, patient selection is critical. In the Literature, the criteria given are: primary coxarthrosis, medial femoral neck fractures, absence of previous hip surgery, and body mass index (BMI) [9].

Some authors [10] consider that on the basis of the BMI, determined by the weight in kg divided by the height expressed in m^2, the candidates are those patients with a value below 30. We consider the thigh circumference measured at the level of the greater trochanter to be more reliable as a selective criterion. This is because the BMI does not consider the distribution of body fat and does not assess the patient's musculature [11].

Therefore, the inclusion criteria used are: no previous surgery in the hip region, patients with primary coxarthrosis or medial femoral neck fracture, not excessively muscular, with a thigh circumference on the G.T. of up to 80 cm and with a cervical-diaphyseal angle

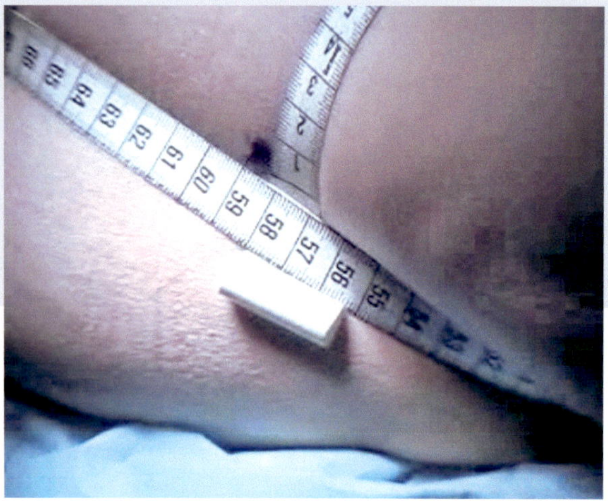

Figure 1
Circumference of the thigh at the level of the greater trochanter

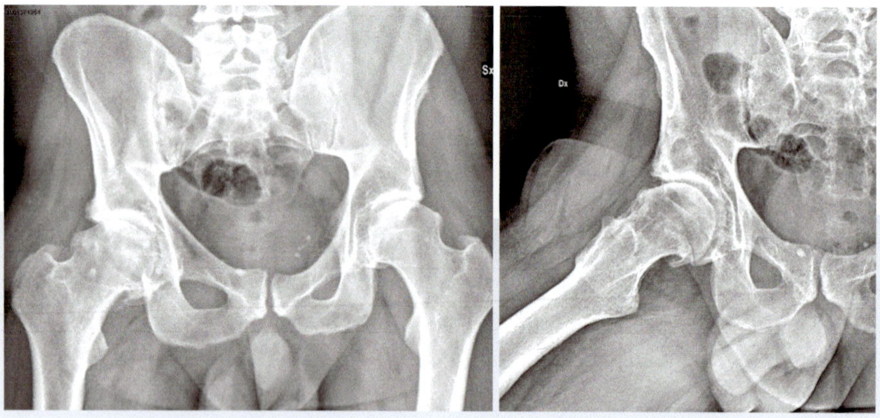

Figure 2
Pre-operative X-ray

(CDA) preferably physiological or valgus (fig. 1). The most difficult cases are those patients with severe osteoporosis, a thigh circumference of more than 80 cm and a varus CDA.
Minimally invasive (DF) approach is contraindicated in patients who have previously undergone other surgical procedures, who have significant anatomical femoral abnormalities or severe dysplastic hips. In these cases, a standard approach is recommended.

Pre-operative planning

Clinical evaluation and proper pre-operative planning allow the appropriateness of surgical approach to be assessed.
The radiographic evaluation provides an assessment of the cervical-diaphyseal angle, the femoral off-set, the femoral neck version, any limb dysmetria and the presence of any anatomical abnormalities (fig. 2).

Surgical technique

We use the protocol with tranexamic acid 15 mg/kg at induction of anaesthesia and three hours after surgery. L2-L3 subarachnoid anaesthesia is performed with hyperbaric Marcaine 1% 15 mg in combination with morphine 150 γ as an adjuvant. During the procedure, Propofol is administered by syringe pump with variable TCI mode (1.2 mg/ml-3.5 mg/ml) and spontaneous breathing control by $EtCO_2$ with nasal detection using a face mask.
This procedure is performed with the patient supine on a standard operating bed, with a pillow in the lumbar region and with the lower limbs parallel. The sterile field is set up only on the affected limb and the procedure performed with the use of standard instrumentation (fig. 3).
To optimise the 'moving window' effect, the incision must be very precise. The apex, the

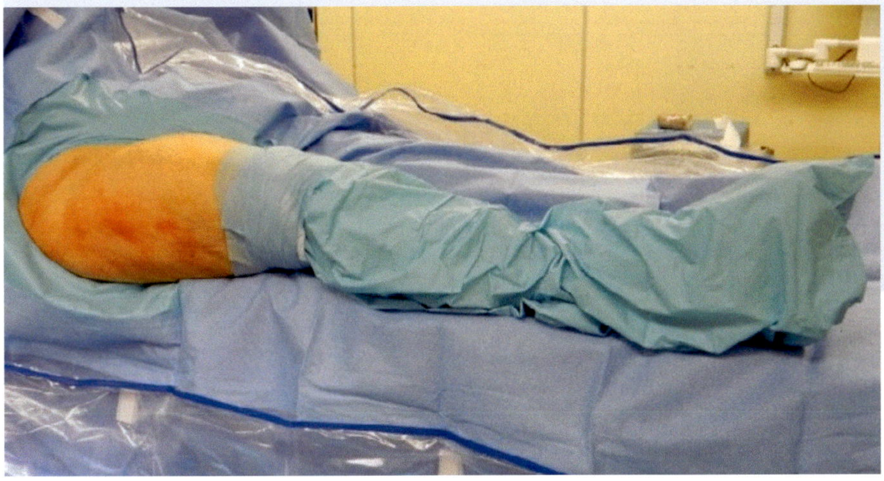

Figure 3
Patient in supine position

posterior border and the anterior border of the greater trochanter are identified. A skin incision of approximately 10 cm is made, slightly curved, 1 cm anterior to the anterior border of the G.T. extending 1/3 distally and 2/3 proximally (fig. 4A). After the incision of the subcutis and fascia, the interstitium between the tensor fascia lata and the gluteus minimus is identified. The vessels present (superior gluteal artery) are cauterized, respecting the superior gluteal nerve (fig. 4B-C) [12]. A Hohmann lever is placed on the lateral side of the capsule to retract the abductors. A second retractor is placed on the medial side of the capsule and a third on the anterior border of the acetabulum (fig. 4D). Exposing the capsule, an inverted T capsulotomy is performed. Using an oscillating saw, the femoral neck is osteotomized in situ and then the femoral head is removed (fig. 4E). To achieve adequate exposure of the acetabulum, Hohmann's retractors are repositioned, one on the anterior rim of the cup, one on the posterior rim and one in the acetabular notch.

Using a straight handle, the cup is reamed (fig. 4F) and then the definitive acetabular component is implanted (fig. 4G). The author uses hemispherical press-fit cups with ceramic or polyethylene inserts.

The femur is then exposed. To achieve optimal exposure, relaxation of the gluteal musculature is required. This is achieved through the administration of propofol in a syringe pump at an average of 1.2 mg/ml and spontaneous breathing control by means of $EtCO_2$ and O_2 administration with FiO_2 of 0.4.

In the case of particularly muscular patients, local infiltration of 10 mg of rocuronium in 5 ml of saline (2 mg/ml) into the minimus and medius gluteus may be helpful, obtaining in 20 seconds a 'customised' relaxation of the muscles involved in the operation and without systemic effects [13].

Bringing the limb into a figure-four position in adduction and external rotation (fig. 5A), a Hohmann retractor is placed at the calcar and a second one is placed on the greater trochanter to retract the gluteal muscles. With a hook, the femur is lifted and a posterior capsulotomy is performed sparing the external rotators. A third Hohmann lever is also placed on the greater trochanter to lift and better expose the femoral canal.

Good exposure of the femur allows proper preparation of the femoral canal using both off-set and straight handles. This also allows the use of various types of both cemented and cementless stems (straight, curved, short and neck-preserving) (fig. 5B).

After preparation of the femoral canal, the definitive stem is positioned. A trial head is used to perform the reduction. Stability, motility and length tests are performed before the definitive head is placed on the prosthetic cone (fig. 5C). Once the implant is completed, the integrity of the abductor musculature is assessed and the joint capsule, fascia and skin are sutured (fig 5D-E).

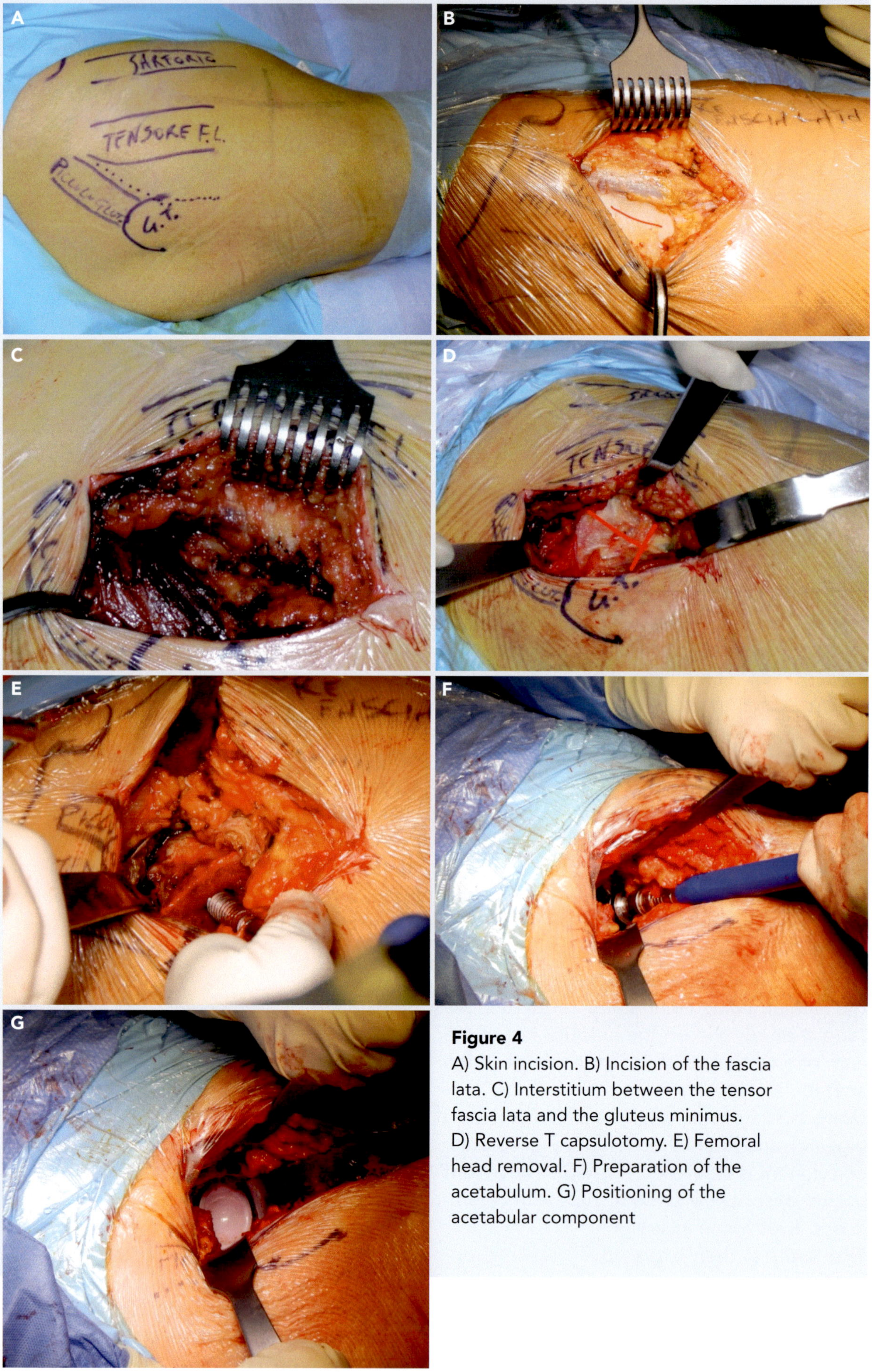

Figure 4
A) Skin incision. B) Incision of the fascia lata. C) Interstitium between the tensor fascia lata and the gluteus minimus. D) Reverse T capsulotomy. E) Femoral head removal. F) Preparation of the acetabulum. G) Positioning of the acetabular component

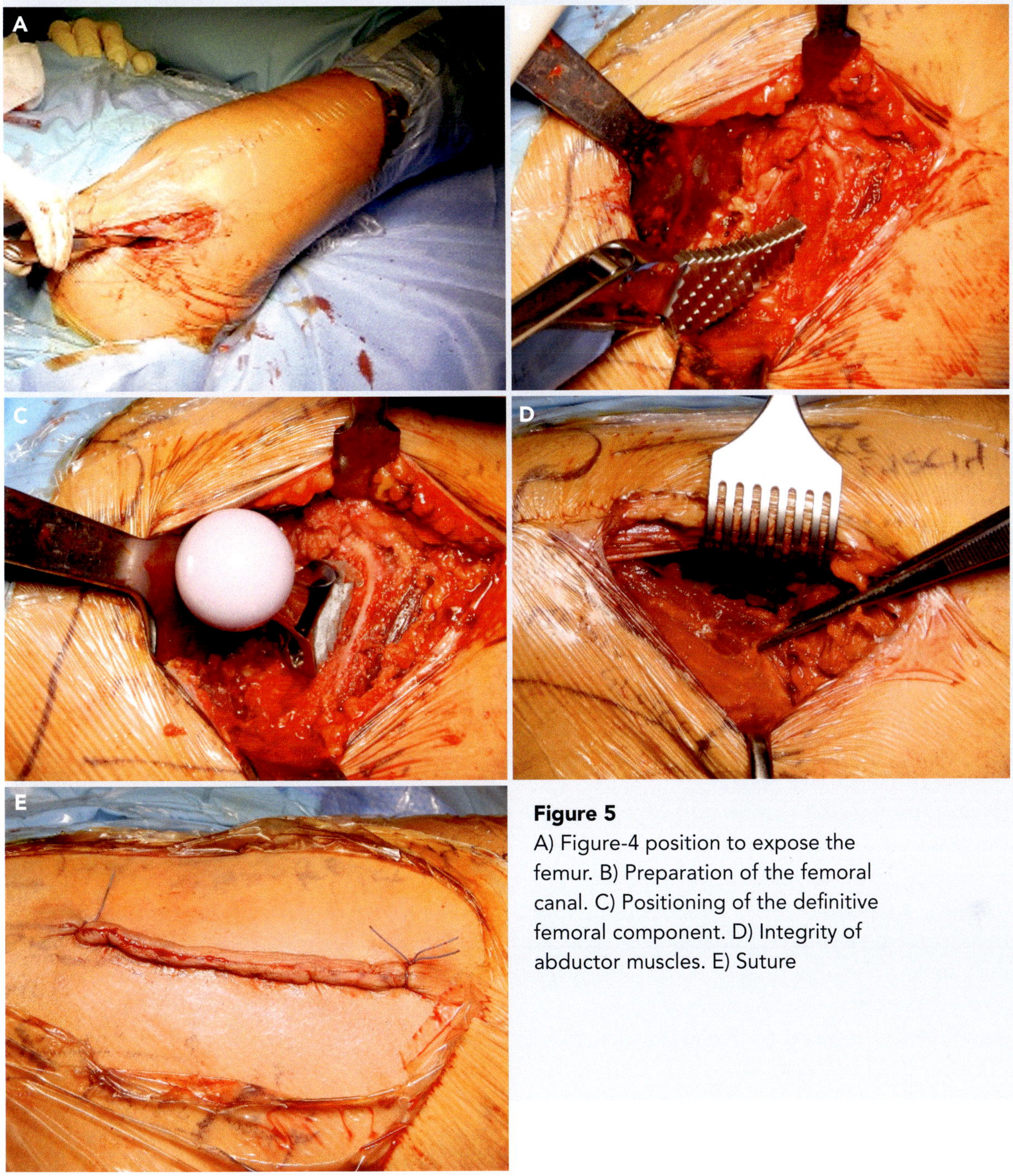

Figure 5
A) Figure-4 position to expose the femur. B) Preparation of the femoral canal. C) Positioning of the definitive femoral component. D) Integrity of abductor muscles. E) Suture

Post-operative care

In the post-operative period, an antithromboembolic prophylaxis is performed, both pharmacological and mechanical (plantar pumps and elastic stockings). In addition, prophylaxis for heterotopic ossifications is performed when indicated. Pain is controlled by continuous intravenous infusion for 24 h.
Post-operative X-rays (fig. 6A-B) are obtained on the day of surgery. This permits rehabilitation to begin immediately, with isometric and isotonic contractions of the gluteal muscles and the quadriceps femoris. Assisted loading with two crutches is permitted on the first day. The average patient stay is 4 days.

Pitfalls and complications

The pitfalls of this surgical approach can be present at each stage of the procedure.

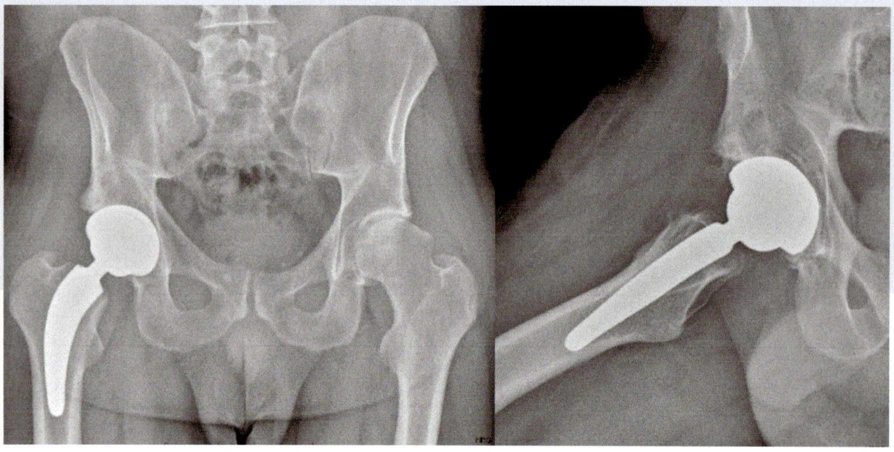

Figure 6
Post-operative X-ray

Preparation of the acetabulum

Special care must be taken when placing the Hohmann retractor on the anterior rim to avoid femoral nerve damage. If straight handles are used, one must avoid levering the femur and reaming eccentrically with the risk of excessively damaging the anterior wall. The use of handles with off-set allows eccentric reaming to be avoided.

Preparation of the femur

During the figure-4 positioning of the limb, if there is not adequate muscle relaxation and a correct posterior capsulotomy is not performed, a fracture of the greater trochanter by excessive pulling of the abductor muscles may occur. This eventuality is more frequent in osteoporotic individuals (fig. 7) [14].
Insufficient exposure of the femur can result in varus positioning of the stem with consequent risk of intraoperative periprosthetic fracture. This is more frequent when using straight stems (fig. 8) [15].
In the case of osteoporotic patients who have undergone ipsilateral knee arthroplasty, the figure-four positioning of the femur can generate torsional forces responsible for supracondylar knee fractures. In these cases, it is recommended to perform the surgery with the patient in lateral decubitus [16].

Soft tissue retraction

In order to avoid the occurrence of post-operative skin pain (fig. 9) or liponecrosis (fig. 10), excessive traction on the skin must be avoided using the 'moving window' concept. To preserve the integrity of the abductor muscles, excessive traction on the retractor should be avoided. It is not uncommon to damage a small portion of the gluteus minimus.
In his practice, the author has experienced the following complications: fracture of the great trochanter occurring in osteoporotic patients with a thigh circumference of more than 80 cm, varus stem placement, intraoperative periprosthetic fracture, periprosthetic ossifications (Brooker 1-2) and skin suffering with liponecrosis.

Conclusions

Various approaches are used for the implantation of a hip prosthesis. Over the years, we have seen a gradual transition from standard approaches, which are not very respectful of the anatomy but are easier for the surgeon, to minimally invasive approaches. With these, efforts have been made to ensure adequate exposure of the joint while respecting the anatomy.
The minimally invasive anterolateral approach, described in this chapter, has real advantages for the patient in terms of greater respect for all anatomical structures not affected by the pathology.
The smaller wound size, the short operation time, the lesser blood loss and the absence of periarticular haematomas protect against early infections.
Respect for abductors does not alter muscle strength and proprioception, reducing load-

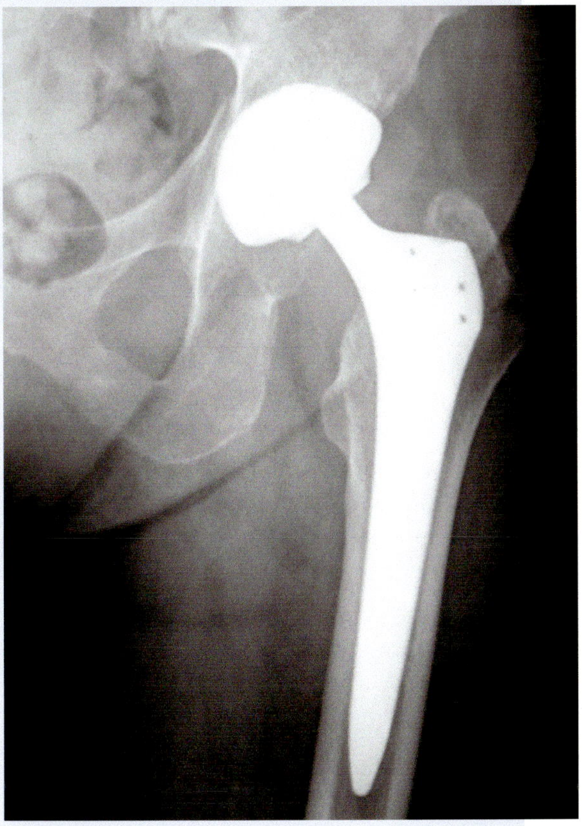

Figure 7 Intraoperative fracture of the greater trochanter

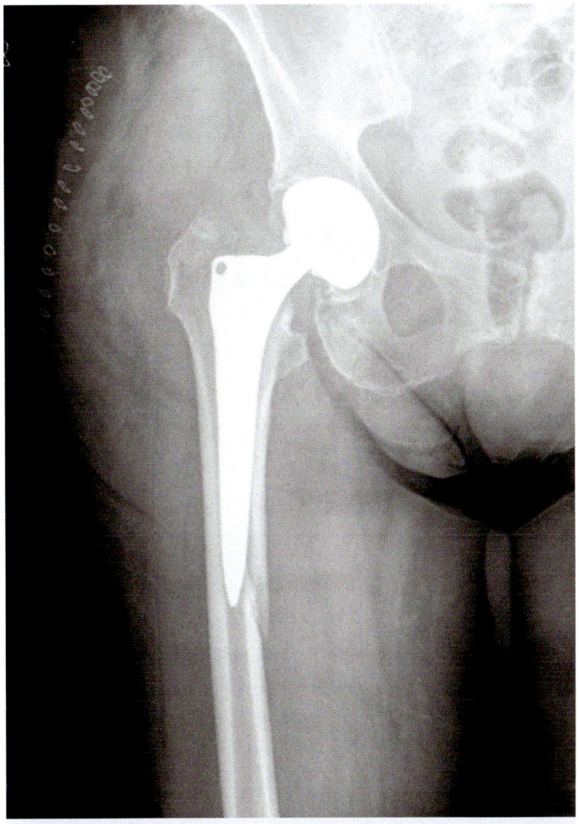

Figure 8
Intraoperative periprosthetic fracture

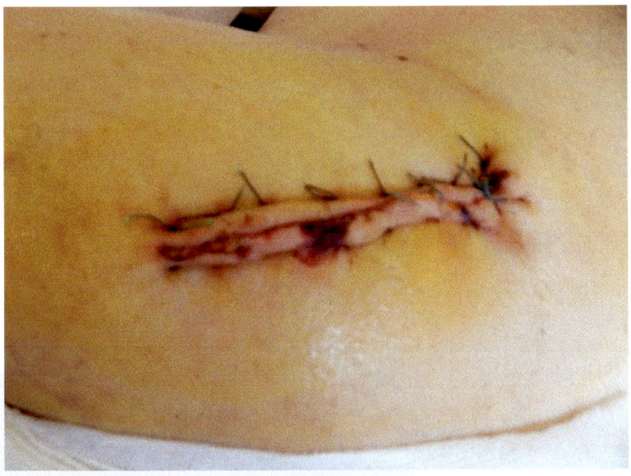

Figure 9 Surgical wound with areas of skin suffering

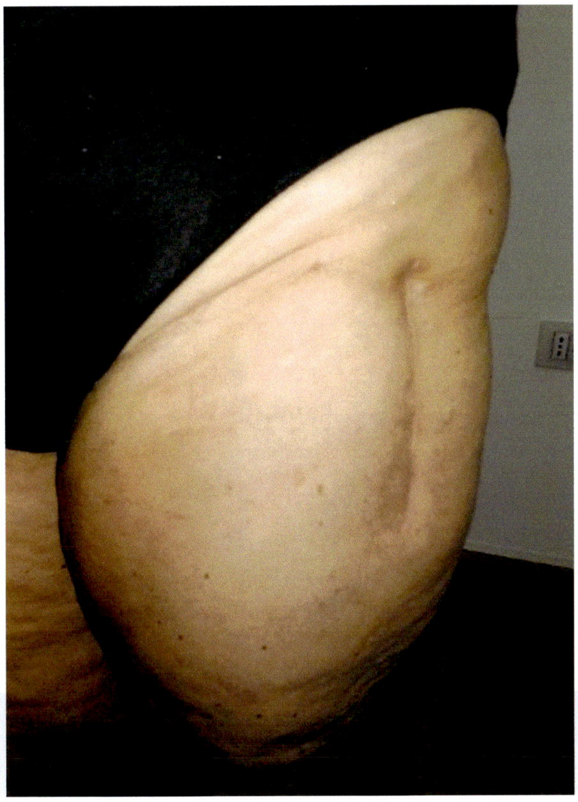

Figure 10
Liponecrosis

ing forces at the head-acetabulum interface and providing greater implant stability [17].
Respect for soft tissue associated with less trauma to the muscles and less blood loss significantly reduced the occurrence of heterotopic calcifications [18]. The absence of post-operative pain and the faster functional recovery have reduced hospitalisation time.
The surgical technique presented does not require a 'dedicated' operating bed and instrumentation, and allows cemented and cementless prostheses to be performed using various types of prosthetic stem.
Like all surgical techniques, anterolateral hip mini-access requires a learning curve that will be shorter the more experience the surgeon has.
We consider patient selection, precision in performing the approach, and cooperation with the anaesthetist to be crucial.

Bibliography

1. Pipino F. Tissue-sparing surgery (TSS) in hip and knee arthroplasty. J Orthop Traumatol. 2006;7:33-35
2. Wojciechowski P, Kusz D, Kopeć K, Borowski M. Minimally invasive approaches in total hip arthroplasty. Ortop Traumatol Rehabil. 2007;9(1):1-7.
3. Tang Z. Minimally invasive total hip replacement. Issues Emerg Health Technol. 2004;(60):1-4.
4. Smith-Petersen MN. Approach to and exposure of the hip joint for mold arthroplasty. J Bone Joint Surg Am. 1949;31A(1):40-46.
5. Watson-Jones R. Fractures of the neck of the femur. Br J Surg. 1936;23:787.
6. Hardinge K. The direct lateral approach to the hip. J Bone Joint Surg Br. 1982;64(1):17-19.
7. Gibson A. Posterior exposure of the hip joint. J Bone Joint Surg Br. 1950;32-B(2):183-186.
8. Edmunds CT, Boscainos PJ. Effect of surgical approach for total hip replacement on hip function using Harris Hip scores and Trendelenburg's test. A retrospective analysis. Surgeon. 2011;9(3):124-129.
9. Chimento GF, Sculco TP. Miniaccesso nella protesi totale d'anca. Tecniche di chirurgia ortopedica. Vol.2, n.2-116-119,2002.
10. Bray GA. Overweight is risking fate. Definition, classification, prevalence, and risks. Ann N Y Acad Sci. 1987;499:14-28.
11. Grano GF. Minimally invasive antero-lateral approach in primary hip prosthetic surgery: notes of surgical technique: Medit J Surgery Med. 2002;10:59-62.
12. Ince A, Kemper M, Waschke J, Hendrich C. Minimally invasive anterolateral approach to the hip: risk to the superior gluteal nerve. Acta Orthop. 2007;78(1):86-89.
13. Vincenti E, Todesco A, Grano G. Rocuronium as selective local musclerelaxant in orthopedic surgery. Orthop Musc System Curr Res. 2017:6:2.
14. Iwata H, Sakata K, Sogo E, Nanno K, Kuroda S, Nakai T. Total hip arthroplasty via an anterolateral supine approach for obese patients increases the risk of greater trochanteric fracture. J Orthop. 2018;15(2):379-383.
15. Herndon CL, Nowell JA, Sarpong NO, Cooper HJ, Shah RP, Geller JA. Risk Factors for Periprosthetic Femur Fracture and Influence of Femoral Fixation Using the Mini-Anterolateral Approach in Primary Total Hip Arthroplasty. J Arthroplasty. 2020;35(3):774-778.
16. Bertin KC, Röttinger H. Anterolateral mini-incision hip replacement surgery: a modified Watson-Jones approach. Clin Orthop Relat Res. 2004;429:248-55.
17. Glaser D, Dennis DA, Komistek RD, Miner TM. In vivo comparison of hip mechanics for minimally invasive versus traditional total hip arthroplasty. Clin Biomech (Bristol, Avon). 2008;23(2):127-134.
18. Hürlimann M, Schiapparelli FF, Rotigliano N, Testa E, et al. Influence of surgical approach on heterotopic ossification after total hip arthroplasty - is minimal invasive better? A case control study. BMC Musculoskelet Disord. 2017;18(1):27.

CHAPTER 13

The posterolateral minimally invasive approach in hip arthroplasty

Guido Grappiolo, Francesco La Camera, Riccardo Ruggeri

Hip Diseases and Replacement Surgery Unit, Humanitas Clinical and Research Center - IRCCS, Rozzano, Milan, Italy
Livio Sciutto Foundation Biomedical Research in Orthopaedics Onlus, Campus Savona, Italy

Introduction

The natural tendency to evolve the strategies inherent in hip arthroplasty has led us to revisit the traditional surgical approaches by minimising the dissection of soft tissues and the detachment of muscle insertions. The theoretical advantages are obvious, but on a practical level there are technical difficulties. These are related to the type of implant used and the not easy learning curve of such techniques. The posterolateral approach is in our hands the easiest to perform.
Applying the femur-first technique allows us optimal and precise control of component positioning and almost complete muscle sparing. In our opinion, the posterolateral approach is perfectly adaptable to the evolution in terms of minimally invasive. The almost complete sparing of the gluteus medius associated with that of the fascia lata, thanks to a transmuscular approach involving the anterior fibres of the gluteus maximus, makes recovery remarkably rapid. This also increases post-operative joint stability, especially if the posterior muscular wall is reconstructed (either with transosseous sutures or with reinsertion of the bone with the quadratus inserted).

Indications and contraindications

According to the philosophy of our school, there are no absolute contraindications to minimally invasive surgery applied to posterolateral access in hip arthroplasty. Mini-invasiveness is intended as complete muscle sparing of the gluteus medius, the 'engine of the hip', as correct planning, choice and positioning of the implant, as optimal patient management in terms of perioperative procedures and rapid recovery.
Even in the most complex cases such as severe dysplasia, arthrodesis, periarticular deformities, where ancillary interventions such as tendon and ligament releases, osteotomies are involved, our concept of mini-invasiveness remains valid. All this is aimed at preserving the gluteus medius and the femoral and acetabular bone stock.

Pre-operative assessment

Clinical assessment

The patient generally complains of pain and progressive functional limitation at the hip.
Clinical assessment involves a physical examination and administration of specific questionnaires (Proms). Adjacent joints are evalu-

ated for correct functional assessment and appropriate surgical indication.

Imaging assessment

Radiographs

X-ray of pelvis and hips with 'false profile' (Lequesne) projection are the first level examinations. Lower limb and spinal X-rays may be requested for further investigation.

Computed tomography (CT)

CT scan with 3-D reconstruction may be required for the evaluation of bone components, particularly the acetabular component, in complex cases.

Magnetic resonance imaging (MRI)

MRI is not routinely obtained, however could be useful to evaluate osteonecrosis.

Timing for surgery

As soon as the patient's clinical condition allows surgery. Delayed intervention could be more demanding due to muscular impairment or bone deformities.

Preparation for surgery

Pre-operative planning

Digital or analogue, the planning is necessary to study which type of implant best suits the patient's anatomy without altering joint relationships and if necessary to provide lengthening to correct dysmetria. Moreover, the planning is also useful to instruct the operating room staff.

Surgical equipment

- Complete MIS set with trial components.
- Drill and saw.
- Scalpels and osteotomes.
- High resistance non-absorbable suture and metallic cerclage.

Patient anaesthesia and positioning

Typically peripheral anaesthesia (peridural or spinal) is associated with sedation (upon patient request).

Patient is positioned in lateral decubitus with flexed hips and knees and the contralateral limb immobilised. External landmarks are used for positioning the acetabular component. The pelvis must be firmly stabilised perpendicular to the operating table. This is so that the pelvis does not roll forward with adduction of the hip or retraction of the femur during implantation of the acetabulum. The leg on the opposite side is flexed 45° at the hip and 90° at the knee, helping to stabilise the patient's position. It must be ensured that the table is in a flat position, as the inclination of the acetabulum is partly determined by its orientation in

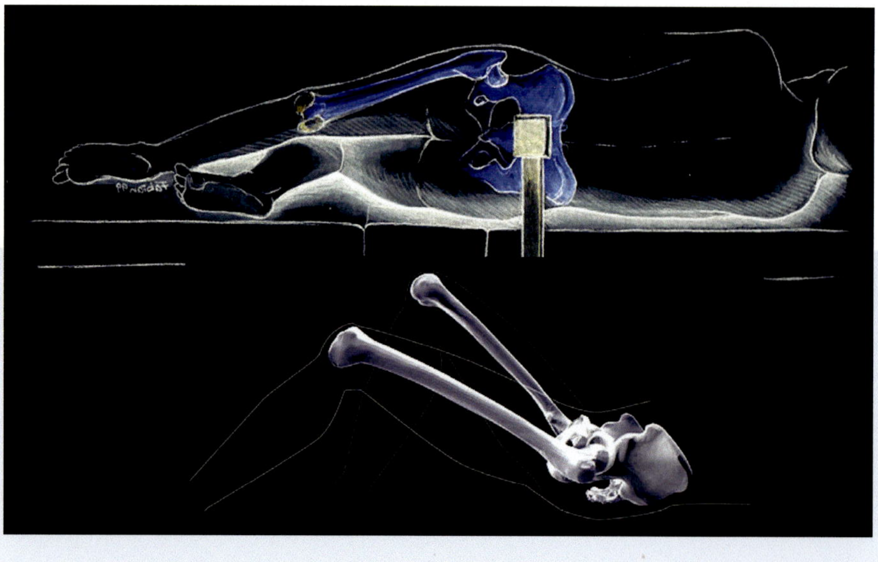

Figure 1 This image shows the position of the patient in right lateral decubitus for left hip surgery

relation to the table (fig. 1).
Use soft pad to protect all bony prominences.
Prepare the surgical field and drape it widely.
The first surgeon stands posteriorly to the patient, the assistants anteriorly and the scrub nurse next to the first surgeon.

Further preparation

- Short term antibiotics protocol 20 minutes prior to surgical incision.
- Administration of 1 g of tranexanic acid according to the bloodless surgery protocol.

Surgical technique

Approach and exposure

- We perform a minimally invasive posterolateral approach associated with the 'femur first' technique for the positioning of the implants.
- Surgery begins with an 8-cm to 12-cm rectilinear incision starting from the tip of the greater trochanter and extending distally and proximally along the diaphysis of the femur (fig. 2). In case of varus neck the incision could be a bit posterior.
- Use electrocautery to extend the incision through the subcutaneous fat until the fascia is reached.
- Incise the fascia lata in line with the skin incision and apply the Charnley retractor.
- Separate the gluteus maximus muscle bluntly in line with the muscle fibers.
- Placement of a Homann retractor below the gluteus maximus muscle and above the piriformis tendon at the level of the femoral neck (fig. 3).
- Localisation and section of the piriformis tendon and 7-shaped posterior capsulotomy (fig. 4).
- Piriformis-sparing is not mandatory in MIS technique (in case of sparing piriformis tendon just remember that exist an anatomical aberration of sciatic nerve that could spare in two branches across piriformis).

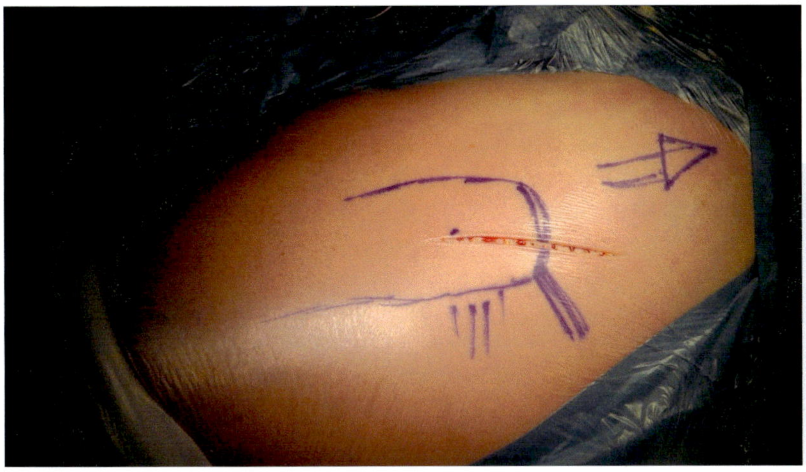

Figure 2 Surgical incision. The arrow indicates the proximal end

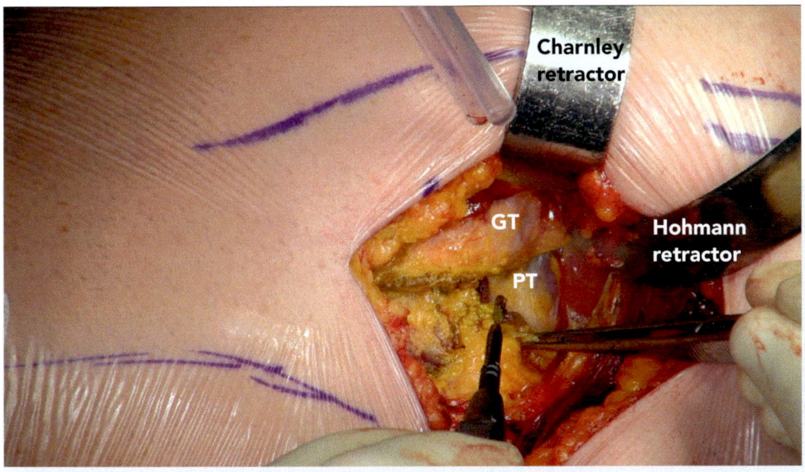

Figure 3 Exposure of the capsule. GT: greater trochanter. PT: piriformis tendon

13

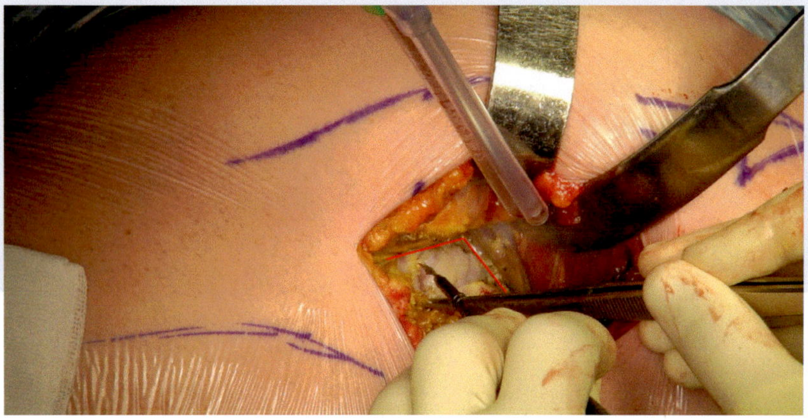

Figure 4 Red line indicates 7-shaped capsulotomy

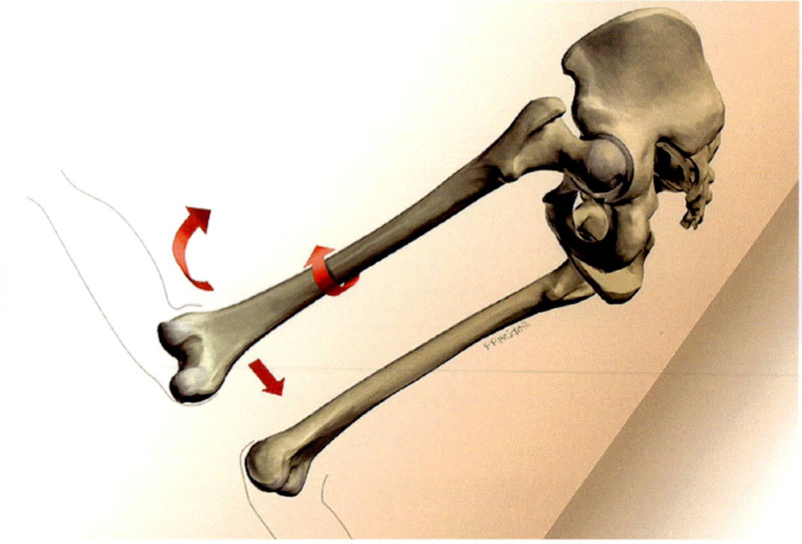

Figure 5 Posterior dislocation manoeuvre

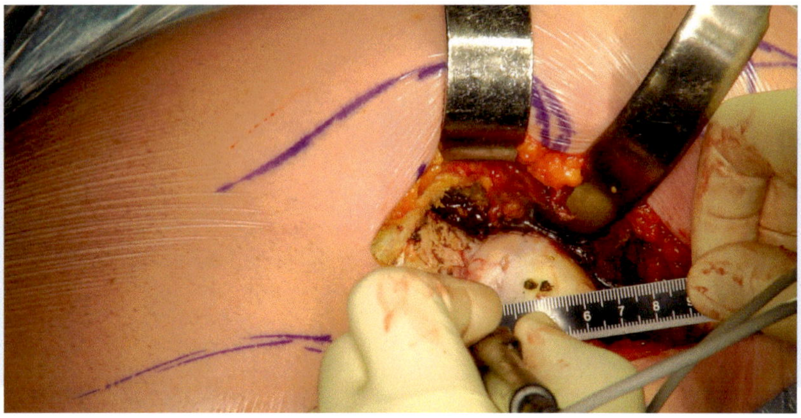

Figure 6 This image shows the native offset measurement. This will be compared with the measurements taken during planning

- Partial or total sectioning of the extrarotator muscles (quadratus femoris, obturator externus, gemellus inferior, obturator internus, gemellus superior muscles) depending on the degree of their retraction.
- Hip luxation with combined manoeuvre of internal rotation, flexion and adduction (fig. 5).
- Exposure of the femoral head, identification of the centre of rotation, measurement of the vertical offset (distance between lesser trochanter and centre of rotation) and horizontal offset (distance between piriformis fossa and centre of rotation) and osteotomy level (fig. 6).
Check of these measurements with those of the planning.

Femur preparation

- Osteotomy of the femoral neck after measurement of the osteotomy level, according to the pre-operative plan.
- The distal osteotomy line is parallel to the intertrochanteric line, the height is determined by the type of implant chosen (fig. 7).
- Femoral head extraction.
- Place the hip in 60° of flexion, 40° of adduction and 40° of internal rotation.
- Placement of the retractors for femoral exposure: a Muller retractor in the posteromedial neck region and a Hohmann retractor in the gluteus medius-minimus muscle interval to retract and protect the gluteus medius fibres.
- Start of canal preparation in the posteromedial neck portion, with initiator or gouge depending on the chosen instrumentation.
- Manual introduction of the first broach with an anteversion of 10°-15° in relation to the transepicondylar axis of the knee (fig. 8).
- Gradual manual insertion of the broaches until the final size is reached according to the measurement given in the pre-operative plan. Subsequent introduction of the trial neck.
- Measurement of the distance between the lesser trochanter and medial angle of the trial neck (vertical offset) and between the piriformis fossa and lateral angle of the trial neck (horizontal offset).
- Removal of the trial neck.

Acetabular preparation

- Correct positioning of the centre of rotation creates the conditions necessary to restore the hip to its 'physiological' function. However, with the anatomical alterations associated with the various pathological condi-

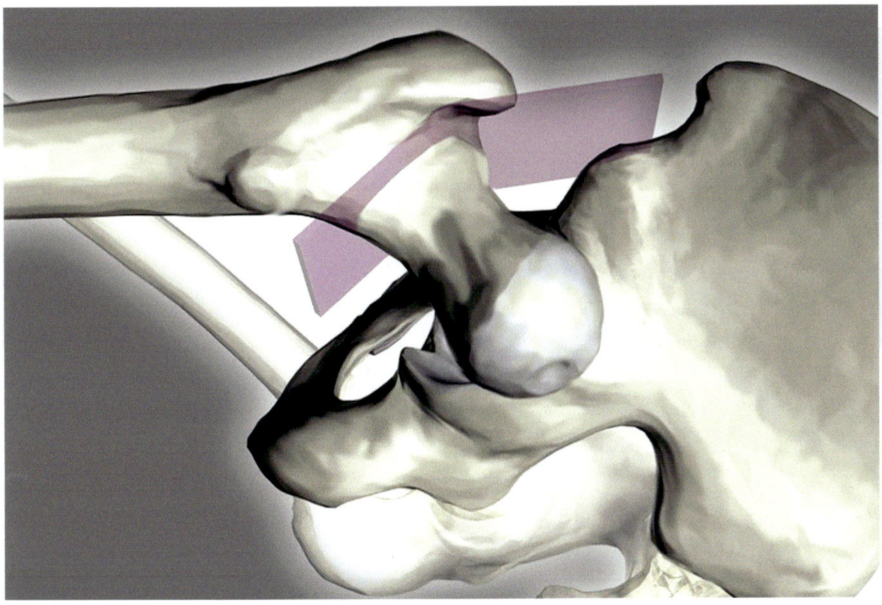

Figure 7
Anatomical layer of the femoral head osteotomy

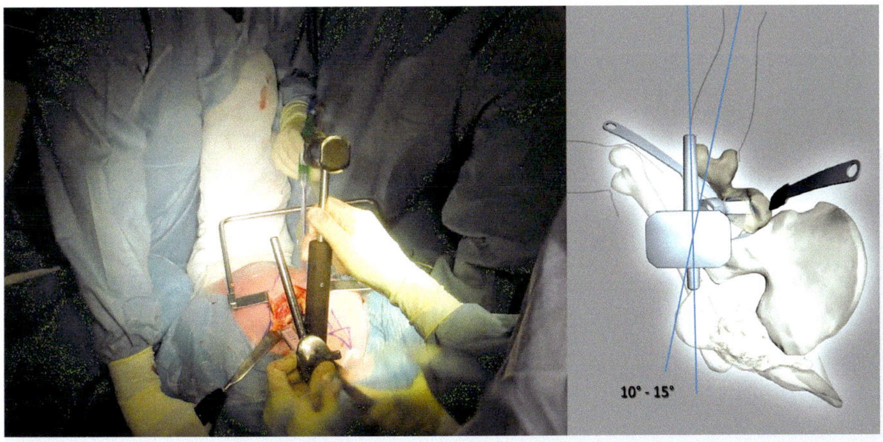

Figure 8
Intraoperative assessment of femoral stem anteversion

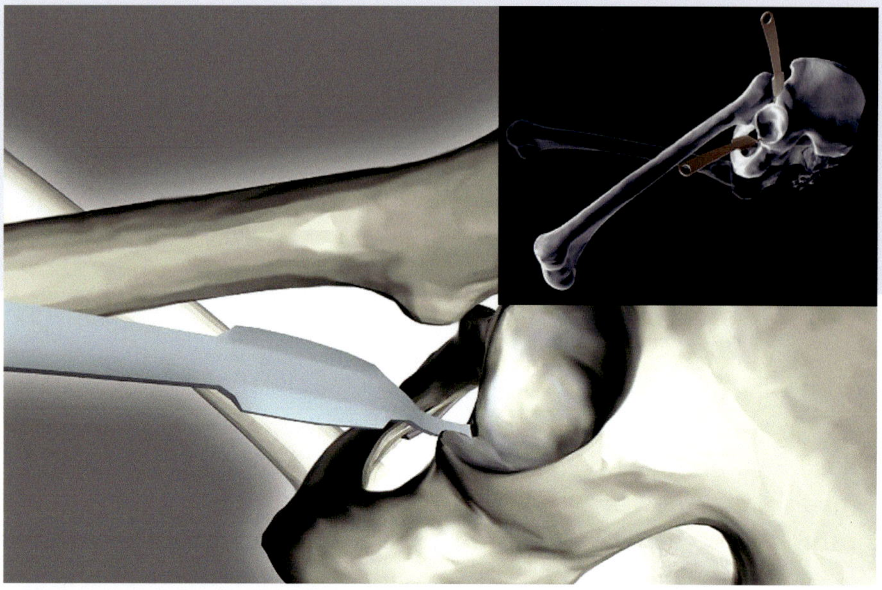

Figure 9 Positioning of the Hohmann retractors for exposure of the acetabulum

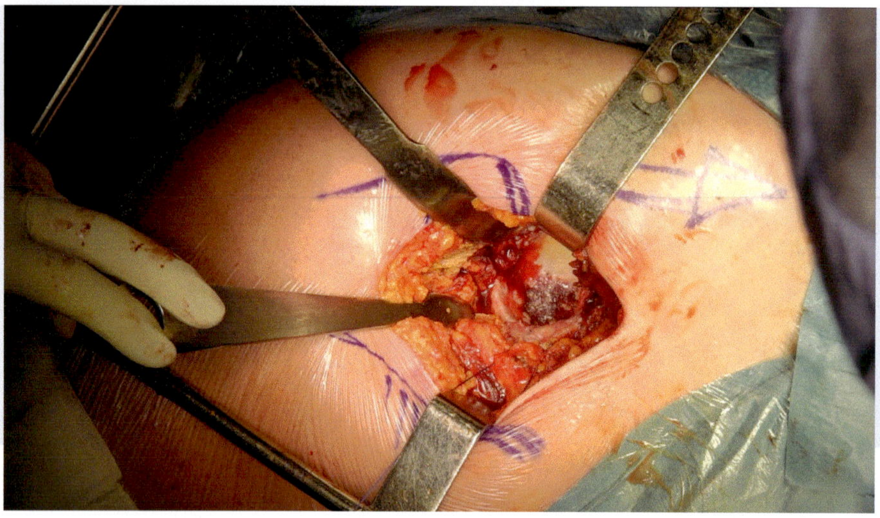

Figure 10 In this image, the exposed acetabulum can be appreciated. Note the suture stitch on the posterior capsule acting as a retractor

tions that can be treated with a prosthesis, the cup position always remains a compromise. By reaming the acetabulum, the position of the prosthesis' centre of rotation can be optimised, depending on the available bone substance.
- Leaving the trial broach in the femur, the acetabulum is prepared.
- The acetabulum is exposed by retracting the femur anteriorly with a Hohmann No. 7 retractor on the anterosuperior margin of the acetabulum and anterior migration of the femur (fig. 9). The retractor is not placed above the anterior acetabular wall to avoid contact with the neurovascular structures anterior to the acetabulum.
- To better expose the acetabulum, the release of the reflected head of the rectus femoris is performed if it is very tight.
- Using a stitch and suture the posterior capsule flap is retracted posteriorly (fig. 10) to protect the sciatic nerve and better expose the acetabulum.
- Release of the inferior capsule.
- Positioning of a straight Hohmann inferiorly at the level of the ischiatic notch.
- Removal of the acetabular labrum.
- Using a gouge and hammer, remove the osteophyte, if present, in the pulvinar region.
- Reaming of the acetabulum using 2 mm increasing diameter sizes, starting with the one approximately 8-10 mm smaller than the final size predicted in the pre-operative plan.
- If the quadrilateral lamina has been reached during reaming, the floor of the acetabu-

lum is covered with bone fragments produced by the reaming.
- Positioning of the acetabular cup with 40°-45° of inclination and 10°-15° of anteversion, taking into account the version obtained with the stem.
- Checking the contact between the cup and the acetabular floor.
- Removal of osteophytes and soft tissues from the acetabular contour to allow introduction of the liner.
- Introduction of the linear trial liner into the implanted acetabular cup.

Trial reduction

- Introduction femoral trial neck and head of appropriate length as planned in the pre-operative plan.
- Trial reduction and evaluation of the combined anteversion according to the femur first technique: after the reduction, we place the limb in neutral abduction, then internally rotate the limb until the leg forms an angle of 37° with the horizontal plane. In this way we compensate for that 37° which is the value we have identified as the ideal sum of femoral antitorsion and cup abduction. In this position the cutting diameter of the hemispheric head is parallel to the diameter of the cup and indicates the fact that we are in a safe zone (fig. 11).
- If the combined anteversion is not satisfactory, optimisation can be attempted with the use of constrained liners or cup repositioning can be performed.
- Anterior and posterior stability, flexion, abduction and adduction manoeuvres are performed.
- If stability is optimal and no conflicts are identified, definitive prosthetic implantation is performed.

Final implant

- Positioning of the final acetabular liner and checking its effective engagement with the metalback. Before insertion it is necessary to check whether marginal osteophytes in the acetabulum and any remnants of the capsule may interfere with the correct positioning of the liner.
- The stability of the trial broach is checked both rotationally and longitudinally, if there is movement at the bone-metal interface, the size is increased by one if possible.
- Removal of the trial broach and manual introduction of the stem until it locks into the femoral canal, the introduction is completed using hammer (fig. 12).
- Measurement of the distance between the lesser trochanter and medial angle of the prosthetic neck (vertical offset) and between the piriformis fossa and lateral angle of the prosthetic neck (horizontal offset).
- Insertion of the trial head and reduction.
- Control of stability, joint mobility and muscle tension.
- Trial head removal and definitive head implantation.

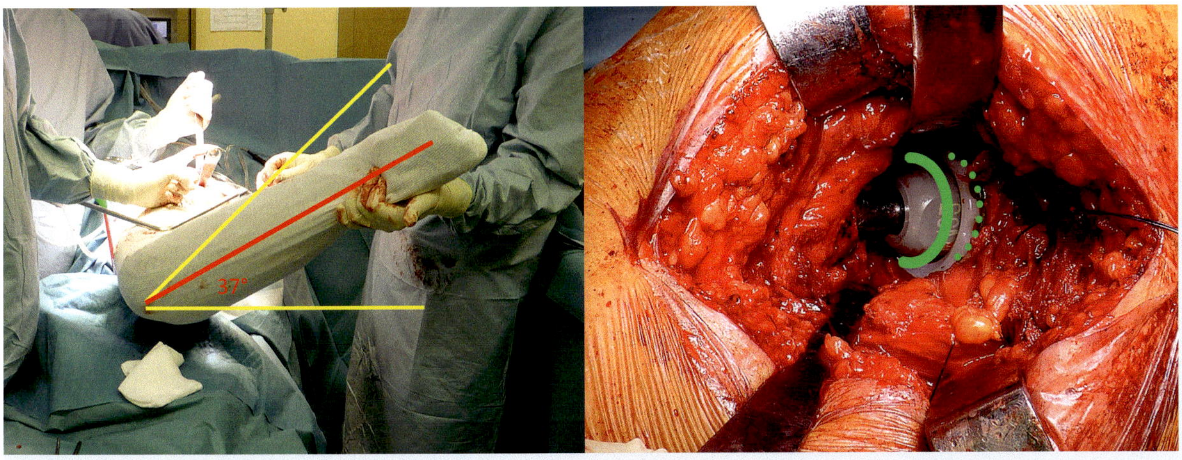

Figure 11 Intraoperative assessment of combined anteversion

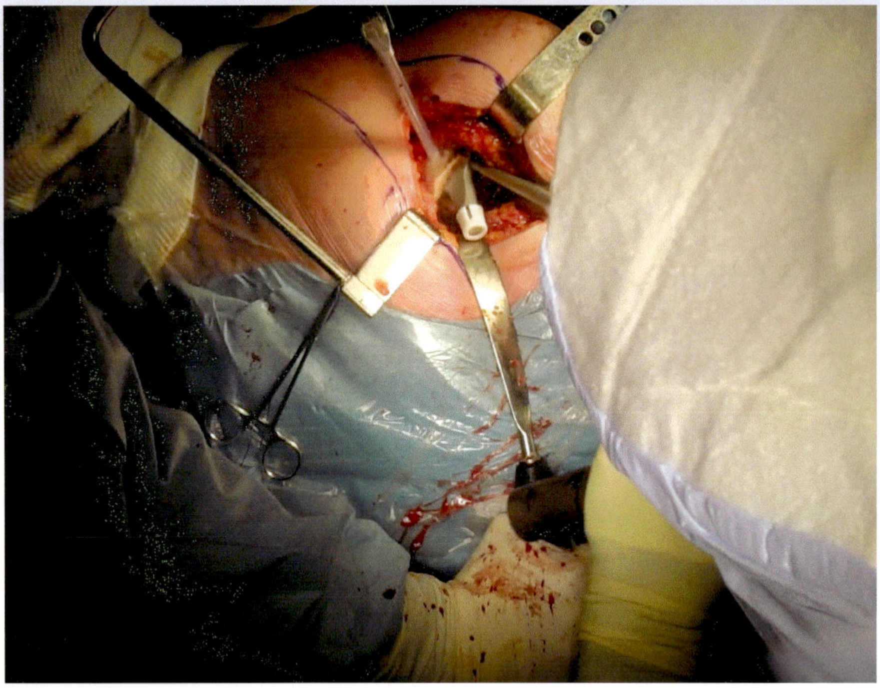

Figure 12
Implantation of the definitive stem

Choice of implant

Several factors are taken into account when choosing the prosthesis to be implanted, including the following: bone quality, patient's age, activity level, morphological characteristics of the femur and acetabulum, any pre-operative dysmetria. The objective is to recreate a correct anatomy, providing adequate femoral fixation to allow proper osseointegration and avoiding conflicts.
We generally go for short uncemented stems (fig. 13) in case of good bone stock and young age. We reconstruct the anatomy using the specific stem design, size and depth, so we do not often use stems with high offset. In the case of poorer bone quality, we turn to conventional cementless stems (fig. 14). In the case of severe osteoporosis, advanced age with a high risk of bleeding we use short cemented stems (fig. 15). In cases of severe dysplasia we use conical stems to correct the pathological version of the femoral neck.
For the acetabular component we generally use conventional modular cups or low-profile cups in the case of acetabular dysplasia to avoid conflict with the anterior soft tissue. The most commonly used bearing couple is ceramic-polyethylene enriched with vitamin E, while ceramic-ceramic is the choice in very young patients. Double mobility is reserved for patients with severe muscle deficits or neurological diseases. We no longer use metal-on-metal bearings.

Closure

Our technique does not involve the use of drainages.If there is no excessive tension, the posterior capsule is reconstructed and the external rotators are reinserted with intraosseous sutures (fig. 16). Close fascia, subcutaneous layer and the skin in standard fashion, apply advanced dressing.

Post-operative management

Immediately after surgery the patient takes control X-rays in the operating room.
On the day of surgery the patient walks with aids. The following day the rehabilitation programme begins. After 3/5 days the patient is discharged home.
Medications: low dose heparin or NAO for DVT prevention (usually for 30 days), pain killers (e.g. acetaminophen and opioids) and local cryotherapy several times a day.

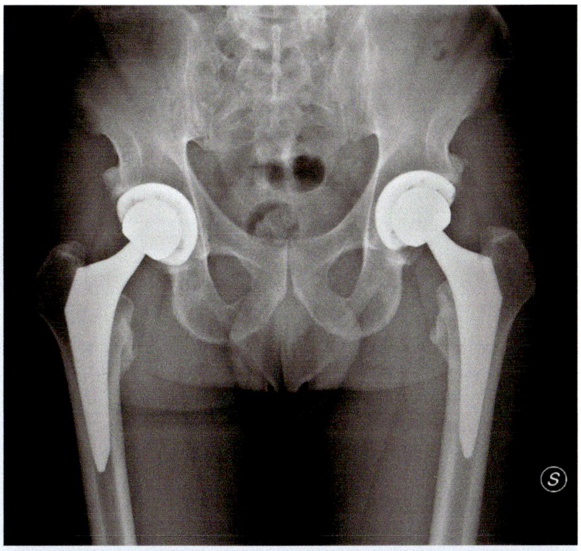

Figure 13 Bilateral prostheses with tissue-preserving short stems and ceramic-polyethylene bearing are shown in this figure

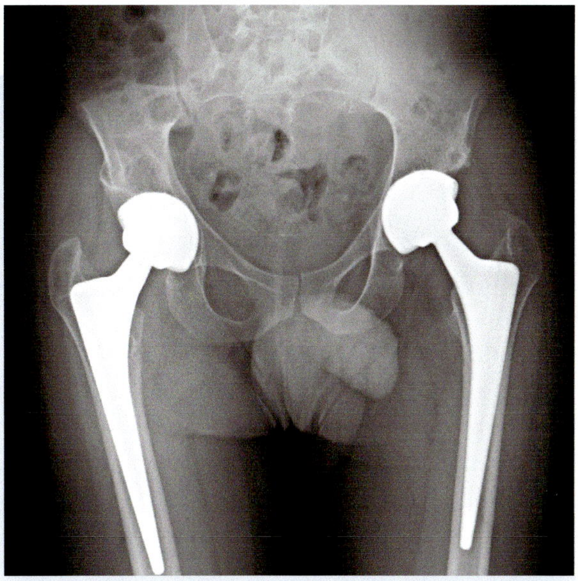

Figure 14 Bilateral prosthesis with straight stems and ceramic-on-ceramic bearing

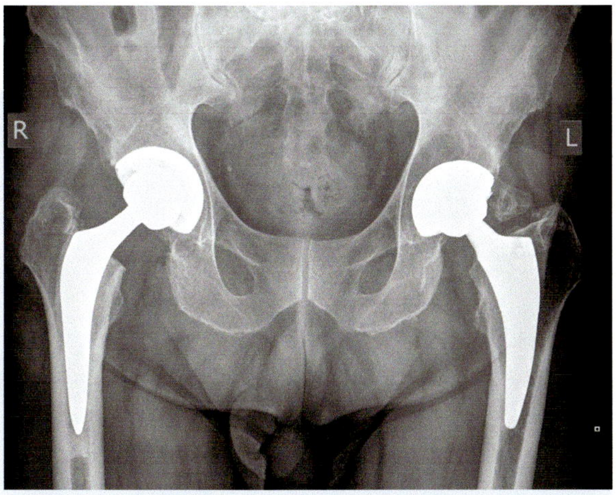

Figure 15 Right hip prosthesis with cemented short stem. Note the stem size and bone sparing which are comparable to an uncemented short stem

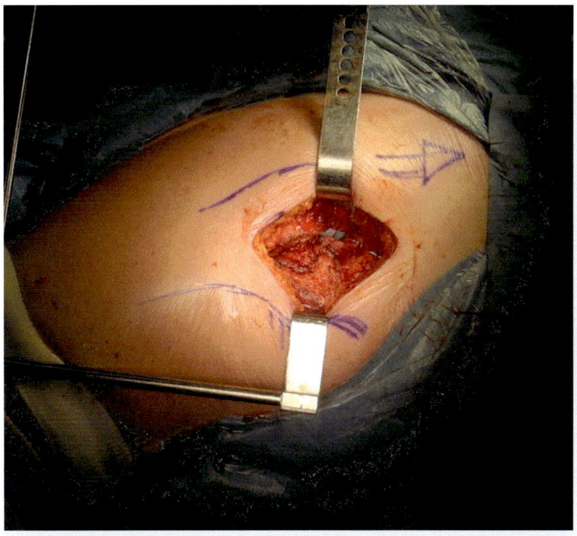

Figure 16 In this image, the capsule closure and external rotators can be appreciated

Outpatient follow-up

The patient is educated from enrolment on the importance of clinical and radiographic follow-up over time.
Clinical evaluation is assessed at 15 days, 4 weeks, 6 months after surgery and annually thereafter.

Radiographic evaluation is performed at 4 weeks, 6 months, 1 year after surgery and then on an annual basis. Radiographs are examined for stem and cup position, bone density and restoration of morphometric parameters.
From the first follow-up appointment, patients complete several PROMS.

Complications

The complications of this specific surgery are related to the reduced visibility associated with tissue sparing. Reduced visibility associated with the surgeon's lack of experience can lead to an increase in complications.
The most common complications are haematoma, intraoperative fracture, heterometry of the operated limb, dislocation, sciatic nerve injury, peri-prosthetic calcifications and thromboembolism.

Haematoma

Commonly caused by injury to the first perforating branch of the deep femoral artery at the insertion of the gluteus maximus (during release for deformity in flexion) or to the branches of the obturator artery (when osteophytes are removed from the lower margin) or by the incision to release the transverse ligament. Prevention is through adequate hemostasis and treatment includes correction of predisposing factors (coagulopathy, medication), compression dressing. The use of drainage is not part of our technique as no differences in use have been observed.

Intraoperative fracture

May occur during preparation of the femur or during implantation of the definitive stem. This is generally due to characteristics of the bone or an incorrect or aggressive surgical technique. It usually occurs in the calcar region and can sometimes extend into the meta-diaphyseal region. It can be treated immediately with metal cerclage. In our case history there is no difference in the medium to long term compared to prostheses without this complication.

Heterometry

According to literature data, it has been assessed that lengthening is tolerated up to a maximum of 6 mm. Beyond this measurement it may become symptomatic and excessive lengthening may cause limping or even sciatic nerve injury (> 2.5-4 cm). Careful pre-operative planning in combination with intraoperative measurements and femur first application are the most accurate method for limb length equalisation. Shortening is rarer but possible and generally better tolerated than lengthening.

Dislocation

The risk of dislocation after primary hip arthroplasty is reported to be between 2-5%. More than half of all dislocations occur within the first three months after surgery. Factors predisposing to instability include component malpositioning (excessive ante or retroversion, inadequate offset or head centre), inadequate soft tissue tension, abductor insufficiency, impingement of the neck or femoral component on the pelvis, trauma, extreme limb position, and small head size. In our case series, this event does not exceed 0.3 % of cases of primary minimally invasive hip arthoplasty, but is slightly higher in revision and complex cases. Treatment generally involves at least one attempt of reduction under narcosis with a brace and restrictions for 1 month if no mobilisation or malpositioning is evident. Otherwise, revision is performed, changing components or using dual mobility systems.

Sciatic nerve injury

Literature reports a frequency ranging from 0.5 to 4 %. The sciatic nerve can be damaged during exposure (most at risk in protruded hips, revisions, dysplasia, external rotation deformity, head and neck resorption, due to soft tissue retraction on the posterior aspect of the acetabulum, subgluteal haematoma or excessive stretching (> 4 cm)). Complete recovery is observed in only a few patients. In our case series, the incidence of this complication is around 0.1 % and basically only occurs in complex cases.

Heterotopic ossification

It occurs in up to 10 % of cases. Only a very small percentage require surgical removal, and they are generally asymptomatic. It is most common in post-traumatic arthrosis and in patients with a previous history of heterotopic ossification. The common site is the adductor area and the iliopsoas and gluteus medius muscles in the form of calcification approximately 3-4 weeks after surgery. Our prophylaxis includes NSAIDs (indomethacin or etoricoxib) or low-dose radiotherapy (500 cGy) (pre-operative and post-operative).

Thromboembolism

The thromboembolic event after total hip replacement has been consistently reported to be between 0.1 and 0.2 per cent, regardless of the drug used for prophylaxis. Improved perioperative care, pain management and early mobilisation drastically reduced the incidence of thromboembolic phenomena. In our case series, we observed that major thromboembolic adverse events are in most cases associated with paradoxical embolism from a patent foramen ovale.

Bibliography

1. Loppini M, Longo UG, Caldarella E, Rocca AD, Denaro V, Grappiolo G. Femur first surgical technique: a smart non-computer-based procedure to achieve the combined anteversion in primary total hip arthroplasty. BMC Musculoskelet Disord. 2017;18(1):331.

2. La Camera F, Loppini M, Della Rocca A, de Matteo V, Grappiolo G. Total Hip Arthroplasty With a Monoblock Conical Stem in Dysplastic Hips: A 20-Year Follow-Up Study. J Arthroplasty. 2020;35(11):3242-3248.

3. Loppini M, Grappiolo G. Uncemented short stems in primary total hip arthroplasty: The state of the art. EFORT Open Rev. 2018;3(5):149-159.

4. Grappiolo G, Blaha JD, Gruen TA, Burastero G, Spotorno L. Primary total hip arthroplasty using a grit-blasted, press-fit femoral prosthesis.Long-term results with survivorship analysis. Hip Int. 2002;12(2):55-72.

5. Loppini M, Pisano A, Ruggeri R, Della Rocca A, Grappiolo G. Pelvic tilt and functional acetabular position after total hip arthroplasty: an EOS 2D/3D radiographic study. Hip Int. 2022;11207000211073668.

Robotic arm assisted total hip arthroplasty using minimally invasive posterolateral approach: surgical technique

Fabio Catani, Filippo Selleri, Enrico Bertugli, Luca Bianchi, Alessandro Berni, Andrea Marcovigi

Department of Orthopaedics and Traumatology, Modena University Hospital, University of Modena and Reggio-Emilia, Italy

Introduction

The postero lateral approach to the hip was firstly described in 1867 by Bernhard von Langenbeck as a surgical approach to the hip joint for the treatment of septic arthritis and war wounds [1,2]. Emil Theodor Kocher modified Langebeck's approach by extending it in a caudal direction for treatment of pelvic fractures [3].

Gibson, Moore and Southern in 1950 described [4-5] the posterolateral approach as we know today. Over the decades It has undergone several modifications to minimize soft tissue damage. Nowadays, it is the most widespread approach to perform total hip arthroplasty [6]. The reasons stand in substantial advantages: it's safe and quick, gluteus medius is not detached, it allows good visualization of both acetabulum and femur, it could be extended proximally and distally as needed and it requires only two surgeons. This approach was historically burdened by high dislocation rates [7], ranging from 1% to 5% [8-14], but modern literature has shown lower dislocation rates to when performed sparing soft tissue [15-19].

The described procedure is the result of the adjustments made on a minimally invasive posterolateral approach to suit robotic arm-assisted surgery. This means a shorter skin incision, but focusing mainly on soft tissue sparing. Piriformis tendon preservation increases implant stability. Furthermore, robotic surgery allows optimal positioning of prosthetic components and restoration of soft tissue tension, further decreasing dislocation rate.

Patient selection

Minimally invasive posterolateral approach can applied on all patients undergoing total hip arthroplasty. However, there are factors that could make the procedure more demanding: high BMI, especially in gynoid obesity, acetabular protrusion and ankylotic arthritis. In those patients, there will likely be the need for a more extensive approach, at least regarding skin and fascia. However, even if those patients are more demanding, piriformis tendon might be spared. Acetabular protrusion and ankylotic arthritis may require ostephytes removal or in situ osteotomy in order to perform hip dislocation.

When using Computer Assited Surgery or Robotic Arm- Assisted Surgery, early osteophytes removal could make the acetabular matching less accurate, so it should be performed only if strictly necessary. For the same reason also in situ osteotomy should be avoided if possible, but in our experience, leaving at least half of the femoral head is sufficient to achieve a satisfactory registration; obviously the described procedure will make registered points closer one each other and could reduce accuracy.

Pre-operative planning

The described surgical procedure is based on our experience with the Mako Robotic Arm-Assisted System (Stryker Orthopaedics, Kalamazoo, MI, USA). Mako is a semi-active, image based closed robotic system [20].

All patiens perform a CT scans following a customized protocol. Afterwards scans are sent to an engineering team of segmentation specialists to get accurate measurement of patient's anatomy and create a 3D model of the hip joint.

Acetabular and femoral component sizing and templating are performed on TC 3D reconstruction and on 2D X-Ray simulation; the planning software automatically provides the surgeon with Hip Length, Global Offset, and Combined Anteversion (the sum of stem anteversion and cup anteversion) (figg. 1-3).

Femoral stem position is then adjusted on tranverse plane to match 15° in anteversion, or to the closest value to 15° compatible with femoral anatomy (fig. 4).

Initial cup position is set to 40° in inclination and 20° in anteversion, then adjusted checking eventual anterior, posterior o superior uncoverage. The latest version of the planning software enables pelvic tilt simulation.

Sacral slope is measured on pre-operative lateral view pelvis X-Rays with the patient in standing and sitting position, then inserted in the software, which automatically calculate Cup anteversion and inclination in supine, standing and sitting position (fig. 5). When facing a fixed pelvis (Sacral Slope difference < 10°) the use of a dual mobility cup

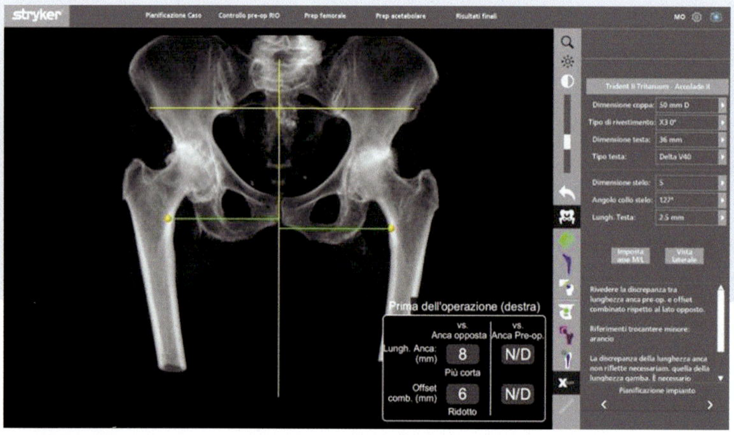

Figure 1 Mako pre-operative planning: a 2D X-Ray reconstruction based on CT is displayed. Pre-operative hip length and offset in respect to contralateral hip are provided

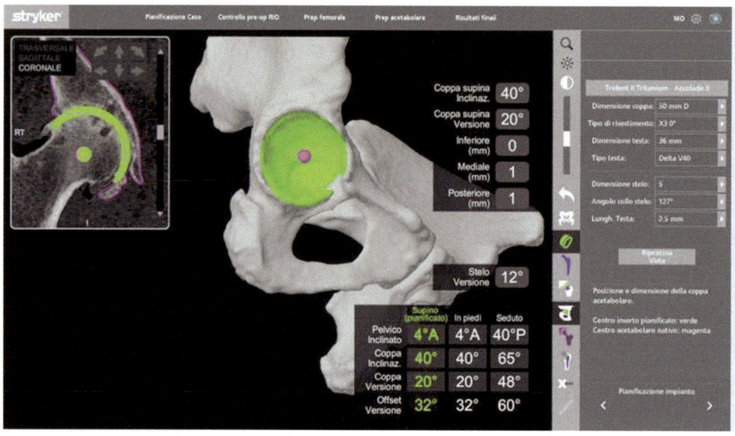

Figure 2 Cup position is defined on 2D and 3D CT reconstruction. Cup inclination and anteversion are measured in respect to CT spatial coordinate system in the first column, and calculated upon sacral slope changes in standing position (second column) and in sitting position (third column)

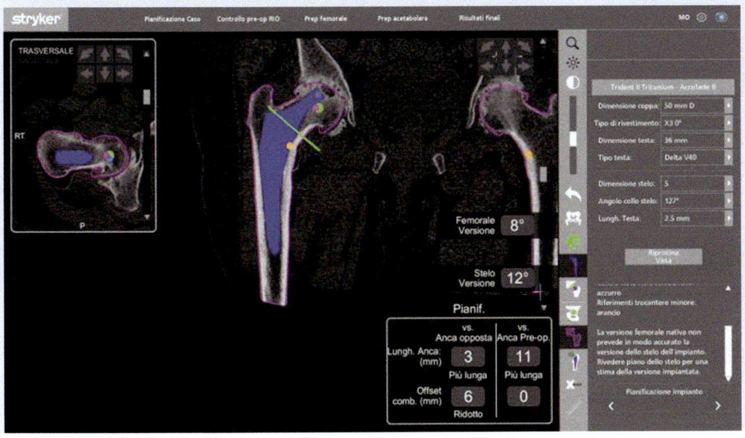

Figure 3 Stem sizing is evaluated on 2D CT reconstruction, post-operative simulated results are provided for stem anteversion, hip length and hip offset in respect to contralateral and pre-operative measurements

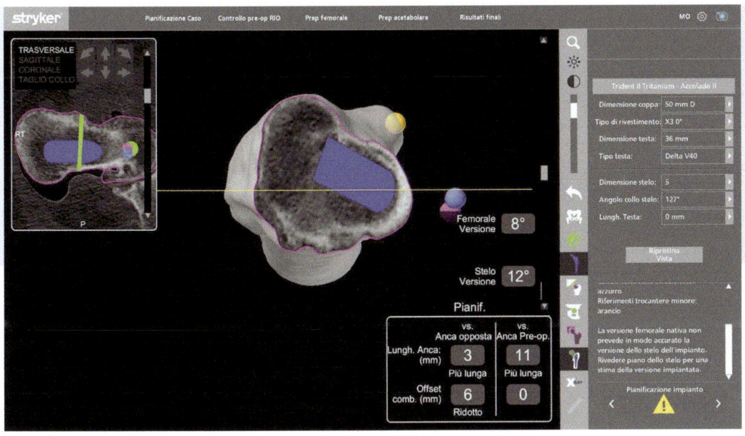

Figure 4 Transversal view is also possible to simulate neck resection, planning also box chisel position

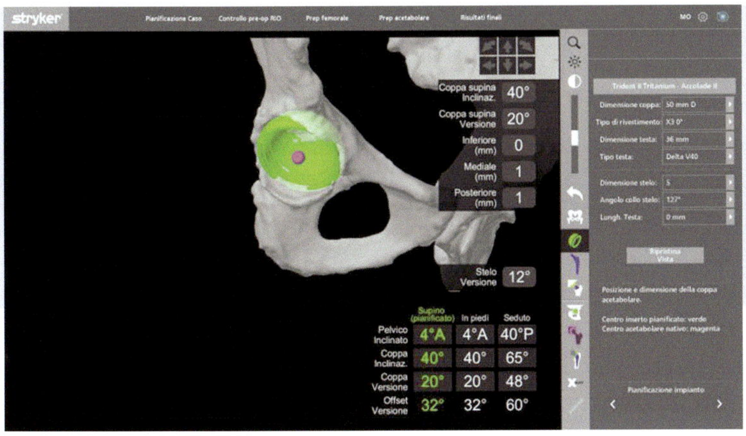

Figure 5 After stem planning combined anteversion is checked with the different pelvic tilt values; cup position could be modified accordingly

could be suggested [21].

A Range of Motion simulator is then available to check implant impingement in with the pelvis in standing and sitting position (figg. 6-7).

Routinarly we simulate 3 movements: rising from a low sitting (100° of flexion, 5° of abduction and 15° of internal rotation with the pelvis in a sitting position), shoe tying (90° of flexion, 5° of adduction and 15° of internal rotation with the pelvis in a sitting position) and (5° of extension, 5° of adduction and 30° of external rotation with the pelvis in a standing position) [22].

When implant-involving impingement is detected, stem or cup anteversion may be adjusted to fit to patient's spino-pelvic parameters. If bone on bone or implant on bone impingement is detected, osteophytes removal, or the use of a longer prosthetic head

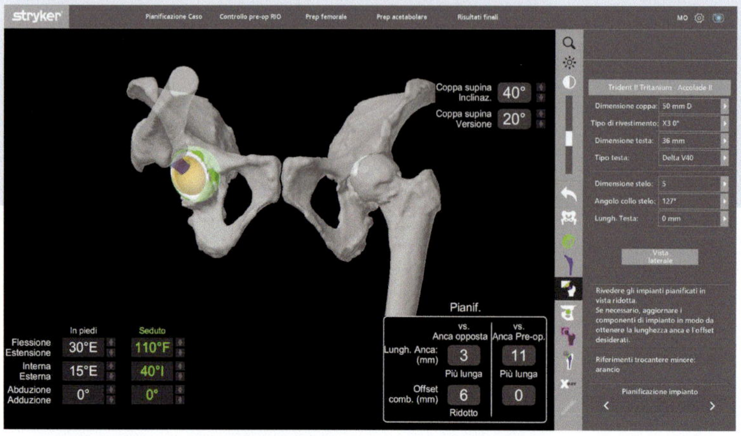

Figure 6 The range of motion simulation is used to check for anterior impingement in hip flexion and internal rotation

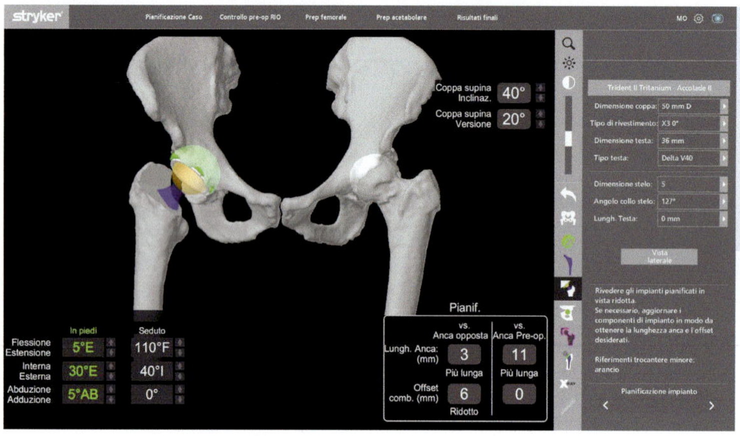

Figure 7 The range of motion simulation is used to check for posterior impingement in hip extension and external rotation

may be planned. However, reducing combined anteversion in a hypermobile pelvis could be risky because a hypermobile pelvis could be the compensation effect of a stiff hip, replacing the hip might reduce pelvic movement [23].

Operative room set up and patient positioning

A standardized and optimized set up during Mako THA will greatly aid the surgical flow. The patient is positioned on the surgical table in lateral decubitus. Pelvis is stabilized with a posterior bump at the level of sacrum and an anterior one at the Anterior Superior Iliac Spine. Attention should be paid to avoid anterior or posterior slope of the pelvis.

Bone prominences are protected using padding. Belly is also protected from the bump if needed. Both Anterior Superior Iliac Spine and Iliac crest has to be easily palpable.

The operative limb must be free to move on every plan during surgery, flexion of the hip must be at least 90°, to allow adequate testing of the stability of the implant.

Lead surgeon and first assistant will stand behind the patient, the second assistant will stand in front of lead surgeon. Mako System Specialist will stand behind the lead surgeon with the computer interface. The camera will aim the surgical field from the head of the surgical table leaving space for anesthesiologic assistance.The robotic arm should be placed as close as possible to the anterior side of the patient, at the back of the second assistant, aligned with the anterior superior iliac spine of the patients (fig. 8).

Patient's skin is carefully disinfected and the surgical field is draped including iliac crest and anterior superior iliac spine for pelvic array placement. For this reason, surgical draping should be positioned as close as possible to the bump pudding closely surrounding the superior half. After completing

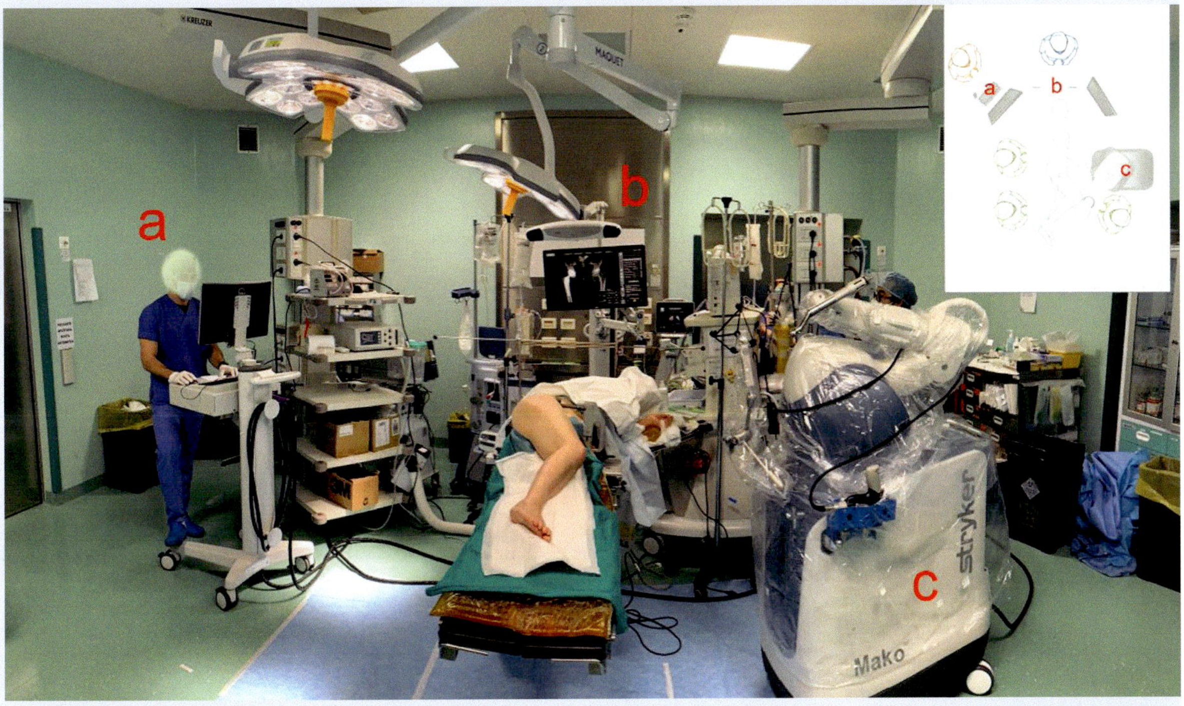

Figure 8 Operating theater set-up: robotic control consolle (a) is placed posteriorly to the patient; the camera (b) is placed at the head of the patient, having care to leave enough space for anesthesiological maneuvers; the robot (c) is placed anteriorly to the patient

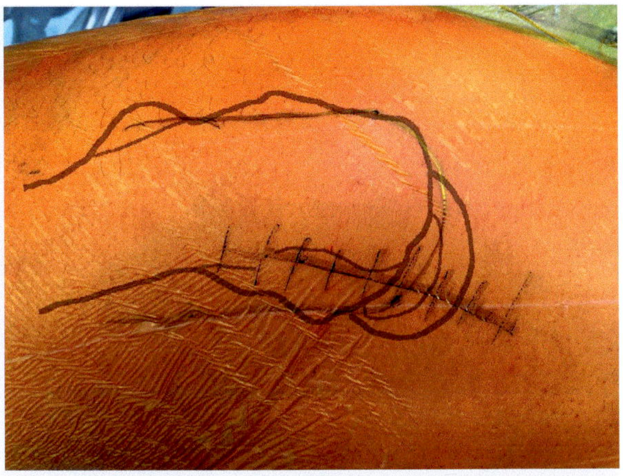

Figure 9 Surgical approach: the patient is positioned with the hip slightly flexed. The incision is performed at the posterior aspect of greater trochanter starting 3-4 cm distally from the apex and proceeding posteriorly for 8 cm

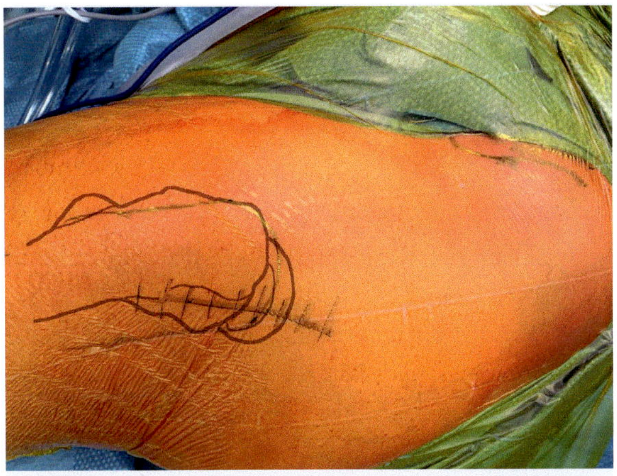

Figure 10 When preparing the surgical field, iliac crest should be left completely free for pelvic array pins positioning

the draping procedure, the skin is covered with a iodine adhesive sheet (figg. 9-10). Robotic arm calibration required for safety and accuracy reason by the software is performed by the scrub nurse or an assistant. It can be performed either before the patient enter the operating room of after the completion of the draping. Room traffic greatly affects the speed of the process because robotic arm has to be visible by the camera.

Pelvic array placement

In order to decrease the surgery time with open wound, we suggest performing pelvic array placing before skin incision or, as experience increases, by the second assistant while the lead surgeon starts main surgery.
In order to position the pelvic array, two pins have to be placed in the ileum crest. The ideal position for a pin placing is as perpendicular as possible to the iliac crest, otherwise iliac crest surface could be slippery. Also, the two pins should be parallel one with each other to insert the array holder. Double pin guide helps in achieving a compromise for perpendicularity. We suggest to perform two single stab incision in order to insert the pin guide through the skin to iliac crest bone (fig. 11). Medial and lateral border of iliac crest are palpated with the pin guide, then a pin is slightly hammered in the bone through the guide. The pin is therefore screwed with the drill. The second pin is positioned in the same way with the same guide, assessing again medial and lateral border of the iliac crest before hammering the pin.
The pin guide is removed and pin stability assessed. A third stab incision is performed between the former to allow direct contact of the array holder with the iliac crest bone. A third pin could be placed through a hole in the middle of the array holder and this third incision but we do not feel the need of more stability.
Then, the array holder is fixed with the middle part in direct contact with the bone thought the third incision, with, possibly, a third pin as further guide.
The array itself is placed but still not fixed to reduce visual obstruction during femoral registration (fig. 12).
A gauze is wrap around the array holder to reduce hypothetical contamination to the primary surgical wound.

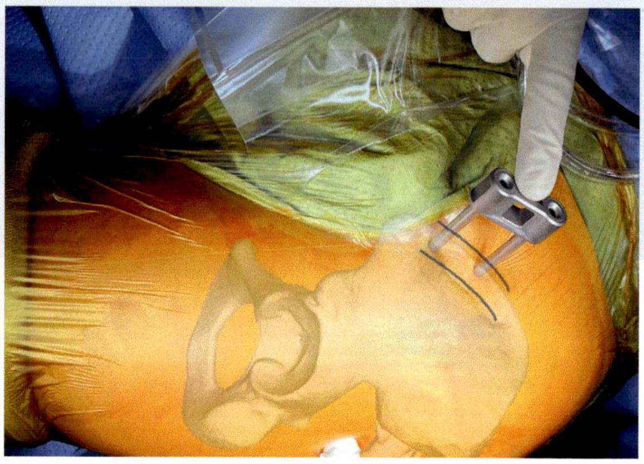

Figure 11 Pelvic pins positioning: pelvic array is held in position by 2 pins. Screw pins are inserted in the most anterior aspect of tibial crest with the use of a specific guide

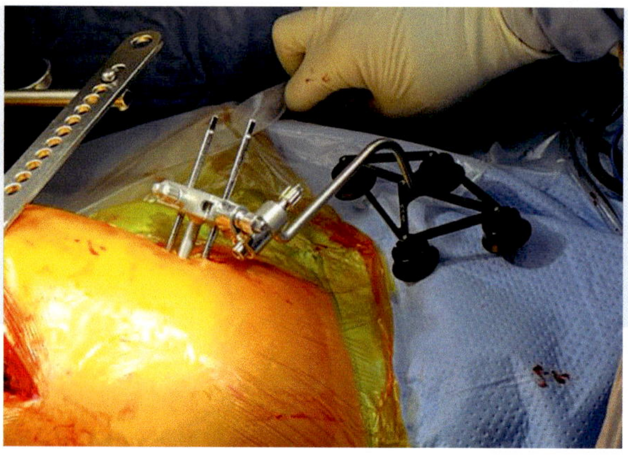

Figure 12 Pelvic array holder is fixed on the positioned screw pins, but pelvic array is left hanging to facilitate femoral calibration and preparation

Surgical procedure and intra operative planning

Surgical approach

The apex, the anterior and posterior margin of greater trochanter are marked with a stencil: the incision should run between the two third anterior and the third posterior, in a straight line distally for 3-4 cm and slightly curved proximally following gluteus maximus fibers for 5-6 cm (fig. 10).

The dissection of the subcutaneous fat could be performed either with electric scalpel or with surgical knife. It is of utmost importance to dissect along the whole skin incision and perpendicularly to the skin (fig. 13).

Especially in gynoid obese patients, grater trochanter palpation should be performed during dissection to avoid a posterior dissection.

The hip is abducted and the fascia layer is incised in line with gluteus maximus fibers which are therefore bluntly dissected and a Charnley retractor is placed (fig. 14).

Then the hip is extended and internally rotated with the knee flexed to protect sciatic nerve and to better expose trochanteric bursa which is then removed with an electric scalpel. Gluteus medius is retracted anteriorly then short extra rotator muscles can be visualized and piriformis tendon identified (fig. 15). A small incision between piriformis tendon and superior gemellus is performed and a Hohmann retractor positioned to protect the former. Tenotomy of conjoined tendon (superior gemellus, internal obturator, inferior gemellus) and capsulotomy can be performed separately or with a single incision just posterior to the posterior aspect of the greater trochanter (fig. 16). In order to limit the bleeding, ascendant branch of medial circumflex artery, that is located at the level of the proximal margin of quadratus femori should be cauterized in advance. The proximal part of the quadratus femori is incised, then the hip can be dislocated posteriorly. Soft tissue from trochanteric fossa and from femoral neck is removed (fig. 17). A small hole is performed with a Kirshner wire in the outer part of the posterior aspect of the greater trochanter to facilitate the positioning of the femoral array base (fig. 18). Attention should be paid to place the array in the posterior column of the proximal femur metaphysis where can be seen from the camera, both in reduced and in dislocated position, without impingement with the skin (fig. 19).

The checkpoint is placed slightly distal to the femoral array screw (fig. 20) and consequently the femoral anatomy is acquired with the probe. The osteotomy level is checked with the same probe and marked with electric scalpel (fig. 21), the femoral array is removed from his base, blunt Hohmann retractors are placed around the neck and osteotomy is performed with an oscillating saw. If necessary, the osteotomy is completed with a large osteotome.

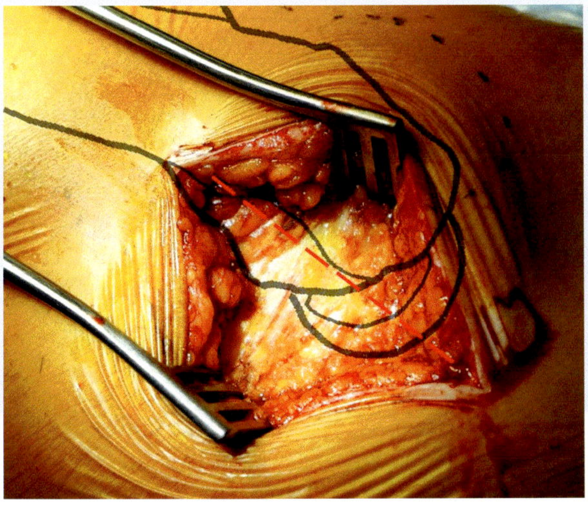

Figure 13 Fascia dissection follows the same direction of skin cut. Since at this time is easier to identify greater trochanter, especially in obese patients, fascia could be incised more anteriorly or posteriorly

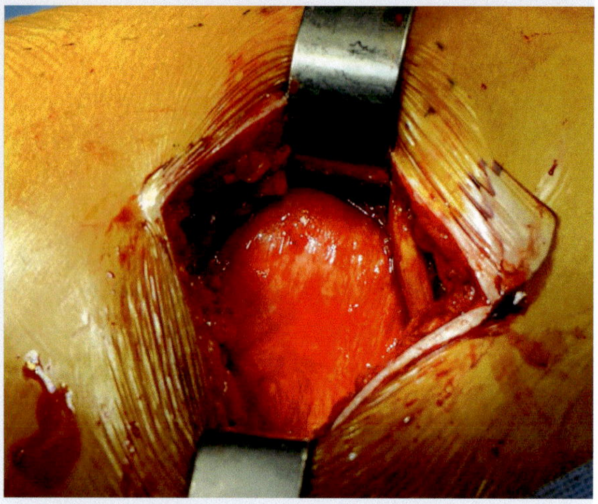

Figure 14 Trochanteric bursa. Accurate bursectomy is fundamental fora a good exposition and helps prevent post-operative bursitis relapses

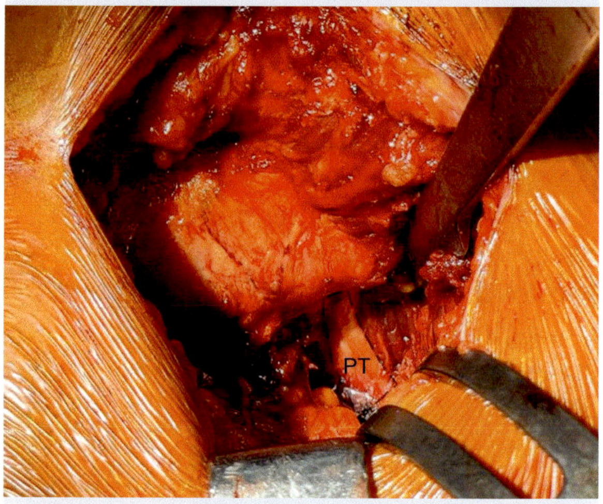

Figure 15 Short External Rotators. Externale rotators trochanteric insertions are exposed and Piriformis Tendon (PT) is identified and preserved for the whole intervention

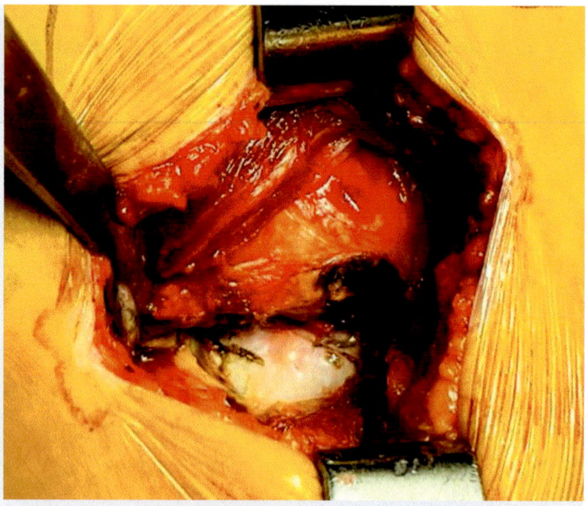

Figure 16 Complete capsulotomy is performed, having care to avoid to damage Piriformis tendon at the proximal edge

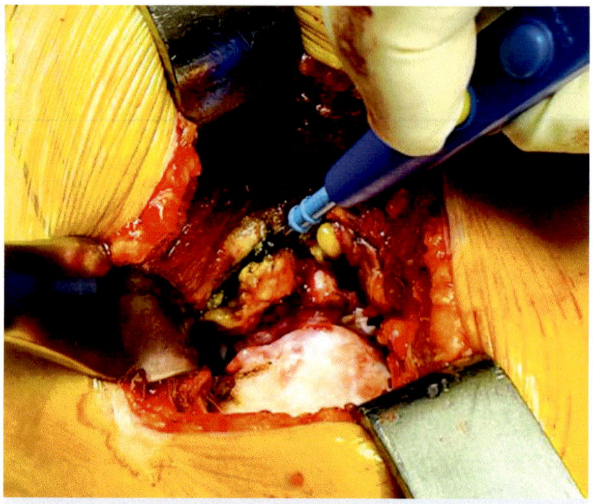

Figure 17 Femoral neck has to be accurately exposed and every residue of capsule and synovia has to be removed in order to facilitate calibration for robotics

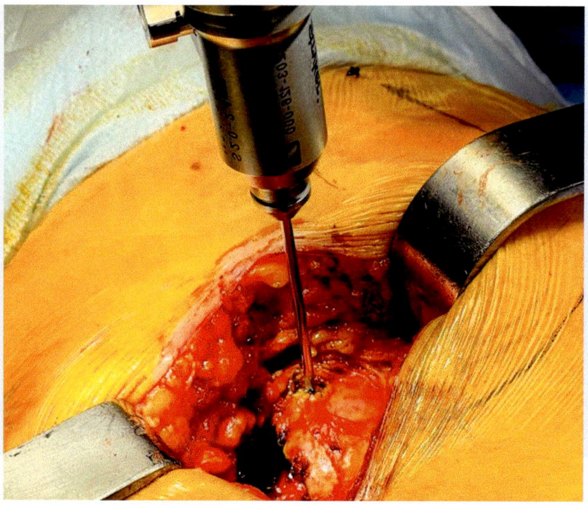

Figure 18 Femoral Array preparation. Femoral array screw is positioned on the posterior aspect of greater trochanter, where it meets the distal 1/3 of the femoral neck. To facilitate screw insertion, cortical bone is drilled with a 2-2.5 mm Kirschner wire

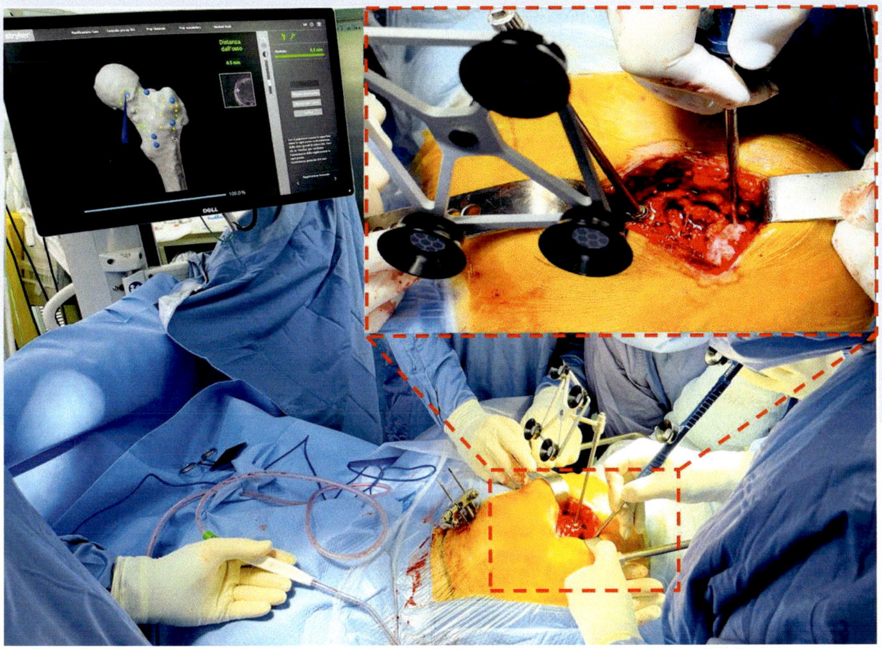

Figure 19 Femoral array post-opshould be oriented toward the camera; during calibration contact between the femoral array and the retracted tissues should be prevented, to avoid array malpositioning

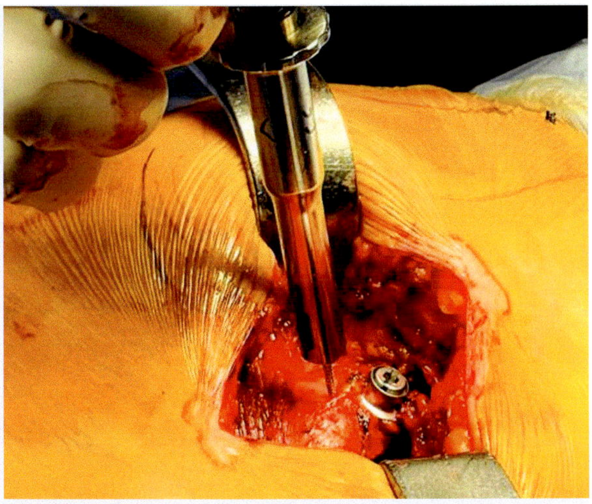

Figure 20 Femoral checkpoint positioning

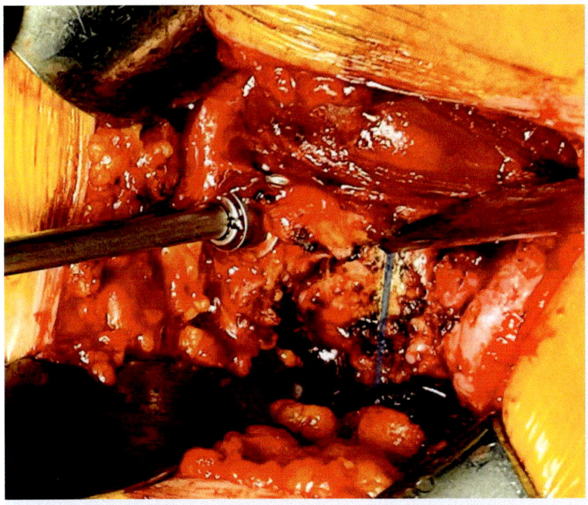

Figure 21 Neck resection landmark. Neck resection line is identified with the probe traced with electrocauterization, following pre-operative planning

Femur first

A femoral elevator is positioned at the base of the neck and a Homan retractor is placed in the lateral aspect of the greater trochanter to protect gluteus muscles, then the hip is flexed, internally rotated and adducted. In order to facilitate the orientation of the femoral stem, the patient's leg must be positioned perpendicular to the ground. Remaining soft tissue is removed from the neck and from the trochanteric fossa.

The anatomy of the medullary canal at osteotomy level can be compared with robotic planning on the monitor and posterior cortex can be used as a reference point for the positioning of the box osteotome. Femoral broaching is then performed with progressive broaches (fig. 22). Stem version can be checked at any moment: the broach handler is removed and the broach left in place, a trial neck is positioned (fig. 23), the hip is extended with neutral adduction and rotation and the femoral array positioned. Attention must be paid in order to avoid skin impinge-

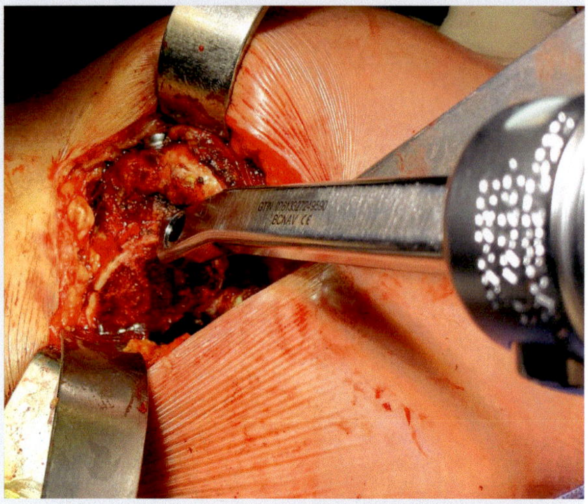

Figure 22 Box chisel entry point is determined following 3D planning

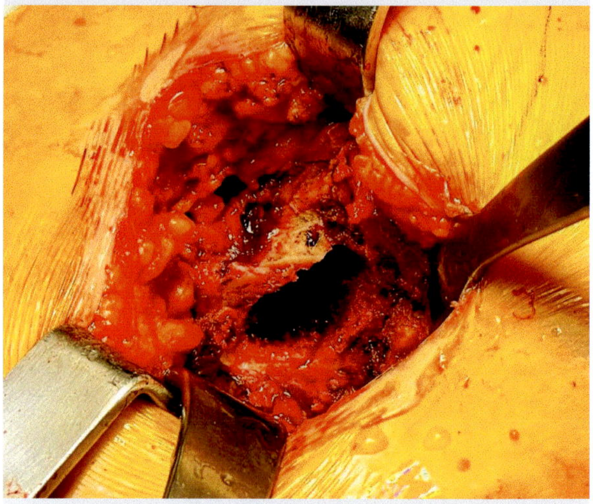

Figure 23 Femoral broaching is also performed following transverse view on 3D planning

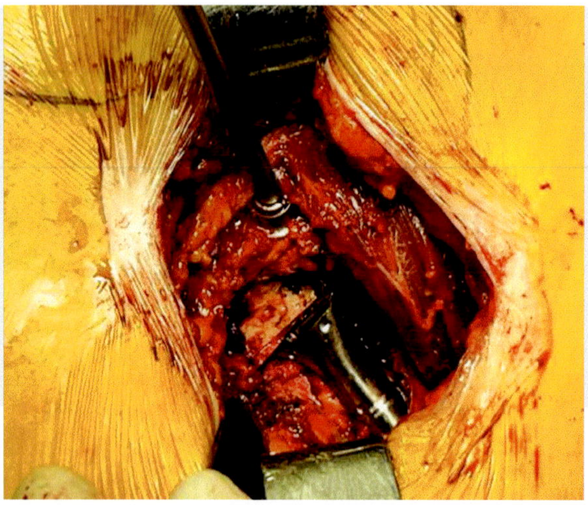

Figure 24 Trial broaches are then checked for length, offset and anteversion calibrating the three holes on trial neck

ment with femoral array otherwise the array itself might move. If the prosthesis trial neck does not fit due to impingement with femoral neck bone, the dedicated reamer should be used.

We suggest checking femoral version at least twice: with the broach one size smaller than planned and with planned size. Always check when in doubt. The femoral array is removed, femoral elevator positioned and broach remove with his handler (fig. 24).

Acetabular time

The final fixation of the pelvic array is performed (fig. 25) and a femoral retractor is placed over the anterior aspect of the acetabulum with the hip in neutral flexion and slight internal rotation. Steinman pins or Hohmann retractors are placed where needed, usually one superior and one posterior to the acetabular rim.

Pelvic checkpoint should be positioned proximally to the superior margin of the acetabulum, but small incision usually prevents its right placing and its removal. For this reason, we suggest registering the checkpoint on the base of the pelvic array.

Pulvinar and acetabular labrum are removed and acetabular matching is performed with the probe (fig. 26).

Acetabular planning can be checked and modified according to femoral version and

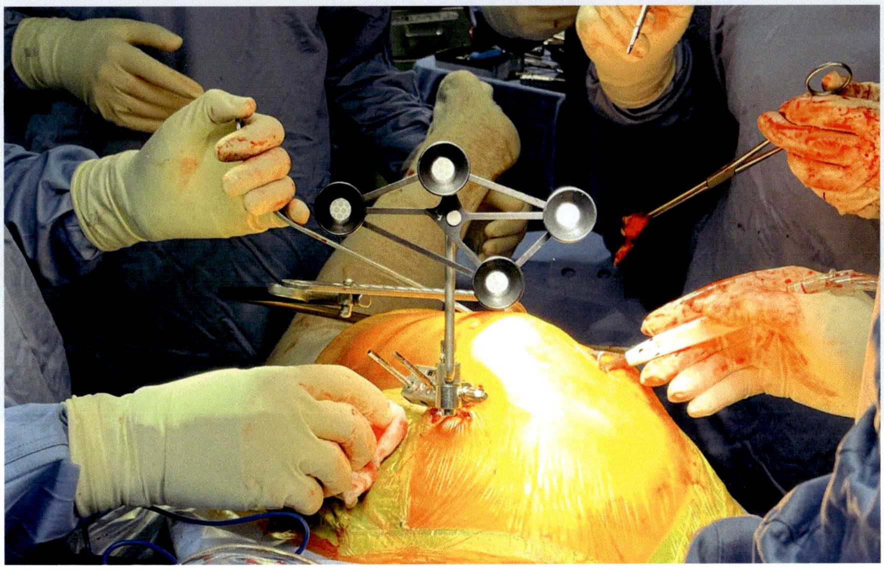

Figure 25 After finishing femoral preparation pelvic array is fixed in its final position

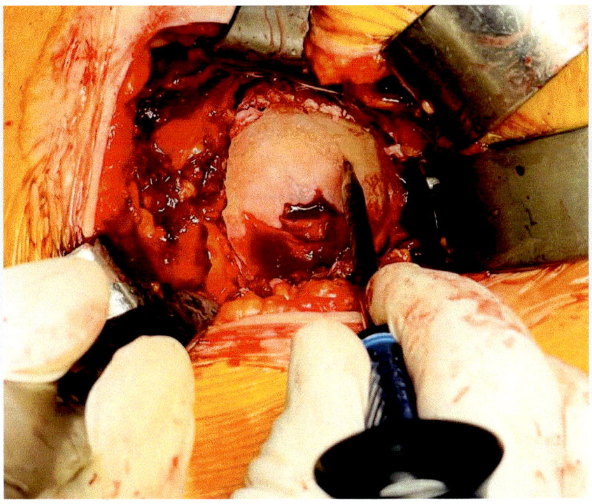

Figure 26 Acetabular calibration is performed with the specific probe

intraoperative findings.
A reamer basket is positioned by hand to double check the size. Osteophytes can be removed if necessary to allow correct reamer positioning.
The robot is then approached to the operating table, the reamer engine and the reamer basket are connected to the robotic arm. Once positioned the reamer in the acetabulum, version and inclination can be checked in real time on the monitor and reaming can be performed according to planning. The system allows reaming with 15° of freedom with respect to the planned position of the cup (fig. 27). The reamer is therefore removed, abundant saline irrigation performed and the reamed acetabulum is eye checked. If the result is satisfactory, a trial cup can be used to utterly verify the reaming. On the back table the chosen definitive cup is assembled to the impactor meanwhile the reamer is removed from the robotic arm. The impactor is connected to the robotic arm which is then freed in order to allow the definitive cup to be positioned close to the acetabulum. Once the cup and the acetabulum are close enough, the robotic arm can be engaged. This allows the robot to set the arm direction according to the version and inclination planned. The cup is finally impacted in the pelvis with the hammer (fig. 28). During the impaction, the robot

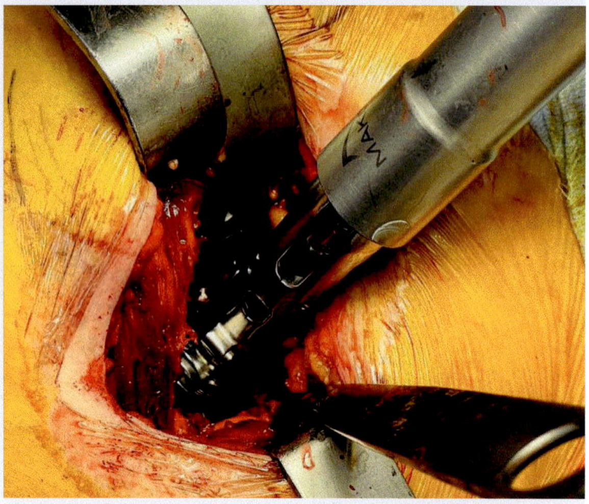

Figure 27 Acetabular reaming is guided by the robotic arm. A complete acetabular exposure may be avoided, since ream orientation is determined by the robotic guidance; in so doing, soft tissue stress may be reduced

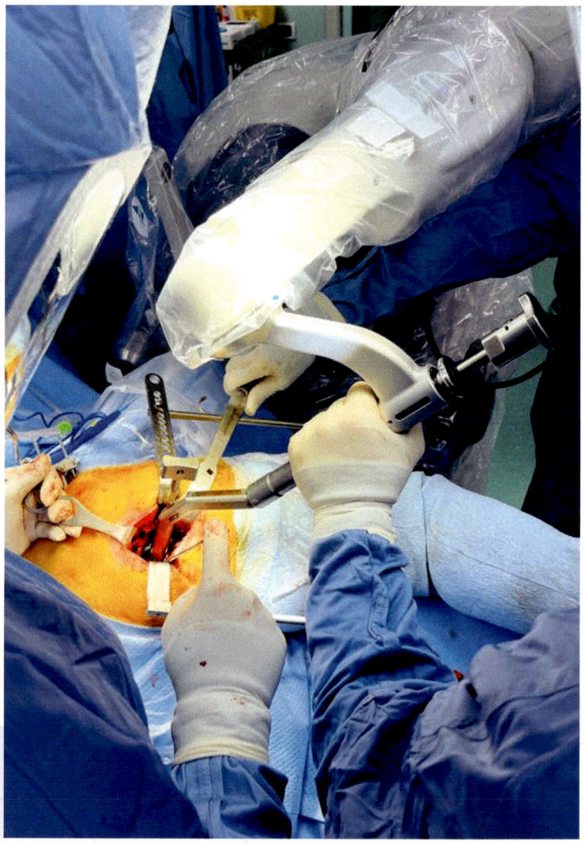

Figure 28 Cup impaction guided by the robotic arm

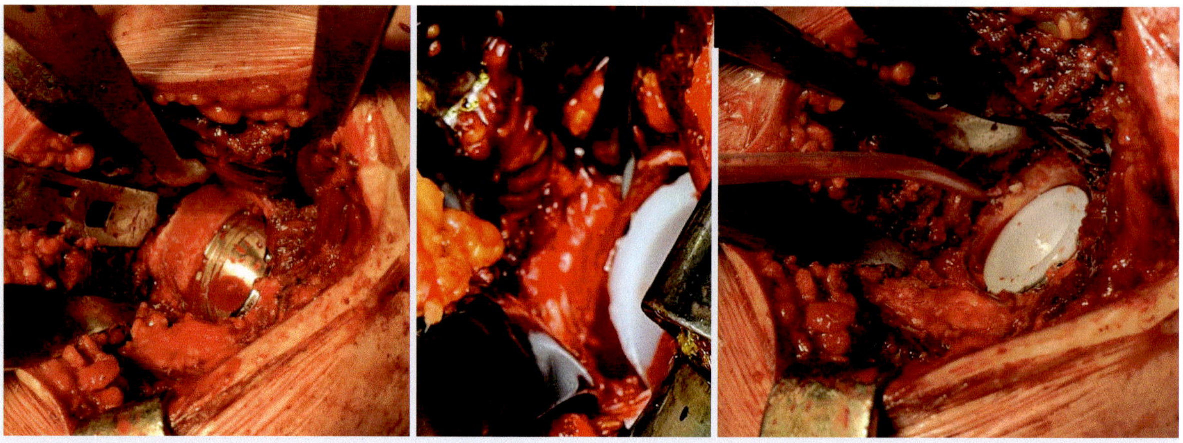

Figure 29 Osteophytes removal. Acetabular rim is easily accessible with the described approach

engineer register progressively the distance between the cup and the bottom of the acetabulum which can be seen on the monitor during the procedure. The handler is then disconnected and the robot moved away.
Cup plug is placed, if needed, screws can be positioned. If presents, osteophytes should be removed before positioning the insert or the liner in the case of dual mobility (fig. 29). After impaction of the insert, inclination and version of the cup can be checked registering with the probe 5 points on the outer margin of the insert/liner. The transverse ligament of acetabulum is an important landmark for verifying in the field the correct anteversion of the acetabulum

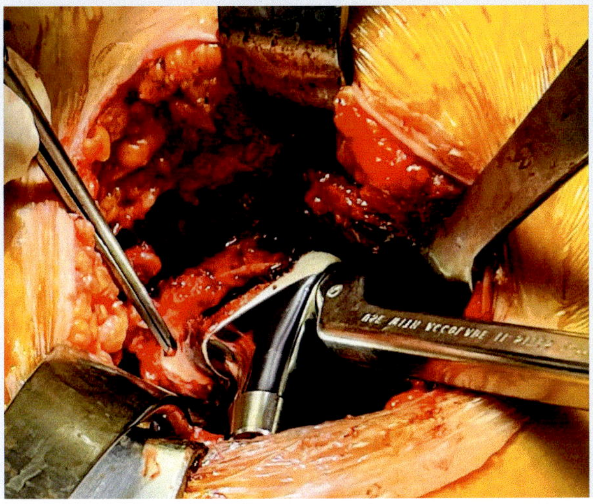

Figure 30 Stem is positioned following the mark made on cortical bone and based on pre-operative plan

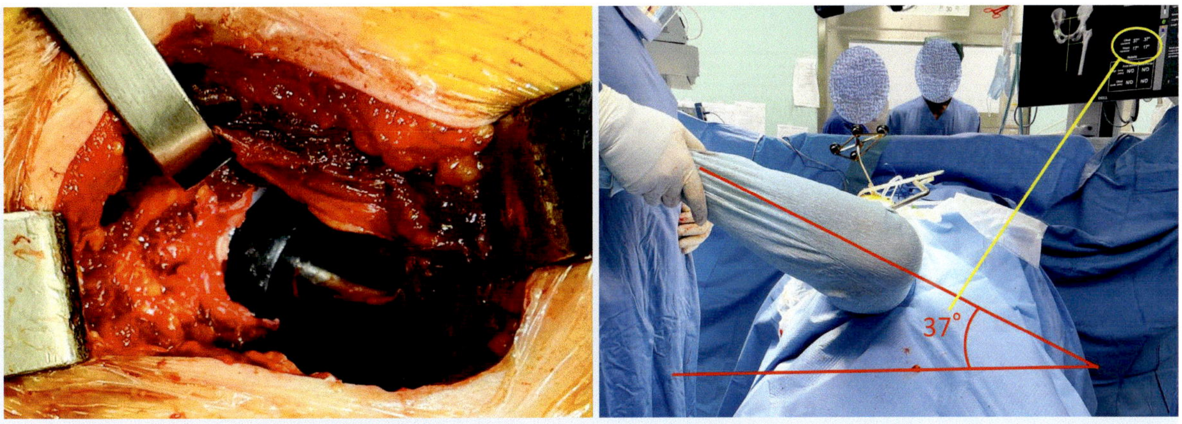

Figure 31 Components position is checked with Ranawat's manouver

Final components

Exposed the femur once again, if previously satisfied with the broaching, final stem can be implanted (fig. 30). If not, planning can be checked again for leg length, offset and combined version (which were registered previously). Also, 3D movements for impingement con be verified. Cemented stem could also be an option allowing accurate positioning for version, length and offset. However, the array for cemented stem positioning requires the widening of the wound due to the need to keep both femoral and stem array simultaneously in place (also without skin impingement for femoral array). After positioning the final stem, trials with heads can be performed (figs. 31-32). After trial head placing and hip reduction, femoral array should be positioned and hip center acquired via circular motion. Attention to not mobilize femoral array during this procedure should be paid. Leg length and offset can be check clinically and on monitor such as 3D model for impingement in both sitting and standing position. Head length can then be changed in the software and if satisfying, final head implanted.

The array is then removed, hip dislocated and final head impacted. The hip is reduced again and final data registered though femoral array positioning (a new hip center may be acquired).

Femoral checkpoint and array base are now removed. If pelvic checkpoint were placed, it should have been removed after insert/liner impaction.

An intraarticular drainage can be positioned according to surgeon preference. Fascia is sutured and wound is closed by layer. Pelvic array is then removed and skin sutured.

CASE REPORT 1

A) Pre-operative X-ray. Hip dysplasia (DDH). S.G. 65 years old, male. Right THA 8 years ago; B) Pre-operative planning. C) Robotic surgery report. D) Post-operative X-ray.

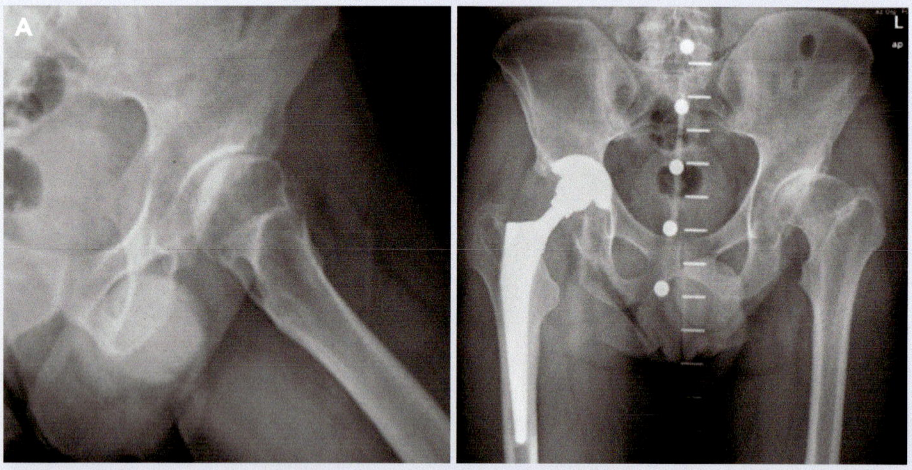

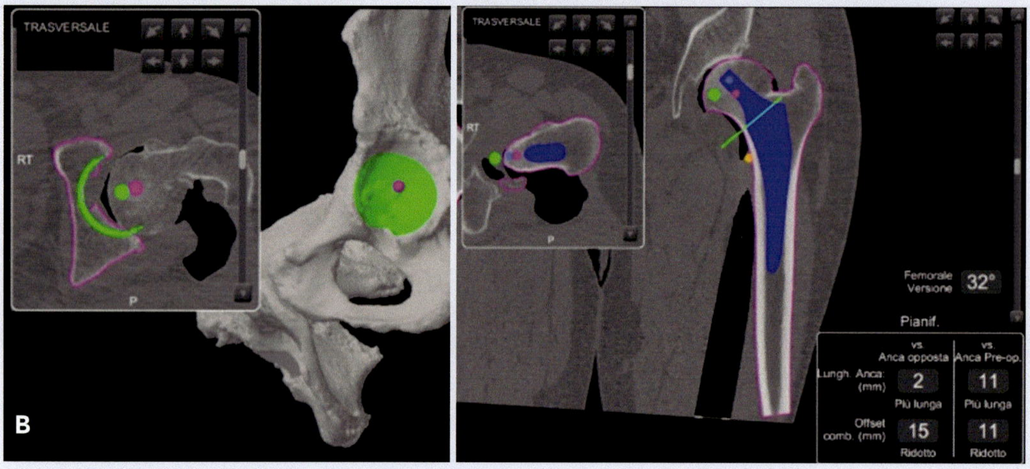

C **Femoral version 32° - straight stem**

Before THA	VS opposite	VS pre-op
Hip lenght (mm)	-9	-
Combined offset (mm)	-3	-

Planned Stem size 5, cup 52 mm	VS opposite	VS pre-op
Hip lenght (mm)	+2	+11
Combined offset (mm)	-15	-11
Stem version (°)	19	
Cup version (°)	17	
Combined version (°)	36	

Final results Stem size 6, cup 50 mm	VS opposite	VS pre-op
Hip lenght (mm)	+4	+13
Combined offset (mm)	-16	-13
Stem version (°)	21	
Cup version (°)	17	
Combined version (°)	38	

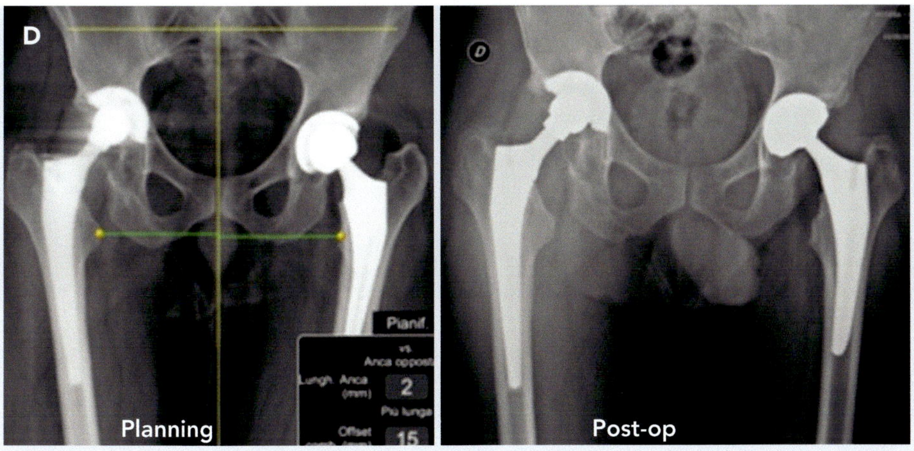

CASE REPORT 2

A) Pre-operative X-ray. Femoral head and pelvis avascular necrosis. M.L. 71 years old, female. Rapidly progressive AVN. B) Pre-operative. Straight uncemented stem, press-fit dual mobility cup + acetabular omologous cancellous bone graft. C) Robotic surgery report. D) Post-operative X-ray. Straight uncemented stem, press-fit dual mobility cup stabilized with 2 screws + acetabular omologous cancellous bone graft.

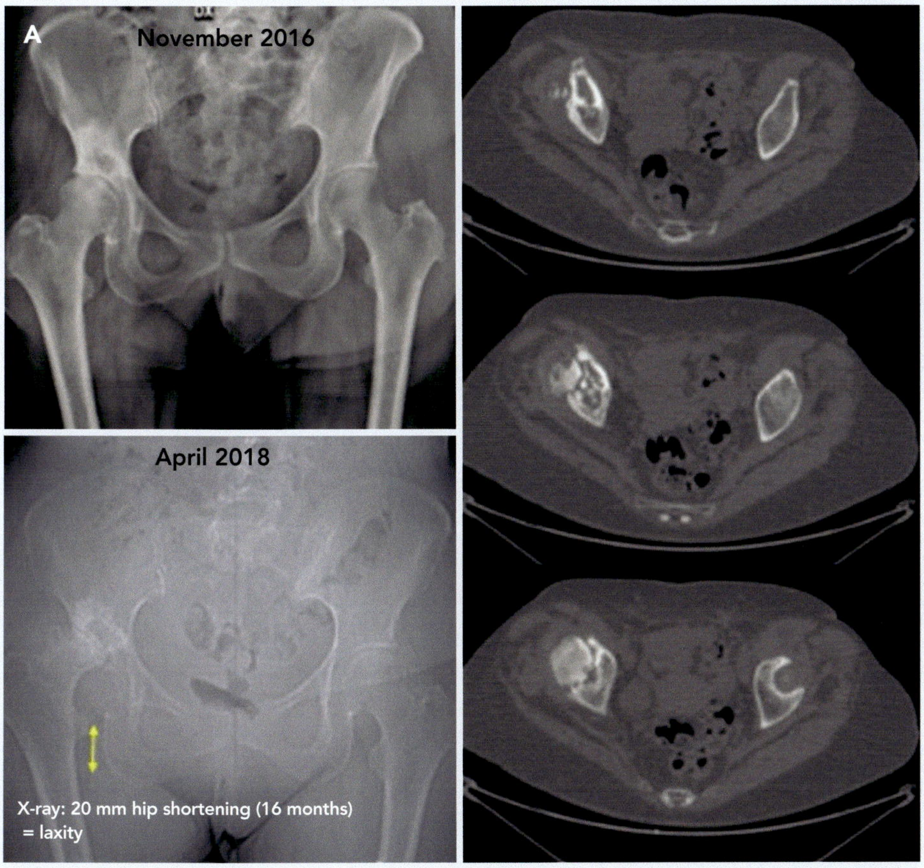

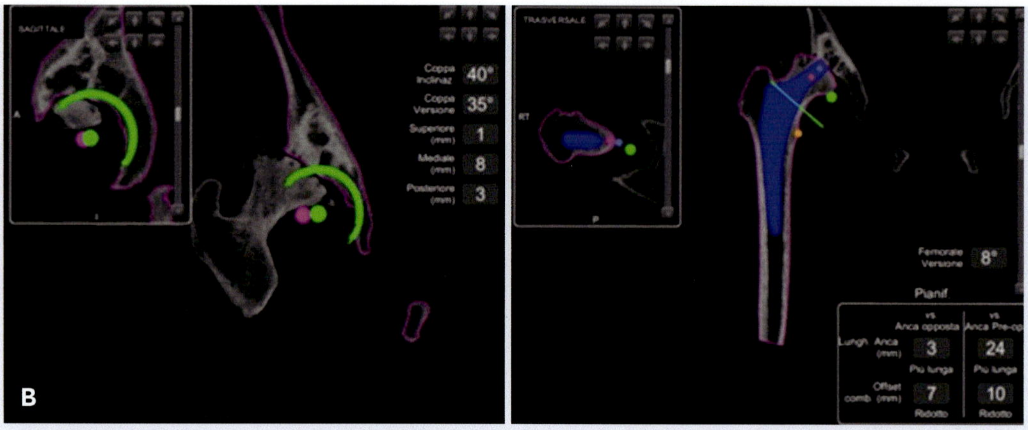

C **Femoral version 8° - straight stem**

Before THA	VS opposite	VS pre-op
Hip lenght (mm)	-22	-
Combined offset (mm)	+3	-

Highly compromised proximal femur anatomy

▼

Risk of discrepancy between FNV and SV

▼

High importance of intraoperative stem version measurement

Planned Stem size 4, cup 48 mm	VS opposite	VS pre-op
Hip lenght (mm)	+3	+24
Combined offset (mm)	-7	-10
Stem version (°)	-7	
Cup version (°)	35	
Combined version (°)	28	

Final results stem size 4, cup 48 mm	VS opposite	VS pre-op
Hip lenght (mm)	+1	+23
Combined offset (mm)	-4	-7
Stem version (°)	-7	
Cup version (°)	36	
Combined version (°)	29	

Planning Post-op

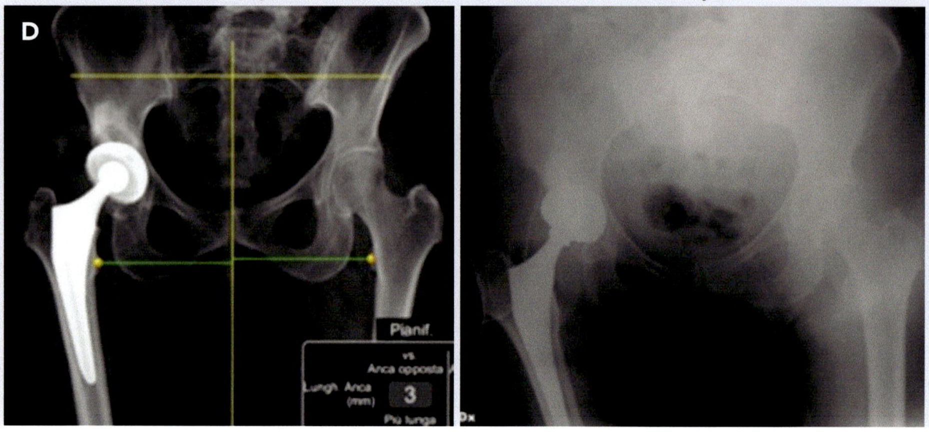

CASE REPORT 3

A) Pre-operative X-ray. AVN left hip. B.S. 82 years old, female. Osteoporotic bone. Right THA 7 years ago. B) Pre-operative planning. C) Robotic surgery report. D) Post-operative X-ray

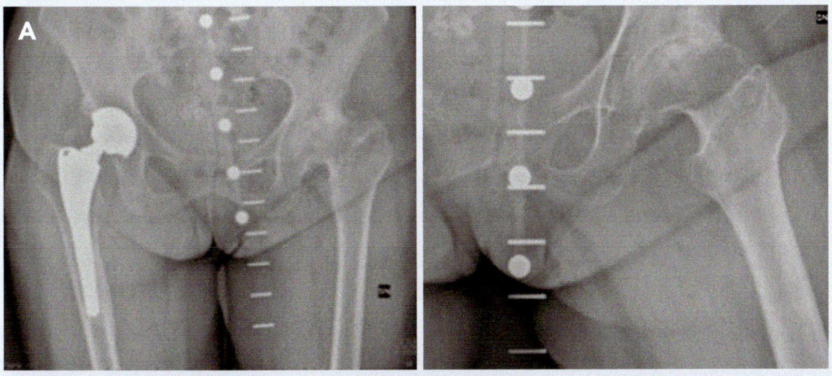

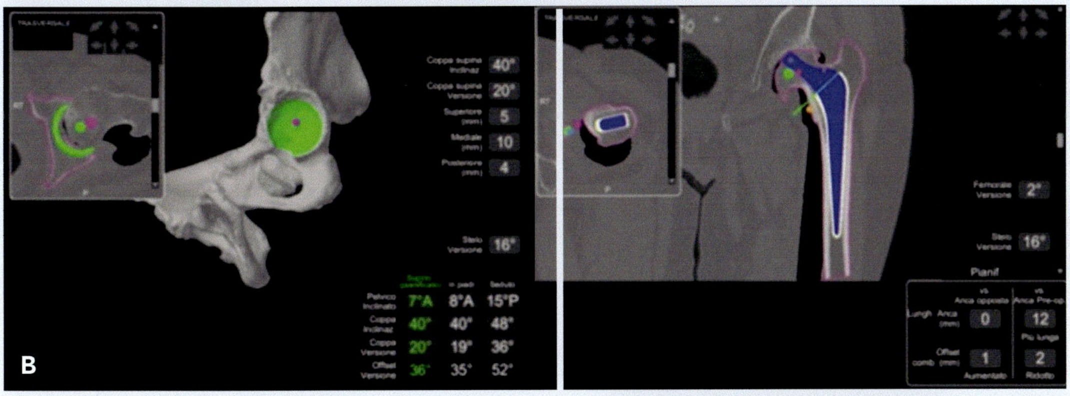

C **Pre-op femoral version 2°**
Planned femoral version 16°

Before THA	VS opposite	VS pre-op
Hip lenght (mm)	-12	-
Combined offset (mm)	+3	-

Planned Stem size 9, cup 54 mm	VS opposite	VS pre-op
Hip lenght (mm)	0	+12
Combined offset (mm)	+1	-2
Stem version (°)	16	
Cup version (°)	20	
Combined version (°)	36	

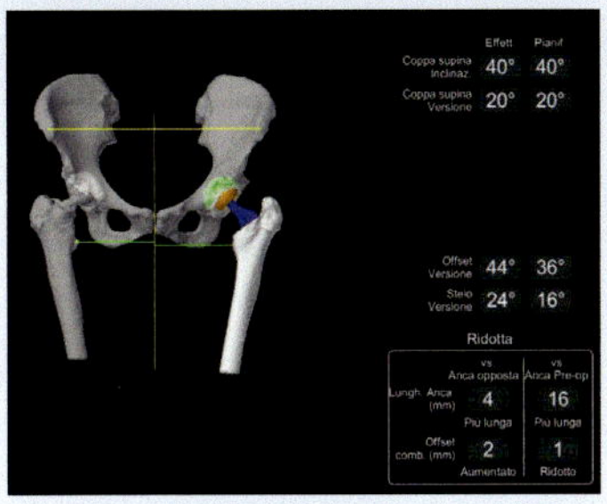

Final results Stem size 8, cup 54 mm	VS opposite	VS pre-op
Hip lenght (mm)	+4	+16
Combined offset (mm)	+2	-1
Stem version (°)	24	
Cup version (°)	20	
Combined version (°)	44	

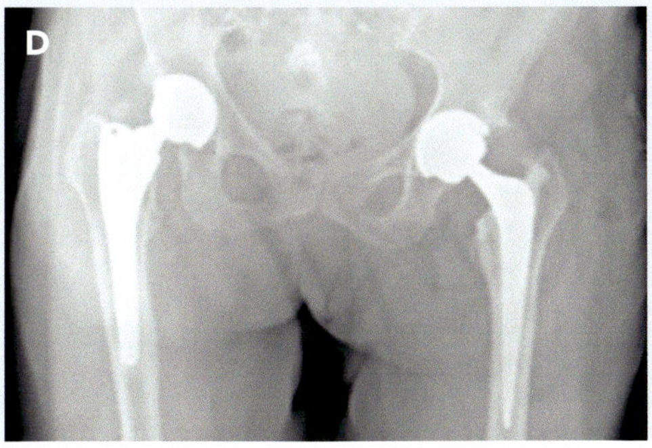

Discussion

Total hip arthroplasty can be performed using a variety of surgical approaches. Choosing the optimal surgical approach may improve the outcomes minimizing the risks. However, there is still disagreement regarding which is the most suitable approach for a certain type of patient: as a matter of fact, no approach is the most suitable one for everyone.

Recent studies have shown similar functional outcomes using posterolateral approach and anterior direct approach 3 months after surgery. However, lower rates of limping, less satisfaction, heterotopical ossifications [24-25] and residual pain were shown when compared to lateral direct approach.

The main advantage of postero lateral approach, compared to lateral, is the sparing of the abductor mechanism, expecially gluteus medius, avoiding post-surgical Trendelenburg gait.

The main concern about this via is still the high dislocation rate as demostraded in the past by various authors (1-5%) [8-14]. Many surgeons have reported lower dislocation rates when repairing posterior soft tissue (0.5-2%) [26-30]. However, the revision rates following dislocation are still higher compared to other approaches as shown by Dutch national registry [30-31] (1.1-1.5% compared to 0.5-0.6% for anterior and lateral approaches), probably due to the failure of the repaired external rotators [32-34]. For this reason we spare piriformis tendon instead of repairing it as shonw by Kim in a retrospective study comparing dislocation incidence in three groups of patient: external rotators not repaired (5.3%), repaired external rotators (3.9%) and spared piriformis (0%) [18].

Biomechanical studies demostrate that the piriformis tendon overlies the femoral head posteriorly, mechanically limits excessive internal rotation on weight-bearing, and acts as an external rotator and abductor of the hip in flexion, stabilizing the head in the socket [35]. However, there is still no consensus whether muscle sparing decreases dislocation rate.

Dutch registry reports higher revision rates in anterior approach for aseptic loosening of femoral stem and for periprosthetic fractures [31]. The main reason is the more demanding femoral exposition. Differently, posterolateral approach allows good visualization of both femoral and acetabular sides, minimizing intra-operative and post-operative complications. Moreover, it could be easily extended both proximally and distally if in the need of complication handling. Anyway, there is no statistical significative difference in the revision rates for all causes.

The minimally invasiveness minimize muscolar trauma, allows quicker recovery time and decrease post-surgical pain, blood loss and has a better cosmetic appearance [36-37].

Between 1st may 2014 and 31st may 2019, we performed robotic arm-assisted THA with the Mako Rio System (Stryker, Mahwah, NJ, USA) on 394 patients using minimally invasive posterolateral approach. We reported only one case of atraumatic dislocation and one case of traumatic dislocation after a fall from the stairs. Both cases were single episodes and they did not require revision surgery. Dislocation rate of 0.5% and revision rate for dislocation of 0% is remarkably lower than reported in literature.

Conclusions

Robotic-arm assisted THA using minimally invasive posterolateral approach allows to optimize the advantages of posterolateral approach, minimizing recovery time, surgical pain and soft tissue damages.

Recently introduced 4.0 Mako Software also allows to evauate spino pelvic movements in relation to component positioning.

Dislocation rate is significantly decreased mainly due to the accuracy in component positioning and to posterior soft tissue sparing.

Robotic surgery is the tool to accurately achieve the planned combined version, which is today the most effective way to prevent dislocation together with posterior tissue sparing as stated by Dorr et al. [38-40]. Further studies are necessary to evaluate the role of pelvic balance in preventing dislocations.

In conclusion, minimally invasive posterolateral approach is a safe and suitable approach in selected patients for routinary robotic THA.

Bibliography

1. Langenbeck B: Chirurgische beobachtungen aus dem kriege, Berlin, 1874, Hirschwald.
2. Langenbeck B: Ueber die schussfracturen der gelenke und ihre behandlung, Berlin, 1868, A. Hirschwald.
3. Kocher T. Operative surgery, 3rd English ed, transl by Siles HJ, Paul CB, London, 1911, Black.
4. Gibson A. Posterior exposure of the hip joint. J Bone Joint Surg Br. 1950;32-B(2):183-186.
5. Moore AT. The self-locking metal hip prosthesis. J Bone Joint Surg Am. 1957;39-A(4):811-827.
6. Chechik O, Khashan M, Lador R, Salai M, Amar E. Surgical approach and prosthesis fixation in hip arthroplasty world wide. Arch Orthop Trauma Surg. 2013;133(11):1595-1600.
7. Woo RY, Morrey BF. Dislocations after total hip arthroplasty. J Bone Joint Surg Am. 1982;64(9):1295-1306.
8. Sariali E, Leonard P, Mamoudy P. Dislocation after total hip arthroplasty using Hueter anterior approach. J Arthroplasty. 2008;23(2):266-272.
9. Matta JM, Shahrdar C, Ferguson T. Single-incision anterior approach for total hip arthroplasty on an orthopaedic table. Clin Orthop Relat Res. 2005;441:115-124.
10. Mulliken BD, Rorabeck CH, Bourne RB, Nayak N. A modified direct lateral approach in total hip arthroplasty: a comprehensive review. J Arthroplasty. 1998;13(7):737-747.
11. Sheth D, Cafri G, Inacio MC, Paxton EW, Namba RS. Anterior and Anterolateral Approaches for THA Are Associated With Lower Dislocation Risk Without Higher Revision Risk. Clin Orthop Relat Res. 2015;473(11):3401-3408.
12. Aggarwal VK, Elbuluk A, Dundon J, et al. Surgical approach significantly affects the complication rates associated with total hip arthroplasty. Bone Joint J. 2019;101-B(6):646-651. doi:10.1302/0301-620X.101B6.BJJ-2018-1474.R1
13. Kwon MS, Kuskowski M, Mulhall KJ, Macaulay W, Brown TE, Saleh KJ. Does surgical approach affect total hip arthroplasty dislocation rates?. Clin Orthop Relat Res. 2006;447:34-38.
14. Sierra RJ, Raposo JM, Trousdale RT, Cabanela ME. Dislocation of primary THA done through a posterolateral approach in the elderly. Clin Orthop Relat Res. 2005;441:262-267.
15. Maratt JD, Gagnier JJ, Butler PD, et al. No Difference in Dislocation Seen in Anterior Vs Posterior Approach Total Hip Arthroplasty. J Arthroplasty. 2016;31(9 Suppl):127-130.
16. Jolles BM, Bogoch ER. Posterior versus lateral surgical approach for total hip arthroplasty in adults with osteoarthritis. Cochrane Database Syst Rev. 2006;2006(3):CD003828.
17. Chiu FY, Chen CM, Chung TY, Lo WH, Chen TH. The effect of posterior capsulorrhaphy in primary total hip arthroplasty: a prospective randomized study. J Arthroplasty. 2000;15(2):194-199.
18. Kim YS, Kwon SY, Sun DH, Han SK, Maloney WJ. Modified posterior approach to total hip arthroplasty to enhance joint stability. Clin Orthop Relat Res. 2008;466(2):294-299.
19. Kayani B, Konan S, Thakrar RR, Huq SS, Haddad FS. Assuring the long-term total joint arthroplasty: a triad of variables. Bone Joint J. 2019;101-B(1_Supple_A):11-18.
20. Jacofsky DJ, Allen M. Robotics in Arthroplasty: A Comprehensive Review. J Arthroplasty. 2016;31(10):2353-2363.
21. Eftekhary N, Shimmin A, Lazennec JY, et al. A systematic approach to the hip-spine relationship and its applications to total hip arthroplasty. Bone Joint J. 2019;101-B(7):808-816.
22. Patel AB, Wagle RR, Usrey MM, Thompson MT, Incavo SJ, Noble PC. Guidelines for implant placement to minimize impingement during activities of daily living after total hip arthroplasty. J Arthroplasty. 2010;25(8):1275-81.e1.
23. Berliner JL, Esposito CI, Miller TT, Padgett DE, Mayman DJ, Jerabek SA. What preoperative factors predict postoperative sitting pelvic position one year following total hip arthroplasty?. Bone Joint J. 2018;100-B(10):1289-1296.
24. Bischoff R, Dunlap J, Carpenter L, DeMouy E, Barrack R. Heterotopic ossification following uncemented total hip arthroplasty. Effect of the operative approach. J Arthroplasty. 1994;9(6):641-644.
25. Morrey BF, Adams RA, Cabanela ME. Com-

parison of heterotopic bone after anterolateral, transtrochanteric, and posterior approaches for total hip arthroplasty. Clin Orthop Relat Res. 1984;(188):160-167.
26. Kwon MS, Kuskowski M, Mulhall KJ, Macaulay W, Brown TE, Saleh KJ. Does surgical approach affect total hip arthroplasty dislocation rates?. Clin Orthop Relat Res. 2006;447:34-38.
27. Pellicci PM, Bostrom M, Poss R. Posterior approach to total hip replacement using enhanced posterior soft tissue repair. Clin Orthop Relat Res. 1998;(355):224-228.
28. Suh KT, Park BG, Choi YJ. A posterior approach to primary total hip arthroplasty with soft tissue repair. Clin Orthop Relat Res. 2004;(418):162-167.
29. White RE Jr, Forness TJ, Allman JK, Junick DW. Effect of posterior capsular repair on early dislocation in primary total hip replacement. Clin Orthop Relat Res. 2001;(393):163-167.
30. Yamaguchi T, Naito M, Asayama I, Kambe T, Fujisawa M, Ishiko T. The effect of posterolateral reconstruction on range of motion and muscle strength in total hip arthroplasty. J Arthroplasty. 2003;18(3):347-351.
31. Zijlstra WP, De Hartog B, Van Steenbergen LN, Scheurs BW, Nelissen RGHH. Effect of femoral head size and surgical approach on risk of revision for dislocation after total hip arthroplasty. Acta Orthop. 2017;88(4):395-401.
32. Masonis JL, Bourne RB. Surgical approach, abductor function, and total hip arthroplasty dislocation. Clin Orthop Relat Res. 2002;(405):46-53.
33. Stähelin T, Drittenbass L, Hersche O, Miehlke W, Munzinger U. Failure of capsular enhanced short external rotator repair after total hip replacement. Clin Orthop Relat Res. 2004;(420):199-204.
34. Stähelin T, Vienne P, Hersche O. Failure of reinserted short external rotator muscles after total hip arthroplasty. J Arthroplasty. 2002;17(5):604-607.
35. Roche JJ, Jones CD, Khan RJ, Yates PJ. The surgical anatomy of the piriformis tendon, with particular reference to total hip replacement: a cadaver study. Bone Joint J. 2013;95-B(6):764-769.
36. Chimento GF, Pavone V, Sharrock N, Kahn B, Cahill J, Sculco TP. Minimally invasive total hip arthroplasty: a prospective randomized study. J Arthroplasty. 2005;20(2):139-144.
37. DiGioia AM 3rd, Plakseychuk AY, Levison TJ, Jaramaz B. Mini-incision technique for total hip arthroplasty with navigation. J Arthroplasty. 2003;18(2):123-128.
38. McKibbin B. Anatomical factors in the stability of the hip joint in the newborn. J Bone Joint Surg Br. 1970;52(1):148-159.
39. Dorr LD, Malik A, Dastane M, Wan Z. Combined anteversion technique for total hip arthroplasty. Clin Orthop Relat Res. 2009;467(1):119-127.
40. Yoshimine F. The safe-zones for combined cup and neck anteversions that fulfill the essential range of motion and their optimum combination in total hip replacements. J Biomech. 2006;39(7):1315-1323.

CHAPTER 15

The anterior approach in proximal femur medial fractures

Alberto Ricciardi*, Beatrice Ricciardi*, Alessandro Geraci**

*Department of Orthopaedics and Traumatology, Venice Hospital, ULSS 3 Serenissima/Veneto, Italy
**Department of Orthopaedics and Traumatology, San Valentino of Montebelluna Hospital, Treviso, ULSS 2 Marca Trevigiana/Veneto, Italy

Introduction

Femoral neck fractures are typical of the elderly patient. In fact, they can occur as a result of the peculiar anatomical conformation of the proximal femoral epiphysis, the ageing process and the consequent increased fragility of the bone (osteoporosis) or as a consequence of traumas in which the 'vis lesiva' is extremely scarce.
The task of the orthopaedic traumatologist is to restore the functionality of the coxofemoral joint as quickly as possible. This is to minimise immobility, + to patients who often suffering from cardiovascular disease, could lead to complications that are sometimes unresolvable and could quickly lead to death [1].
For this reason, in addition to early treatment [2], it is also advisable to use minimally invasive surgery that allows the joint to be exposed through small incisions without damaging the muscles that represent the motor of the hip.
Respect for the regional anatomy allows a post-operative phase characterised by almost no pain. This allows functional re-education to begin quickly. In this context, we are convinced that the treatment of femoral neck fractures in the elderly patient using the anterior surgical approach is the best possible solution. As early as the second day after surgery, if the general conditions are good, the patient is able to walk again with the aid of crutches.
In fact, this surgical approach not only allows the joint to be exposed through a small incision (about 8-10 cm), but it is the only truly anatomical approach. The surgeon accesses the hip joint with absolute respect for muscular and neurovascular structures.

Epidemiology

Femoral neck fractures in the elderly are an increasing disease and are considered one of the major causes of morbidity and mortality worldwide. These fractures are also becoming increasingly important in terms of healthcare-costs.
The close correlation between age and incidence is well documented, with some studies showing double the incidence rate for each year after the age of 50.
Currently in Italy there are about 55,000 fractures per year with an M:F ratio of 1:3. The rate doubles when adjusted for age group, with a downward trend in this ratio due to greater attention to osteoporotic pathologies in women than in men [3]. Women have a 4 times higher risk of fracture after the menopause [4].
Even belonging to one race rather than ano-

ther seems to favour the onset of osteoporosis: white and Asian women are more affected than African women [5]. In the United States, the majority of the population over the age of 50 has either very low bone density or marked osteoporosis [6]. In South America, the increase in the incidence of osteoporosis is also equalling European and US levels [7]. In our country, more than 55,000 femoral neck fractures occur annually due to bone fragility caused by osteoporosis, with a clear prevalence (72%) in women [8-9].
Such a high number of femur fractures can be considered as a real pandemic that, due to the ageing of the population (the over-65s in Italy represent 18.6% of the total population), is intended to increase further in the next few years. According to the latest estimates, it seems that in the next 40 years, without any targeted therapeutic measures on the population at risk, we will witness a doubling of the incidence of fragility fractures. In detail, according to current forecasts, the worldwide increase in the number of hip fractures in the coming decades is estimated at 6.5 million. Of these, 4.43 million will occur in Asia, Latin America, and the Middle East, while in the United States, considering the constant age-specific incidence, it is expected to increase from 238,000 cases in 1986 to 512,000 in 2040. In Japan, a doubling of fractures is even expected by 2025.
There are two main predisposing factors for femoral neck fractures in the elderly: an altered bone quality, hence bone strength (osteoporosis), and a higher incidence of fall injuries [10].

Classification of proximal femur fractures

These fractures are mostly characteristic of old age or senility, and are generally caused by an indirect mechanism, through minor trauma. The behaviour of the limb at the moment of impact is important, because it influences the occurrence of one type of fracture rather than another. The stresses are in fact transferred to areas of lower resistance of the bone tissue, made weaker by the presence of osteoporosis. In lower limb trauma, the reason why such a fracture occurs is basically because the lateral femoral cortex becomes thinner as you get closer to the epiphysis (figs. 1-2) [11].
Furthermore, in that area, since the trabeculae of the femoral neck are unidirectional, they represent a "locus minor resistant" to trauma.
This is determined by the particular anatomical structure of the femoral neck, which has a trabecular structure. Within this, three important trabecular systems of resistance can essentially distinguish. Between these systems, there is a triangular zone, known as Ward's zone, in which the skeletal structure is less resistant. The fragile area where fracture can occur is this [12]. These fractures are much more frequent in the elderly due to the concomitant presence of a reduction in mineral density and the number of trabeculae, characteristics of senile osteoporosis.
As regards to the vascularisation of the epiphysis it is necessary to consider that it derives essentially from the following arteries (fig. 3):

- the anterior circumflex artery which supplies the great trochanter and sends a branch to the femoral head. This runs in the anteroinferior part of the neck;
- the posterior circumflex artery which supplies the posterior part of the femoral epiphysis and the greater trochanter;
- the round ligament artery, that feeds the fovea region, runs in the round ligament and has a secondary role in the vascularisation of the head. This vessel is usually obliterated in old age [13].

The posterior superior retinacular arterial system provides the major blood supply to the epiphysis. These vessels pass through the femoral neck contained within the joint capsule and supply the lateral epiphyseal vessels at the junction of the femoral head and neck.
They penetrate the bone and supply the femoral epiphysis with blood. As the femoral epiphysis or neck separates from the femoral head, the femoral metaphysis dislocates superolaterally and the femur rotates externally. This causes distal stretching of the posterior-

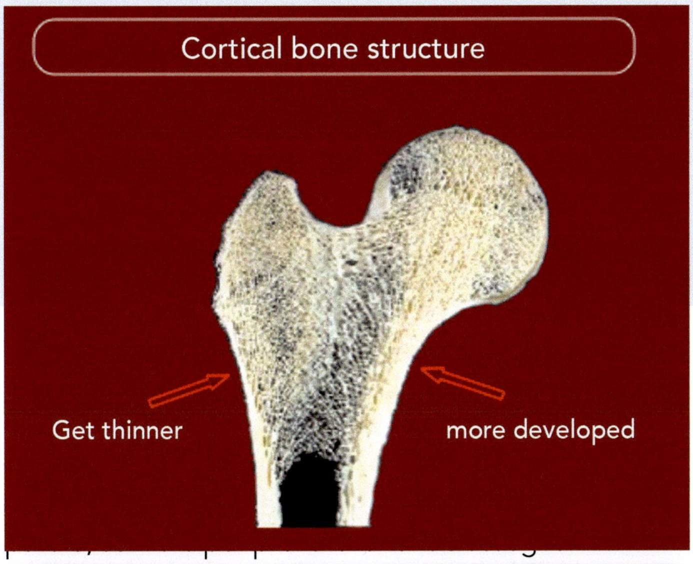

Figure 1
Cortical bone structure of the proximal femoral epiphysis

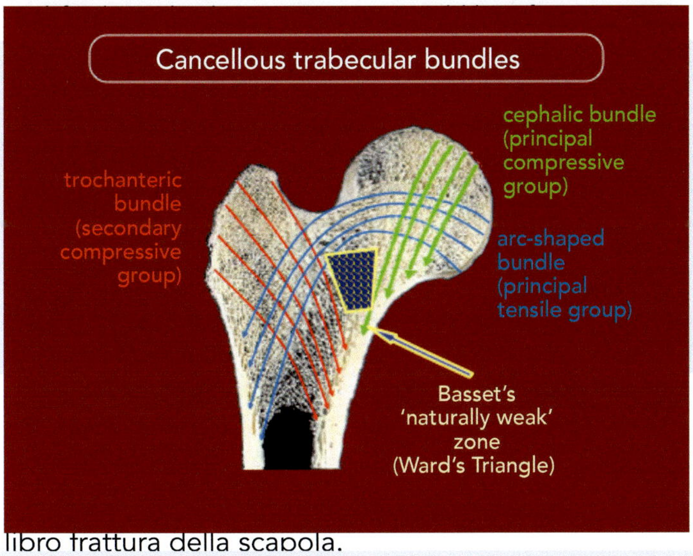

Figure 2
Spongy/cancellous trabecular structure of the femoral epiphysis

libro frattura della scapola.

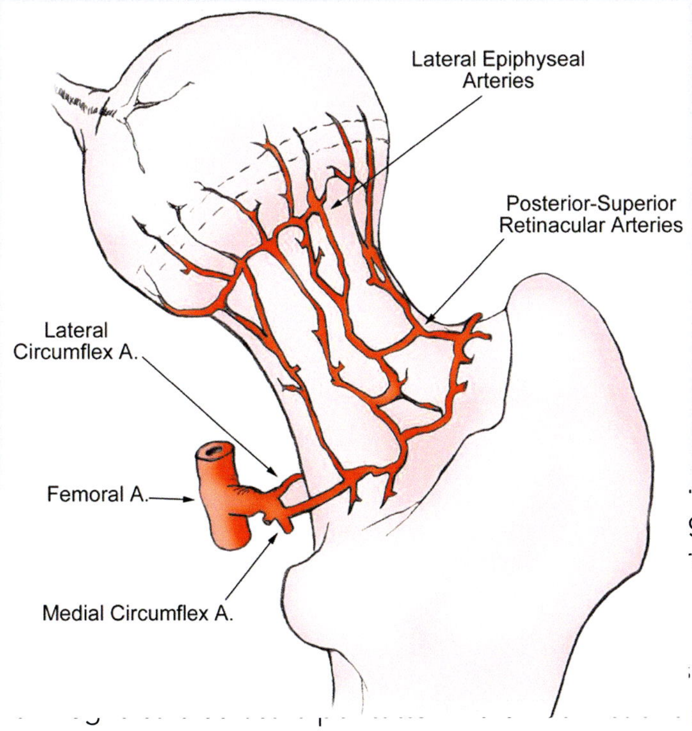

Figure 3
Visualization of the normal arterial supply of the femoral head from a posterior view. From: De Bac S. Radiologia ortopedica. Osteonecrosi asettica della testa del femore

gnare il foglio stile da usare per tutto il
attura della scapola.

stile da usare per tutto il libro frattura
capola libro scapola prova di testo ge-
parole, scrivere per provare la font e

superior retinacular arteries and proximal stretching of the lateral epiphyseal vessels. This is associated with a subsequent kinking or rotation of the lateral epiphyseal vessels, compromising the blood supply to the epiphysis. If these conditions persist, osteonecrosis may develop in the femoral head.
There are three main groups:
1. extracapsular lateral fractures, trochanteric and subtrochanteric (55%);
2. medial intracapsular fractures of the femoral neck (44%);
3. femoral head fractures (1%).
Medial fractures, due to this peculiar vascularisation, generally have a poor prognosis and, therefore, in the elderly patient (age >65 years) require replacement treatment (prosthesis).

Classification

Different classification systems for medial femoral neck fractures have been suggested. The system based on an anatomical classification divides femoral neck fractures into three regions: subcapital, the most frequent, transcervical and basicervical. Since the subcapital and transcervical regions are intracapsular, the fracture characteristics in these regions will be different from those in the basicervical region, which are extracapsular. Intracapsular fractures have a high risk of osteonecrosis, which is a much rarer complication in the case of an extracapsular basicervical fracture.
The classification system suggested by Pauwels is based on the angle of inclination of the fracture line (fig. 4) [14].
- Type I: fracture line inclined at 30° compared to the horizontal.
- Type II: fracture line inclined at 50° compared to the horizontal.
- Type III: fracture line inclined at 70° compared to the horizontal.

The most popular classification system for femoral neck fractures was introduced by Garden in 1961. Fractures are divided into four types based on the fracture displacement visible on antero-posterior radiographic examination (fig. 5) [15-16].
To complete, we also report the AO (Arbeitsgemeinschaft für Osteosynthesefragen) classification system [17] which gathers these fractures in group 31B. The 31 indicates fractures of the proximal end of the femur and the B the femoral neck subgroup. Continuing with the AO classification, B1 fractures are subcapital fractures with moderate displacement, B2 are transcervical fractures and B3 are displaced subcapital

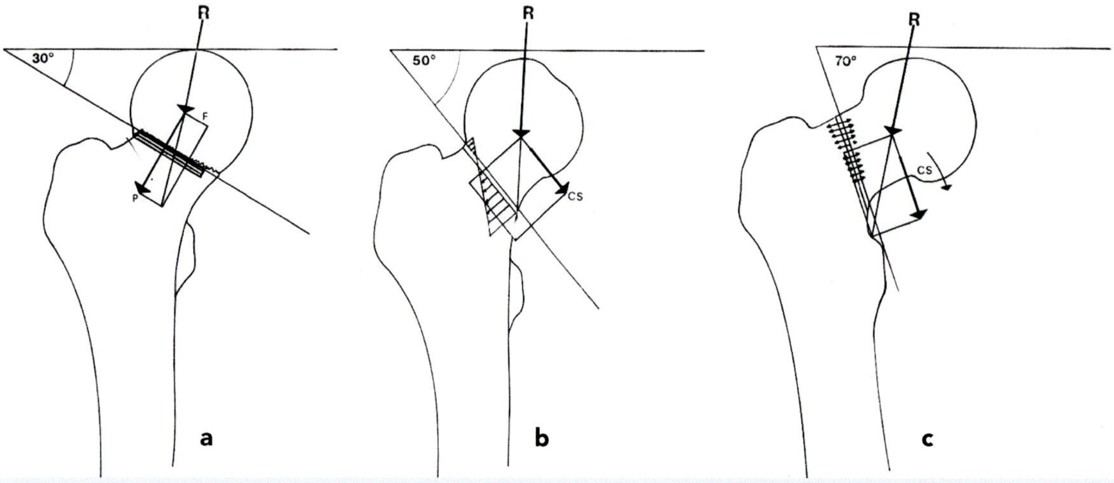

Figure 4 Pauwels' scheme: a) when the fracture forms an angle of less than 30° it is stable because uniform compression is exerted on the fracture plane of the neck; b) when the angle is between 30° and 50° the pressure forces move towards the internal side of the femoral neck. Shear forces appear which tend to rotate the femoral head (cs); c) for an angle greater than 70° the shear forces increase. At the same time, some forces come into action and tend to bring the femoral neck into varus, displacing the fracture surfaces of the upper part of the neck. (Ricad R. and Molè L.).
From: Gui L. Fratture e lussazioni. Aulo Gaggi Editore. Bologna 1973, Vol IV.

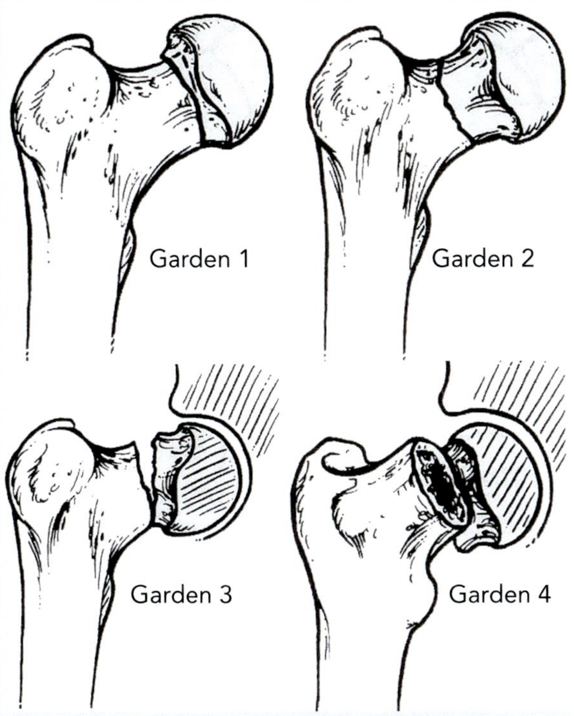

Figure 5
Garden femoral neck fracture classification system

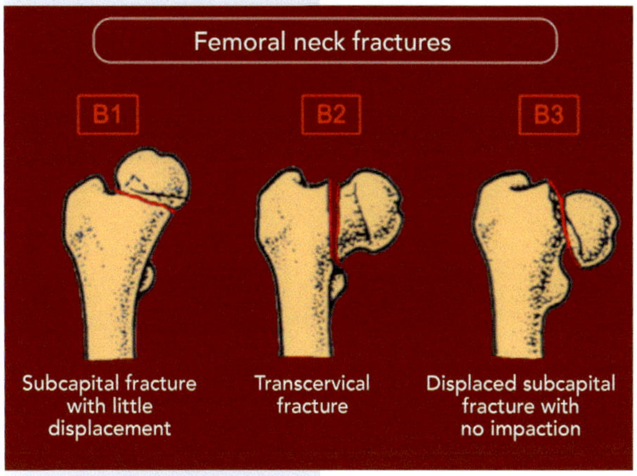

Figure 6 AO classification system for femoral neck fractures

fractures. Further subgroups describe in detail the type of fracture and the displacement severity (fig. 6).

The anterior approach in femoral neck fracture treatment

Proximal medial femur fractures in patients over 65 are treated with prosthetic replacement of the injured joint. Over the years there has been an evolution of prosthetic implants in terms of design and biomaterials, while the surgical approaches have basically remained those described long ago in the literature.
The orthopaedic surgeon must focus on techniques that lead to an early functional recovery. This is also in compliance with the Ministry of Health guidelines that oblige the surgeon to treat these fractures within 48 hours of admission to hospital.
For this reason, it is essential to rigorously spare the peri-articular tissues during surgery, thus avoiding excessive blood loss during the operation and in the recovery period.
Therefore, minimally invasive hip surgery (MIS) has become increasingly popular.
The concept of minimally invasive surgery is linked not only to soft tissue preservation (skin, muscles, vessels and nerves) but also to bone conservation. Currently, there are minimally invasive prosthetic models that permit minimal use of bone stock.
Although there is no universally accepted definition of a 'minimally invasive surgical approach', the aim remains clear: to minimise tissue trauma in order to shorten the recovery period, enable fast functional recovery and minimise hospitalisation time.
Reducing hospitalisation time is important not only to reduce healthcare costs but also to prevent that a prolonged time in hospital could result in a rapid psychophysical decline of the elderly patient.
The surgical technique we use is based on the so-called modified Hueter anterior approach. Before implanting the final femoral component, the reduction of the trial implant is obviously carried out. Then the stability, mobility and length tests are done,

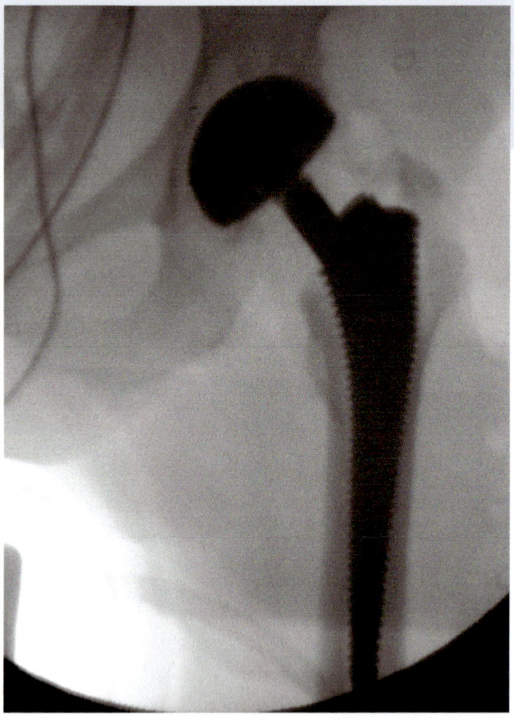

Figure 7
Fluoroscopic evaluation

and finally the radiographic assessment (fig. 7). Once the test results are satisfactory, the implantation of the definitive components can proceed. When the implantation is completed, the joint stability and limb length are tested again.

Type of prosthesis: partial or total, cemented or uncemented

Considering healthcare costs, the most logical criteria to follow when choosing which prosthesis to implant, partial or total, would probably be the chronological one.
One could therefore indicate 65 as the discriminating age below which the surgeon should implant a total prosthesis and above that a partial prosthesis.
However, in our opinion, biological age is undoubtedly the most appropriate criteria. This is because it is now common to encounter patients over seventy who are still active not only in everyday life but also in sports.
These patients therefore deserve a total implant that allows them to maintain their quality of life.
Initially, even with a partial prosthesis, the patient is able to carry out all daily life activities and many sports. However, we believe that, in the long term, the stress produced by the implant on the cup leads to inflammation of the acetabulum (cotyloiditis) with clinical symptoms of pain and functional limitation.
In addition, if the patient continues to stress the implant, the cup itself degenerates.
A revision surgery would then become necessary. Therefore, the choice of a prosthesis based purely on chronological criteria would also be wrong in terms of healthcare costs.
Currently, for the 'replacement' in medial femoral neck fractures, orthopaedic surgeons have at their disposal prostheses that can be divided into the following categories (fig. 8).

- Bi-articular prosthesis: a system consisting of three components, stem (cemented or uncemented), head and movable liner. The stem and head (metal or ceramic) are those of normal total prosthesis. The movable liner consists of a polyethylene cap with a metal coating. Therefore, there are two levels of mobility: between the head and the polyethylene and between the metal cup and the acetabular bone.
- Total hip prosthesis: a system that completely replaces the hip joint, consisting of a medullary stem (cemented or uncemented) and a head that articulates with the aceta-

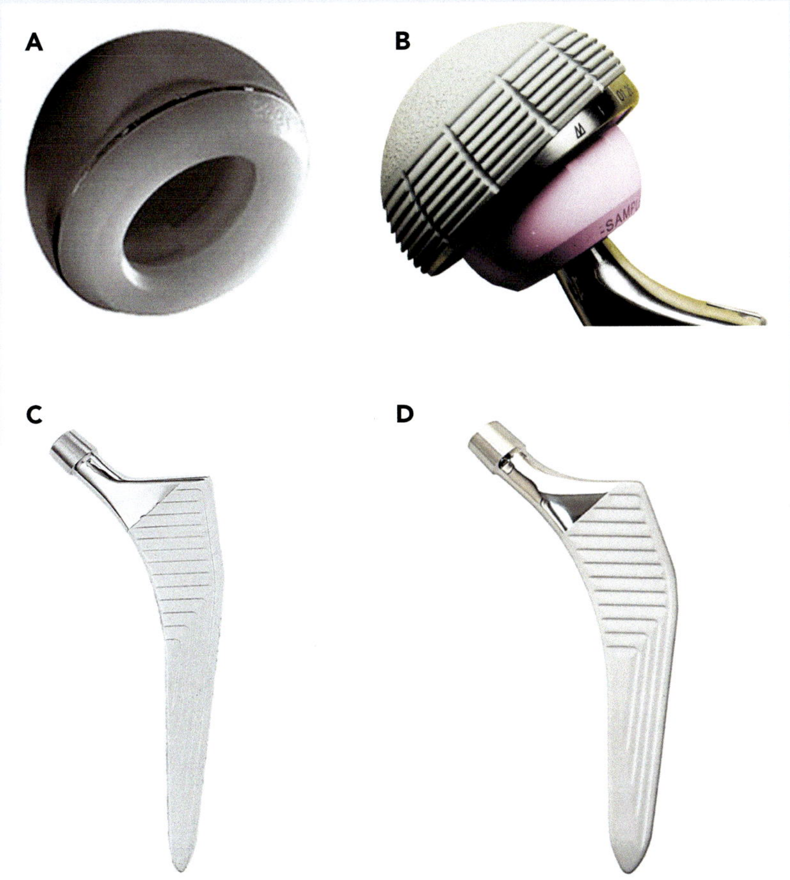

Figure 8 A) Biarticular/ Dual Mobility cup. B) Total hip prosthesis. C) Quadra femoral stem. D) AMIStem femoral stem. Courtesy of Medacta International SA

bular component integral with the pelvis.
Normally, press-fit cups and uncemented stems [18] are used, cement is used only when the bone quality is very poor.

Personal case history Materials and methods

Between March 2009 and September 2013, 369 hip replacements using the AMIS technique were performed on our department in patients with femoral neck fracture. The patients were divided into two groups (Group A and Group B). Group A consisted of 236 patients (137 females and 99 males) with a mean age of 86 years (range 80-95). Group B consisted of 133 patients (87 females and 46 males) with a mean age of 66 years (range 54-78) (tab. 1).
The inclusive criteria were a femoral neck fracture type 2,3,4 of the Garden classification. No exclusion criteria were used. Uncemented prosthetic implants were used on all patients. In group A a PHA (partial hip arthroplasty) was implanted, in group B a THA (total hip arthroplasty). The surgical approach was the same on all patients: The Hueter approach. All procedures were performed by the same surgeon. The patients were placed in supine decubitus on an 'OPT 80' orthopaedic table from Trento Factory with the aid of the 'AMIS Mobile Leg Positioner' positioning device. The table allows the extension, rotation and traction of the lower limb to be operated on, allowing easy access to the femoral diaphysis for implantation of the stem. The skin incision is made approximately 2 cm inferiorly and 2 cm laterally to the anterior-superior iliac spine and extended distally for 8-10 cm parallel to an imaginary line between the anterior-superior iliac spine and the head of the fibula. Radioscopy is used during surgery to guide component placement during both PHA and THA procedures.
The same post-operative protocol was used for all patients. The therapeutic protocol included 'short' antibiotic prophylaxis (2 g of

Table 1 Distribution of patients who underwent prosthetic surgery using the AMIS technique

	Group A	Group B
	PHA	**THA**
Mean age	86 years	66 years
Women	137	87
Men	99	46
Total	**236**	**133**

Cefazolin half an hour before surgery) and antithrombotic prophylaxis with low-molecular-weight heparin until weight-bearing gait was resumed. Analgesia was provided through the application of a slow-release system (supervised by the anaesthesiologist) without parenteral narcotics. The surgical drain was removed on the second post-operative day by the doctor on duty. Rehabilitation treatment started on the second day. Patients were transferred to the rehabilitation ward in our hospital after seven days (+/two days) or to the long-term care ward after 10 days (+/ three), and received the same standardised rehabilitation treatment. The average length of hospital stay was four weeks (+/-one week) During their stay, patients had 30 minutes of physiotherapy treatment per day.

The main objectives of rehabilitation were to improve joint mobility and recover muscle strength to allow a rapid return to normal daily activities. Patients were encouraged to walk without any aid as soon as possible. The evaluation included the following parameters: duration of surgery, intra-operative complications, blood loss, post-operative pain, duration of hospitalisation. A clinical follow-up was performed at 1, 3 and 6 months after surgery and data such as pain, function of the new joint, general health status, blood transfusions performed, complications and residual joint crackling were recorded. The level of hip pain was assessed using the visual analogue scale (VAS) 0-10. Specific hip joint function data were analysed using the Harris Hip Score (HHS) and the WOMAC index. The radiographic positioning of the implant was also assessed by examining the cup (inclination, anteversion), stem (centrality in the diaphyseal canal), any dysmetria and the off-set.

Results

The average duration of surgery for a partial hip replacement was 41 minutes (30 to 55 minutes). The average duration of surgery for group B was 62 minutes (51 to 106 minutes). Intra-operative complications were two intertrochanteric fractures and one subtrochanteric fracture in group A, three intertrochanteric fractures in group B. These fractures were all stabilised with a cerclage or a plate. Haemoglobin values were recorded on the first and third post-operative days and compared with preoperative values: 151 patients in group A and 96 in group B required a blood transfusion.

There were 10 superficial infections in group A and 4 in group B. All infections regressed within three months after adequate antibiotic therapy. In three patients we observed a sensory deficit in the lateral region of the thigh (hypoesthesia and dysesthesia): 1 case in group B and 2 cases in group A. These were probably due to a stretch of the lateral femoral cutaneous nerve during surgery. All three cases resolved 6 months after surgery.

There were also 6 cases of haematoma in the different groups that were treated by incision and drainage (4 in group A and 2 in group B). There were three cases of dislocation, in group B only. Two of these were resolved by closed reduction and application of a pelvic brace, and only one required revision surgery and the replacement of the pelvic component.

The VAS, HHS, and WOMAC scales were used to assess outcomes during the follow-up period. Pain levels from the VAS assessment were lower in patients treated with PHT. The HHS and WOMAC values were better overall

Table 2 Clinical results in the two groups

Group A (PHA)	After 1 months	After 3 months	After 6 months
VAS	5	3	3
HHS	61	71	77
WOMAC	62	51	37

Group B (THA)	After 1 months	After 3 months	After 6 months
VAS	5	3	2
HHS	66	78	87
WOMAC	60	46	25

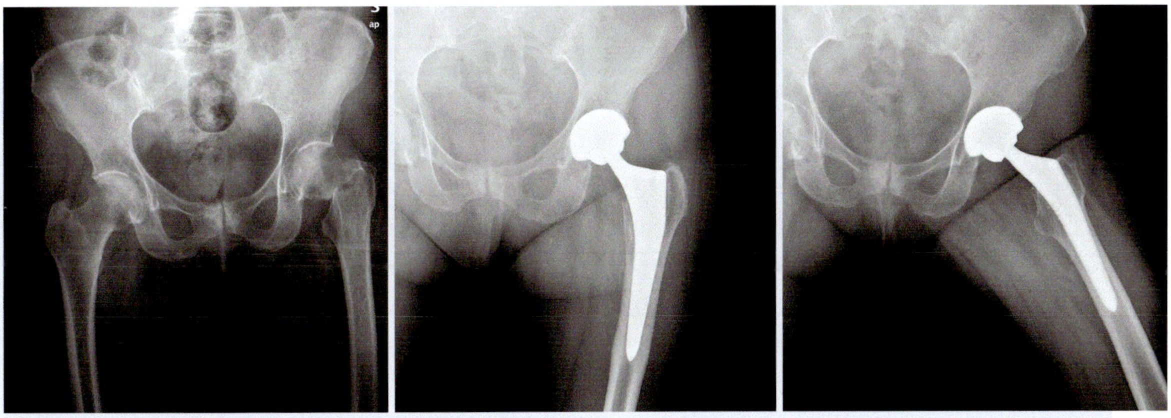

Figure 9 75-year-old female. Total hip arthroplasty, two-year post-operative follow-up

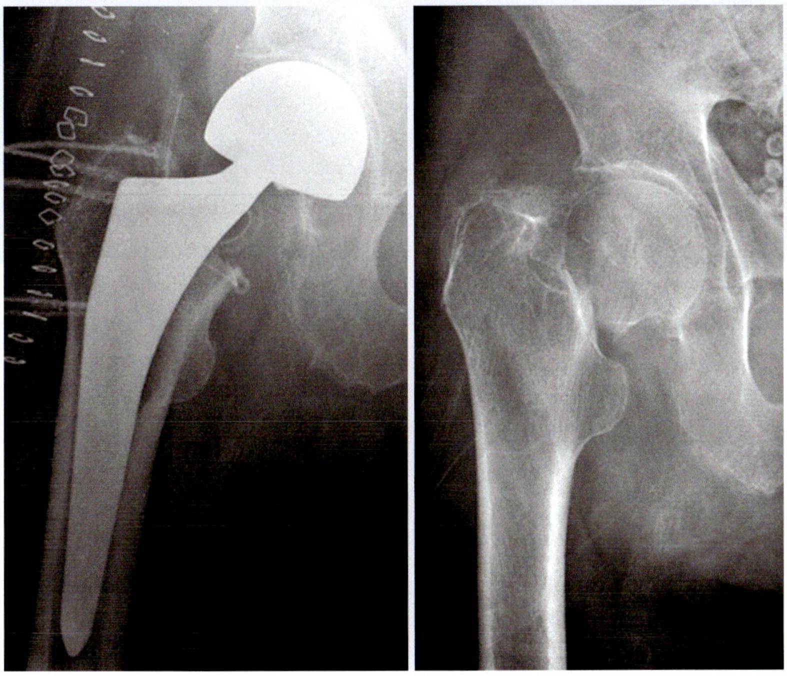

Figure 10
83-year-old male. Biarticular partial hip arthroplasty, post-operative follow-up

in group B (tab. 2). In patients treated with THA we found a wider ROM (Range Of Motion), especially for internal and external rotation movements of the hip, and a better quality of the movement (figs. 9-10).

Complications

Regarding the most critical complications of prosthetic surgery, infections and thromboembolism, the data currently in our possession show that there are no substantial differences with other surgical procedures.
Among the complications of the surgical site, in our experience we report three cases of prosthesis dislocation.
This is a small number compared with the total number of operated patients, and all occurred at the beginning of the learning curve. This observation is consistent with the current literature [19]. Matta et al. [20] reported a dislocation rate of 0.61% in their study with more than 4000 patients. A study by Restrepo [21] showed only 4 dislocations out of 2386 patients treated with total joint replacement (0.15%). Jewett et al. [22] reported 0.9%. In our experience the percentage is 0.3%.
Many authors attach great importance to the positioning of the cup for the stability of the prosthesis. They acknowledge a 'safety zone' consisting of 10-20° of anteversion and 40+10° of inclination. Respecting this safety zone would greatly reduce the risk of dislocation [23].
Anterior approach facilitates the fulfilment of these safety indices. Having the patient in the supine position and the excellent visualisation of the acetabulum, allows the surgeon to have a better reference in positioning the cup.
Hip replacement surgery can have complications affecting the peripheral nervous system. The incidence of injury to a peripheral nerve during a first replacement surgery varies between 0 and 3% [24].
Generally speaking, the cause of nerve injury can be found in direct trauma, tension, ischaemia, thermal damage from cement polymerisation, electrocautery or compression from haematoma. However, 40% of cases are unexplained [25].
The direct anterior approach may put the lateral femoral cutaneous nerve [26] and the femoral nerve at a higher risk of injury than the lateral and postero-lateral approaches. Injury, 'stupor', of the femoral nerve after the anterior approach has also been mentioned by other authors.
In this regard, we believe that one of the causes of this temporary impairment may be the action of the Hohmann retractor. Specifically, the one positioned anteriorly on the acetabular rim below the iliopsoas muscle can act by compressing the femoral nerve against the fascial structures. Another cause may be excessive traction of the limb during implant reduction movements.
Fortunately, femoral nerve injury seems to have a good prognosis and usually resolves completely within a few months.
In our experience, we have seen four cases of femoral nerve stupor that resolved completely within six months of surgery.
Another potential intraoperative complication is periprosthetic fractures. These can occur in the femur or the acetabulum, but most affect the femoral segment. In cemented implants, the incidence of fractures ranges from 0.1 to 3.2%, whereas in cementless implants the incidence is much higher, ranging from 4.1 to 27% (fig. 11).
Femoral fractures are caused by the excessive mechanical stress on the bone exerted by the rasps during the preparation of the canal and in particular during the introduction of the femoral stem. They can be favoured by general predisposition factors, such as poor bone quality or pre-existing alterations in the femur anatomy. Usually the fracture affects the proximal third of the femur, more rarely the middle or distal third [27].
In many cases, the fracture is not detected during surgery because it is minimal and hardly visible on radiographic examination. Schwartz et al. in a study of 1318 uncemented hip replacements found 39 femur fractures, of which only half were diagnosed during surgery.

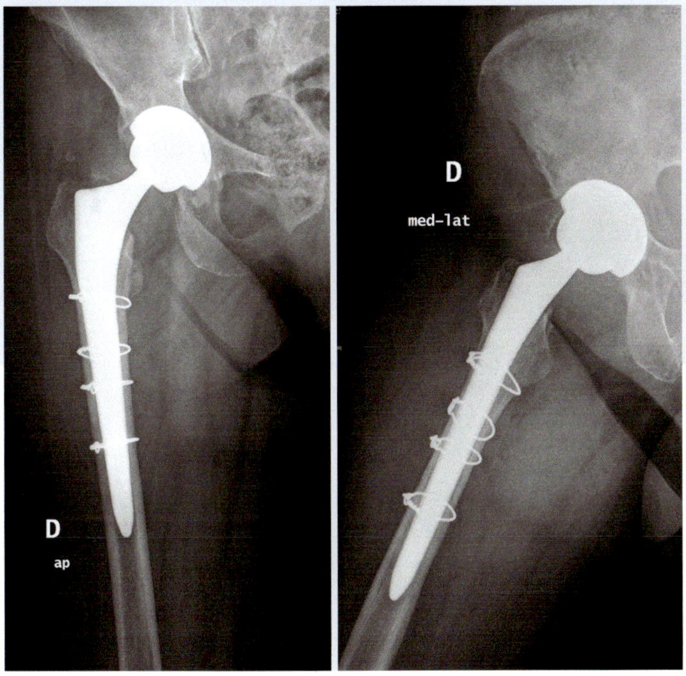

Figure 11
Intraoperative fracture: cerclage and long revision stem

Through the anterior approach, a fracture of the femoral diaphysis is usually the direct result of external rotation torsion. If the fracture is extended and the prosthesis is not stable, it is advisable to replace the prosthetic stem with a longer implant that exceeds the fracture point distally.
In order to minimise this risk, the external rotation, extension and adduction movements of the hip must be carried out with extreme caution and attention, reducing traction to minimum.
Nevertheless, if a femoral fracture does occur, it can be reduced and stabilised by widening the incision distally and laterally. This allows the femoral diaphysis to be exposed without causing injury to the quadriceps femoris muscle when performing the osteosynthesis (cerclage/plate).
The minimally invasive nature, as already mentioned, offers a statistically significant reduction in blood loss, as also shown in studies by Wentz et al. [28], Goldstein et al. [29] and Chimento et al. [30].
Many authors consider obesity an absolute contraindication. On the contrary, we consider the anterior approach to be the preferred choice in obese patients.
This is because the anterior approach allows easy access to the joint due to the partial or complete absence of adipose tissue in that particular region (below the ASIS in the upper quarter of the thigh). Below we report one of the cases operated in our Operating Ward (fig. 12).
In our opinion, a relative contraindication is represented by the patient with large muscle masses. In these cases, it is advisable to perform a larger skin incision (about 15 cm) to be able to spread the muscles more easily and without damaging them (figs. 13-14).

Conclusions

The hip joint can be approached anteriorly, laterally and postero-laterally. The advantages and disadvantages of each surgical approach have been well documented in the literature and the choice depends largely on the surgeon's training.
The anterior approach is internervous and does not include dissection of muscles or tendons. The lateral approach involves de-

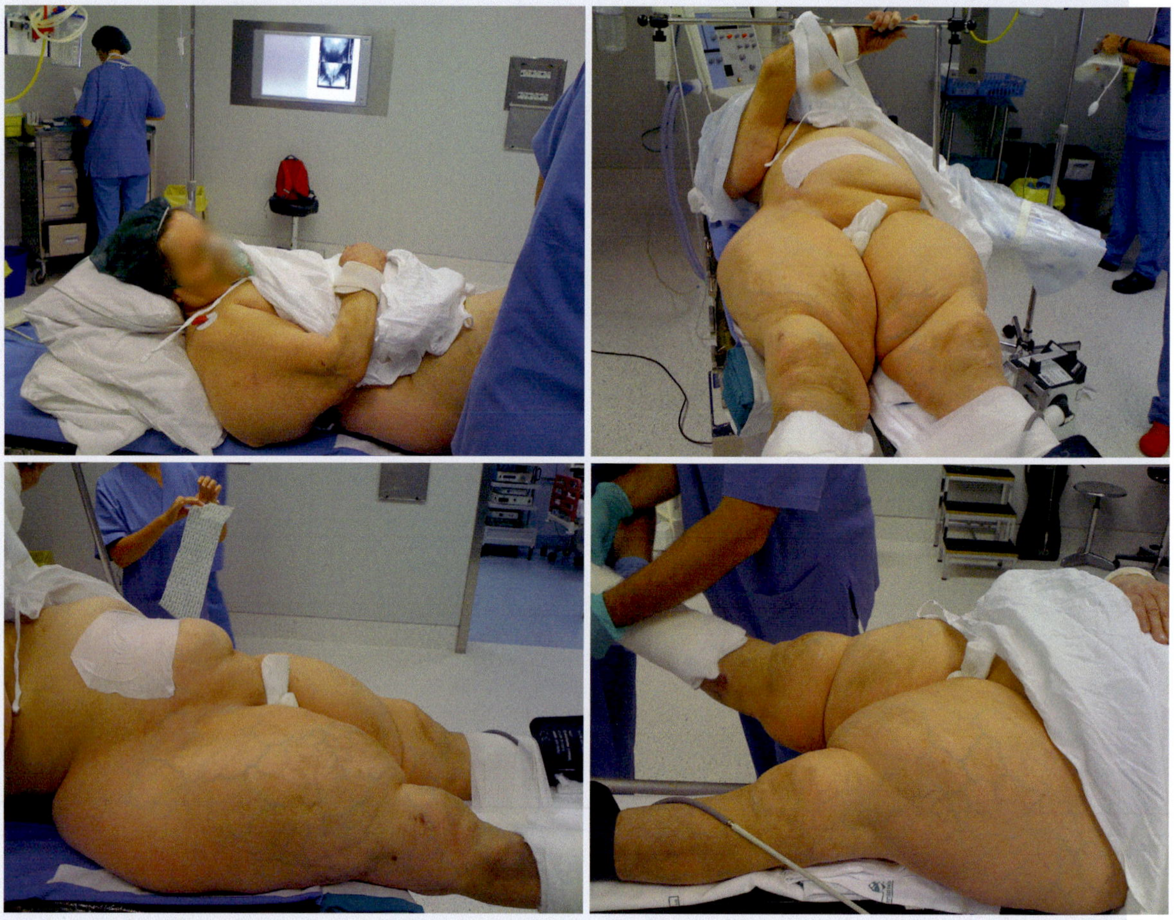

Figure 12 52-year-old female, bilateral femoral head necrosis

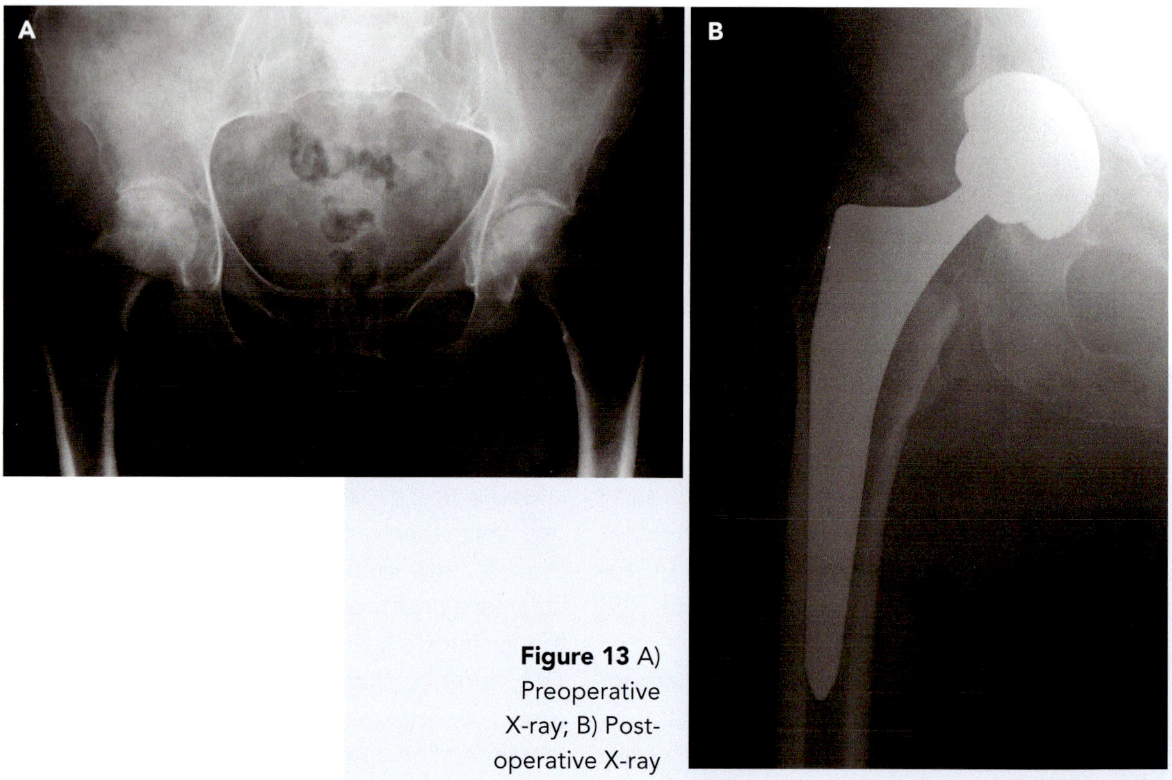

Figure 13 A) Preoperative X-ray; B) Post-operative X-ray

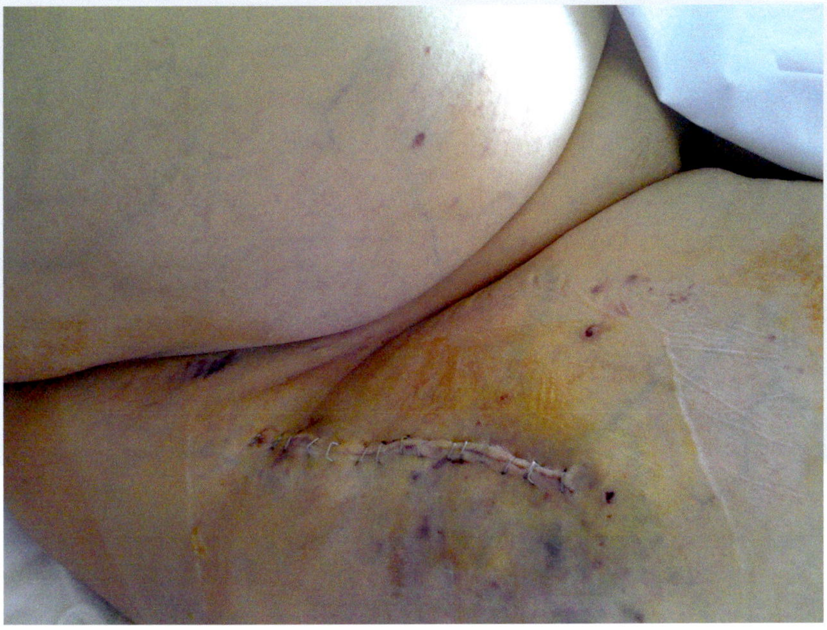

Figure 14
Surgical skin scar

taching the gluteus medius and gluteus minimus muscle from the greater trochanter. In the posterior approach, the rotator muscles are detached.
The AMIS (Anterior Minimally Invasive Surgery) technique has therefore become widely adopted as it allows the surgeon to position the prosthetic components while respecting the periarticular tissues (muscles - vessels – nerves) [31].
The possibility of using minimally invasive approach has also been favoured for the development of new instrumentation 'dedicated' to this approach (self-retaining retractors, Hohmann levers with specially created curves) as well as new prosthetic designs, in particular short, curved and with a meta-diaphyseal grip stems.
In this regard, we consider the Medacta AMIS Mobile Leg Positioner positioning device to be fundamental, which allows to manage the lower limb with simple manoeuvres and with a minimum effort for the surgical team.
In fact, this device allows, once the osteotomy of the femoral neck has been performed, to expose the femoral meta-diaphysis through a movement of external rotation, extension and adduction of the hip with a minimum traction of the limb itself.
It is important to emphasise, that in our experience the device is not used to pull the limb but only to perform those movements described above which are sufficient to expose the femoral canal. Traction on the limb should be minimal. The surgeon accompanies and promotes the exposure by performing a periarticular lysis of the pubo-ilio-femoral ligaments. In this way it is possible to use the minimally invasive anterior approach in complete safety.
The practical advantages of the anterior approach can be seen in the immediate post-operative functional recovery due to the partial or complete absence of pain, in the absolute respect for the anatomy of the region and in the reduced blood loss. The excellent exposure of the acetabulum also allows the surgeon to perfectly position the cup component according to the anatomical axes (inclination and anteversion), thus eliminating the risk of prosthesis dislocation [32].
In our experience, most patients are able to regain full weight bearing as early as the second post-operative day. Furthermore, depending on their age and general condition, they can be off crutches as early as a few

days after surgery [33].

Finally, we believe that the anterior approach completely fulfils the fundamental characteristics of a surgical approach:

1) allow easy access to the affected district;

2) respect the anatomical structures whose correct functioning will be essential for the success of the implant;

3) offer the best possible view of the operating field;

4) allow additional procedures such as augmentation, osteotomy and osteosynthesis;

5) be aesthetically acceptable.

Bibliography

1. Raaymakers EL. Fractures of the femoral neck: a review and personal statement. Acta Chir Orthop Traumatol Cech. 2006;73(1):45-59.
2. Hagino T, Maekawa S, Sato E, Bando K, Hamada Y. Prognosis of proximal femoral fracture in patients aged 90 years and older. J Orthop Surg (Hong Kong). 2006;14(2):122-126.
3. Marinoni EG, Cossio A, Rossi A. Le fratture mediali del collo del femore nell'anziano. In: Marinoni EC, De Nicola U. Osteoporosi: le nuove prospettive in ortopedia e traumatologia, Springer Milan, 2006;75-88.
4. Cheng H, Gary LC, Curtis JR, et al. Estimated prevalence and patterns of presumed osteoporosis among older Americans based on Medicare data. Osteoporos Int. 2009;20(9):1507-1515.
5. Bohannon AD. Osteoporosis and African American women. J Womens Health Gend Based Med. 1999;8(5):609-615.
6. Bone Health & Osteoporosis Foundation (BHOF) https://www.bonehealthandosteoporosis.org (formerly NOF, the National Osteoporosis Foundation).
7. Riera-Espinoza G, Epidemiology of osteoporosis in Latin America, Salud Publica Mex. 2008.
8. Dati SDO 2006 ISS.
9. Tarantino U, Resmini G. La gestione delle fratture da fragilità. Raccomandazioni per chirurghi ortopedici. Springer, 2011.
10. Dolinak D. Review of the significance of various low force fractures in the elderly. Am J Forensic Med Pathol. 2008;29(2):99-105.
11. Gui L. Fratture e lussazioni. Aulo Gaggi Editore, Bologna 1973, Vol. IV.
12. De Bac S. Radiologia ortopedica. Osteonecrosi asettica della testa del femore, 2012.
13. Pauwels S. Biomechanics of the normal and diseased hip. Springer, Berlin, Heidelberg, 1976.
14. Garden RS. Low-angle fixation in fractures of the femoral neck. J Bone Joint Surg Br 1961,43;647-663.
15. Garden RS. Stability and union in subcapital fractures of the femur. J Bone Joint Surg Br 1964, 43;630-647.
16. Muller ME, Nazarian S, et al. The AO classification of fractures of long bone. Springer, 1990.
17. Gierer P, Landes J, Grubwinkler M, Gradl G, Lob G, Andress HJ. The femoral neck fracture in the elderly patient - cemented or cementless hip arthroplasty? Zentralbl Chir. 2002;127(6):514-518.
18. Siguier T, Siguier M, Brumpt B. Mini-incision anterior approach does not increase dislocation rate: a study of 1037 total hip replacements. Clin Orthop Relat Res. 2004;(426):164-173.
19. Matta JM, Shahrdar C, Ferguson T. Single-incision anterior approach for total hip arthroplasty on an orthopaedic table. Clin Orthop Relat Res. 2005;441:115-124.
20. Restrepo C, Mortazavi SM, Brothers J, Parvizi J, Rothman RH. Hip dislocation: are hip precautions necessary in anterior approaches?. Clin Orthop Relat Res. 2011;469(2):417-422.
21. Jewett BA, Collis DK. High complication rate with anterior total hip arthroplasties on a fracture table. Clin Orthop Relat Res. 2011;469(2):503-507.
22. Hassan DM, Johnston GH, Dust WN, Watson G, Dolovich AT. Accuracy of intraoperative assessment of acetabular prosthesis placement. J Arthroplasty. 1998;13(1):80-84.
23. Rossi P, Salvi V, Sibelli P, Boux E. Le complicanze neuro vascolari. GIOT 1996, 22 (Suppl 1):1129-1135.
24. Sunderland S. Nerves and nerve injuries. Churchill Livingstone, London, 1978, 155-155.
25. Bhargava T, Goytia RN, Jones LC, Hungerford MW. Lateral femoral cutaneous nerve impairment after direct anterior approach for total hip arthroplasty. Orthopedics. 2010;33(7):472.
26. Toni A, Ciaroni D, Sudanese A, et al. Incidence of intraoperative femoral fracture. Straight-stemmed versus anatomic cementless total hip arthroplasty. Acta Orthop Belg. 1994;60(1):43-54.

27. Wenz JF, Gurkan I, Jibodh SR. Mini-incision total hip arthroplasty: a comparative assessment of perioperative outcomes. Orthopedics. 2002;25(10):1031-1043.
28. Goldstein WM, Branson JJ, Berland KA, Gordon AC. Minimal-incision total hip arthroplasty, J Bone Joint Surg Arm, 2003;85-A(Suppl 4):33-8.
29. Chimento GF, Pavone V, Sharrock N, Kahn B, Cahill J, Sculco TP. Minimally invasive total hip arthroplasty: a prospective randomized study. J Arthroplasty. 2005;20(2):139-144.
30. Dora C, Kalberer F. Muscular damage after total hip arthroplasty: conventional versus minimally invasive anterior approach. AOA 2008, Australia, Hobart.
31. Siguier T, Siguier M, Brumpt B. Mini-incision anterior approach does not increase dislocation rate: a study of 1037 total hip replacements. Clin Orthop Relat Res. 2004;(426):164-173.
32. Berger RA, Jacobs JJ, Meneghini RM, Della Valle C, Paprosky W, Rosenberg AG. Rapid rehabilitation and recovery with minimally invasive total hip arthroplasty. Clin Orthop Relat Res. 2004;(429):239-247.
33. Franchin F. La protesi d'anca di primo impianto. Springer-Verlag, 2003.

CHAPTER 16

Hip replacement using the minimally invasive anterior technique. Our experience

Sergio Candiotto*, Stefano Concheri**, Vittore Costa***, Antonio Camporese*, Salvatore Gravinese*, Jacopo Tagliapietra*, Alberto Procura*, Matteo Cengarle*, Giulio Edoardo Vigni***

*Hip and Shoulder Surgery Unit, Abano Terme General Hospital, Padua, Italy
**Department of Orthopaedics and Traumatology, S. Antonio Hospital, Padua, Italy
***Hip and Prosthetic Surgery Unit, Humanitas Gavazzeni Hospital, Bergamo, Italy
****Department of Orthopaedics and Traumatology, University of Palermo, Italy

Introduction

The use of minimally invasive surgical techniques, in the broader context of the modern 'philosophy' of tissue sparing surgery, has attracted increasing interest and widespread use in general clinical practice in recent years. Orthopaedic surgery has been no exception to this. Numerous surgeons have in fact progressively changed their therapeutic orientation, using minimally invasive techniques in the various fields of modern orthopaedic and trauma surgery (arthroscopy, MIPO, etc.). Still relatively important, however, is the dissent towards mini-invasiveness in prosthetic surgery in general and in hip surgery in particular.

The push towards minimally invasive surgery was not, however, supported by 'aesthetic' motives (fig. 1), as it might seem to a superficial and simplifying analysis. Rather, the real motivations were the observation of improved clinical outcomes and reduced complications compared with traditional surgical procedures.

The increasingly recognised and appreciated advantages are: shorter operation time, reduced blood loss and transfusion requirements, easier post-operative pain control, shorter length of hospital stay, easier functional recovery, faster return to high activity levels, reduced complication rate, and lower overall economic cost.

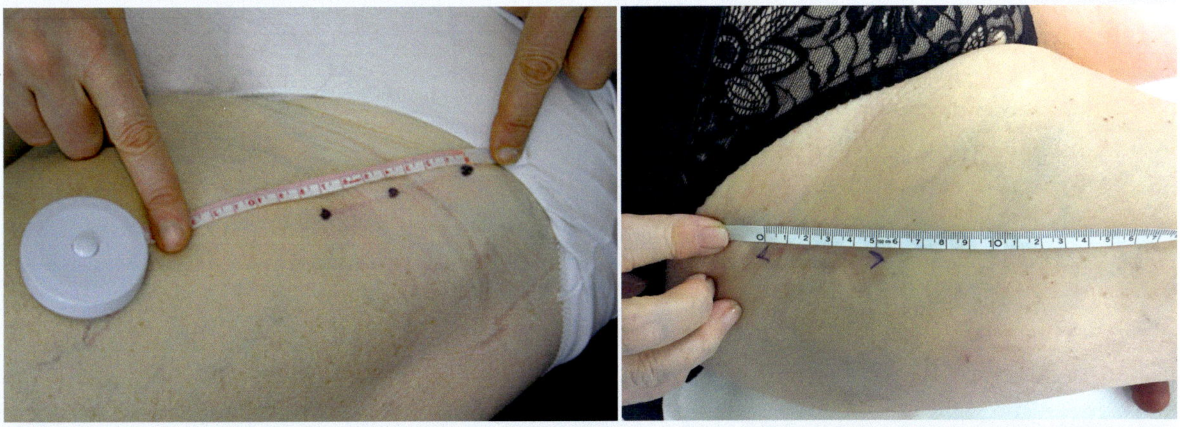

Figure 1 Example of surgical scars after hip replacement surgery performed using the minimally invasive anterior technique

However, certain aspects of surgical pathophysiology, more recently identified and appreciated, make the advantage of minimally invasive techniques even more convincing. Particular attention is nowadays paid to the problems of the so-called enzymatic-metabolic 'signalling' associated with tissue damage, which is always variably produced by the surgical act. These are true biochemical alterations in intercellular communication and direct expressions of surgical damage and stress.

This metabolic imbalance turns out to be closely related to the 'weight' and 'duration' of the surgical act and to the extent of tissue damage (particularly of muscle tissue). It reflects on the entire organism with significant immunohistochemical and metabolic changes (increase in catabolic hormones and reduction in anabolic ones, increase in thromboplastin-like factors with alterations in the haemostatic balance in a pro-thrombotic direction, loss of muscle tissue with increase in CPK and free myoglobin, relative immunodepression, adrenal hyperactivity with increase in catecholamines, glycocorticoids and blood glucose, increase in cardiac work).

In this respect, it is of particular interest to be able to minimise muscle damage by choosing operating techniques that do not require either detaching or incising muscles. This advantage, combined with less bleeding (reduced damage, facilitation of haemostasis, reduced duration of the operation, volumetric reduction of the 'surgical dead space', etc.), reduces the deleterious immunohistochemical network produced by the surgical act.

Muscle and blood necrobiotic degradation factors and the amount of thromboplastin-like factors are thus advantageously reduced in minimally invasive surgical techniques and are now the cornerstones of modern surgical approaches. More recent studies even tend to detect favourable variations in the chemical factors of inflammation. These are expressed by lower values of IL6, IL8 and TNF alpha, which also potentially correlate with the degree of tissue damage, especially muscle damage.

However, the steepness of the learning curve, which involves even the most experienced surgeons, and the significant incidence of complications in the early stages of surgical training must be acknowledged and adequately illustrated.

Our experience

Our experience with anterior minimally invasive approach hip replacement surgery began in 2005, without the use of a traction device. The first 47 cases were in fact performed with the 'free hand' technique. This phase, however, allowed us to experience a certain difficulty in performing the operation in a significant number of patients. The difficulties were mainly encountered in the presence of coxofemoral dysmorphism (coxa vara, protrusio acetabuli, dysplasia), joint stiffness or relevant muscle masses or obesity.

This experience later led us to prefer the use of the limb positioning-traction device, as we were able to quickly appreciate its great advantages, even though it required an important learning phase for its correct and safe use (fig. 2) (A-leg positioner/Medacta; B-Apon-Gar/Zimmer; C-Hana/Mizuho-OSI/Lima).

In particular, the traction in the neutral position of the limb (during cervical femoral osteotomy and femoral head extraction) and the fundamental combined movement of extension and external rotation of the limb associated with the automatic release of traction (during the subsequent femoral prosthetic preparation and implantation) constitute the valuable contribution made by the traction apparatus. This is now an indispensable benefit for us.

Over time, the choice towards the minimally invasive technique has progressively increased. Today, approximately 98% of patients in our department undergo hip replacement surgery using the minimally invasive anterior approach. As experience has grown and we have become more aware of the advantages (and limitations) of the technique, we have been able to adopt it on an increasing number of patients. Today, we are able to treat even the most complex and difficult patients

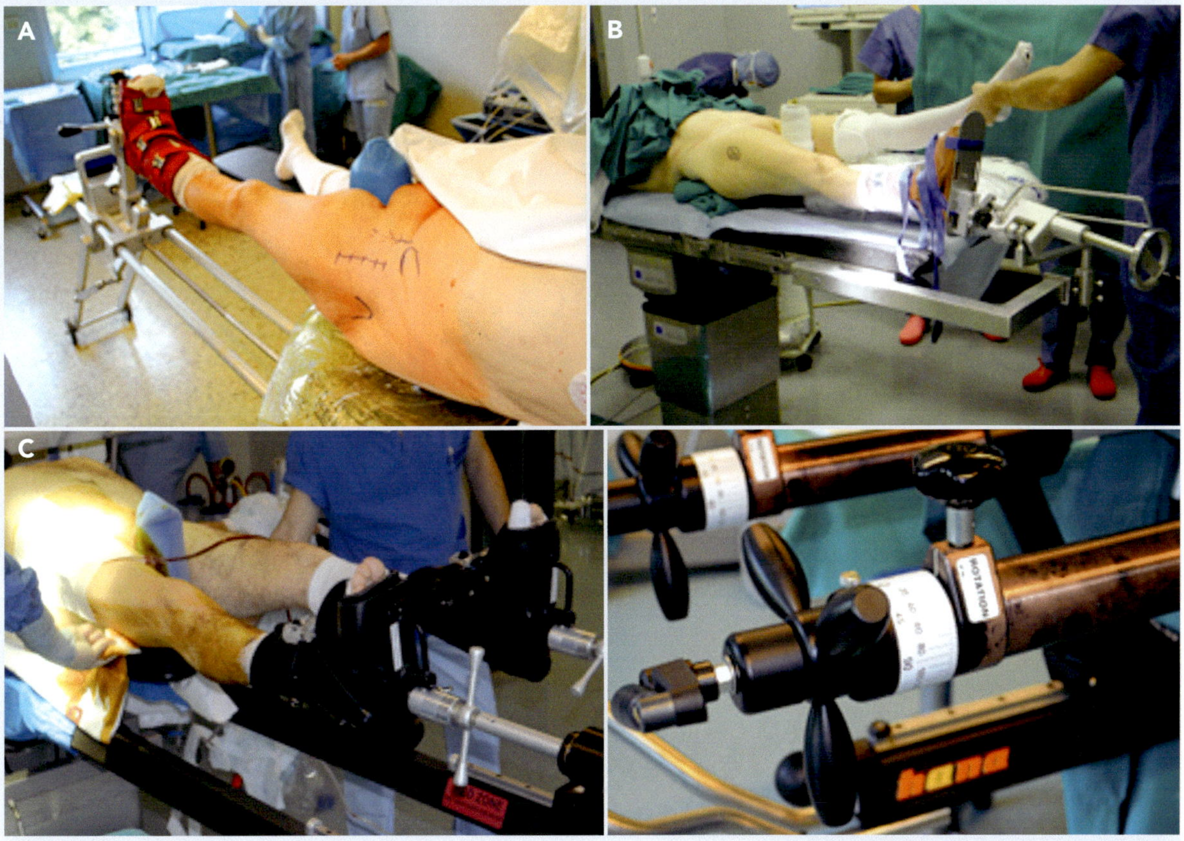

Figure 2 Traction-position beds used in our clinical practice. A) Leg Positioner/Medacta; B) Apon-Gar/Zimmer; C) Hana/Mizuho-OSI/Lima

with this technique. These include those with the following critical features: physical structure (weight, height, muscular trophism, etc.), severe hip dysmorphism (dysplasia, varus, coxa profunda or protrusa, etc.), a particularly high surgical risk, such that the operation would be contraindicated if performed with standard surgical access routes.

We were also able to apply various types of stems, which belong to the 'medium' category and can be applied without difficulty using the minimally invasive anterior approach. (fig. 3) In addition, anaesthetists are more willing to subject 'difficult' patients to surgery when the chosen technique is minimally invasive.

This is due to a faster operation and less surgical stress recorded (blood loss, need for transfusions, use of drugs for pain control, faster resumption of sitting, orthostasis and walking with weight-bearing allowed).

As of 31 December 2021, in different wards but still using the same basic technique, the authors of this chapter were able to report a total of 4787 procedures (tab. 1). In 125 cases (2.6%) we operated on femoral neck fractures using this technique. The remaining cases were coxarthrosis, either primary or secondary, or necrosis of the femoral head. The same radiographic 'severity' of the arthropathy admitted to minimally invasive surgery gradually increased as the surgeons' experience refined and the learning curve was completed.

The female sex accounted for 2729 cases (57%), the male for 2058 (43%). The average age was 53 years (minimum 22, maximum 98). The right side was prevalent (56% of cases). We operated on 18 large obese patients, appreciating the surprising facilitation granted by the minimally invasive anterior surgical technique (fig. 4).

The field of possible use of the minimally invasive surgical technique in hip prostheses is very extensive. It must be related to the surgeon's technical skills, which will be progressively refined, thus making the minimally invasive approach possible in increasingly

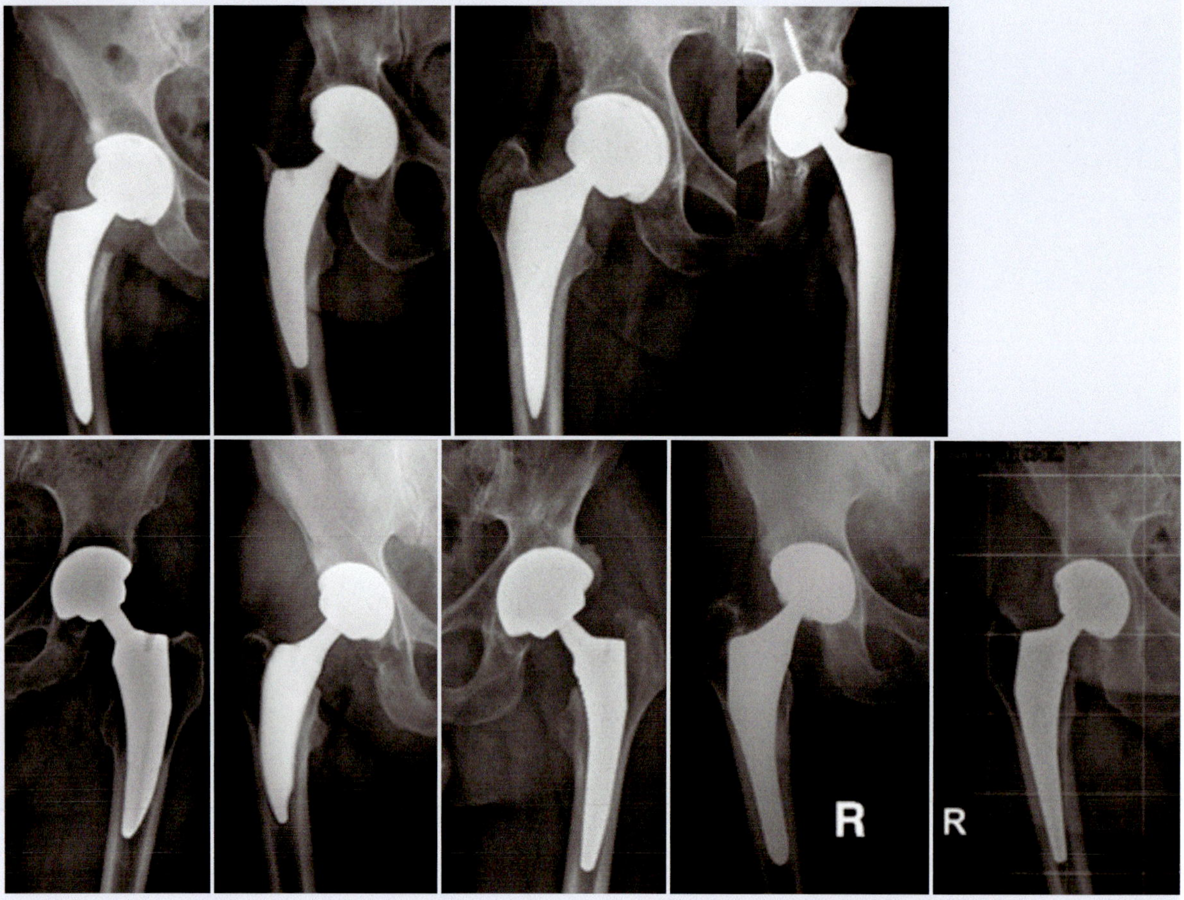

Figure 3 Types of stems that we implant using the anterior minimally invasive technique

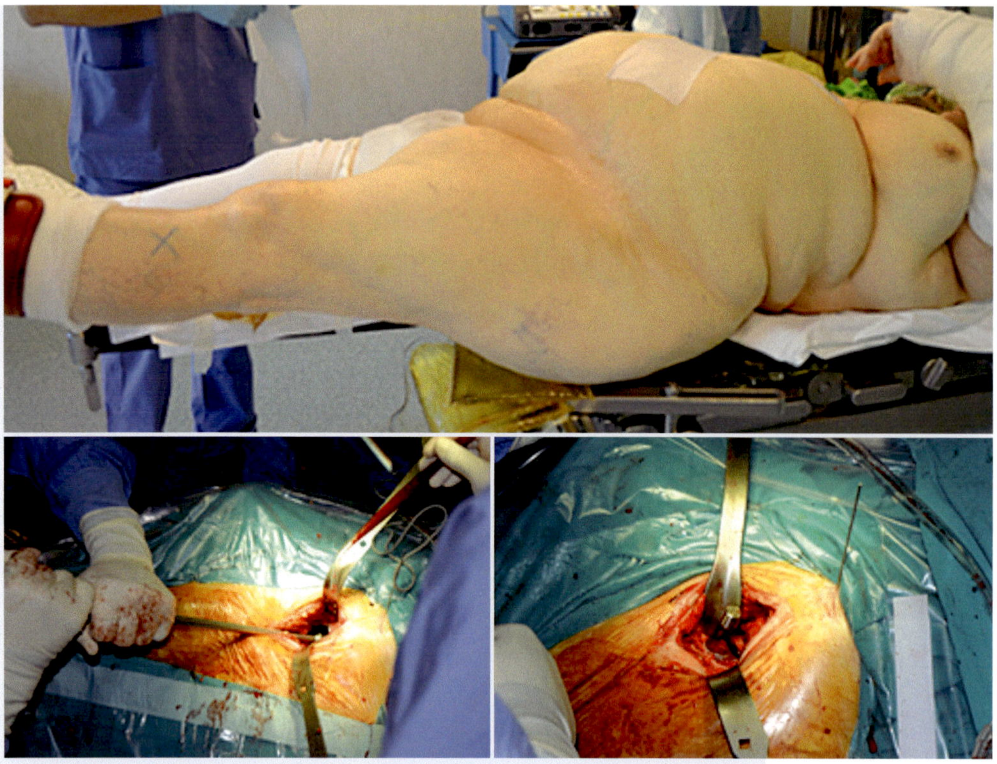

Figure 4 Example of an obese patient undergoing left hip replacement using the minimally invasive technique

Table 1 Report

Implanted prostheses	Nr of procedures
STEM	
Amistem	2.315
Quadra	164
Minimax	185
Masterloc	130
Fitmore	1.758
Avenir Complete	94
Gts	2
Taperloc microplasty	68
Abg II	47
Minima	24
CUP	
Mpact	2.278
Versafit	516
Trilogy	1224
Continuum	301
G7 PPS	397
Trident	47
Delta TT	24
MATERIALS	
Cer/Cer	4.579 (95%)
Cer/PE	208
TOTALE IMPLANTS	**4.787**

complex cases.
In the initial stages of learning, especially if a more experienced tutor is not present, it is prudent in any case to 'choose' clinically and radiographically 'easier' patients (figs. 5-7).
Then, as skills and experience mature, more challenging cases can be addressed, such as obese patients, particular and difficult coxofemoral morphologies (dysplasia, varus, protrusio) or patients in need of large prosthetic sizes (figs. 8-12).
As far as obese patients are concerned, the simplification produced by the minimally invasive technique has also been confirmed in other clinical experiences.
An anterior surgical incision of 8/9 cm has proved to allow the surgery, avoiding the longer incisions of the standard traditional approaches. Above all, it spared the area of greatest presence of adipose tissue. This is important because of the known difficulties and complications that this can present, such as: liponecrosis, scarring difficulties, infections and thromboembolic risks (fig. 13).
Individuals with a particular build (weight, height and muscle mass) may also be suitable for this technique, but it will be necessary that the anaesthetist ensures adequate muscle relaxation (fig. 14).
In 95 of our patients, surgery was performed on both hips. (fig. 15). Of these, in 51 cases, the second procedure was performed 4 to 5 months after the first. In 44 cases, however, it was possible to perform a prosthetic replacement of both hips at the same time, thanks to experience and increased surgical skill. Also thanks to the support of the anaesthetists and the encouragement of the rehabilitators, patient satisfaction was recorded. In fact, they solved the problem bilaterally in a single surgical procedure, avoiding a second operation and an additional rehabilitation phase after a few months (figs. 16-17).
Cervical femoral fractures are very good candidates for the minimally invasive technique, especially in cases of advanced age or particular comorbidities. Another interesting element that should not be ignored is that these fractures are usually placed in the so-called 'emergency room'. This detail allows younger colleagues to learn the minimally invasive technique under the supervision of a more experienced surgeon (fig. 18).
Some particular conditions may benefit from this technique, which is less invasive and does not sacrifice muscle tissue. This is the case in the following patients: in polio patients (where less muscle damage facilitates functional recovery), in the presence of particular comorbidities (such as rheumatoid disease, where the minimally invasive technique appears less stressful and less risky) (fig. 19), in post-traumatic hip ankylosis (fig. 20) and in very young patients (fig. 21).
Minimally invasive surgery may present some technical difficulties in particular conditions, such as varus cervical diaphyseal angle, cervical shortness, coxa profunda and certain

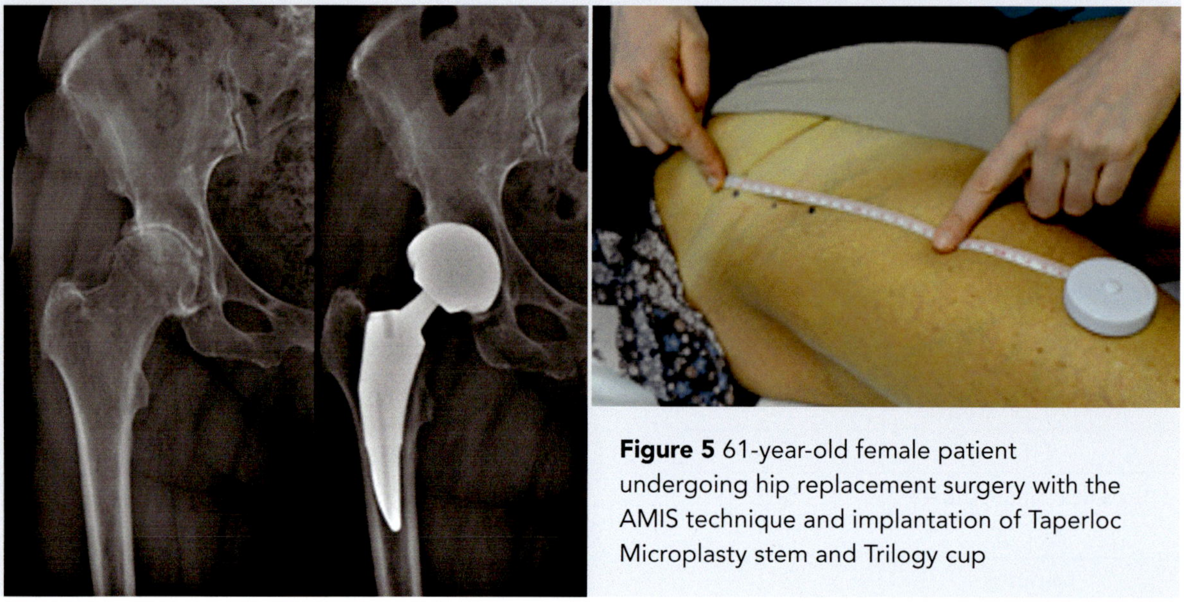

Figure 5 61-year-old female patient undergoing hip replacement surgery with the AMIS technique and implantation of Taperloc Microplasty stem and Trilogy cup

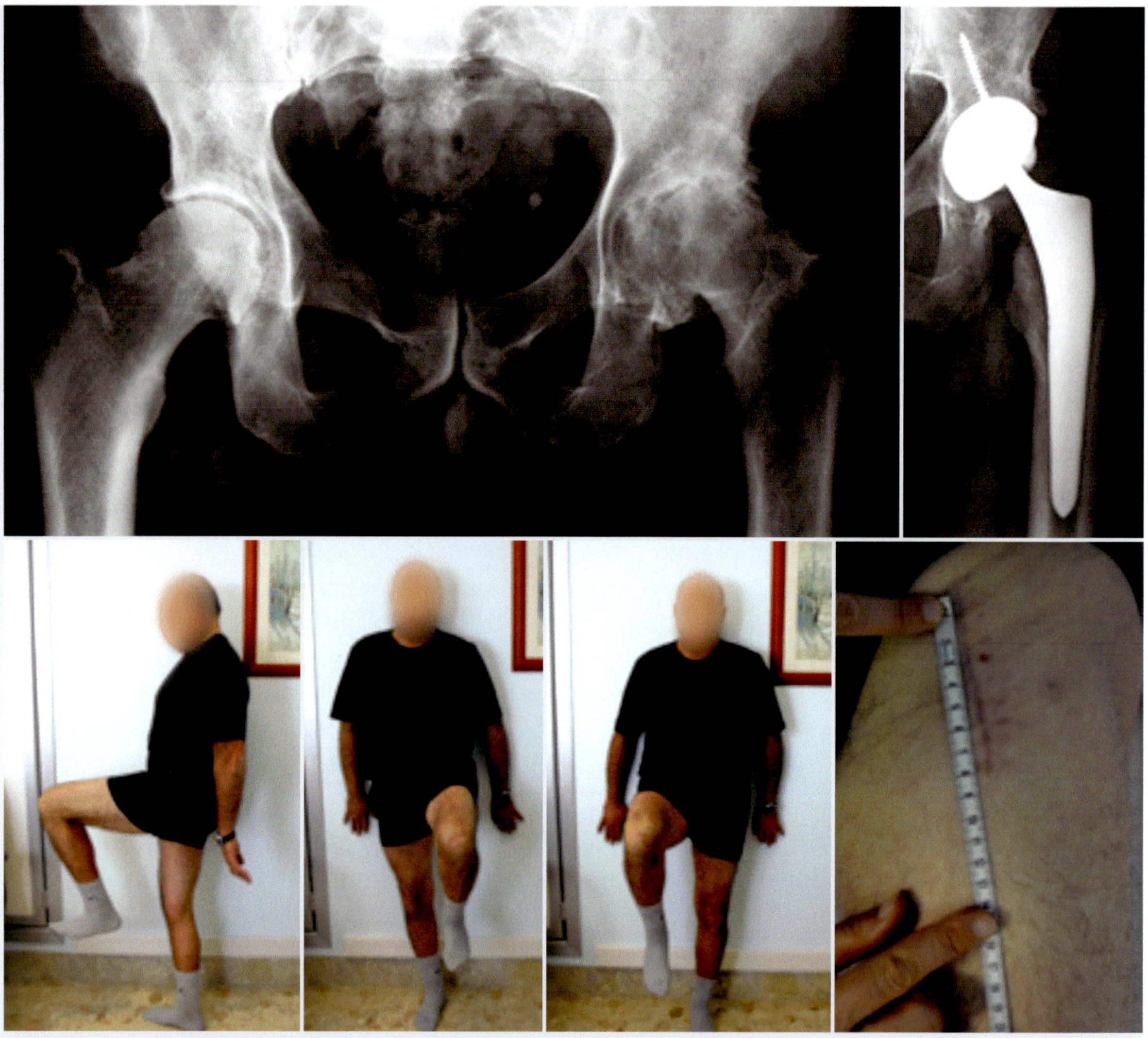

Figure 6 A 58-year-old male patient who underwent hip replacement surgery using the AMIS technique and implantation of a Versafit cup and Quadra stem

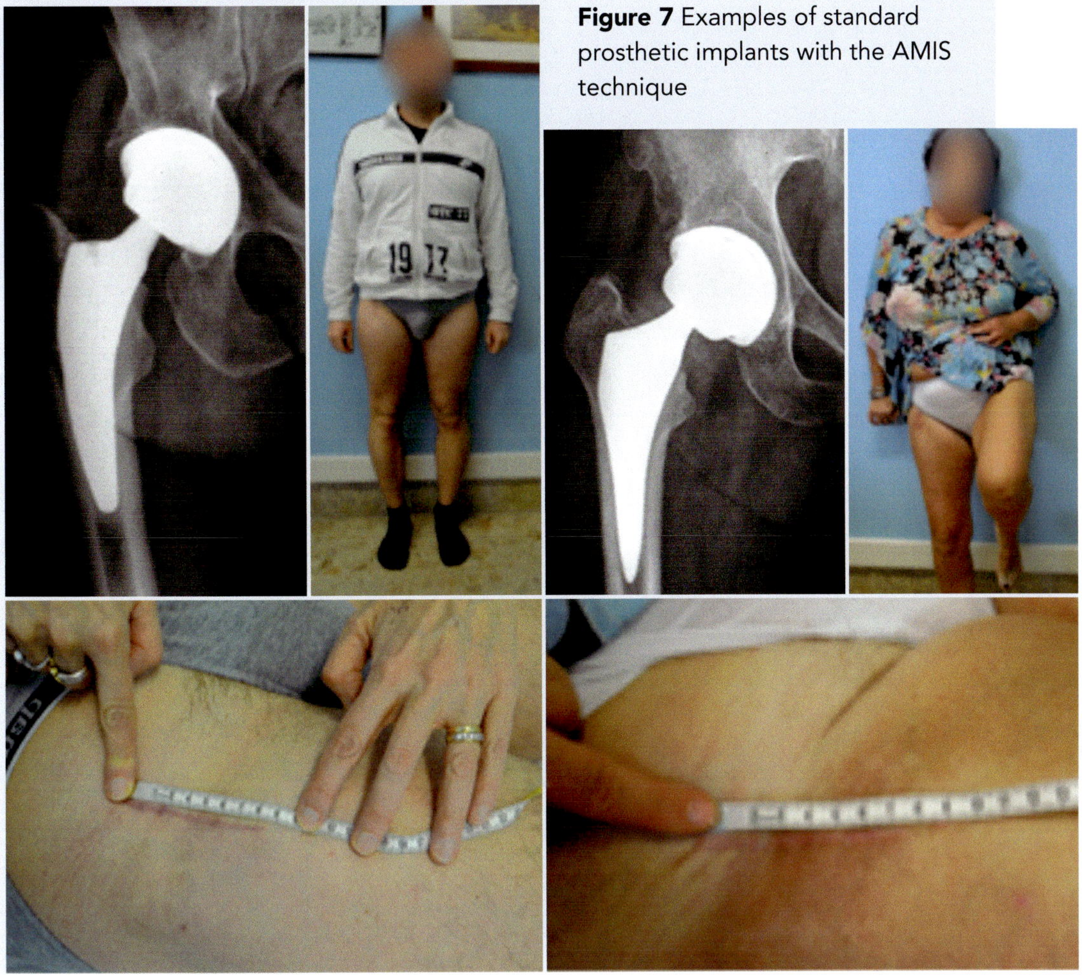

Figure 7 Examples of standard prosthetic implants with the AMIS technique

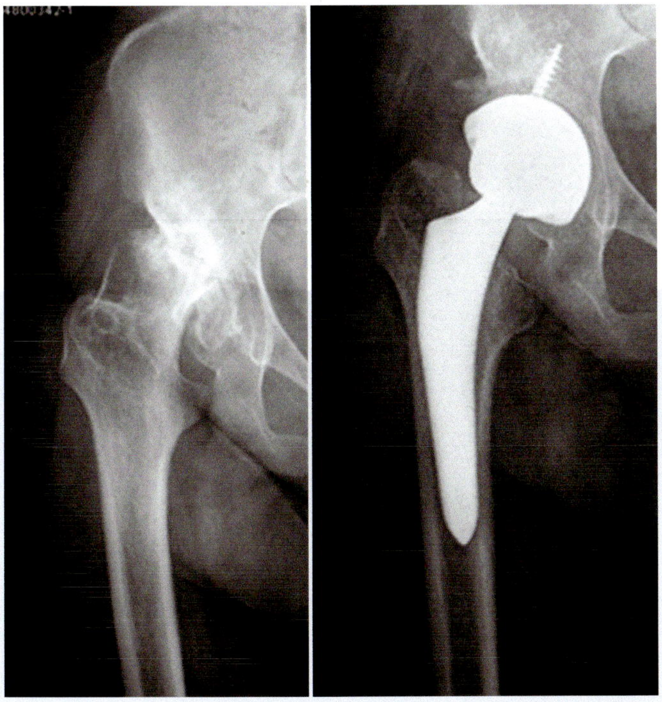

Figure 8 Female patient, 52 years old, suffering from right hip arthropathy secondary to high-grade dysplasia. The patient underwent hip replacement surgery using the AMIS technique

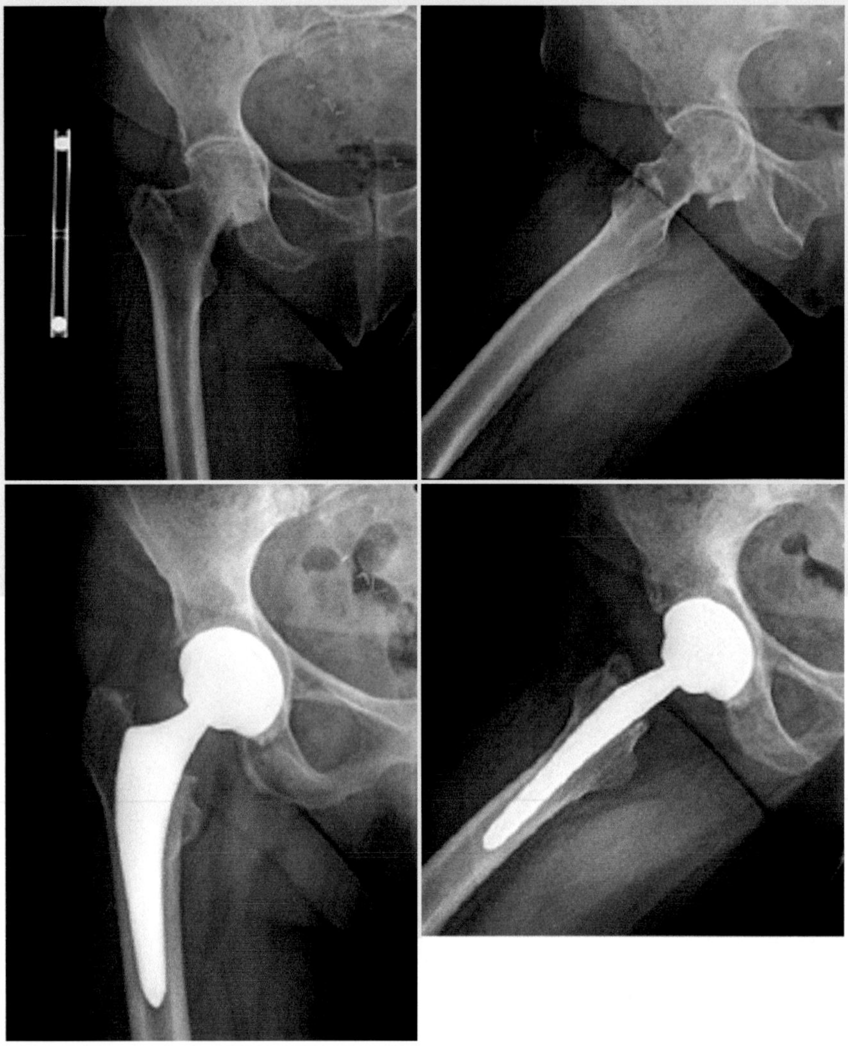

Figure 9 Example of coxa profunda undergoing anterior minimally invasive hip replacement surgery

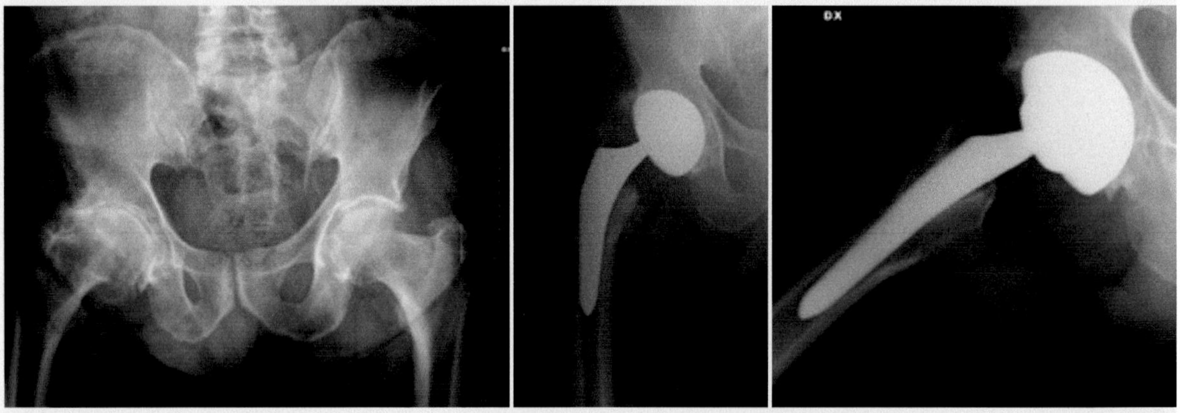

Figure 10 Example of bilateral coxa vara undergoing right hip replacement surgery with the AMIS technique

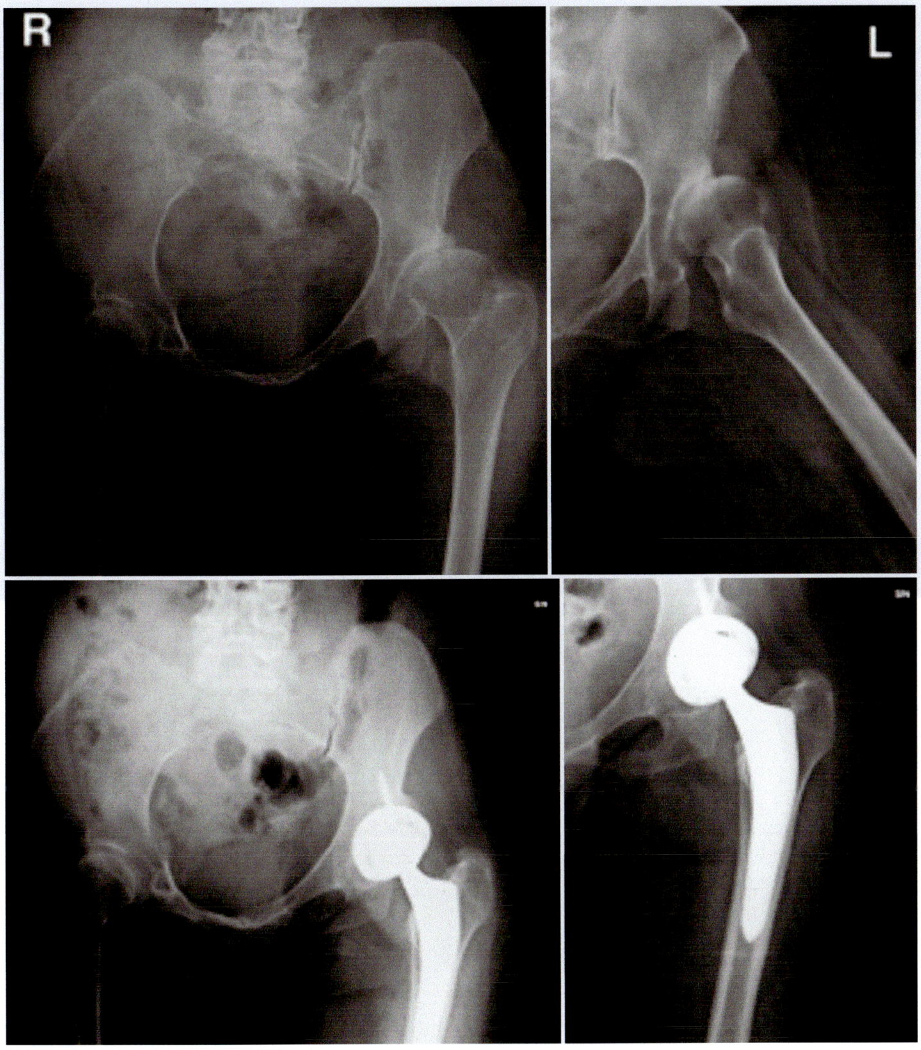

Figure 11 Left subluxating coxopathy secondary to marked pelvic tilt in right lower limb polio outcomes

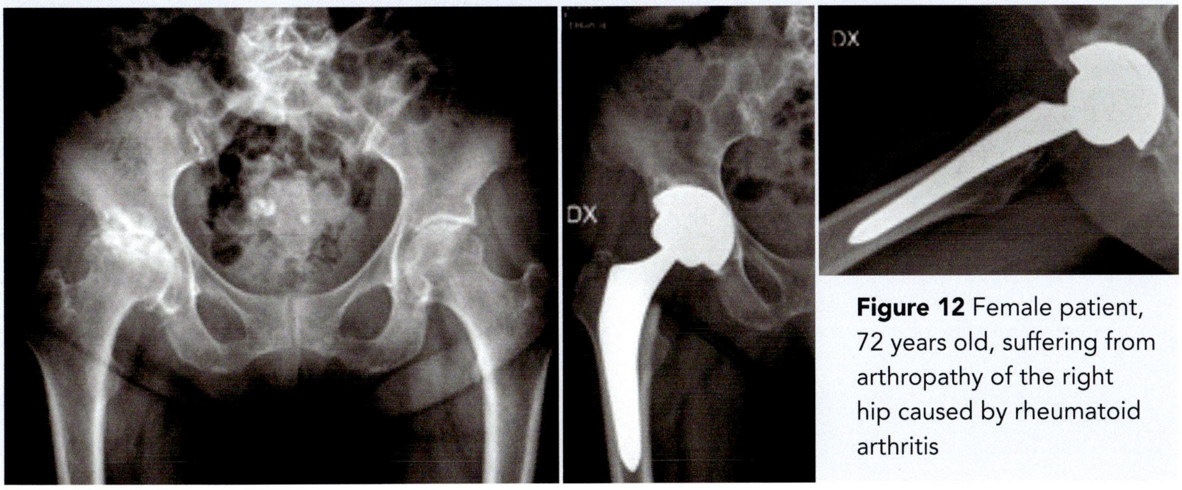

Figure 12 Female patient, 72 years old, suffering from arthropathy of the right hip caused by rheumatoid arthritis

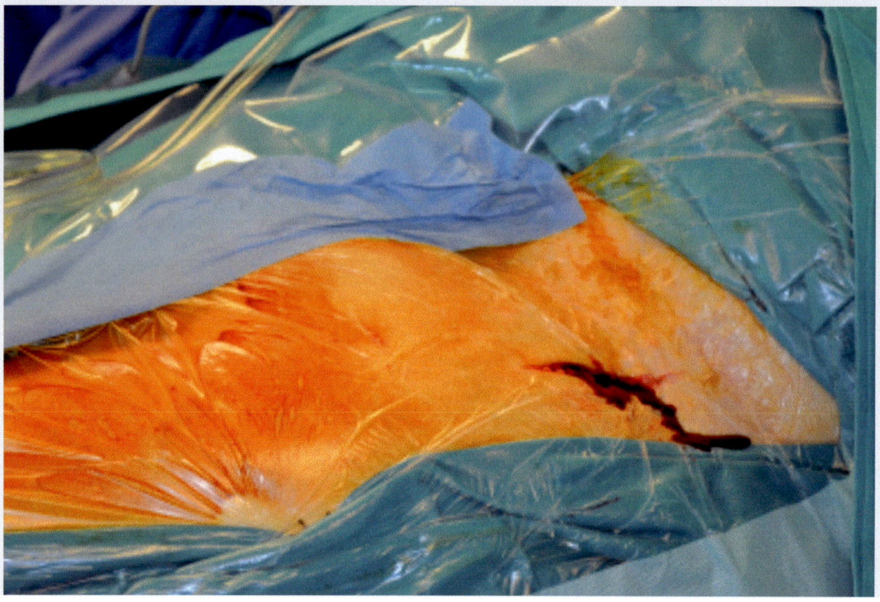

Figure 13 Image of an obese patient undergoing hip replacement surgery with the minimally invasive anterior technique

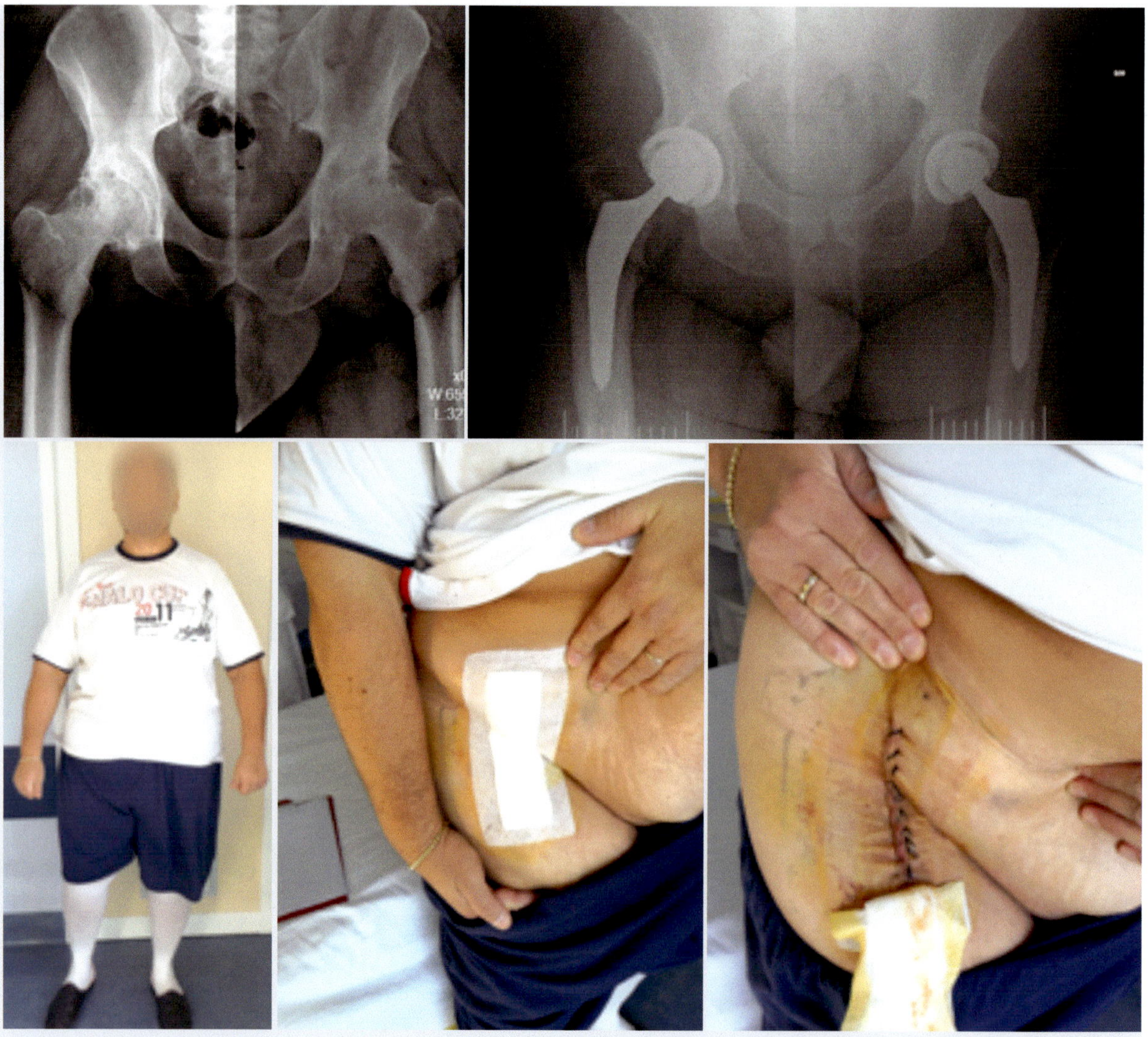

Figure 14 51-year-old obese male patient (187 cm x 170 kg) undergoing bilateral hip replacement surgery with the AMIS technique (right in 2017 and left in 2018)

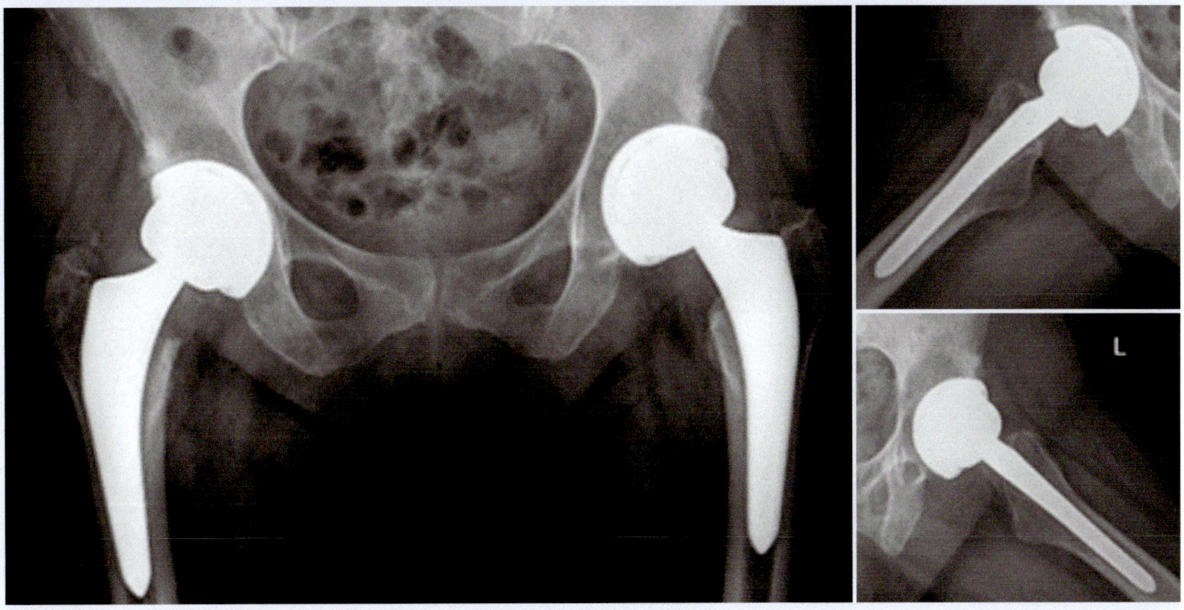

Figure 15 Example of bilateral prosthetic replacement performed separately: on the right in April 2018 and on the left in November of the same year

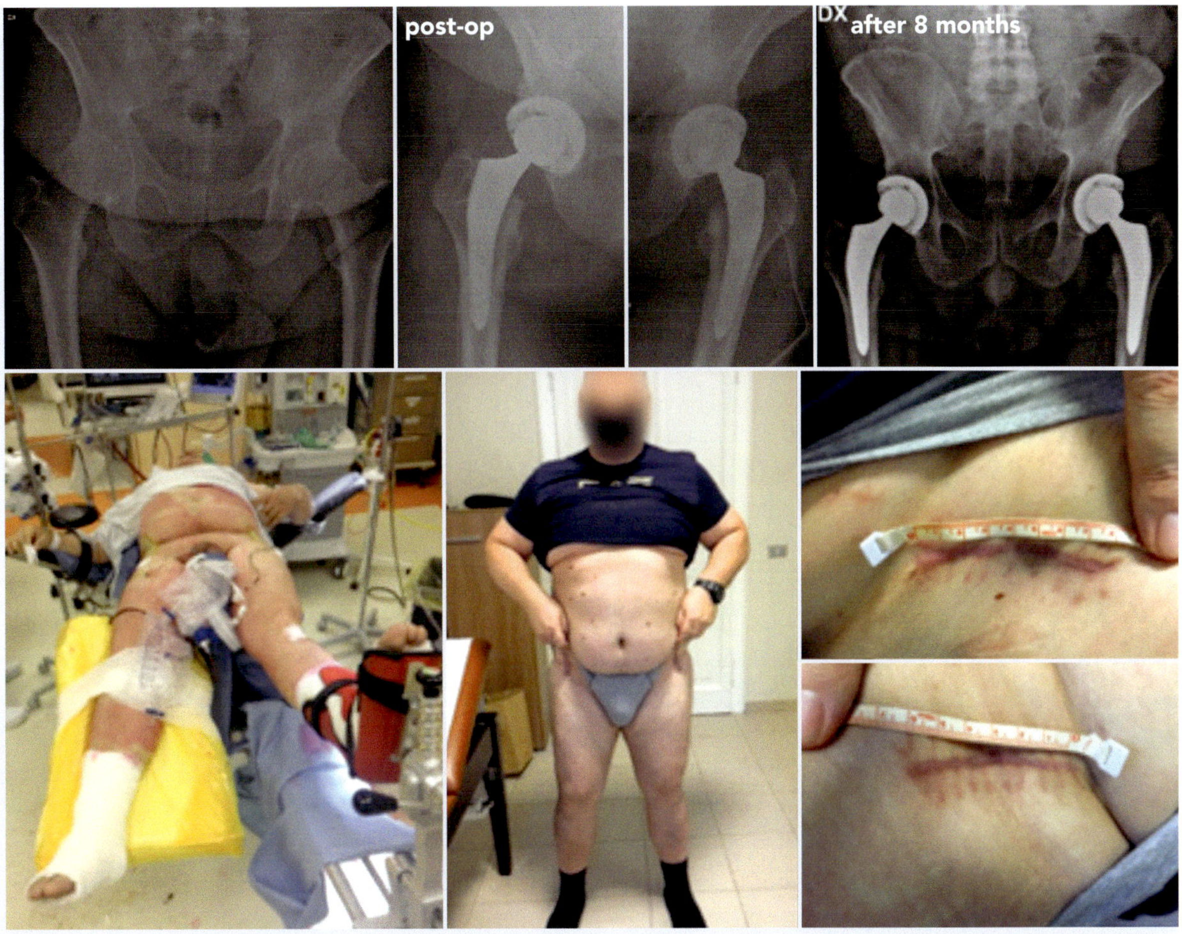

Figure 16 43-year-old male patient (188 cm x 135 kg). Bilateral prosthetic replacement surgery was performed in the same surgery in September 2021

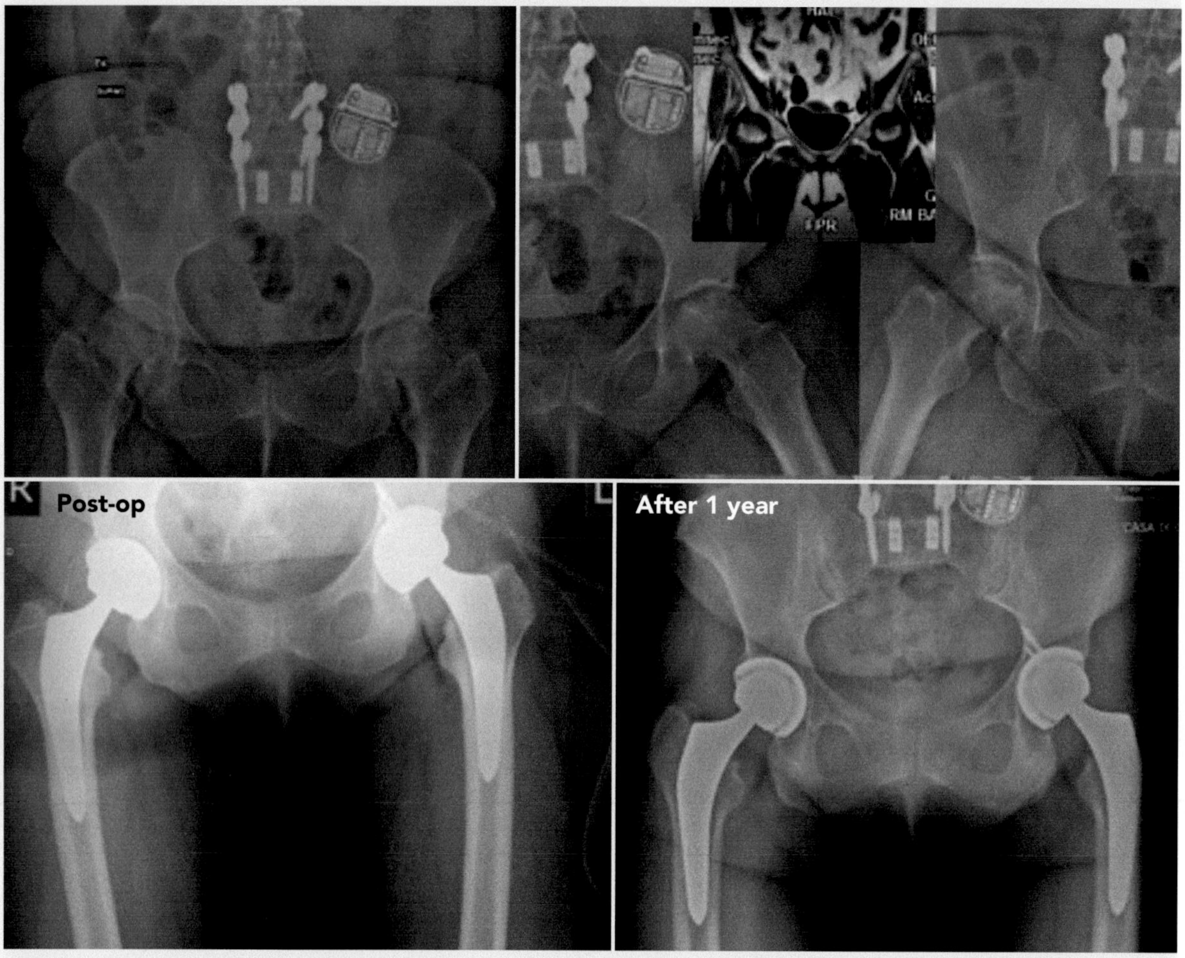

Figure 17 41-year-old female patient (95 kg x 172 cm) who had undergone multiple spinal operations for spondylolisthesis of L5 on S1. The patient has bilateral femoral head necrosis, probably secondary to prolonged treatment with corticosteroids for chronic back pain and bilateral sciatica. The placement of the vertebral stimulator can be observed. The patient underwent bilateral hip replacement using the minimally invasive anterior technique in the same surgery

forms of acetabular dysplasia. Generally, these conditions produce a 'shortening' of the hip, with a reduction in capsular volume and inevitable joint stiffness.

The most delicate phase of the operation is in fact the femoral 'exposure', which is normally achieved by external rotation and extension of the limb. The anatomical situation, capsular shortening/thickening and short external rotator muscle shortness/stiffness, may impede the advancement of the femur, holding the greater trochanter behind the posterior cup wall. This situation, which generally adds to joint stiffness, can make surgery more challenging. Therefore, it may require deeper sedation to increase muscle relaxation or sometimes conversion to general anaesthesia in order to obtain sufficient extension of the limb and avoid dangerous trochanter-acetabulum conflicts (fig. 22).

We adopt a particular technique to facilitate the passage-advancement of the greater trochanter over the posterior acetabular rim. Generally, the extension of the limb is carried out with a reduced external rotation of the limb, so that the greater trochanter is placed more lateral to the acetabulum. Once brought to the maximum extension allowed by the traction apparatus, we carefully increase the external rotation to the appropriate degrees (130-150°). This allows the advancement and 'exposure' of the femoral neck, relying on the easier and less risky passage-advancement of the greater

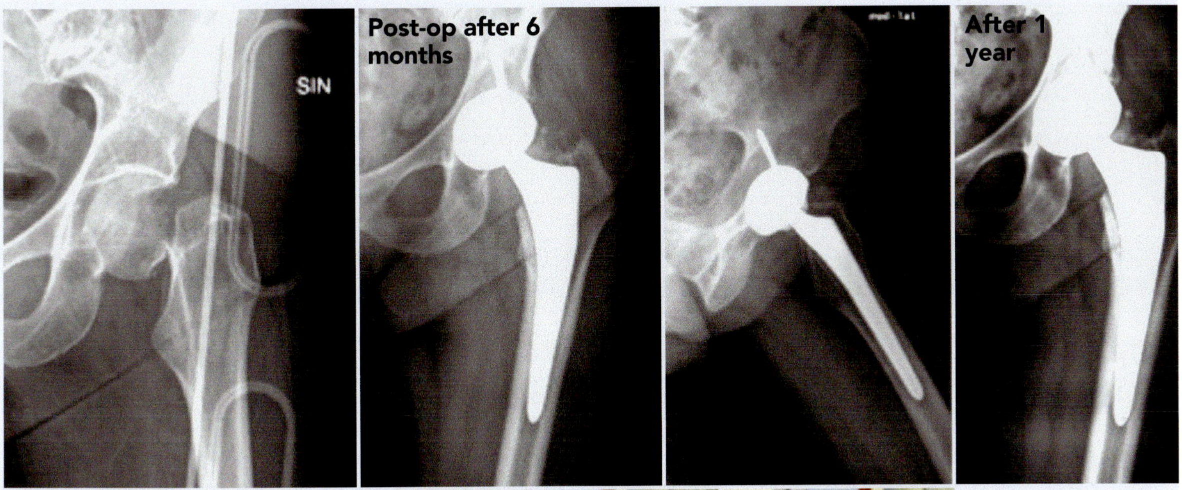

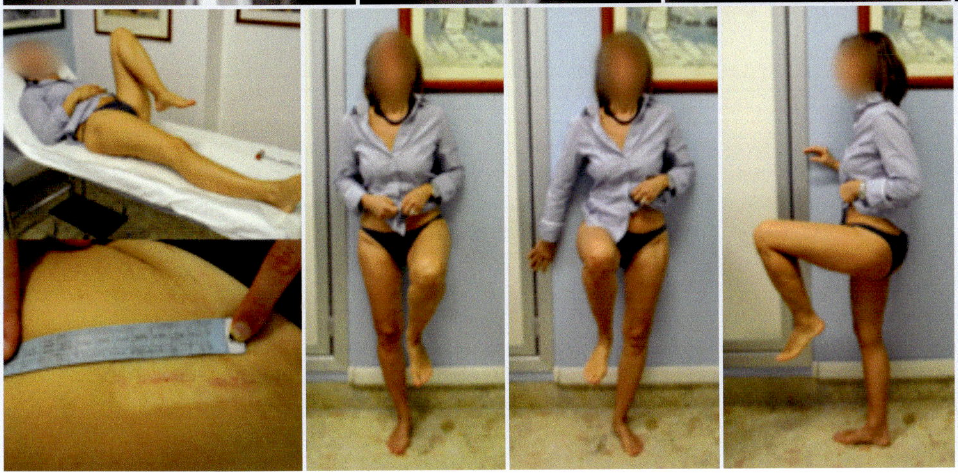

Figure 18 58-year-old patient with a left femoral neck fracture undergoing hip replacement with the anterior minimally invasive technique

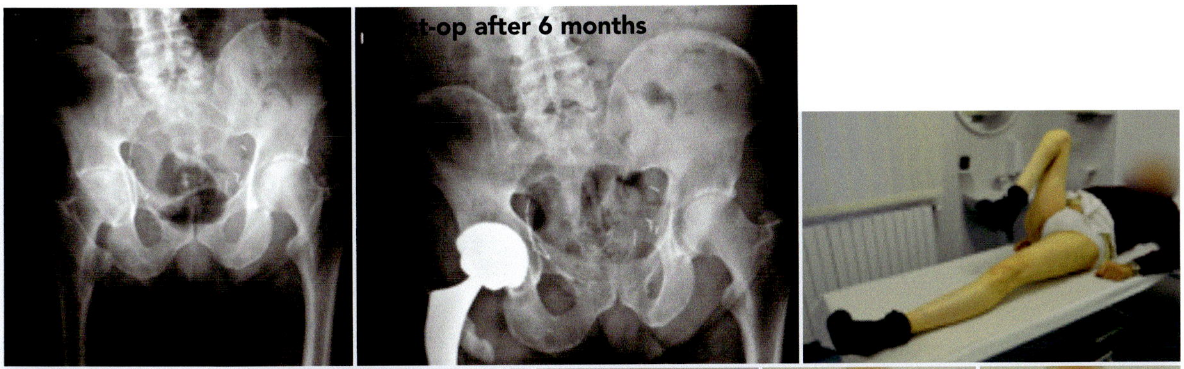

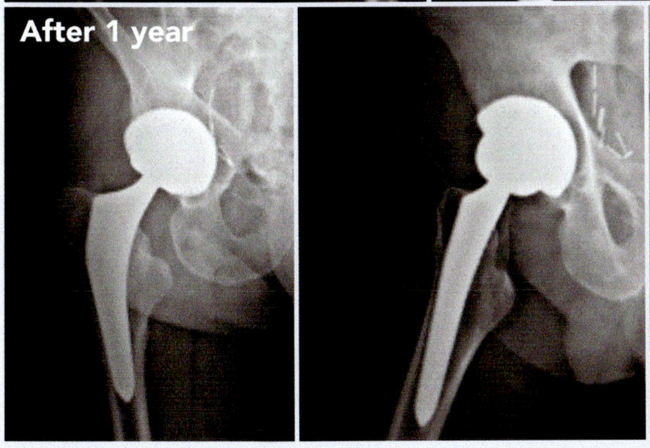

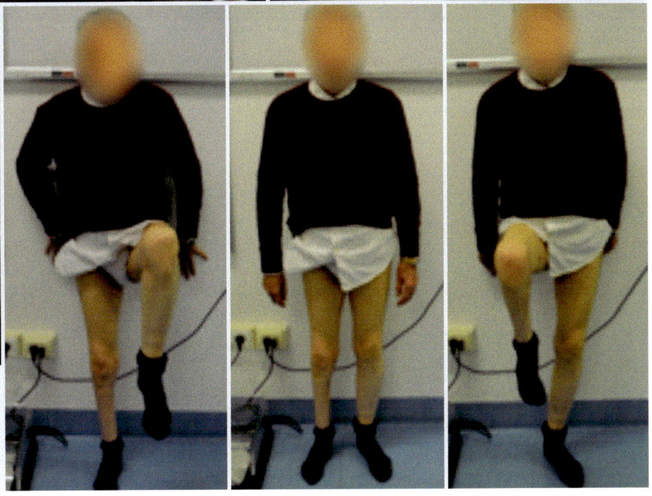

Figure 19 Right coxarthrosis in a patient with polio outcomes (steppage gait)

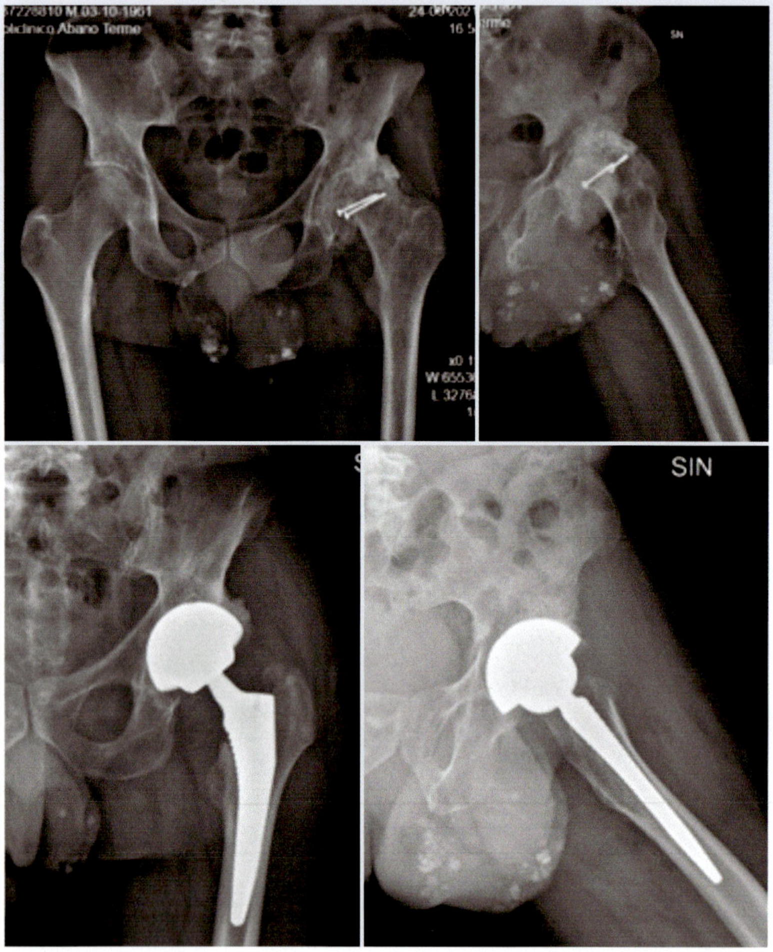

Figure 20 Flexion ankylosis of the left hip in a 55-year-old male patient. The current clinical scenario is an outcome of femoral head fracture, treated with wide posterior surgical approach at the age of 14 years

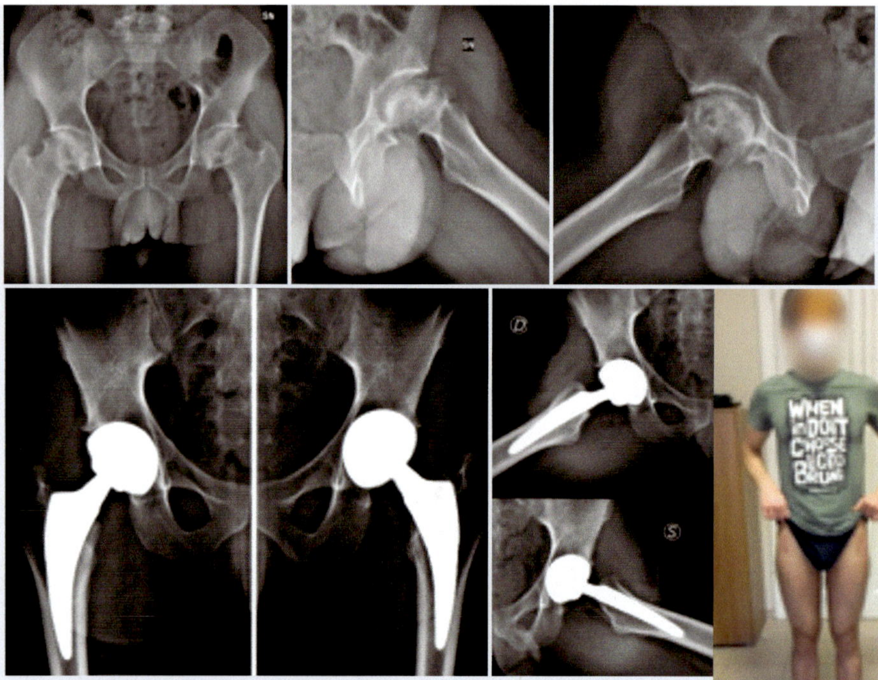

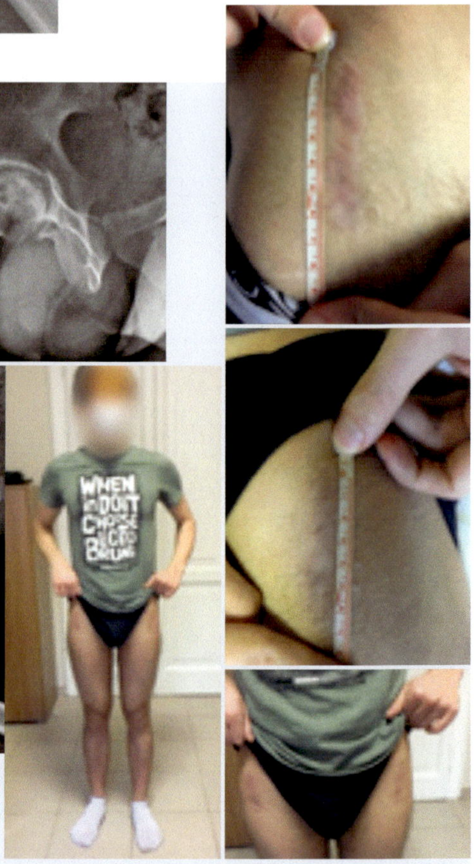

Figure 21 A 22-year-old male patient suffering from systemic lupus erythematosus and on cortisone therapy since the age of 15. This treatment resulted in bilateral femoral head necrosis. The patient underwent bilateral hip replacement surgery at two separate times (right December 2020 and left June 2021)

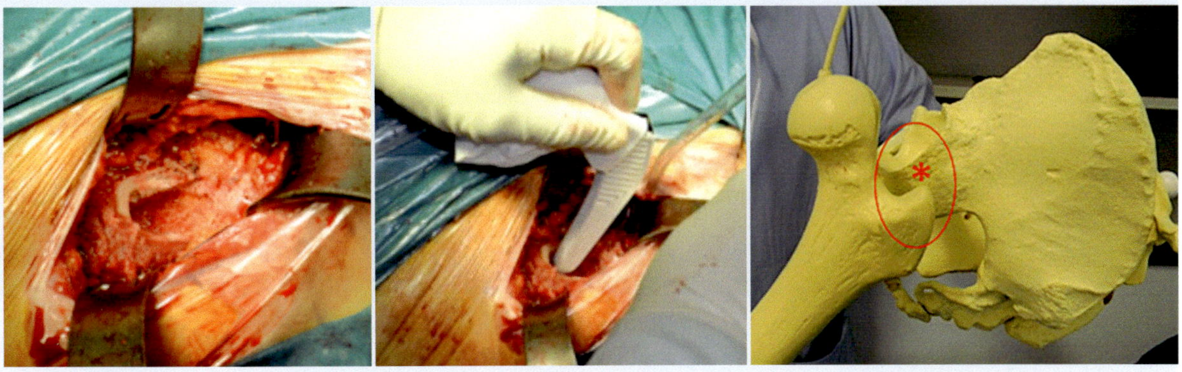

Figure 22 An adequate 'exposure' of the femur is necessary for the preparation of the femoral diaphyseal canal and for the smooth introduction of the prosthetic stem. The femur must be in anteposition and maintain marked external rotation throughout the femoral phase. It is necessary for the greater trochanter to pass the posterior acetabular margin without 'conflicts' that could lead to femoral fractures. To achieve this with relative safety, we usually complete the external rotation of the femur (150° generally) with the limb already extended

trochanter in front of the acetabulum.

Mention should be made of the 'anaesthesiological' aspects of the minimally invasive surgical technique, since we usually operate with subarachnoid anaesthesia (currently used in about 92% of cases, while the remainder are under general anaesthesia).

The cooperation with the anaesthetist is very important. Sometimes, we may ask our colleague to administer additional drugs in the 'femoral' phase, to facilitate the disengagement of the gran trochanter from the posterior cup wall and the advancement-exposure of the femoral neck. In 3% of cases, the procedure started with general anaesthesia, as this was the recommended procedure, the one imposed by particular clinical conditions or the one requested by the patient. In 5% of cases, however, there was an intraoperative switch to general anaesthesia with a laryngeal mask (two thirds of patients) or by intubation (one third of cases).

Complications

We reiterate emphatically that the minimally invasive technique is not an easy procedure, quick to learn and free of difficulties or complications. After an initial approach to the minimally invasive technique, many younger surgeons give up learning and perfecting the technique. This phenomenon is caused by the steepness of the learning curve and the significant number of risks or complications that may occur in the first 150-200 operations. In fact, most complications occur in the early stages of learning this surgical technique, even for surgeons already experienced in traditional techniques. It should be pointed out that surgeons dedicated to the minimally invasive technique should have solid experience of traditional techniques. However, one can appreciate a significant reduction in intra- and post-operative complications compared to traditional techniques, when related to the global number of procedures.

The incidence of complications tends to progressively decrease as surgeons' experience grows.

In addition, complications are in fact the same as in standard techniques, but in much lower percentages. It is necessary, however, to point out three specific additional problems that we believe can be correlated with this surgical technique:

- lateral cutaneous nerve suffering;
- subfascial haematoma caused by the transverse branch of the anterior descending artery (originating from the circumflex lateral artery, a branch of the deep femoral artery);
- a temporary post-operative pelvic obliquity with transient pseudo-lengthening of the limb.

Instability of the prosthesis

There were 9 (0.2%) cases of prosthetic dislocation in the immediate post-operative period. Spinal anaesthesia was used in all these cases. In six cases the condition occurred preoperatively, when the patient was moving from the surgical bed to the stretcher. In these cases, extemporaneous reduction was performed. Then, having verified the stability of the implant after the restoration of muscle tone, the patients proceeded with the normal rehabilitation programme. In two cases, however, a recurrence of the dislocation led to surgical revision with the implantation of a longer head. This procedure solved the problem definitively (fig. 23). In another case, the cup had to be replaced due to an abnormal orientation (increased anteversion). This was the cause that had led to two dislocation episodes.

Periprosthetic fracture

We have so far recorded 26 fractures (0.5%): 8 of the great trochanter, 4 of the femoral calcar, 3 of the cup, 11 with femoral diaphyseal involvement. In 20 cases we proceeded to surgical stabilization: in 14 cases this took place in the same operating session and in 6 cases several days later. (fig. 24). In the other 6 cases (e.g., infraction of the greater trochanter, infraction of the fundus of the cup), no osteosynthesis was performed. We waited for spontaneous healing and asked the physiotherapist to slow down the functional recovery phase by postponing loading until the radiographic check at day 45 after surgery.
Special mention should be made of the greater trochanter, which, in the position with the limb extended and in external rotation (necessary to allow 'exposure' (advancement) of the femur and preparation of the diaphyseal canal and subsequent insertion of the stem) is in contact with the posterior acetabular wall. If this is overhanging (failure to resect the acetabular osteophytosis, protrusio acetabuli, etc.) or if there is muscle or capsular contracture/retraction, it may happen that the greater trochanter fails to pass over the posterior acetabular rim during extension, inevitably creating the conditions for its possible fracture.
This is the most delicate phase of the surgical procedure, where the surgeon has to 'clear' the path of the greater trochanter during extension (acting on the capsule and possibly on the muscle insertions) and ask for the assistance of the anesthesiologist.

Haematoma during surgery

We count 24 cases (0.4%) of clinically relevant haematoma, confirmed by ultrasound examination. In 2 cases, surgical evacuation of the hematoma was necessary (fig. 25). In three cases, the interventional radiologist

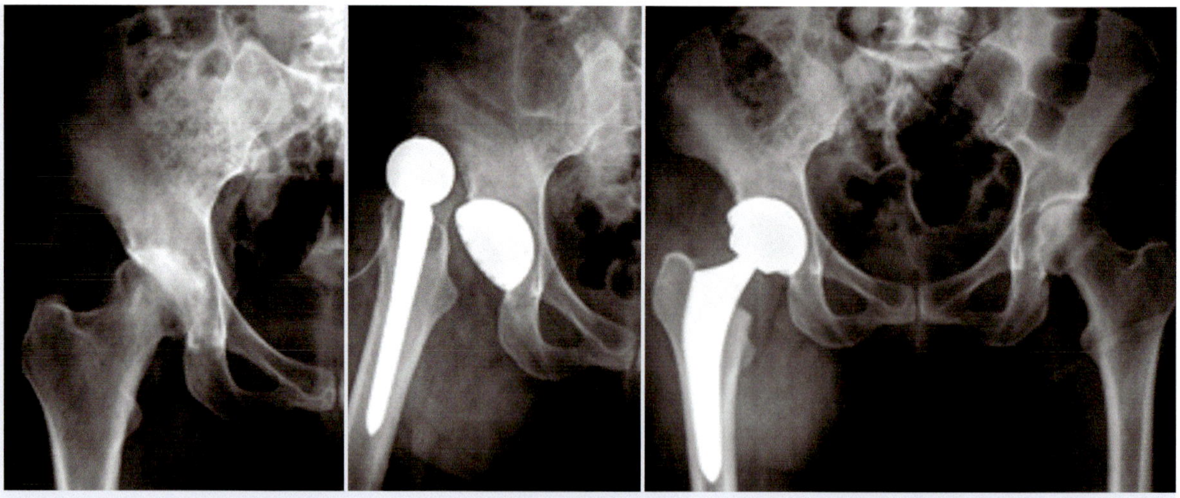

Figure 23 Example of dislocation of the prosthesis in the immediate post-operative period. In this case, revision with insertion of a head with a longer neck was necessary

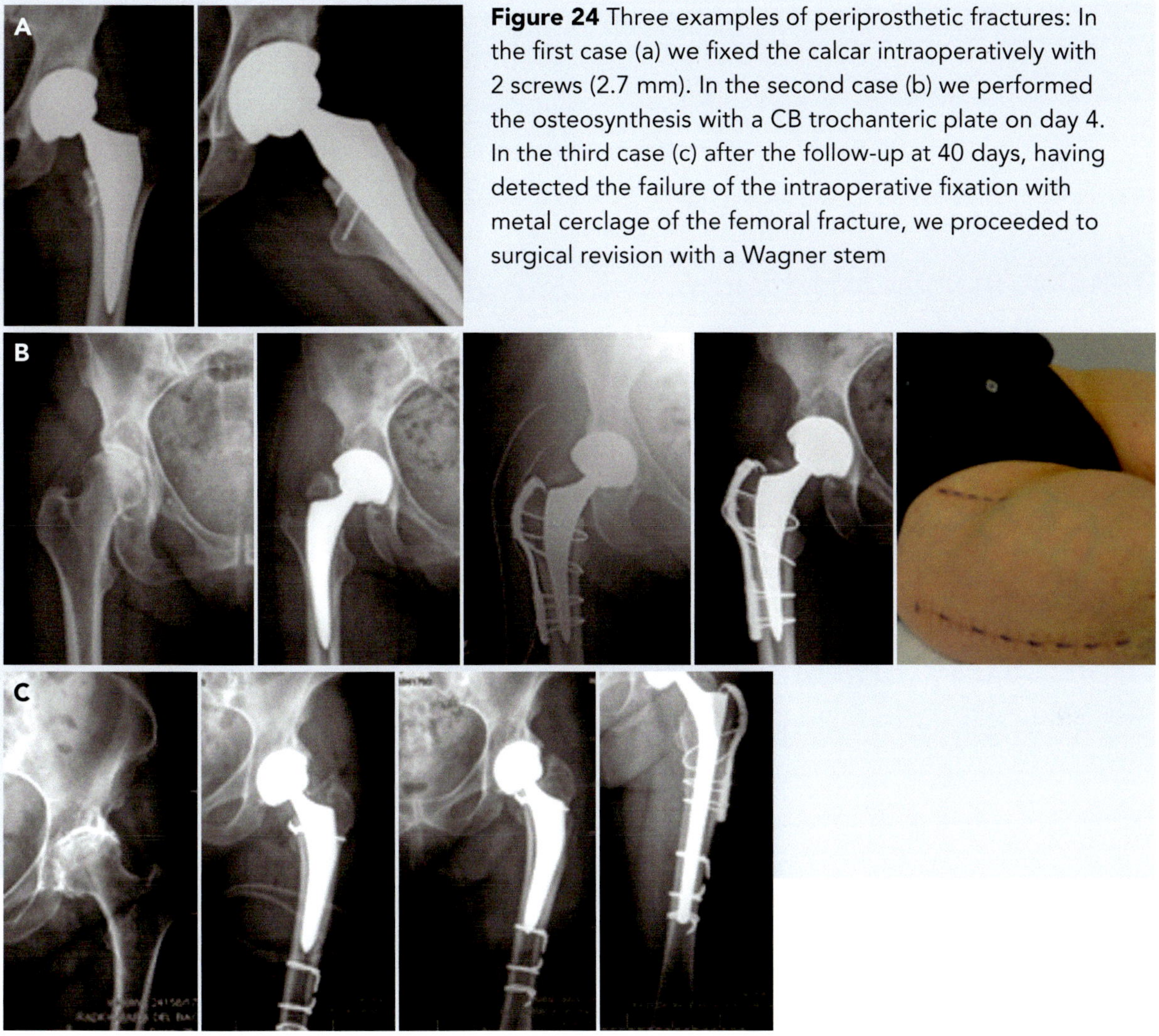

Figure 24 Three examples of periprosthetic fractures: In the first case (a) we fixed the calcar intraoperatively with 2 screws (2.7 mm). In the second case (b) we performed the osteosynthesis with a CB trochanteric plate on day 4. In the third case (c) after the follow-up at 40 days, having detected the failure of the intraoperative fixation with metal cerclage of the femoral fracture, we proceeded to surgical revision with a Wagner stem

performed a selective percutaneous embolisation of a bleeding circumflex femoral vessel (fig. 26). In order to avoid this problem we recommend to always ligate the small branches of the transverse artery (fig. 27). In fact, we exclude relying solely on electrocoagulation of the vessels. These are located just in front of the capsular plane, where we incise to perform the arthrotomy. Electrocoagulation alone poses the risk of a possible reopening of the vessels when pressure values are restored after the operation or due to the action of antithrombotic drug therapy.

Other vascular lesions

Apart from haematomas from a post-surgical complication of the lateral circumflex branches, which must always be tied, we have so far recorded no lesions of the vessels of the iliac-femoral arterial axis. On the other hand, in terms of venous compartment issues, we have never recorded DVT of the major axis (femoral, popliteal and posterior tibial). This fact appears to us to be of great clinical significance. We believe that this is attributable to the reduced surgical aggressiveness, the brevity of the surgical procedure and the rapid recovery of standing and walking. In some cases, we have identified thrombosis of the small veins of the calf (sural, peroneal), which were managed with ultrasound follow-up as indicated by the angiologist.

Involvement of the lateral cutaneous nerve of the thigh

It is necessary to distinguish a form of irritation due to the surgical manoeuvres of traction-compression by the retractors from the scenario of a true nerve injury similar to Roth's meralgia paresthesica.

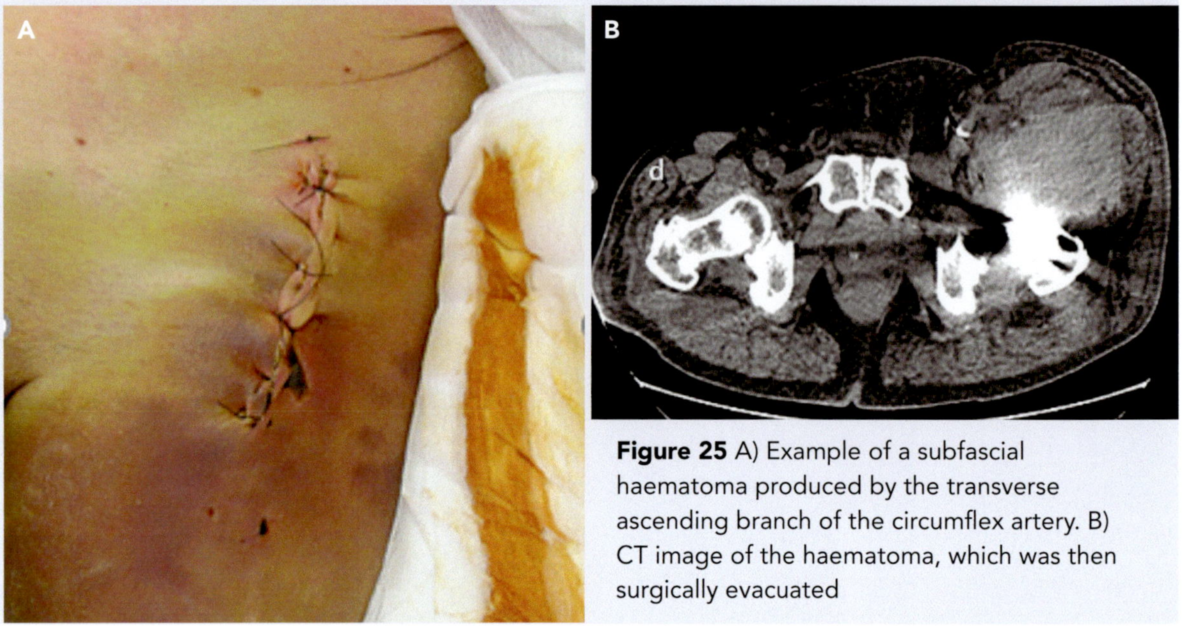

Figure 25 A) Example of a subfascial haematoma produced by the transverse ascending branch of the circumflex artery. B) CT image of the haematoma, which was then surgically evacuated

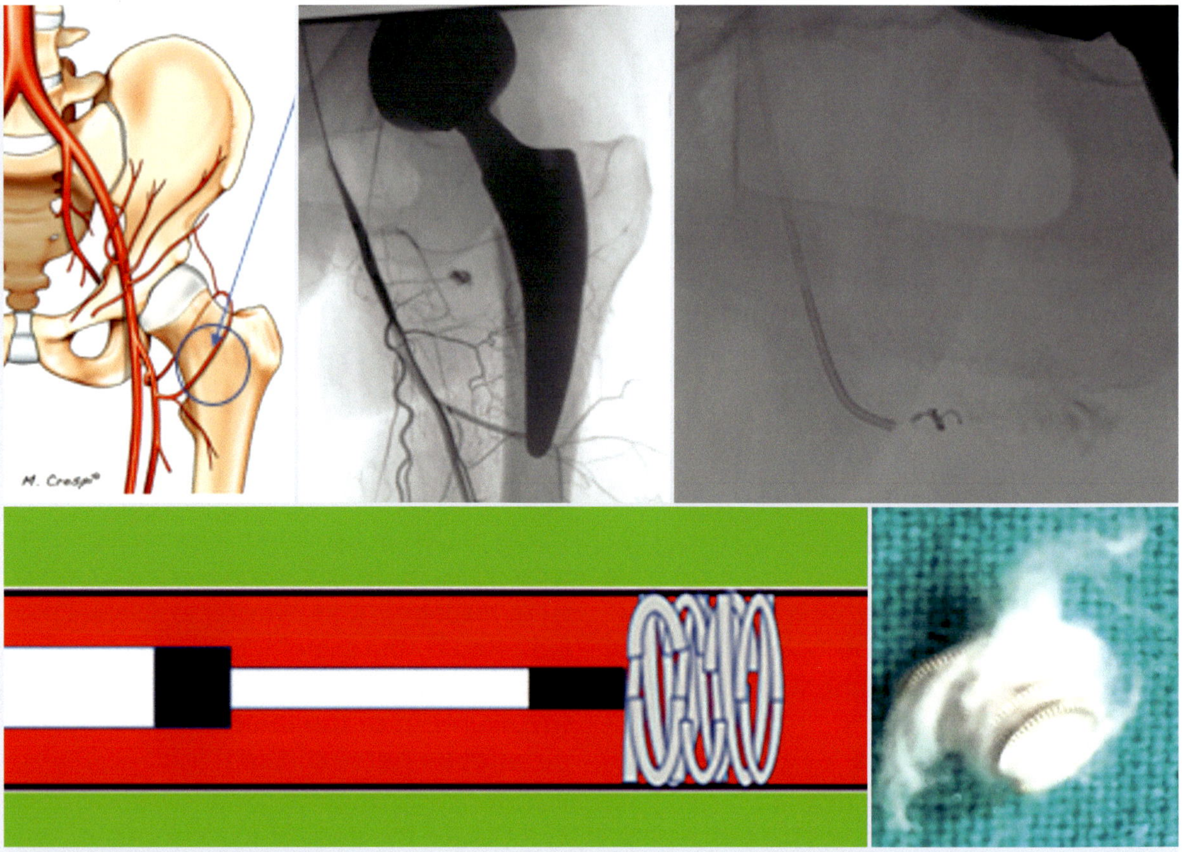

Figure 26 Example of arterial embolisation using hair coils introduced with percutaneous endovascular technique. The procedure was performed by our interventional radiology department (Dr. Marco Manzi)

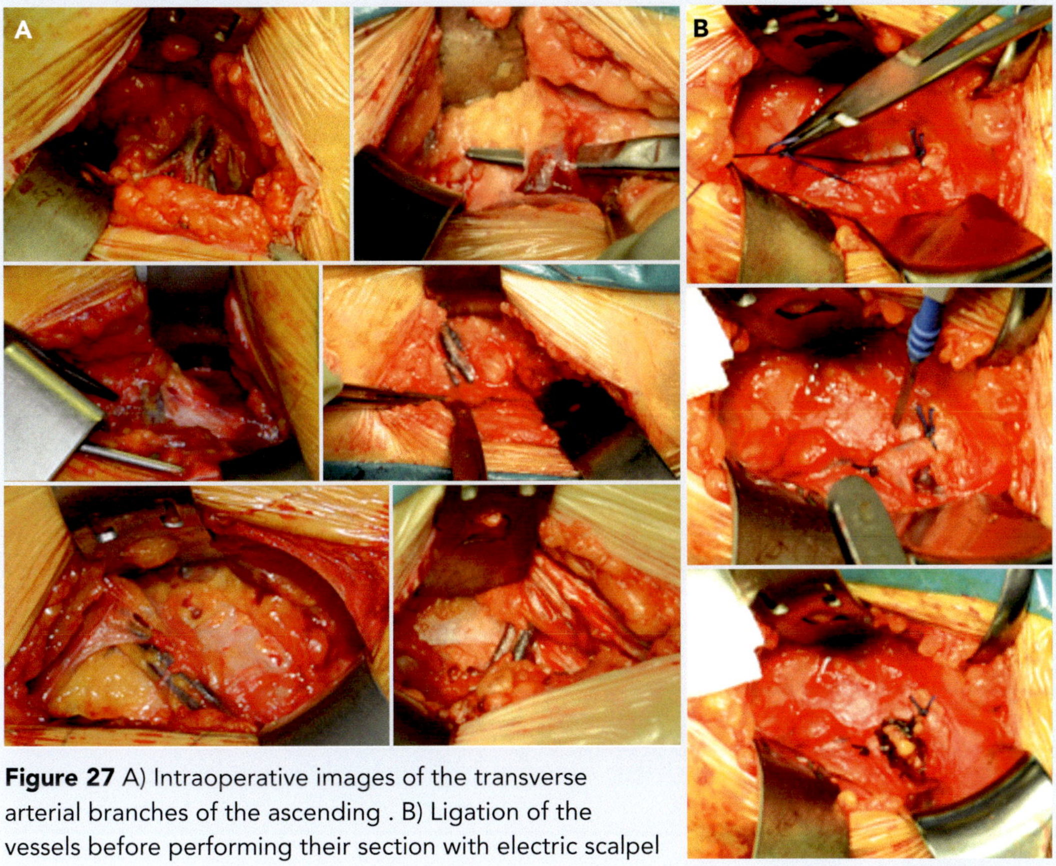

Figure 27 A) Intraoperative images of the transverse arterial branches of the ascending . B) Ligation of the vessels before performing their section with electric scalpel

The former occurs especially during extension of the limb and is usually a mild/moderate condition that is reversible within about 6-12 months.

In anatomical studies, several abnormalities of origin, conformation and course of the LCN nerve are recognised. These are conditions that can help to understand and explain post-operative dysesthesias without LCN nerve injury.

We are unable to provide a precise number of cases that revealed signs of LCN nerve suffering. However, in the skin area of the thigh belonging to the LCN nerve, we can assume that hypoesthesia was present in approximately 27-28% of patients after surgery.

In almost all of these patients, there was a gradual reduction of the affected skin area and progressive alleviation of the complaints, until they disappeared or were subjectively irrelevant. This is due to the well-known compensatory process mediated by the contiguous skin innervation (femoral and genitofemoral), or due to the patient's adaptation. Over time, the patient becomes unable to pay attention to the area of hypoesthesia, which also tends to be progressively 'reduced' (a phenomenon that also occurs in other areas of orthopaedic surgery).

However, on clinical examination, we detected areas of definite hypoesthesia in the cutaneous territory of the LCN nerve in 85 cases (1.5%). On the other hand, this problem had not emerged in the patient interview and never affected the patient's favourable opinion of the clinical outcome.

Nine cases (0.2%), evaluated during the outpatient activity, presented clinical symptoms and electrophysiological data that were indeed similar to the so-called Roth's meralgia paresthesica (numbness, tingling and burning). Two were treated surgically with partial improvement. Seven cases, on the other hand, have so far required no treatment other than pharmacological, infiltrative and physiokinesitherapy, with a good clinical outcome.

Residual hypoesthesia, which is usually tolerated or not recognised by the patient, is quite different from the rarer Roth's paresthesia meralgia and in our opinion should be distinguished from it.

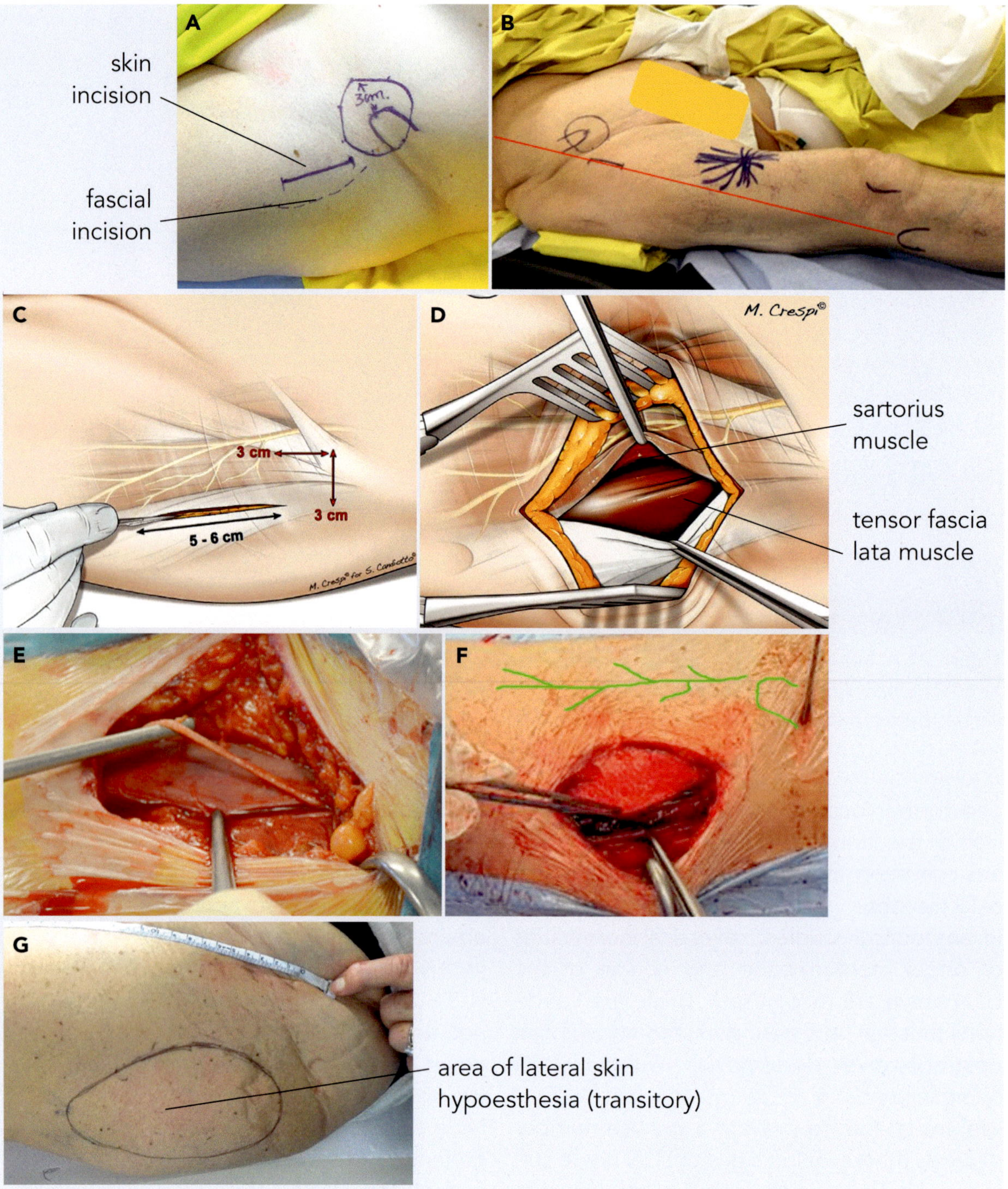

Figure 28 A) Skin incision placed 3 cm laterally and 3 cm distal to the ASIS to avoid the dangerous zone. The incision is directed towards the femoral head (B). C) Anatomical view of the skin incision and the more lateral fascial incision. The fascia is then separated from the tensor muscle and retracted, with a protective action for the FCL nerve endings. D) We show the finding of a nerve branch that can be traced back to the branches of the LCN nerve which, in this case, runs in the muscle interstitium used during surgery. E) We show how our technique involves the lateral section of the fascia lata. This is retracted medially to allow the deeper layer to be reached by passing through the muscle interstitium between sartorius and tensor. As mentioned, the medial retraction results in a reduced risk of damaging the LCN nerve branches. F) The patient three months after the minimally invasive anterior left hip replacement surgery shows an area of lateral skin hypoesthesia, without pain or functional impairment

In order to avoid injury to the LCN and its branches, or to reduce its incidence and extent, the skin incisional is made lateral and distal to the ASIS by about 3 cm and is directed towards the head of the fibula (fig. 28 A-B). Once the fascial plane is reached, we absolutely avoid laying it 'bare' with the periosteal elevator or dissecting the adipose tissue medial to the skin incision.

We usually incise the fascia lata more laterally than the line corresponding to the muscular interstice between sartorius and tensor fascia lata. Retracted (raised) and medialised the fascial flap, we locate the passage between the aforementioned muscles and deepen. We rely on the protection of the LCN nerve branches by the fascial flap interposed as protection between the medially retracted sartorius muscle and the nerve structures, thus avoiding direct injuries (lacerations, sections, etc.) (fig. 28 C-D).

We must remember that the sartorius muscle is actually wrapped in a sheath of the fascia lata ('tubularised'). Therefore, the medial retraction of the sheath that surrounds it, together with the fascial flap, tends to lift, move and protect the nerve structures.

Furthermore, we consider the suturing of the fascia lata crucial. For us, this should be done with thin stitches very close to the dieresis line. This is to avoid encapsulation of branches or terminal filaments of the nerve in the suture. However, the problems associated with the numerous variants of lateral cutaneous nerve branches must always be considered.

In such cases, the possible nerve damage belongs to the phenomena of stretching-compression of the nerve by the retractors. This is usually therefore modest, limited and transient because it is not anatomical (fig. 28E).

After an initial phase in which we used the Charnley retractor, we switched to using three different retractors (fig. 29). This ensured a more cautious, controllable and intermittent tension on the soft tissue, which we perceived as a lower risk of injury.

Other peripheral nerve injuries

We have recorded only one case of transient paresis of the femoral nerve. We believe it occurred in the extension of the limb due to the action of the medial retractor or compression of the degenerated and sclerotic Poupart inguinal ligament. No damage occurred to the sciatic nerve.

Skin suffering from the surgical incision

In 7 cases (0.16%) we encountered problems with the surgical wound. These all occurred at the beginning of each surgeon's surgical experience. The problems were as follows: areas of circumscribed necrosis of the margins, dehiscence, delayed healing. In 6 cases, we recurred to skin plastic surgery under local

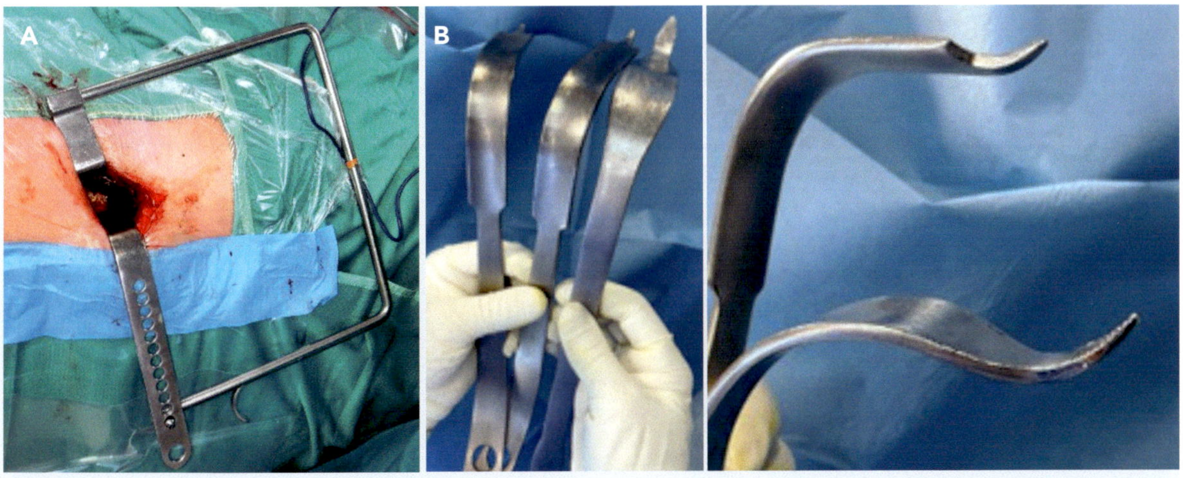

Figure 29 A) Use of the Charnley retractor in the initial phase of our AMIS experience. B) The retractors that we routinely use today allow adequate anatomical exposure and a safer and more manageable control of soft tissue 'tension'

anaesthesia, in order to avoid the long times of spontaneous healing or the risk of infectious overlap (fig. 30).

Prosthetic infection

We can count five cases of post-surgical infection (0.1%). In one case, the post-surgical haematoma, drained twice in the operating theatre, was complicated with Pseudomonas Aeruginosa infection. This episode forced a 2-stage surgical revision (explantation and spacer implantation, subsequent prosthetic revision). The other two cases were reoperated 5 months later. One case, suffering from SA, was treated with spacer implantation and definitive prosthetic revision. The other case was treated with a one-stage revision after evaluation of laboratory data (S. Hominis) and SPECT/TC. Two cases resolved with an early joint wash-out and a targeted, prolonged antibiotic therapy.

Heterotopic ossifications

Minimally invasive anterior hip prosthetic surgery is widely acknowledged to be the least at risk for the development of heterotopic ossifications, due to the less tissue damage produced. Almost all our patients also regularly undergo post-operative prophylaxis with NSAIDs for 3 weeks (excluding certain categories, such as nephropathic patients, etc.). In fact, we have so far recorded a real and strong reduction in the statistical incidence and extent of ossifications.

From a previous review of 1510 patients, 32 (0.2%) had only small epitrochanteric or paracetabular ossifications, without clinical symptoms or therapeutic needs.

Among the cases treated with the minimally invasive anterior technique, we report only one case of voluminous ossification in a male patient. This developed in the sartorius muscle and required surgical removal.

Dysmetria of the lower limbs

È un effettivo e importante problema legato alla tecnica che prevede l'utilizzo dei dispositivi di trazione: (tradurre e lasciare inserito)

In fact, the leg positioner does not allow the simple comparison of limb length using patellar or medial malleolus alignments.

In our experience great importance is given to the pre-operative assessment. We carry out an accurate measurement of the distances from the ASIS to the medial malleolus and from the umbilicus to the medial malleolus, which can provide us with the actual lower limb length, if measured correctly and compared. The lumbopelvic structure (lumbar lordosis, rotation, version or tilt of the pelvis, possible presence of homologous or heterologous lumbar scoliosis) must also be carefully studied.

A correct pre-operative planning, an accurate technical execution of the surgery and some intra-operative extemporary solutions (in our experience we usually refer to the distance between two Kirschner wires placed on the ASIS and the tibial tuberosity) greatly limit the risk of producing an excessive dysmetria (fig. 31).

However, the main commitment is to en-

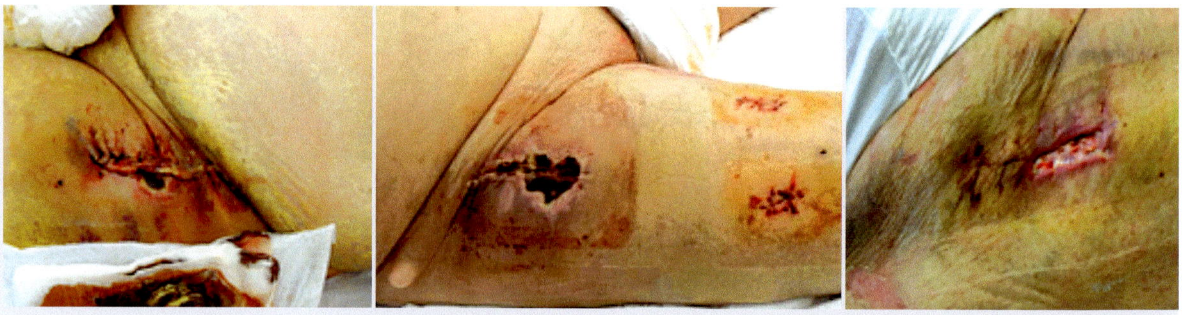

Figure 30 Example of skin suffering in the surgical scar of anterior minimally invasive approach cases. The rare cases reported by us occurred in the early stages of our minimally invasive surgical experience due to excessive traction by the retractor

sure the stability of the prosthetic implant, sometimes usefully resorting to a 'controlled' lengthening of the prosthetic modularity and, consequently, the limb.

Common clinical experience generally justifies lengthening of up to 1-1.5 cm, if they are aimed at providing secure stability for the prosthetic implant. These must, however, take place in compliance with the correct orientation of the cup and stem and without any particular modification of the offset and lever-arm. In the legal sector there is a tendency today to consider lengthening beyond 2 cm as unacceptable.

Using the traction bed technique, we observed a particular phenomenon, induced by the manoeuvres of the leg positioner. With the pelvis supported and immobilized by the perineal support, we believe that the longitudinal traction followed by the extension and external rotation of the limb can produce an abnormal pelvic tilt-rotation towards the operated side. This situation tends to persist for some time after surgery. A sort of 'pelvic embalance' that is sometimes clinically observable (inspective and palpatory) and may give the perception of a pseudo-extension of the operated limb (figs. 32-33).

In some cases, an actual elongation produced by the surgical procedure can be added to the static imbalance of the pelvis. The combined effect of these two phenomena can produce situations that are challenging to manage, both in terms of rehabilitation and patient acceptance. Furthermore, patients sometimes do not understand the variables related to their postural alterations.

Generally, however, we have noticed a resolution of the pelvic imbalance within 5 to 6 months, thanks also to the rehabilitation programme.

Other important conditions that can make it difficult to identify and realise the correct limb length are the presence of: bilateral forms of coxarthrosis, homologous or heterologous lumbar scoliosis, changes in static posture with pathological variations in the pelvis version.

In our case history, we report 3 cases (0.06%) of significant hypermetria, over 15 mm, which

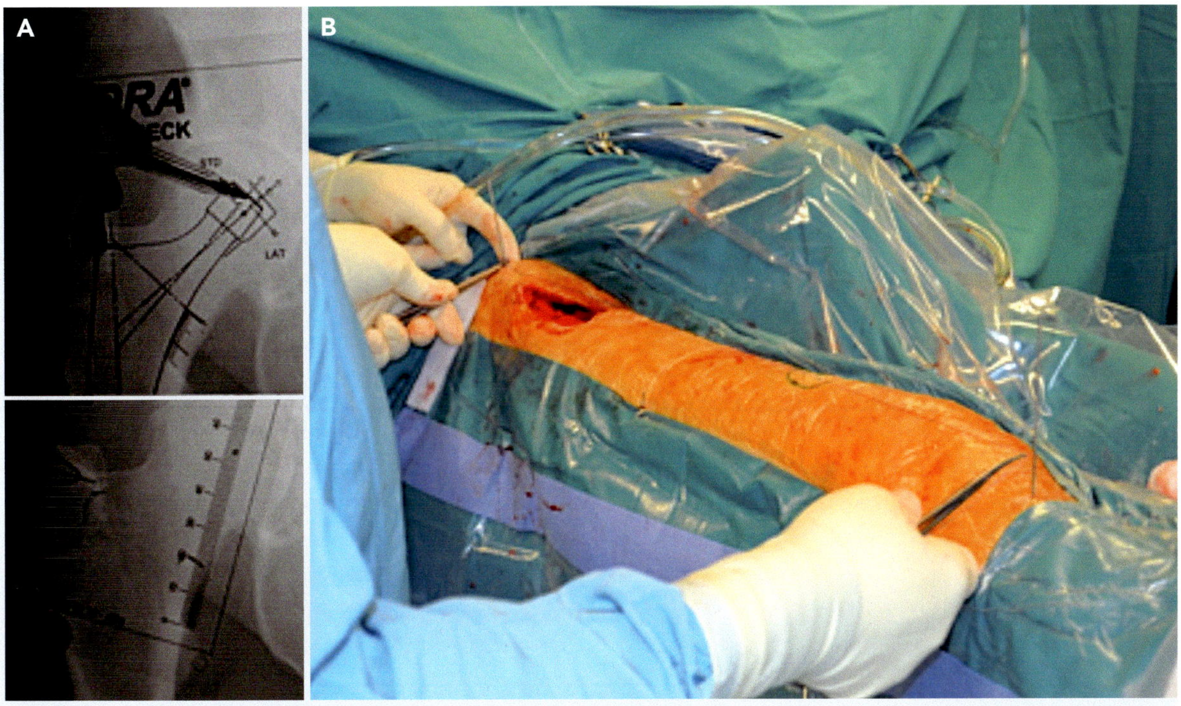

Figure 31 A) Pre-operative planning. B) Length measurement with a wire placed between two kirschner wires introduced one near the ASIS and one on the tibial tuberosity. The comparison of the measurement before the osteotomy of the femoral neck and after the insertion of the prosthesis will give us important indications about the length

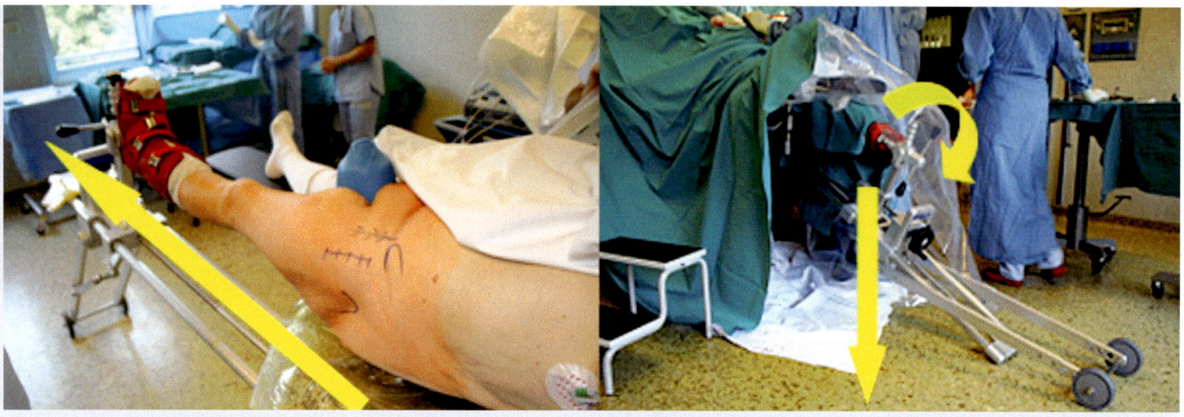

Figure 32 The externally rotated and extended limb can create the conditions for the post-operative 'pelvic embalance'. This can lead to abnormal pseudo-elongation of the limb

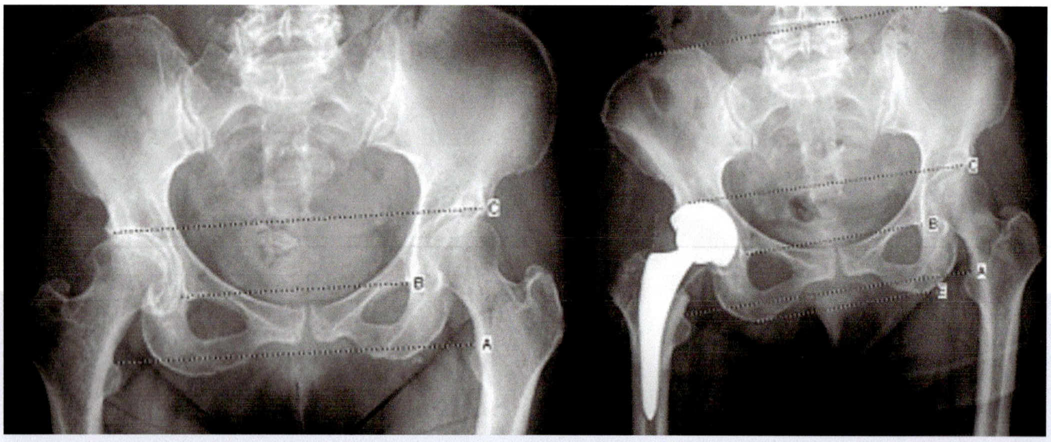

Figure 33 Example of pseudo-extension of the operated limb produced by the post-op pelvic tilt. It is usually reversible and occurs as a result of the traction, extension and external rotation of the limb produced by the leg positioner. However, the limb length assessed with the position of the radiological landmarks is correct

were not justified by necessary adaptations of the prosthetic modularity. However, these all belonged to the initial period of our surgical experience.

Considerations

The concept of minimally invasive surgery is fluid and constantly evolving. Perhaps we would find less criticism regarding meaning and use of minimally invasive surgery if we adopted C.S. Ranawat's expression of 'reduced tissue trauma surgery or RTTS'.
In this way, no one would be able to question the main objective of surgery: to perfectly execute the planned technique for the specific case and to limit the damage to the tissues involved, especially muscle tissue. This does not refer to the mere and simple length of the skin incisions, but to the constant effort to reduce the extent of the surgical approach in all anatomical planes and to decrease the surgical time. Surgical extension, surgical timing and blood loss are therefore the key concepts of the minimally invasive procedure.
At the moment, however, we still have to consider the data reported in the literature. These, evaluated only 6 to 12 months after surgery, show comparable clinical results between standard and minimally invasive techniques.
The case histories, prevailing in the literature so far, admit various advantages obtainable with modern minimally invasive techniques but still tend to emphasise a higher incidence

of complications and difficulties in performing surgery. However, the recognised advantages are: shorter hospital stay, less blood loss, easier post-operative pain control, faster rehabilitation phase and functional recovery, lower direct and indirect costs.
We believe that the literature is conditioned by a few factors. First of all, it must be considered that there are still few centres and surgeons who practice and are familiar with this complex surgery. In this context, the surgical volumes of each hospital and surgeon are a fundamental statistical element for a correct assessment of the outcomes and validity of the technique. Then, we have a shorter follow-up compared to standard techniques, as almost all cases of minimally invasive surgery were performed within the last 10 to 12 years. We can rely on a large number of patients treated with a standardised technique. Therefore, it is our firm belief that the results obtainable with minimally invasive surgery are much better than the alternatives. Moreover, the results are also particularly appreciated by patients, whose post-operative management is 'easier'. We also report a marked decrease in complications typical of hip replacement.
While we are aware of the statistical limitations, we are convinced of the advantage of minimally invasive techniques, which, however, must be acquired, matured and practised frequently. Like any surgical field, it is the frequency of surgery that contributes to the training of the surgeon and the hospital, making both safe and reliable.
The positive opinion of physiatrists and physiotherapists, who are entrusted with the recovery of our patients, is a strong encouragement. The data in their possession, compared with those of patients treated with traditional techniques, and the evidence from instrumental examinations (MRI, CT, ultrasound and gait-analyses) are a strong incentive to continue developing minimally invasive surgical procedures.
We look forward to the future and definitive affirmation of minimally invasive surgery. This will probably come in 10-15 years and, at that time, we will have many surgeons specialised in minimally invasive surgeries and a large number of these procedures. Moreover, this will be accompanied by evidence of other favourable factors, in addition to those already identified in the short- and medium-term follow-ups.
In conclusion, we hope that the appreciation for the benefits that prompted surgeons to embrace this modern surgery will grow in the future. These are a longer 'effective life' of the prosthesis, a reduction in revisions, fewer infectious complications, and a better quality of life for patients.

CHAPTER 17

Clinical management of minimally invasive hip arthroplasty

Francesco Melan

Operative Unit of Orthopaedics and Traumatology, Hospital of Adria, Rovigo, ULSS 5 Polesana/Veneto, Italy

Introduction

The minimally invasive surgical procedure for hip arthroplasty has shown many positive aspects, both for the patient and the orthopaedic surgeon. Nowadays, it is being evaluated and compared with the lateral and posterolateral approaches, which are currently the most widely used by most orthopaedists [1].
Once initial perplexity has been overcome and adequate manual dexterity has been developed (by gaining experience in specific courses or with the initial guidance of a tutor), the direct anterior mini-invasive approach will be appreciated for its considerable benefits. These will be for the patient both in the medium and in the long term and especially for 'fragile' patients [2].
The main benefits of the direct anterior approach will therefore be highlighted below. In addition, I will describe the steps that characterise the clinical management of the direct anterior approach that is usually carried out at the hospital where I practice.

Patient information

When people affected by coxarthrosis seek advice from an orthopaedic surgeon, they are often psychologically prepared for hip replacement surgery. Despite repeated medical, physical or infiltrative treatment, these patients have been suffering for months or years from pain and functional limitation due to the pathological condition.
Patients, especially younger ones, are increasingly seeking information on the Internet or from relatives or friends who have been through the same pathology. Therefore, they tend to be familiar with implant materials and often also with surgical techniques. Consequently, they are particularly interested in those techniques that offer a better analgesia and a faster and more complete recovery [1-3].
During the orthopaedic consultation, the patient asks for information on: the type of surgery recommended (general technical characteristics and duration); the most suitable surgical approach; the possibility of using homologous or autologous blood transfusions, with or without the possibility of a predeposit; the type of anaesthesia and hospital stay; the use of medical auxiliary devices (type and duration of use); the rehabilitation to be carried out in the ward or at home; the weight bearing and the recovery period.
After an initial phase in which the patient collects the information received, during the preadmission day, all the necessary information is provided again to the patient. Then, with

all the information gathered, the surgeon has to assess, together with the anaesthetist, the surgical risk and its extent.
Once this second phase has been successfully completed, we proceed to what is known as 'patient enrolment'. Once the 'therapeutic advice' has been understood and accepted, the patient can contact the surgical facility department with serenity and confidence. Then proceed with the registration to schedule the operation. It is now common practice that the patient's clinical assessment begins about a month before surgery and includes one or more days of pre-hospitalisation.

Pre-admission

Each orthopaedic department shares, with its surgical department, a protocol of blood tests, ECG, chest and pelvis X-rays, as well as an anaesthesia consultation and other specialist visits.
After this initial phase, it is appropriate to indicate autologous blood donation. This is to avoid donations of homologous blood, even if it is from a controlled and suitable donor, and to contain hospital costs for homologous transfusion centre.
Autologous donation is usually recommended up to the age of 75, but not beyond that. This is because after this age the bone marrow is not so ready to provide reticulocytes and therefore erythrocytes in a short time.
Autologous blood donation is not recommended for patients with heart disease, cerebral ischaemia or in patients with kidney or liver disease. However, the decision should be made in consultation with the physician of the blood transfusion service on the basis of our clinical indications. If autologous donation is possible, at least three 400 ml blood bags should be collected (usually once a week). The transfusion centre may freeze the whole blood or preferably separate the concentrated red blood cells from the plasma, which should be reinfused within 35 days. After this time, the preparation spontaneously haemolyses and is therefore no longer effective.
It is commonly believed that there are also economic advantages in using autologous blood. In fact, while the donation of homologous blood costs about 190 euros to a blood transfusion centre, the preparation of an autologous blood transfusion costs about 92 euros. Social cost must also be added: the homologous blood donor is entitled to a (paid) day of leave from work. Moreover, by donating and receiving your own blood, there is no risk of infectious disease transmission. Therefore, wherever possible, autologous donation is always preferred [3]. However, recent literature is unanimous in considering the anterior approach to be advantageous in terms of intra- and per-operative blood loss, thus requiring less haemotransfusion [4-5].
We consider it very useful that the patient is sent to the physiotherapy centre for a short meeting with the specialists who will care for him/her after the surgery. The physiatrist and physiotherapist will inform the patient on the recovery time, the initial, intermediate and ost-operative phases.
Patients will also be informed about the possibility of starting gait
re-education (with a walker, or with crutches either with partial or full weight-bearing, according to a schedule determined by the surgeon). Active and passive physio kinesiotherapy exercises should be explained to the patient, the gym should be shown and individual or group exercise instructions given. The patient will learn that with the anterior approach technique he/she can start a few days of physiotherapy during the hospital stay and be quickly discharged from the hospital. Patients will continue their rehabilitation at home or at the gym as an outpatient, without prolonging hospitalisation time which is always unwanted [6-7].
Following this process, the patient will feel that the person and the pathology are central to the team's efforts, and will feel reassured and protected.
At the end of this preparatory phase, which is essential for the patient's and the surgeon's confidence, after having answered all the patient's questions in a complete and detailed manner, the patient must sign an informed consent form.

Admission and preparation for surgery

The patient enters the ward in the morning the day before surgery. In the morning, on an empty stomach, blood tests are repeated. Even if they had already been carried out about a month before, they are done to check the values. A request for homologous blood bags is then made. These are necessary if the patient has not made an autologous donation, or are required in order to have them in case of need.
The nurse who receives the patient will record the patient's personal data, the pathology, the reason for admission and the side to be operated on. An identification bracelet will be put on the patient's wrist which will be kept throughout the entire period of hospitalization. This day will be dedicated to the care of hygiene and nutrition of the patient. In particular, in the afternoon an enema will be used to stimulate intestinal evacuation. This is to avoid possible complications due to the slowing of intestinal transit induced by anaesthesia and antalgic drugs (especially opioids) used during and after surgery.
After this, the patient will have a shower with disposable antiseptic soap provided by the nurse, to remove as much skin germs as possible, and clean clothes will be worn.
It will be necessary to remove any cosmetic products applied for aesthetic reasons (nail varnish or lipstick). These are a breeding ground for germs and at the same time do not allow observation of the mucous membranes or the nail bed, thus preventing assessment of the oxygenation status of the blood.
The skin of the surgical part is then depilated, i.e. all around the inguinal area, up to the pubic bone, the umbilicus and the outer and front side of the thigh. In the morning before entering the operating theatre, an iodine dressing should be applied on the surgical part (except in cases of specific allergies).
It is preferable for the patient to have a very light meal the evening before surgery. In addition, total abstention from liquids and solids from midnight onwards is mandatory to avoid vomiting during the operation.
If a patient is being treated with acetyl salicylic acid, ticlopidine, warfarin or other anticoagulants, the medication should be discontinued five to ten days before the planned date of surgery. At the same time, thromboembolic prophylaxis with low molecular weight heparin will begin and continue for about a month after surgery.
After a few days, when bleeding from the surgical site has been excluded, acetylsalicylic acid or ticlopidine can be reintroduced. In the case of warfarin, on the other hand, low molecular weight heparin can be discontinued when the INR is between 2.5 and 3 and the patient's previous treatment schedule is restored.
If a patient is not on anti-platelet or anticoagulant therapy, anti-thromboembolic prophylaxis can be started the evening before surgery with low molecular weight heparin and continued for a month, with weekly platelet monitoring (possible thrombocytopenia).
Alternatively, a new type of oral anticoagulant, such as dabigatran, apixaban or rivaroxiban, can be used. These should be taken daily after surgery, at six hours or the next day, depending on the drug used, for thirty days. There is no longer any need to monitor platelets or clotting times.
On the day of surgery, the patient will be taken to the Recovery Room for anaesthetic preparation. A large vein in the arm will be cannulated on the contralateral side of the surgery site for infusion therapy. The antibiotic will then be intravenously administered at least half an hour before surgery to ensure maximum diffusion. Finally, anaesthesia is administered.
Depending on the clinical condition and the presence of any pathologies, the anaesthetist will prefer spinal anaesthesia or general anaesthesia with a laryngeal mask or endotracheal tube.
Once all these procedures have been completed, the surgical phase begins.

The post-operative period

At the end of surgery, the patient returns to the Recovery Room. Here the patient will stay for about one to two hours, in order to have continuous and careful monitoring of vital parameters and general condition. This is to reduce the risk of complications during the immediate post-operative period.

Positioning of the operated limb

When the patient returns to the ward, the nursing staff will again assess all vital parameters and check the correct positioning of the operated limb. This should be with the leg placed on a foam valve or soft cushion, in slight flexion and abduction of the hip. This position favours the relaxation of the hip flexor muscles, relatively stretched by the surgical procedure, and has an antalgic function.

An ice pack is placed on the dressing covering the surgical wound. This is to prevent local post-operative oedema, while at the same time contributing to a mild analgesic action. Suction drainage, if present, will be checked at intervals of at least thirty to sixty minutes during the first six hours.

However, it can be said that with the minimally invasive anterior technique, blood loss is usually very small compared to the lateral and posterior approaches. The average post-operative blood loss is 150-200 cc [8].

Four to six hours after surgery, follow-up blood tests should be done with particular attention to the blood count. Autologous pre-deposit blood bags should be returned gradually in the immediate post-operative period. Plasma with coagulation factors will be administered first, then the bags of concentrated red blood cells will be alternated.

If the post-operative blood count and subsequent controls give values close to normal, the bags should be returned within 24 to 48 hours. It should be considered that the more haemodiluted the patient's blood is in the perioperative phase, the lower the risk of pulmonary thromboembolism.

The drainage should usually be removed twenty-four hours after surgery, when the suction of serum fluid has ceased. This will also reduce the risk of transdermal infection.

Post-operative pain

Using the minimally invasive anterior technique, muscles and tendons are not detached, but only pulled apart using special retractors. This minimises the algogenic stimulation of the deep planes and therefore results in less pain for the patient in the clinical practice [9].

In the immediate post-operative period, the patients' assessment of the extent of pain is surprising, although expected thanks to the care and respect for the tissues that characterises this approach.

In fact, even taking into account how sensitivity to pain is personal and therefore variable, the operated patient, using the anterior approach reported mild to moderate pain on a pre-established scale. On the contrary, when the lateral or posterolateral approach was used, the values reported were between moderate and high. In this scenario, a reduced use of analgesic drugs becomes possible, with clear advantages for the user and the healthcare provider.

Usually the application of an elastomeric pump for forty-eight hours is sufficient for pain control. This is usually prepared with four vials of tramadol or ketorolac, one vial of ranitidine and one vial of droperidol. In addition, the periprosthetic bone region can be infiltrated with abundant local anaesthetic and then an intramuscular analgesic catheter can be placed [10-11].

Although this last method is based on a known and tested protocol, and therefore feasible, it has two disadvantages which can be a source of problems for the patient.

The first is the large amount of local anaesthetic liquid needed to obtain the antalgic effect (with the consequent possible general side effects).

The second disadvantage is the antalgic catheter, which is in fact an additional direct communication, besides the drainage, between the surgical site and the outside. However, it will be up to the surgeon, before making a choice, to evaluate the anaesthetist's opinion, considering all possible implications and variables.

Post-operative mobilisation

The anterior surgical approach is performed in the anterior part of the hip joint, taking care to preserve all muscles. Thus, only the anterior capsular region is opened, which significantly reduces the risk of dislocation [12].
During the day after surgery the patient should be monitored with blood tests and control X-rays (if not already performed at the end of surgery). Any drainage that may have been applied is then removed and dressed. It is considered appropriate and useful to have the patient wear a class II compression stocking. This is an additional prevention for deep thrombosis (at the same time promoting the reabsorption of post-operative oedema). On the contralateral limb an elastic knee sock is worn.
Once these operations have been completed, the patient is helped to sit at the bedside and then moved to the chair. At this point, gradual active kinesis of the quadriceps, knee and ankle is started. With the help and assistance of the physiotherapist, the patient can, with the necessary caution, reach an upright position and take a few steps. At first the patient starts (preferably) with the use of a walker, then with two anti-brachial supports, initially allowing a minimum load for the newly operated limb. Later, upon indication of the orthopaedic surgeon, a gradually progressive weight-bearing is implemented. This type of surgical procedure, since the post-operative pain is mild or even absent, allows many patients (young or old, with a normal weight or overweight) to regain spontaneous gait and walking in a surprisingly short time. As this approach passes between the muscles, the integrity of the entire district involved is preserved. The irritation of the nerve fibres which run in the muscle belly and reach a high concentration at tendon level is therefore greatly limited [13-16]. No other surgical procedure achieves such a high percentage of people who are able to walk again almost immediately and bear weight on the operated limb without fear and with confidence. This is not to take anything away from the prosthetic implant. Its geometry is the mechanical safety that allows immediate weight-bearing. On the other hand, it is well known that the fate and durability of an implant is closely linked to good osseointegration between bone and prosthesis. In particular, it is important how this takes place, the sooner the better and especially if there is no micro-movement.
This is the reason why the patient is generally advised to apply a partial and progressive load on the operated limb. Two anti-brachial supports are indicated for twenty to thirty days, then only one for about another month on the contralateral side.
After discharge, the patient can cycle on an exercise bike or in a swimming pool and continue physical rehabilitation at home or in a gym. Statistics show and confirm that, with this surgical technique, the recovery of spontaneous walking is very quick. In addition, the period required to achieve complete rehabilitation is, in all cases, considerably shortened. This has extremely significant effects. From a personal point of view, it offers the patient a surgery with mild or no post-operative pain and a quicker return to functional activities. From a social point of view, it requires fewer days in hospital and a shorter average rehabilitation time. It therefore guarantees a much earlier return to society and to normal living and working habits, with a considerable reduction in social and health costs.

Physiotherapy

Patients undergoing mini-invasive anterior hip replacement in the department where I operate follow rehabilitation protocols shared with the physiatrist and physiotherapist.
They are the key figures in the rehabilitation process and must therefore be adequately informed of both the patient's general clinical condition and the surgical approach used. In fact, depending on the anatomical structures affected during surgery, the timing of recovery varies and is modulated.
Once the necessary assessments have been completed, the physiatrist and physiotherapist determine the rehabilitation treatment plan, which has the following objectives dur-

ing hospitalisation:

1. recovery of joint function and muscle strength;
2. recovery of autonomy in postural transitions and transfers;
3. recovery of standing and walking with anti-brachial supports;
4. recovery of the ability to move up and down stairs with the use of supports.

On the first day after surgery the suction surgical drainage is removed. After dressing and wearing the compression stocking, the patient is entrusted to the care of the physiotherapist. Who will recommend, while maintaining the supine position, exercises of:

1. active/passive assisted mobilisation of the hip and knee, never exceeding the pain limit;
2. mobilisation of the ankles;
3. gradual isometric contractions of the gluteus and quadriceps;
4. training in postural transitions, from supine to sitting;
5. training for transfers.

This phase is fundamental for the continuity of rehabilitation. In fact, through these exercises, the patient can assess the entity of the (feared) post-operative pain and identify its limit.

Thanks to the proprioceptive function and the low level of pain ensured by the surgical approach, the patient is able to immediately cooperate in the recovery and re-education action [17-19].

After successfully completing this phase, the physiotherapist encourages the patient to move from a supine position to a sitting position. Assisting the patient in this transition, the physiotherapist verifies that in this position the patient is able to efficiently control the trunk and does not experience any problem with postural adaptation. At this point the upright position can be reached.

After which, with the initial aid of a walker or two anti-brachial supports, the patient can resume walking. Finally, following the surgeon's instructions, full weight bearing on the operated limb will be allowed. At the end of this first re-education session the patient is brought back to bed with the instruction to repeat (when possible) the isometric exercises independently.

Specifically, he can continue with active or passive (with a Continuous Passive Motion device) joint mobilisation exercises of the hip, knee and ankle.

On the second day after surgery, the exercises of the first day should be repeated with the following variables:

- increase the amount of time spent sitting, encouraging knee and ankle mobilisation;
- progressive increase in walking distance (being cautious not to cause excessive fatigue to the patient).

On the third day after surgery, all the exercises previously learned should be repeated and the following exercises introduced:

- abduction and flexion-extension exercises, to be performed in a standing position and with a fixed anchorage;
- lateral movement exercises, to be performed in standing position and with a fixed anchorage.

From the fourth to the eighth day after the surgery, all previously learned exercises must be repeated and the following exercises are introduced:

- using the re-education ladder with an anti-brachial support and support of the non-engaged hand on the handrail;
- use of the re-education ladder with two anti-brachial supports;
- exercise bike with a targeted approach, using a slightly high saddle position at first and gradually moving to a suitable position in the following days.

Once discharged, the patient can continue physical rehabilitation on an outpatient basis. The main objectives of the programme are:

1. total recovery of muscle strength;
2. total recovery of joint capacity;
3. recovery of a correct walking pattern with pelvis and column in axis;
4. discontinuation of support aids;
5. the achievement of autonomy in the normal relational and working activities.

In order to establish indicative terms, it can be stated that:

- usually the rehabilitating patient uses two anti-brachial supports for three to four

weeks and switches to the use of only one (on the contralateral side) for as many weeks;
- driving a car is 'recommended' as soon as good muscle control has been restored, usually within ten to twenty days of surgery;
- work may be resumed as early as 10 days after surgery in the case of office work, or after at least two months if the patient performs heavy work;
- the return to physical activity and sport varies depending on the specific sport. Specifically: swimming, gymnastics and rehabilitation in water (preferably thermal water) can begin as soon as the surgical wound has healed; cycling can be resumed about a week after surgery; skiing, tennis and running can be resumed at least three months after surgery, being very cautious and avoiding any excessive physical stress.

Sexual activity can be resumed, with appropriate caution, as early as a few days after surgery, since the risk of dislocation linked to a possible excessive accentuation of hip flexion-abduction is not purely theoretical.

Prevention of complications

Infection

Infection prevention begins as early as three months before the surgery. This is in fact the interval that the future patient must be free of dental or other invasive procedures, such as endoscopic procedures. In fact, this type of procedure can entail a high risk of bacterial contamination in the area where the arthroplasty is implanted.

The latter, being a foreign body, ipso facto already stimulates an inflammatory response and acts as a catalyst for the proliferation of bacteria, giving rise to an actual infectious process.

Having said this, it is necessary to specify that the protocol normally used in this surgery for antibiotic prophylaxis, usually during hip arthroplasty surgery, consists of the intravenous administration of:

- two grams of first-generation cephalosporins at least half an hour before surgery begins, to promote optimal perfusion of the drug;
- one gram of first-generation cephalosporins after six hours.

The topic of prosthetic infections has become so important today that an entire chapter would not be enough to be able to adequately discuss this subject. In most cases there are protocols available to the orthopaedic surgeon that have been developed by infectious disease colleagues. However, the number of clinical variables that can make these protocols inadequate is high and, even worse, these risk factors are not always easy to identify. Inevitably, the surgeon is exposed to the unpleasant scrutiny of the medical examiner in the unfortunate event that an infectious process occurs. We therefore believe that the help of the infectious colleague is essential, who will have the complicated role of assessing the patient's 'propensity' for infection, adapting the antibiotic therapy, which is progressively becoming more and more 'custom-made'.

The surgeon, on the other hand, is responsible for the management and clinical evolution of the wound. The presence of any not reassuring alterations (reddening, presence of secretions, haematomas, etc.) must be immediately reported to the infectious disease specialist for any possible therapeutic adjustment. It should also be noted that if the patient has to undergo dental treatment and/or endoscopic procedures after the implantation of the prosthesis, a suitable antibiotic therapy is recommended to be adopted in advance in order to avoid any risk of infection.

Deep vein thrombosis

Deep vein thrombosis is another serious postoperative complication of lower limb arthroplasty. Due to the risk of pulmonary thromboembolism, it can often be fatal.

Promoted by lack of motility and/or prolonged bed rest, should be prevented with a targeted thromboprophylaxis. This should be administered continuously for a period of thirty days after surgery.

Such prophylaxis can follow two protocols:

1. low molecular weight heparin can be

started from the evening before surgery, with (at least) weekly monitoring of blood platelets in order to prevent possible but unlikely thrombocytopenia;
2. start with the new oral anticoagulants (which do not require any blood test) after surgery.

Variable pressure pumps have proved to be a very effective aid in this regard. Using a brace applied to the patient's foot and ankle, exert a gradual intermittent vascular squeeze on the sole of the foot, thus preventing the vascular stasis due to the supine position in bed. The application of this device is most useful in the first five days after the operation and in particular during the hours of rest and at night. Also, as a preventive measure, the use of a class 2 compression stocking on the operated limb and of a contralateral elastic knee-high sock is recommended. These perform a mechanical function that facilitates venous outflow and counteracts the formation of peripheral oedema.

It seems superfluous to emphasise once again how, thanks to this surgical technique, which allows rapid mobilisation of the patient, the risk of deep vein thrombosis is significantly reduced.

Dislocation of the operated hip

The minimally invasive anterior surgical approach ensures that not only the muscles and tendons are respected, but also the capsule. This is incised and then sutured or, if unavoidable, removed only anteriorly.

In this way, the periarticular structures do not suffer or are severely weakened by the surgery. All this is already a first assurance for the stability of the new joint.

However, there are several ways of proceeding and precautions to be adopted in order to achieve the objective of 'stability' of the joint, such as:

1. the cup must be implanted with due inclination (40-50°) and anteversion (about 15°), and the stem with 10/15° anteversion;
2. the search for the best possible equal limb length. In fact, sometimes, in order to obtain a good joint congruence and therefore a better stability of the hip it is inevitable to bend to the necessity of accepting a small difference;
3. begin mobilisation of the limb as early as possible so that the patient can maintain his motor pattern. He will then be facilitated in recovering autonomy in transferring (from bed to chair, from standing to sitting and vice versa) and walking.
4. virtuous behaviour during the first month after surgery:
   - avoid hip flexion beyond 90°;
   - limit flexion-abduction to 45° and forced external rotation;
   - use a low cushion in the sitting position, taking care to occupy the front part of the chair;
   - avoid bending the lower limbs (to pick up objects from the floor, etc.) which can force hip flexion;
   - attach a riser to the toilet;
   - use the shower rather than the bath for personal hygiene;
   - use a long shoehorn.

Heterotopic ossifications

Heterotopic periarticular ossification (HO) is a feared complication and is characterised by a process of bone formation by tissue metaplasia. It is not calcifications, but new bone tissue that can cause pain and severe joint functional limitations. In hip replacement surgery, this is known to occur in 5 to 20% of hip replacements performed with a lateral or posterior approach.

The cause of their origin is debated. To date it seems to be confirmed that the greater the surgical damage to the musculotendinous structures together with the dispersion of bone sawdust in the damaged tissues, therefore with considerable bleeding, the higher the possibility of HO forming.

With the anterior approach, trauma and bleeding are significantly lower than with other surgical approaches. In fact, the percentage of heterotopic ossifications drops to 3-5% on average.

However, medical treatment is recommended to prevent heterotopic ossifications, although there are conflicting opinions in the literature. Non-steroidal anti-inflammatory drugs can be used for one month after surgery, such as ketoprofen or indomethacin.

Follow-ups

The patient usually returns for an outpatient follow-up after about two months with an X-ray of the pelvis and the operated hip in two projections. In addition, the patient will have an X-ray of the lumbosacral spine at least once to analyse any severe pathologies and deformities that may affect walking.
If everything goes according to the planned recovery programme, the removal of elastic stockings and crutches is authorised (very often patients wear crutches as prescribed but already confess to not using them much because of the rapid recovery).
All necessary advice should be given for work and physical activity and the desired resumption of all other physical functions.
Further radiographic and clinical examinations are usually scheduled after six months and then every one to two years at the latest.

Conclusions

After the short learning phase of the minimally invasive anterior hip approach, after previous experience with the direct lateral or posterolateral approach, the surgeon is always favourably surprised by the advantages of the anterior approach. He appreciates the anatomical path between the muscle units, the good anatomical view of both the cup and the femur despite the small incision, even less than eight-to-ten centimetres. He also enjoys the absolute respect of the muscular structures, the minimal blood loss and the certainty of applying a mechanically stable prosthesis.
From a clinical point of view, the reduced severity of pain reported by the patient stands out. This enables the patient to be mobilised at an early stage and encourages a rapid recovery of all his/her functions.
The early discharge from the hospital, compared to other surgical approaches, to be able to return earlier to social and working life and the ability to drive a car and to be quickly independent, are all factors that are appreciated by the patient and gratify the daily work of the orthopaedic surgeon.

Bibliography

1. Chechik O, Khashan M, Lador R, Salai M, Amar E. Surgical approach and prosthesis fixation in hip arthroplasty world wide. Arch Orthop Trauma Surg. 2013;133(11):1595-1600.
2. Barrett WP, Turner SE, Leopold JP. Prospective randomized study of direct anterior vs postero-lateral approach for total hip arthroplasty. J Arthroplasty. 2013;28(9):1634-1638.
3. Huo MH, Parvizi J, Gilbert NF. What's new in hip arthroplasty. J Bone Joint Surg Am. 2006;88(9):2100-2113.
4. Matta JM, Shahrdar C, Ferguson T. Single-incision anterior approach for total hip arthroplasty on an orthopaedic table. Clin Orthop Relat Res. 2005;441:115-124.
5. Laude F et al. Artroplastie totale de la hanche par vie antérieure et son évolution mini-invasive. EMC. 2004,44-667-B.
6. Istituto Superiore di Sanità. Atti del Convegno Nazionale Buon Uso del Sangue, Roma, 2003, Rapporti ISTISAN 04/10, Available at: http//www.iss.it
7. Laffosse JM, Chiron P, Tricoire JL, Giordano G, Molinier F, Puget J. Prospective and comparative study of minimally invasive posterior approach versus standard posterior approach in total hip replacement. Rev Chir Orthop Reparatrice Appar Mot. 2007;93(3):228-237.
8. Wojciechowski P, Kusz D, Kopeć K, Borowski M. Minimally invasive approaches in total hip arthroplasty. Ortop Traumatol Rehabil. 2007;9(1):1-7.
9. Rachbauer F. Minimally invasive total hip arthroplasty. Anterior approach. Orthopade. 2006;35(7):723-729.
10. Siguier T, Siguier M, Brumpt B. Mini-incision anterior approach does not increase dislocation rate: a study of 1037 total hip replacements. Clin Orthop Relat Res. 2004;(426):164-173.
11. Rachbauer F, Krismer M. Minimally invasive total hip arthroplasty via direct anterior approach. Oper Orthop Traumatol. 2008;20(3):239-251.
12. Tang R, Evans H, Chaput A, Kim C. Multimodal analgesia for hip arthroplasty. Orthop Clin North

Am. 2009;40(3):377-387.
13. Kerr DR, Kohan L. Local infiltration analgesia: a technique for the control of acute postoperative pain following knee and hip surgery: a case study of 325 patients. Acta Orthop. 2008;79(2):174-183.
14. Kuchálik J, Granath B, Ljunggren A, Magnuson A, Lundin A, Gupta A. Postoperative pain relief after total hip arthroplasty: a randomized, double-blind comparison between intrathecal morphine and local infiltration analgesia. Br J Anaesth. 2013;111(5):793-799.
15. Bush JB, Wilson MR. Dislocation after hip hemiarthroplasty: anterior versus posterior capsular approach. Orthopedics. 2007;30(2):138-144.
16. Dora C. MRI imaging of the abductor tendons and muscles after total hip replacement in asymptomatic and symptomatic patients. EFORT, 2007.
17. Dora C. Der anteriore Zugang fur die minimal-invasive HTEP. Leading Opinions, 2006.
18. Dora C, Kalberer F. Muscular damage after total hip arthroplasty: conventional versus minimally invasive anterior approach. AOA 2008, Australia, Hobart.
19. Pfirrmann CW, Notzli HP, Dora C, Hodler J, Zanetti M. Abductor tendons and muscles assessed at MR imaging after total hip arthroplasty in asymptomatic and symptomatic patients. Radiology. 2005;235(3):969-976.
20. Zambelli M. Protocollo riabilitativo nell'artroprotesi d'anca per via anteriore. Usl 19, Veneto.
21. Rossi. Protocollo riabilitativo dopo impianto di artroprotesi d'anca (accesso anteriore). Usl di Ferrara, Emilia Romagna.
22. Lesch DC, Yerasimides JG, Brosky JA Jr. Rehabilitation following anterior approach total hip arthroplasty in a 49-year-old female: a case report. Physiother Theory Pract. 2010;26(5):334-341.

Rehabilitation after minimally invasive hip arthroplasty

Alessandro Giovannini, Giuseppe Necci, Lucia Coppola

Rehabilitation and Functional Recovery Department, S. Antonio Hospital, Padua, Italy

Introduction

In recent decades, modern surgery has undergone a great technological development of materials and medical instruments. This has led to the successful experimentation of new surgical techniques that make procedures not only more precise and safer, but also less traumatic. Major orthopaedic surgery, and at the same time prosthetic surgery, has become increasingly sensitive to patients' needs in terms of comfort, complications, pain and functional recovery. Minimally invasive anterior surgical approach for hip arthroplasty, on the one hand, assures respect for the anatomical structures, and therefore less intra- and peri-operative risks for the patient, and, on the other hand, a faster and less demanding recovery and rehabilitation period.

The small size surgical wound (7-8 cm), the almost or complete absence of pain in the immediate post-operative period, the early weight-bearing and the preservation of anatomical structures are determining factors for proceeding with more intensive rehabilitation programmes. This allows a faster return to functional recovery and work activity. There are no standard rehabilitation protocols that can be adapted to every patient. Illustrated below are some work models divided into different phases and periods, which can be modified at any time, in order to make the rehabilitation project 'personalised' for each individual, always respecting the biological healing times.

Clinical assessment

For the physiatrist, the physical examination is certainly the most important and decisive moment in defining a patient's rehabilitation project. The clinical evaluation must be comprehensive and detailed, highlighting the individual's current problems. It has the aim of defining priorities and specificity of objectives, always respecting the patient's general condition and physiological recovery times.

The physiatrist's physical assessment includes the following evaluations.

Muscle strength. The MRC (Medical Research Council) scale is used, inviting the patient to make active movements against the resistance from the examiner (score from 0 to 5).

ROM (range of motion). Involves carrying out active and passive movements in all planes.

Sensitivity. Evaluates the superficial tactile, thermal and pain sensitivity of the limbs, inviting the patient to make a comparison and highlight any differences.

ROT. Superficial (plantar) and deep (bi-tricipi-

FIM: Functional Independence Measure

Personal care
1. Feeding
2. Tidying up
3. Washing
4. Dressing, waist up
5. Dressing, waist down
6. Perineal hygiene

Sphincter control
7. Bladder
8. Bowel movement

Mobility (Transfers)
9. Bed - chair - wheelchair
10. Toilet
11. Bathtub or shower

Locomotion
12. Walk - wheelchair
13. Stairs

Communication
14. Understanding
15. Expression

Cognitive-relational skills
16. Relationship with others
17. Problem solving
18. Memory

Scoring levels
7. Complete self-sufficiency
6. Self-sufficiency with adaptations/ aids
5. Supervision/Adaptations
4. Minimal assistance
3. Moderate care
2. Intensive care
1. Full assistance

Figure 1 FIM Rating Scale

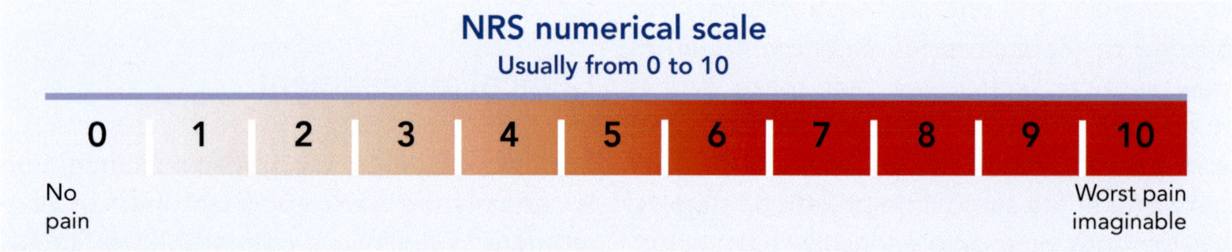

Figure 2 NRS pain scale

tal, patellar, achilleas, mid-plantar) osteo-tendon reflexes.

Lower limbs heterometries. Highlighting any differences in lower limb length by measuring the umbilicus-internal malleolus distance and ASIS-internal malleolus distance.

Walking. Dynamic assessment of the patient while walking with supports, focusing on possible postural defects and motor deficits.

A number of useful evaluation scales are available to the physiatrist, for quantifying pain, health, walking, autonomy and thus defining the Outcomes of rehabilitation treatment. After total hip arthroplasty the most commonly used assessment scales are the following.

FIM (Functional Independence Measure). Examines various activities of daily life (fig. 1) and the score achieved (from 0 to 126) provides an index of the severity of disability.

Barthel. used to quantify the patient's abilities in ADLs through the achievement of a score from 0 to 100.

NRS (Numerical Rating Scale). Quantifies the patient's pain with a numerical scale from 0 to 10 (fig. 2).

Harris Hip Score. Assesses specific items of the coxo-femoral joint (pain, ROM, gait) used to quantify the patient's abilities with a maximum score of 100.

Womac (Western Ontario and McMaster Universities Osteoarthritis Index). Takes into account different aspects related to the coxo-femoral joint (stiffness, pain, function, activities of daily living) with 24 items and a score from 0 to 96.

10-meter Timed Walk test. Assessment of unassisted walking on a 10-meter course; the time taken to walk the central 6 meters, not including acceleration and deceleration, is measured.

Timed up and go test (TUG). Dynamic assessment of mobility and balance; the time taken for the patient to get up from the chair, walk 3 metres, turn around, return to the chair and sit down is measured.

Walking Handicap Scale (Perry and Garrett). A 6-item rating scale that measures walking abilities in the home and in social environment.

Individual rehabilitation project

After the initial clinical assessment, it is time to define the specific rehabilitation plan for the patient undergoing surgery. The individual rehabilitation project (PRI) aims to achieve autonomy in daily life activities, return to home and return to work. The interdisciplinary rehabilitation team (physiatrist, physiotherapists, occupational therapist, operators, nurses) has the task of developing the project synergistically. It will therefore have to define the treatment objectives, the modalities, the most appropriate setting and the necessary timeframe, taking into account the expectations of the patient and family members.

Pre-operative phase

In the rehabilitation project for patients suffering from coxarthrosis, the preparation phase for surgery is becoming increasingly important. It is a more or less long and demanding period aimed at improving the physical condition of the individual. It also instructs the patient on the steps to be taken. In this phase, the patient has important functional limitations and pain is the main element that characterises his physical condition. The objectives to be achieved are related to:

- pain control;
- recovery and maintenance of muscle strength;
- increased cardio-respiratory performance;
- recovery of correct gait pattern and training in the use of walking aids;
- reduction of muscle contractures and bad postures (stretching exercises).

These steps can be achieved through individual physiotherapy programmes in the gym, or, if possible, through repeated cycles of hydrokinesiotherapy, even in groups. Therapeutic exercise in water, at this stage, best meets the needs of the patient with functional limitations. The properties of water, in fact, guarantee the patient a benefit in terms of less stress exerted on the joints, which means a reduction in pain. At the same time, muscle work in water leads to an increased muscle tone and trophism and an increase in cardio-respiratory performance.

In addition to this surgery preparation plan, it is useful to distribute an information leaflet to patients. This should describe the characteristics of the prosthesis and the surgery, as well as what will happen in the days following the operation.

At the end of this initial phase, the patient is ready to face surgery in the best psycho-physical conditions, so as to reduce the risk of complications and make the post-operative rehabilitation period faster and less burdensome.

Post-operative phase

Phase 1: 1st-3rd day

On the first day after surgery the patient lies in bed in supine decubitus with surgical drainage and bladder catheter (fig. 3). At this time the physiotherapist makes the first assessment of the patient and begins to take care of him/her. The AMIS surgical technique, unlike the traditional 'OPEN' approaches, allows early mobilisation of the limb in the first three

post-operative days and the achievement of an upright position with a protected weight-bearing. This is also allowed by the greater comfort and well-being perceived by the patient, essentially due to the partial or complete absence of pain and reduced blood loss.
In this phase we essentially work on:
- activation of the muscle pump of the lower limbs with assisted active foot mobilisation exercises;
- ROM recovery with gradual passive and active assisted mobilisation of the operated limb with flexion-extension exercises of the operated knee and hip (initially only passive, then active-assisted); recovery of a better hip proprioception;
- muscle strengthening with isometric exercises of the quadriceps muscle and the gluteus maximus/medius (fig. 4);
- rehabilitation of postural transitions and sitting position according to anti-luxation rules;
- rehabilitation to stand with early and protected loading (after removal of drains) with a walker or two crutches with forearm support in a three-phases scheme of the first load transfer exercises.

Prevention of post-operative complications

Patients undergoing hip arthroplasty, as with other surgical procedures, have a high

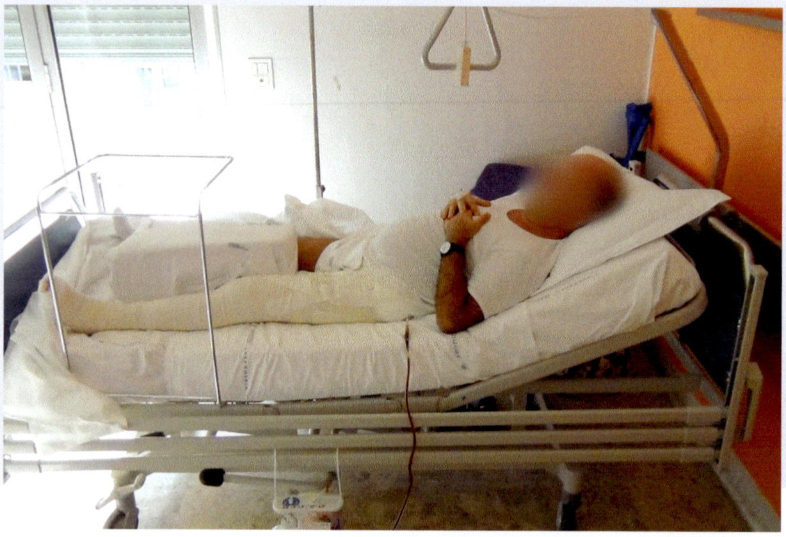

Figure 3 First post-operative day: patient supine with spreading wedge, compression bandage on the operated limb and surgical drain in place

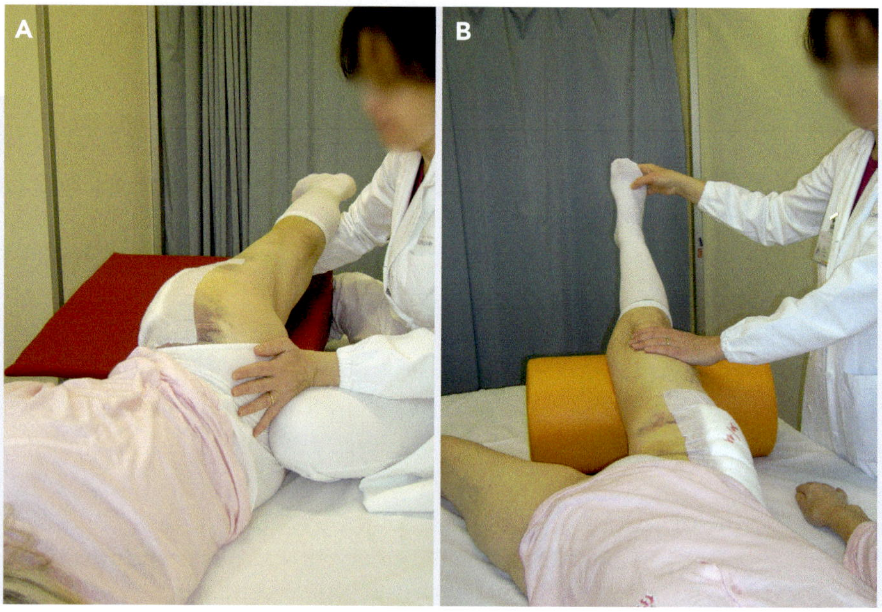

Figure 4 Third post-operative day: the patient performs lateral decubitus assisted exercises for strengthening the abductor muscles (A) and supine decubitus exercises for the quadriceps femoris (B)

risk of developing more or less severe post-operative complications. Among these, we will briefly review the most common complications and the adopted prevention instruments.

Deep vein thrombosis

Deep vein thrombosis (DVT) is the most feared complication. This consists of the formation of small blood clots in the deep venous system of the lower limbs, with serious consequences such as post-phlebitis syndrome and pulmonary embolism. Allurement, prolonged immobilisation, old age, varicose veins, surgery, coagulopathies, etc. are all predisposing factors to the onset of DVT.

Non-specific clinical signs are pain, inflammation, skin redness, swelling. When DVT is suspected, the diagnosis is instrumental by performing ultrasonography (B-mode ultrasound, duplex scanning, echocolordoppler) of the lower limbs, which is the first choice, non-invasive and low-cost method. Our clinical experience shows that the incidence of DVT in patients undergoing AMIS hip arthroplasty is significantly reduced compared to conventional surgical approaches. This is due not only to the preventive mechanisms of deep vein thrombosis consisting of drug therapy (low molecular weight heparins) and the use of elastic stockings with graduated compression or intermittent pneumatic compression, but also to the early mobilisation of the patient.

Oedema

Post-operative low limb oedema can complicate and influence the patient's normal rehabilitation. Pain, swelling and muscle tension can lead to a significant functional limitation for the individual, which sometimes affects the possibility of doing physiotherapy. Once a vascular problem has been excluded, the patient can have a gentle lymphatic drainage of the lower limbs or alternatively the application of neuromuscular taping with draining action (fig. 5).

Dislocation of the prosthesis

The dislocation of the prosthesis consists in the displacement of the prosthetic head outside the cup. This is a less frequent complication with the minimally invasive technique, but it should always be prevented by taking preventive measures for at least 6 weeks after implantation of the prosthesis. In this regard, the patient must strictly follow certain rules of postural hygiene and behaviour:

- do not extend and extra-rotate the hip at the same time (movement at high risk of dislocation for AMIS prostheses);
- do not cross your legs;
- do not flex the hip or trunk more than 90°;
- stand on your side only with a pillow be-

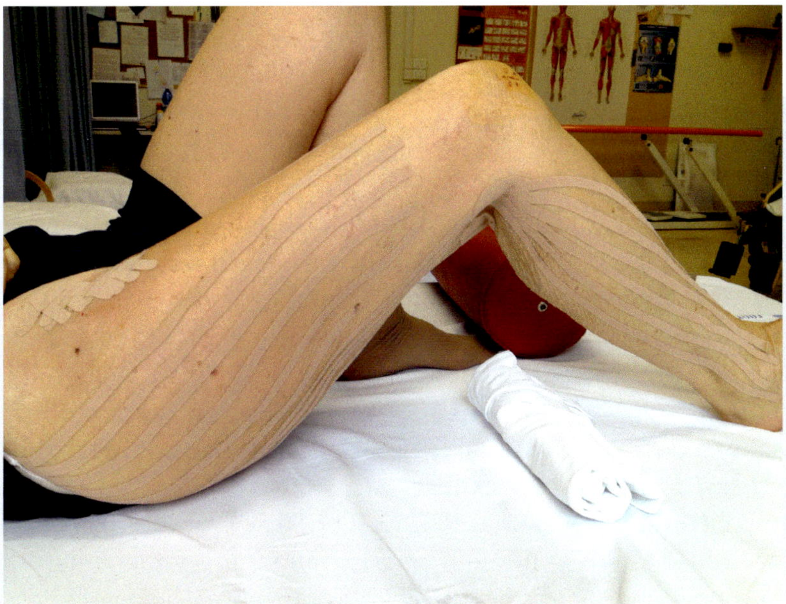

Figure 5
Application of neuromuscular taping for oedema in the lower limb

tween your legs;
- do not make any twisting movements when changing direction.

Pain control

The main objective of minimally invasive surgery is to reduce pain while preserving the muscular anatomy. Based on the assumption that the patient is fine as long as he/she does not feel any pain, a series of precautions must be taken from the immediate post-operative period in order to attenuate if not eliminate pain symptoms. The physiatrist therapies are essentially pharmacological and physical treatment.

Pharmacological treatment is based on the use of different drugs depending on the extent of the pain. In mild pain, paracetamol and NSAIDs (drugs almost always used for this type of intervention) are used. In moderate pain a weak opioid (codeine and tramadol) may be added. In severe pain (usually cancer-related), strong opioids (morphine and the like) are recommended.

There are several physical therapies available for post-operative pain, and they include the following treatments.

Magnetotherapy. It is an electromagnetic field generated by a solenoid crossed by an electric current which produces a pain-relieving effect on the human body due to its anti-edematous and anti-inflammatory action.

Laser therapy. Exploits the effects of the energy generated by laser light sources to produce a biostimulating effect on the tissues with an analgesic, antiphlogistic and anti-edematous action.

Electrotherapy. Different types of current can be used depending on the characteristics of the pain and the concerned part. TENS (mono-biphasic rectangular wave or spike) is generally used for superficial areas and uses the Gate control system (activation of inhibitory interneurons by selective stimulation of A-beta fibres) producing a rapid but short-lasting analgesic effect. Interferential currents (low frequency biphasic) stimulate receptors deeper that act by activating the endorphin system and blocking the conduction of A-delta and C-fibres.

Phase 2: day 4-14

Once the patient has been clinically and surgically stabilized (removal of drains and bladder catheter, post-operative X-ray, normalised blood chemistry parameters), is transferred to the Rehabilitation Department. Here he can continue with intensive rehabilitation treatment, or he can go to outpatient rehabilitation centres. In the first session, a functional assessment is performed by the physiotherapist, who identifies the rehabilitation needs of the specific patient.

In this phase the programme includes:
- recovery of active motility; reaching the zero position of the hip to improve the support and detachment phase of gait;
- reduction of any muscular contractures or tensions through therapeutic cognitive exercises (ETC of 1 degree);
- restoration of a physiological lumbopelvic rhythm;
- muscle strengthening with isometric exercises of the quadriceps femoris muscle, gluteus, ischio-crural, adductor and abductor muscles of the thigh with exercises in supine position, sitting and in lateral decubitus with open kinetic chain;
- stretching of muscle chains;
- continuation of load transfer exercises using one or two scales and simulated stepping; therapeutic exercises to integrate the new joint into the movement, which is also made up of sensations, and feelings. Movement, which is also made up of sensations, perception and body image;
- gait training with protected weight-bearing;
- occupational therapy for the recovery of autonomy in ADLs (dressing/undressing activities, personal hygiene, safe transfers);
- reduction of post-operative oedema with manual lymph drainage and application of neuromuscular taping;
- stair ascent/descent training with aids.

At the end of this period, the patient should be able to carry out the main daily life ac-

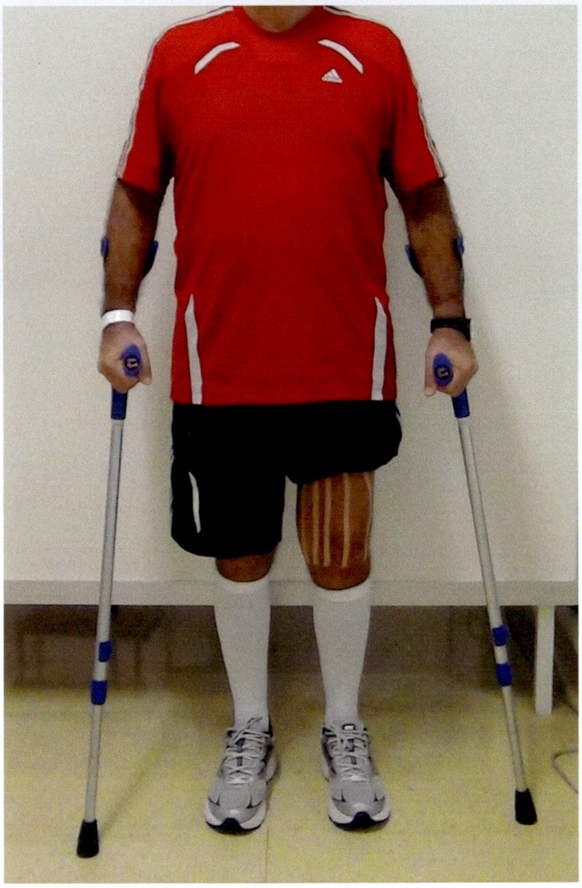

Figure 6 The patient on the fourth post-operative day walks with two anti-brachial crutches

tivities independently. The ROM of the operated hip has to be at least 90° in flexion and 30° in abduction, and the patient must have recovered a good muscles tone-trophism of the lower limbs.

Surgical scar treatment

In our clinical routine practice, it is important to pay particular attention to the surgical scar after the stitch removal. Although there is still no scientific evidence on the influence of the scar on the patient's posture and functional limitations, our physiotherapy treatment is aimed at the prevention and treatment of scar adhesions on the tissues underlying the wound. The presence of skin retraction, redness, oedema, skin hypertrophy on the scar or adjacent skin can cause pain, myofascial tension and thus affect physiotherapy treatment. In our experience it is useful to start with a manual myofascial release treatment for mobilisation of the surgical scar. Then we proceed with the application of neuromuscular taping in a herringbone pattern (Fig. 7). Basically, it involves applying a partially elastic tape, bridging the suture to stimulate the physiological repair processes. The technique recommended by experts is the application of small strips overlapping at a 45° angle, with a slight tension right at wound level. The tape is generally well tolerated, stays in place for a few days, and is unaffected by contact or immersion in water. Clinical results are encouraging, although no efficacy studies are available. Patients' satisfaction is, however, definitely high, because this practice is perceived as a special care for the aesthetic aspect as well.

Phase 3: day 15-30

After two weeks of treatment in the Department of Physical Medicine and Rehabilitation, the patient can be discharged from hospital and continue with an extensive rehabilitation programme on an outpatient basis. At this stage, if there are no complications or contraindications (surgical wounds, urinary

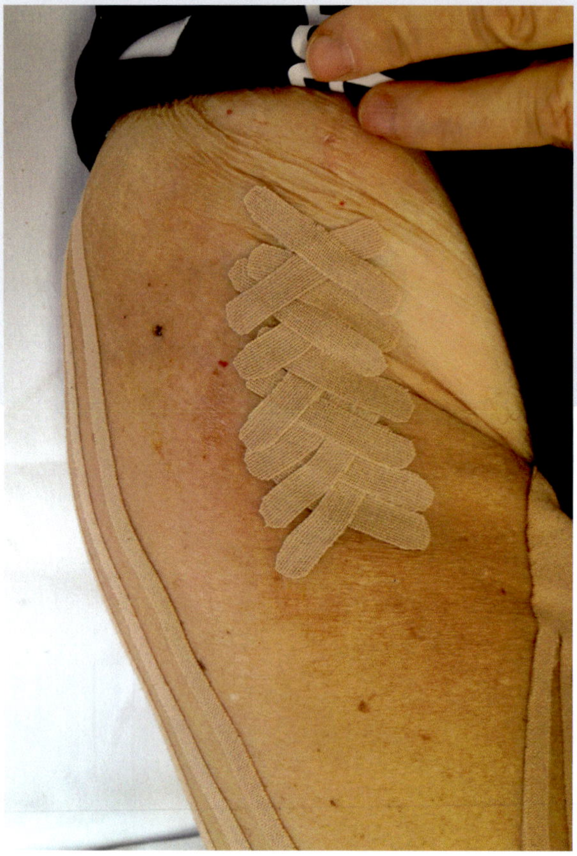

Figure 7
Treatment of the surgical scar with neuromuscular taping

tract infections, skin infections, etc.) a hydro-kinesiotherapy course may be continued for the functional recovery of the operated limb. Alternatively, it is always advisable, after discharge from hospital, to continue the current rehabilitation programme in a physiotherapy centre. At this point it is still necessary to insist on certain objectives:

- recovery of hip ROM through active, passive and assisted mobilisation exercises. Increasingly complex therapeutic exercises to integrate the new joint into the physiological gesture, once sensations, perceptions and body image have changed;
- muscle strengthening of the lower limb by continuing with isometric, counter-resistance (using balls and cushions) and closed kinetic chain exercises;
- proprioceptive training, walking and ascending/descending stairs with aids, until the gradual abandonment of a crutch;
- stretching of the thigh muscles, in particular the anterior region (tensor fascia lata, quadriceps femoris and sartorius) and medial region (adductor muscles), both in lateral and prone decubitus;
- occupational therapy: adapting spaces at home by eliminating all obstacles (carpets, chairs, toys, etc.) that may make walking with aids difficult; adapting the bathroom to make hygiene actions easier and safer (toilet lifts, grab rails, accessible shower, etc.); using aids for getting dressed and undressed (long-handled pliers, sock stretchers, etc.).

Hydro-kinesiotherapy

Patients who have undergone or are undergoing hip replacement surgery can greatly benefit from hydro-kinesiotherapy sessions and movement guided by a physiotherapist in a therapeutic pool (fig. 8). The characteristics of the water useful for therapeutic purposes are temperature, hydrostatic pressure, weightlessness and turbulence. A brief illustration of these aspects follows.

Temperature. The temperature of the therapy pool is usually between 33° C and 35° C, up to 37° C in some thermal pools. At these temperatures, blood flow increases and the body more easily eliminates catabolites produced in the tissues in response to pain. The high temperature also induces muscle relaxation. Even hot, moving water in contact with the skin seems to interfere with the transmission of the pain impulse by acting on the surface mechanoreceptors.

Hydrostatic pressure. Hydrostatic pressure at depth is greater than venous pressure, specifically water exerts a pressure of 73.49 mmHg per metre of depth. This pressure has a squeezing effect on peripheral oedemas, e.g. on the lower limbs of hip replacement patients.

Absence of gravity. This is due to Archimedes' thrust. The body is thus lighter the deeper it is immersed. Reducing, as it does, the gravitational forces on the joints removes the load stress that is the primary cause of pain in hip arthrosis. Every movement, even after the operation, becomes easier if performed slowly and in deep water (fig. 9).

Water turbulence. During movement in water, unlike in air, there is a change in flow resistance. This is determined both by the friction encountered by the body itself against the fluid and by the so-called wake effect. In water physiotherapy, this phenomenon called turbulence is exploited to create resistance to movement and, therefore, achieve greater muscular effort.

Stage 4: 2-3 months after surgery

Two months after surgery it is assumed that the prosthesis is well integrated into the bone and the patient generally undergoes orthopaedic and X-ray follow-up. If the patient has not had any particular problems during this period and the orthopaedic surgeon approves, the last phase of rehabilitation can begin. This consists of:

- progressive suspension of crutches with gait correction and increase in walking time;
- recovery of hip ROM beyond 90° of flexion;
- muscle strengthening by insisting on exercises against resistance and using elastic bands;
- stabilometric platform for re-learning a better response to imbalance and proprioception;
- muscle stretching exercises.

In general, a normal or almost normal social and working life can be resumed after 3 months following the operation, even if some activities and sports take longer. In any case, it is advisable to maintain good muscle tone over time, even only through moderate physical activity (walking, light jogging, cycling, etc.) and to control body weight.

Medical check-ups or physiotherapy treatments at intervals serve to monitor the evolution of the clinical condition. They are also intended to strengthen the health care process, which we recognise as patient educa-

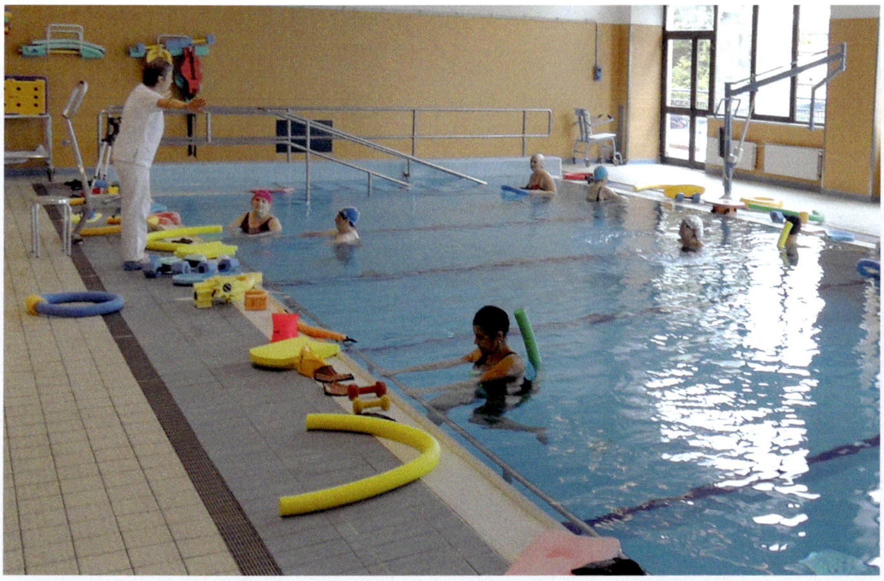

Figure 8
Group hydrokinesiotherapy session in a therapeutic pool

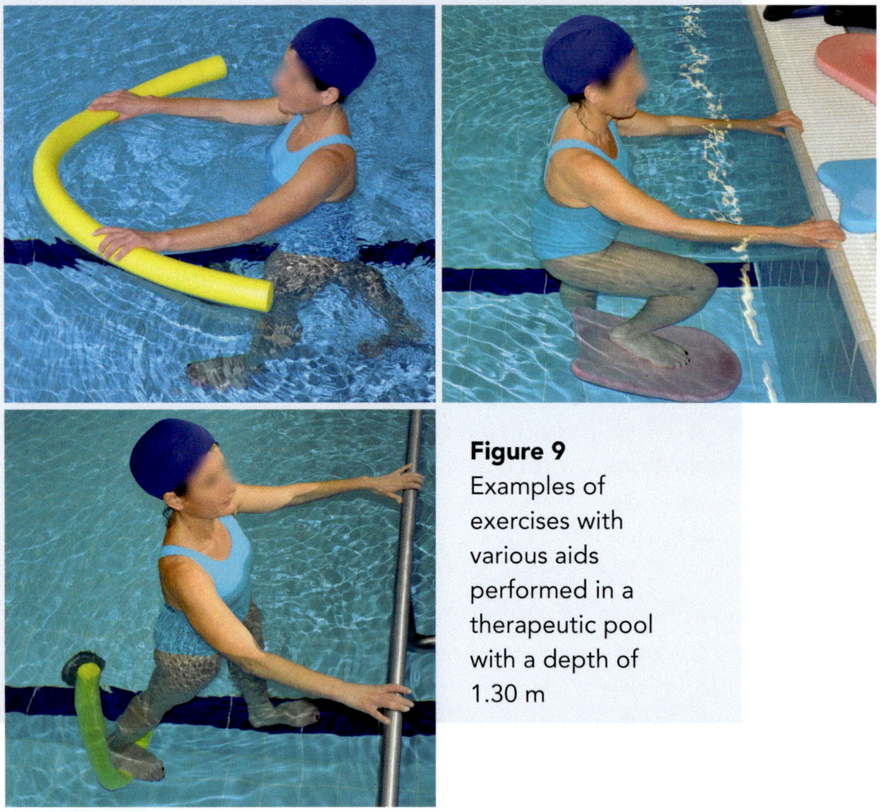

Figure 9
Examples of exercises with various aids performed in a therapeutic pool with a depth of 1.30 m

tion. This is the long-term key to the success of an integrated approach between surgical and rehabilitation teams.

Bibliography

1. Nilsdotter A, Bremander A. Measures of hip function and symptoms: Harris Hip Score (HHS), Hip Disability and Osteoarthritis Outcome Score (HOOS), Oxford Hip Score (OHS), Lequesne Index of Severity for Osteoarthritis of the Hip (LISOH), and American Academy of Orthopedic Surgeons (AAOS) Hip and Knee Questionnaire. Arthritis Care Res (Hoboken). 2011;63 Suppl 11:S200-S207.
2. Barrois B, Gouin F, Ribinik P, Revel M, Rannou F; Société Française de Médecine Physique et Réadaptation (Sofmer). What is the interest of rehabilitation in physical medicine and functional rehabilitation ward after total hip arthroplasty? Elaboration of french clinical practice guidelines. Ann Readapt Med Phys. 2007;50(8):700-699.
3. Berger RA, Jacobs JJ, Meneghini RM, Della Valle C, et al. Rapid rehabilitation and recovery with minimally invasive total hip arthroplasty. Clin Orthop Relat Res. 2004;(429):239-247.
4. Boni A, Coppola L, Costa V, Candiotto S, Giovannini A. Riabilitazione nelle protesi d'anca applicata con tecnica AMIS: riflessioni. 42° Congresso OTODI, 2011, Milano.
5. Blow D. Taping neuromuscolare dalla teoria alla pratica. Edi Ermes, 2012, Milano.
6. Di Monaco M, et al. Rehabilitation after total hip artroplasty: a systematic review of controlled trials on physical exercise programs, Eur J Phys Rehabil Med, 2009, 45 (3):303 17.
7. Giaquinto S, et al. Hydrotherapy after total hip arthroplasty: a follow-up study. Arch Gerontol Geriatr. 2010;50(1):92-95.
8. Giovannini A, Boni A, Coppola L, Costa V, Candiotto S. Artroprotesi d'anca con accesso anteriore AMIS: risultati di uno studio retrospettivo di un focus group sul trattamento differenziale rispetto alle protesi con accesso laterale. MR Giornale italiano di Medicina Riabilitativa. 2011, 25 (suppl. 1 to nr. 5).
9. Hol AM, et al. Partial versus unrestricted weight bearing after an uncemented femoral stem in total hip arthroplasty: recommendation of a concise rehabilitation protocol from a systematic review of the literature. Arch Orthop Trauma Surg. 2010;130(4):547-555.
10. Ibrahim MS, et al. Peri-operative interventions producing better functional outcomes and enhanced recovery following total hip and knee

arthroplasty: an evidence-based review. BMC Med. 2013;11:37.
11. Jung J, Anagnostakos K, Kohn D. Clinical results of minimally invasive total hip arthroplasty. Orthopade. 2012;41(5):399-406.
12. Lilikakis AK, Gillespie B, Villar RN. The benefit of modified rehabilitation and minimally invasive techniques in total hip replacement. Ann R Coll Surg Engl. 2008;90(5):406-411.
13. Leoni V, Daneri G. La riabilitazione nella artroprotesi conservativa d'anca. Eur Med Phy. 2009, 45 (suppl. 1 to n. 3).
14. Mahmood A, et al. Minimally invasive hip arthroplasty: a quantitative review of the literature. Br Med Bull. 2007;84:37-48.
15. Mayr E, et al. A prospective randomized assessment of earlier functional recovery in THA patients treated by minimally invasive direct anterior approach: a gait analysis study. Clin Biomech (Bristol, Avon). 2009;24(10):812-818.
16. Minns Lowe CJ, et al. Effectiveness of physiotherapy exercise following hip arthroplasty for osteoarthritis: a systematic review of clinical trials. BMC Musculoskelet Disord. 2009;10:98.
17. Ogonda L, Wilson R, Archbold P, et al. A minimal-incision technique in total hip arthroplasty does not improve early postoperative outcomes. A prospective, randomized, controlled trial. J Bone Joint Surg Am. 2005;87(4):701-710.
18. Peck CN, Foster A, McLauchlan GJ. Reducing incision length or intensifying rehabilitation: what makes the difference to length of stay in total hip replacement in a UK setting?. Int Orthop. 2006;30(5):395-398.
19. Goebel S, Steinert AF, Schillinger J, et al. Reduced postoperative pain in total hip arthroplasty after minimal-invasive anterior approach. Int Orthop. 2012;36(3):491-498. doi:10.1007/s00264-011-1280-0
20. Schweppe ML, Seyler TM, Plate JF, Swenson RD, Lang JE. Does surgical approach in total hip arthroplasty affect rehabilitation, discharge disposition, and readmission rate?. Surg Technol Int. 2013;23:219-227.
21. Sebečić B, Starešinić M, Culjak V, Japjec M. Minimally invasive hip arthroplasty: advantages and disadvantages. Med Glas (Zenica). 2012;9(1):160-165.
22. Sharma V, Morgan PM, Cheng EY. Factors influencing early rehabilitation after THA: a systematic review. Clin Orthop Relat Res. 2009;467(6):1400-1411.
23. Smith TO, Blake V, Hing CB. Minimally invasive versus conventional exposure for total hip arthroplasty: a systematic review and meta-analysis of clinical and radiological outcomes. Int Orthop. 2011;35(2):173-184.
24. Respizzi S. Il paziente protesizzato di anca e ginocchio. Elsevier-Masson, 2011.
25. Ward SR, et al. Functional recovery of muscles after minimally invasive total hip arthroplasty. Instr Course Lect. 2008;57:249-254.

CHAPTER 19

Gait analysis in hip arthroplasty surgery. Comparison between minimally invasive and standard techniques

Renato Villaminar, Alberto Rigato, Dario Pizzuti, Alberto Rigon

Rehabilitation and Functional Recovery Department, Movement analysis laboratory, Abano Terme General Hospital, Padua, Italy

Gait analysis in patients with coxarthrosis and hip arthroplasty

The systematic review by Ornetti and colleagues [1] highlights how the use of 3D gait analysis has increased in recent decades. Increasingly advanced technologies have thus enabled the accurate measurement of sophisticated movements such as human gait. The real challenge is to use all this information, which currently presents controversies and difficulties in data interpretation as well as limited scientific validation. The review explains how the kinematic parameters of gait analysis are insufficient in predicting outcomes in the treatment of hip and knee osteoarthritis. However, they show a significant reduction in gait velocity, gait length and knee flexion when the knee is affected by arthrosis.

Using gait analysis, Schmidt et al. [2] studied the compensation strategies of patients with unilateral coxarthrosis. Typically, these patients exhibit altered spatiotemporal parameters as well as alterations in kinematics, such as trunk flexion on the affected side. In the study, they showed an increased hip abductor moment of the non-osteoarthritic limb. In addition, the patients' compensation strategies showed a reduction in peak vertical force, a greater angle of progression of the foot, and a reduced ROM of the knee of the limb with coxarthrosis.

The authors hypothesise an increase in the progression of osteoarthritis severity on the healthy limb, and that shifting the load from medial to lateral on the pathological knee could impact the progression of osteoarthritis on that knee.

Several studies analyse gait in patients undergoing surgical hip joint replacement. Among them, Kopec et al [3] evaluated 16 patients before surgery and six months after hip replacement. Almost all kinematic parameters improved after surgery. In particular, the authors emphasise that the parameters improved significantly in the non-operated limb. Therefore, the authors suggested a faster adaptation of the gait to the new biomechanical conditions in the non-operated limb. Despite the excellent clinical results of total hip replacement surgery, the investigated gait parameters always differed from those found in healthy people. This indicates the need for a specific rehabilitation, in particular for correct gait re-education.

A study by Kharma C. Foucher from 2016 [4] investigated whether any characteristics of gait analysis in patients who then underwent total hip replacement (THA) could be associated with a positive or negative clinical post-operative outcome. Many factors associated with a poor outcome after THA are non-modifiable: socio-demographic level, gender, age, comorbidities and psycho-social factors. On the other hand, some biomechanical factors could benefit from rehabilitation. In the study, 11. 3% of the subjects out of a total of 124 were 'non-responders' after THA. The Harris Hip Score (HHS) was predictive of a poor response after surgery. Non-responders presented a higher (better) HHS than responders: the mean was 76.1 vs. 54.2.

However, in support of the HHS, two other variables were found to improve sensitivity and specificity: an inferior hip external rotation moment peak (19% lower than in 'responders') and an increased hip ROM in the sagittal plane (26% higher than in 'responders'). The study thus demonstrated that the pre-operative HHS, hip ROM and hip external rotation moment peak together can identify non-responders after THA with a sensitivity of approximately 71.4% and a specificity of 99.1%.

Felix Stief et al. [5] investigated the extent to which total hip replacement surgery restores the knee adduction moment of the operated limb. The authors compared the joint workloads of the operated patients with those of healthy subjects and the gait characteristics of the operated patients two years after surgery. The results showed a lower II moment of external knee adduction in the end-stance phase compared to controls. This occurred in both the operated and the contralateral limb, indicating a shift in the load distribution on the knee joint from medial to lateral.

However, at the 2-year follow-up, the authors also found a greater hip abductor II moment in their patients compared to healthy controls. This could indicate a good function of the hip adductors in the patients examined in the study.

Rebecca Moyer et al. [6] investigated differences in gait biomechanics in patients undergoing hip replacement with different surgical approaches. A significant increase in gait length was observed in patients with posterior versus antero-lateral surgical approaches in both short-term (≤ 3 months) and long-term (≥ 6 months) follow-up. Furthermore, in the short-term follow-up, a greater increase in hip adduction moment was found in patients operated with posterior approach compared to the lateral approach. However, greater pelvic obliquity after the posterior approach must be considered. This may play a role in the hip adduction moment but could represent a pattern of a less correct gait. In contrast, no significant differences were found in gait velocity and joint ROM.

A 2018 review by Bahl and colleagues [7] compared the biomechanical status of gait before and after surgical hip replacement with the gait of healthy patients. After hip replacement surgery, patients showed improvement in gait velocity, gait length and half-step, single support phase, and hip ROM in the sagittal and coronal planes. However, despite these objective improvements, the operated patients showed a worse performance at 12 months in gait velocity, gait length, single support phase and hip ROM in the sagittal plane, compared to healthy subjects.

In the 2019 meta-analysis and systematic review, Jun-Il Yoo and colleagues [8] compared the gait biomechanics results of patients undergoing hip arthroplasty surgery with direct anterior approach and those operated with antero-lateral approach. Three months after surgery, peak hip flexion and gait velocity were significantly greater in patients operated with the direct anterior approach. There were no significant differences in the two groups with regard to gait, complete cycle, and ROM of the hip in the sagittal plane.

Bahl et al. [9] studied the changes in size and in the pattern of the ground reaction force of the hip, both before and after prosthetic joint replacement surgery. After 6 months, the values of the forces during the first (initial support phase) and second peak (final phase) were similar to pre-operative levels. It should be noted that not all patients showed a two-peak profile, and those with a 'single peak' profile showed reduced gait velocity and less hip flexion-extension.

In the studies included in the systematic review of 2020 [10] , improvement of the dynamic ROM of the hip and knee of the operated limb as well as those of the contralateral limb is shown. In addition, cadence, gait and stride cycle length, gait speed and gait quality improved after total hip replacement surgery. However, when compared to healthy patients, the following deficits were assessed: ROM of the operated lower limb, hip adduction angle, stride and full cycle length, gait speed and symmetry.
A recent article from 2021 by van Drogelen and colleagues [11] showed that a 'pathological' gait pattern before unilateral total hip replacement surgery, in particular evidenced by altered hip flexion-extension (specifically by peak hip extension during the end of the stride) and pelvic tilt, is associated with worse gait kinematics after surgery.

Study on the assessment of gait biomechanics of THA patients operated with anterior minimally invasive approach

Our study aims to evaluate the gait biomechanics of patients undergoing total hip replacement surgery with minimally invasive anterior approach.
The study compares the gait characteristics before surgery with those approximately three and a half months after THA.
The instruments used for the evaluation can identify functional alterations that interfere with gait efficiency or produce specific structural (muscular or articular) overloads.
The comparison between the assessment performed before and after the surgery reveals the effect of the surgery itself on gait, the main function of the lower limbs.
Recognition and quantification of functional alterations, together with clinical evaluation, remain a fundamental target. This makes it possible to elaborate a customised rehabilitation protocol aimed at recovering functional capacity and performance and optimising the outcome of surgery.

Graphical reports

Examples of a report showing some significant graphs of a patient in the study are given below. The left column shows the pre-operative analysis: pelvic tilt, hip flexion-extension, knee flexion-extension, ankle ROM, foot extra-rotation, vertical and antero-posterior GRF. The right column shows the evaluation after hip replacement surgery.
The thicker green line represents the pathological, then operated side, while the thicker red line represents the contralateral side. The grey area represents the normal values plus or minus the standard deviation. The thin green and red lines represent the two limbs in the static evaluation.
As previously described in the results, differences between pre- and post-surgery can be detected in the following factors: pelvic tilt, hip extension ROM, ipsilateral knee and ankle ROM. Furthermore, in the present case, the slight improvement in the external rotation of the ipsilateral foot and the two GRFs can be detected.

Discussion and results

Our study evaluated gait biomechanics in unilateral total hip replacement surgery patients. Thirty-five patients who underwent surgery between November 2019 and March 2021 were included in the study. The surgical approach used for all patients was the minimally invasive anterior approach.
The medical history of the patients included in the study did not include: previous lower limb prosthetic surgery, orthopaedic surgery within the 6 months preceding the gait analysis or a history of inflammatory arthritis/chronic neuromuscular diseases. Furthermore, walking was always possible without the use of walking aids.
The study analysed gait characteristics and collected other data in the entire patient group. Assessments were performed prior to surgery and approximately three months after surgery. The objective was to determine and identify the main biomechanical and

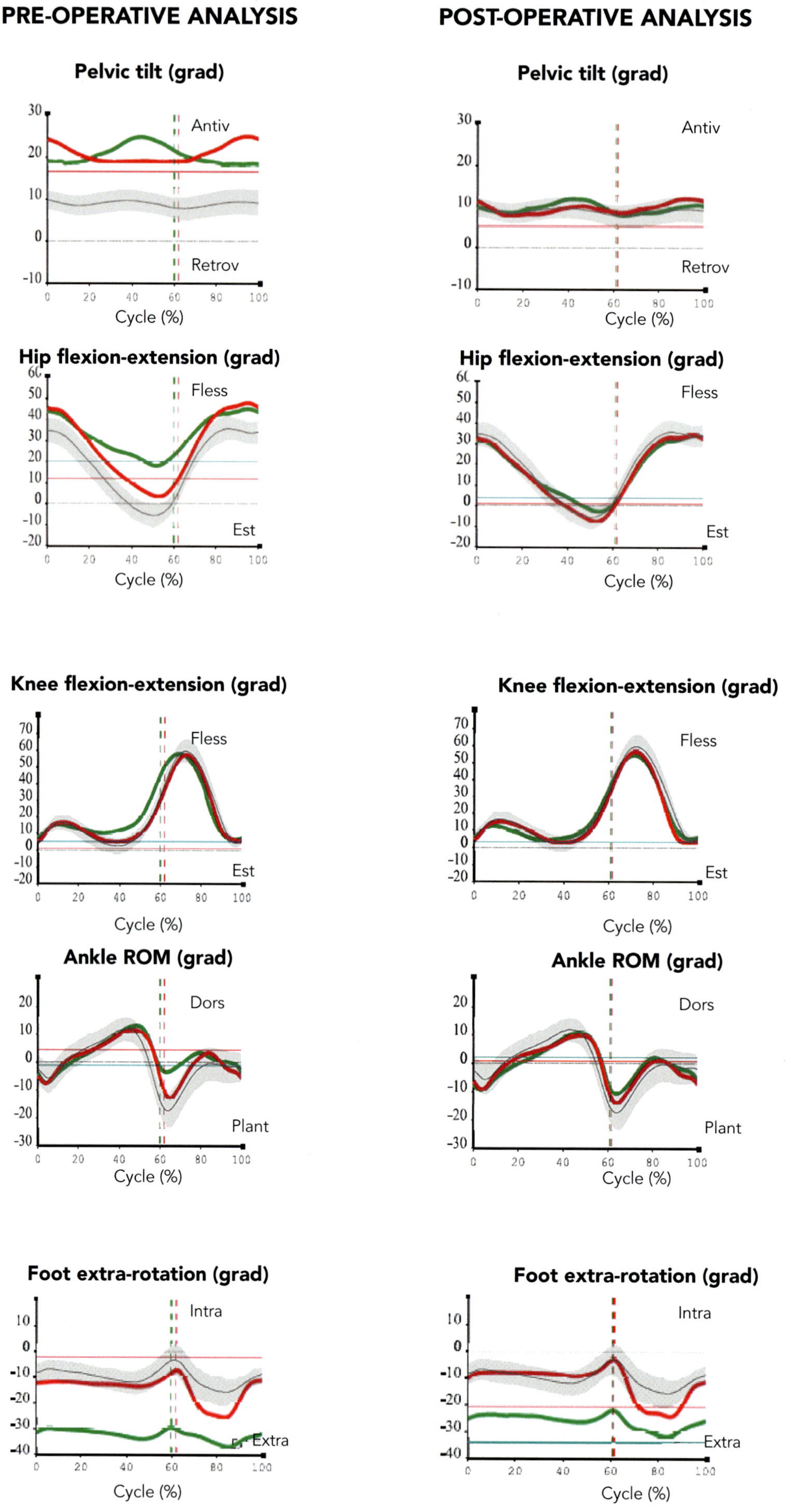
PRE-OPERATIVE ANALYSIS
POST-OPERATIVE ANALYSIS
Pelvic tilt (grad)
Antiv
Retrov
Cycle (%)
Pelvic tilt (grad)
Antiv
Retrov
Cycle (%)
Hip flexion-extension (grad)
Fless
Est
Cycle (%)
Hip flexion-extension (grad)
Fless
Est
Cycle (%)
Knee flexion-extension (grad)
Fless
Est
Cycle (%)
Knee flexion-extension (grad)
Fless
Est
Cycle (%)
Ankle ROM (grad)
Dors
Plant
Cycle (%)
Ankle ROM (grad)
Dors
Plant
Cycle (%)
Foot extra-rotation (grad)
Intra
Extra
Cycle (%)
Foot extra-rotation (grad)
Intra
Extra
Cycle (%)

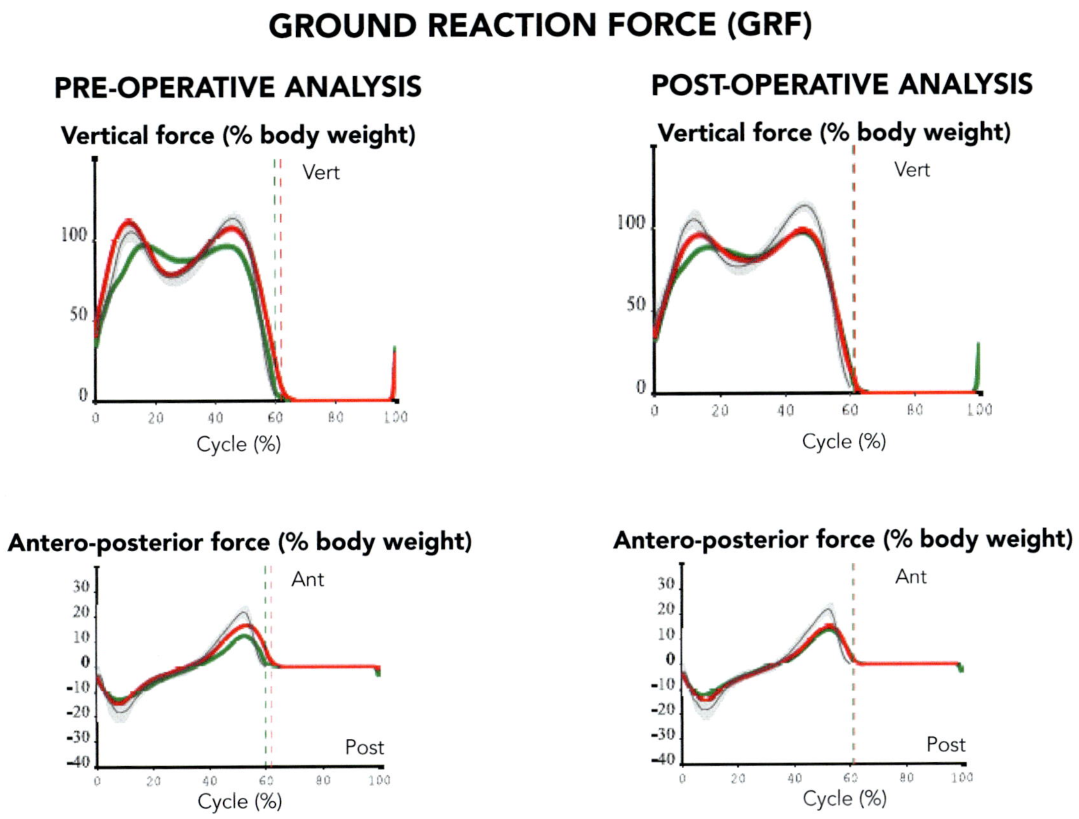

Figure 1 The left column shows the pre-operative analysis: pelvic tilt, hip flexion-extension, knee flexion-extension, ankle ROM, foot extra-rotation, vertical and antero-posterior GRF. The right column shows the evaluation after hip replacement surgery

joint changes along with load abnormalities by comparing the gait analysis findings at the two follow-ups.

As emphasised in the systematic review by Ornetti and colleagues [1], the real challenge is to use the accurate and sophisticated measurements of human gait movements in clinical practice.

In the patients in our study, we confirmed a reduction in spatio-temporal parameters pre-operatively, as also shown by Schmidt et al. [2] in subjects with unilateral coxarthrosis. In fact, 97% of the patients walked with a speed lower than normal before surgery. The average speed of the population is 0.99 m/s, and 58.85 in relation to the height of the subjects (%height/s). Although speed increased significantly after the intervention (p-value < 0.05), it remained below normal for 94% of the subjects, with an average of 1.04 m/s and 62.15 %height/s.

The stride length of the non-operated limb was shorter in 71% of patients pre-operatively and 57% post-operatively.

The percentage of the single support phase was lower than normal for 15 patients (43%) before surgery. It is noteworthy that 63% (22 subjects) presented a lower single support phase of the limb to be operated on compared to the healthy limb. This shows an 'escape step', caused by an attempt to shorten the support on the affected limb (escape from support). The gait cycle was thus 'asymmetrical', as the support phase on one side was shorter than on the contralateral side.

After surgery, only 9 patients had a shorter duration than normal. The 43% of patients, 15, maintained a shorter duration of single support of the operated limb, thus continuing asymmetry in gait.

Schmidt et al. [2] also found that the patients'

compensation strategies showed a reduction in peak vertical force, a greater angle of progression of the foot and a reduced ROM of the knee on the side with coxarthrosis.
The values of the main ground reaction forces during the gait cycle, the 1st peak vertical Ground Reaction Force (GRF), the 2nd peak vertical GRF, the peak posterior GRF and the peak anterior GRF, both pre- and post-operatively and on both sides, remained below normal values.
Furthermore, both before and after surgery, the values of the operated limb were lower than those of the healthy side. However, the difference between the sides was less after surgery.
Our results mirror those of the study by Bahl et al., in which, 6 months after surgery, the value of forces during the first (initial support phase) and second peak (final phase) were similar to pre-operative levels.
In the literature, numerous studies have analysed gait in patients who have undergone surgical hip joint replacement. Among them, Kopec et al. [3] evaluated patients before and six months after hip replacement surgery. Their results are in agreement with ours, although there is a temporal difference in the post-operative follow-up.
Almost all kinematic parameters improved after surgery, even in the untreated limb. However, despite the excellent clinical results of total hip replacement surgery, the gait parameters analysed always differed from those found in healthy people.
The 2018 review by Bahl and colleagues [7] also confirmed an improvement in gait velocity, step and half-step length, single support phase and hip ROM in the sagittal and coronal planes.
However, despite these objective improvements, the operated patients showed a worse performance at 12 months in gait velocity, stride length, single support phase and hip ROM in the sagittal plane, compared to healthy subjects. This confirms our results, although our study presented a shorter post-operative follow-up (< 4 months).
The recent systematic review in 2020 confirmed the improvement in dynamic ROM of the hip and knee not only in the operated limb but also in the untreated one. It also describes an improvement in: cadence, stride length and stride cycle, gait velocity and gait quality. However, when compared to healthy patients, deficits were observed in ROM of the operated limb, hip adduction angle, stride length and gait cycle, gait velocity and symmetry.
When evaluating the knee, we particularly considered the step cycle phase between 10% and 40%. The reason for this is because it is the single support phase in which the knee goes from an initial acceptance of the load in flexion of about 5-20° (between 0 and 10% of the cycle) to full extension reaching about 0°. Pre-operatively, an extension deficit in the loading phase from 10% to 40% of the gait cycle was found for 66% of the subjects (14 patients in the knee to be operated on alone and 9 in both). After the arthroplasty operation, the deficit persisted in 49% of the patients, 10 in the operated knee alone and 7 for both. Dynamic knee extension during gait loading improved in the operated limb from pre- to post-operative. However, this remained below normal.
A feature found in 66% of the population before surgery was external rotation of the foot. In 34% of cases (12 persons) it affected only the side of the operation, in 29% of cases (10 persons) both sides and in one case only the contralateral side. After the operation, 60% of the patients (21 persons) still had this characteristic: 29% (10 persons) only on the side of the operation, 20% (7 persons) bilaterally and 4 patients on the contralateral side.
Even with increased external rotation values compared to normal (v.n. -9.93°), the decrease of the external rotation angle was statically significant with a p-value < 0.05.
Certainly the 2021 study of van Drogelen and colleagues [11] confirmed our results. A 'pathological' gait pattern before unilateral total hip replacement surgery, particularly evidenced by hip flexion-extension and pelvic tilt, is associated with worse gait kinematics after surgery.
In our study, we only considered patients

undergoing hip arthroplasty surgery with a minimally invasive anterior approach. Of great interest is the comparison with other surgical approaches as done by Jun-Il Yoo and colleagues [8] in the 2019 meta-analysis and systematic review. Three months after surgery, peak hip flexion and gait velocity were significantly higher in patients operated with the direct anterior approach compared to the antero-lateral approach. However, there were no significant differences in the two groups in gait, complete cycle and ROM of the hip in the sagittal plane. The study by Jun-Il Yoo and colleagues somewhat confirmed the validity of the anterior approach in terms of outcome.

The study confirmed that approximately 100 days after surgery, some biomechanical abnormalities and functional gait parameters improve. These, however, do not reach normal values, confirming the data in the literature. Various functional alterations naturally have a different impact on the global economy of gait. The evaluation of a single alteration is of limited value if not considered in the complexity of the biomechanics of the gait and the patient.

Pre-operative gait analysis in the laboratory is a very important evaluation. Identifying the most important gait alterations and planning targeted rehabilitation after surgery is essential. This is due to the fact that abnormalities found pre-operatively persist at least 3 months post-operatively, as found in our study, or even longer as reported in the literature.

It remains of fundamental importance to find the causes that lead to the persistence of the alterations even many months after surgery: exclude mechanical limitations of movement, evaluate the adequacy of the rehabilitation protocol (duration, customisation, 'finalisation to the gait function', etc.) and consider the neuroplasticity developed over time in response to experience.

Furthermore, it is important to consider that the biomechanical analysis of gait leads to the prescription of more accurate and customised protocols in order to be able to better assess all functionalities. The modulation of the parameters that define the level of functional performance (duration, velocity, etc.) make it possible to highlight functional alterations that would not be detected at a performance level self-defined by the patient (comfort level walking).

In conclusion, minimally invasive hip replacement surgery has many advantages over traditional surgical approaches as demonstrated both in our clinical evaluation and in the literature.

The advantages are as follows: no pain in the days following surgery, very small scar, rapid restoration of motor activity, considerable stability and improved functional recovery and walking parameters.

In the future, studies with longer follow-ups and evaluating changes in rehabilitation and patient education strategies both before and after hip arthroplasty surgery will be necessary.

Bibliography

1. Ornetti P, Maillefert JF, Laroche D, Morisset C, Dougados M, Gossec L. Gait analysis as a quantifiable outcome measure in hip or knee osteoarthritis: a systematic review. Joint Bone Spine. 2010;77(5):421-425.
2. Schmidt A, Meurer A, Lenarz K, et al. Unilateral hip osteoarthritis: The effect of compensation strategies and anatomic measurements on frontal plane joint loading. J Orthop Res. 2017;35(8):1764-1773.
3. Kopeć K, Kusz D, Sobota G, Nowak K, Mierzwiński M, Nowak M. Gait analysis in patients after unilateral hip arthroplasty. Ortop Traumatol Rehabil. 2015;17(1):39-50.
4. Foucher KC. Preoperative gait mechanics predict clinical response to total hip arthroplasty. J Orthop Res. 2017;35(2):366-376.
5. Stief F, Schmidt A, van Drongelen S, et al. Abnormal loading of the hip and knee joints in unilateral hip osteoarthritis persists two years after total hip replacement. J Orthop Res. 2018;10.1002/jor.23886.
6. Moyer R, Lanting B, Marsh J, et al. Postoperative Gait Mechanics After Total Hip Arthroplasty: A Systematic Review and Meta-Analysis. JBJS Rev. 2018;6(11):e1.

7. Bahl JS, Nelson MJ, Taylor M, Solomon LB, Arnold JB, Thewlis D. Biomechanical changes and recovery of gait function after total hip arthroplasty for osteoarthritis: a systematic review and meta-analysis. Osteoarthritis Cartilage. 2018;26(7):847-863.
8. Yoo JI, Cha YH, Kim KJ, Kim HY, Choy WS, Hwang SC. Gait analysis after total hip arthroplasty using direct anterior approach versus anterolateral approach: a systematic review and meta-analysis. BMC Musculoskelet Disord. 2019;20(1):63.
9. Bahl JS, Arnold JB, Taylor M, Solomon LB, Thewlis D. Lower functioning patients demonstrate atypical hip joint loading before and following total hip arthroplasty for osteoarthritis. J Orthop Res. 2020;38(7):1550-1558.
10. Mendiolagoitia L, Rodríguez MÁ, Crespo I, Del Valle M, Olmedillas H. Kinematic Gait Analysis After Primary Total Hip Replacement: A Systematic Review: Gait After Total Hip Replacement: A Systematic Review. Indian J Orthop. 2020;54(6):767-775.
11. van Drongelen S, Stetter BJ, Böhm H, Stief F, Stein T, Meurer A. Identification of Patients with Similar Gait Compensating Strategies Due to Unilateral Hip Osteoarthritis and the Effect of Total Hip Replacement: A Secondary Analysis. J Clin Med. 2021;10(10):2167.

CHAPTER 20

Instrumental evaluation of periarticular muscles after hip arthroplasty

Lucrezia Tognolo, Daniele Coraci, Stefano Masiero

Department of Neuroscience, Section of Rehabilitation, University of Padova, Italy

Hip joint: functional anatomy and biomechanics

The hip is the proximal joint of the lower limb, surrounded by powerful and well-balanced muscles, allowing a wide range of motion along the three axes: transverse, antero-posterior, and vertical. Hip movements take place at the coxo-femoral joint, a synovial enarthrosis, representing the fulcrum for the coordinated movement of the spine-pelvis complex.

Indeed, recent evidence has shown the crucial role of the so-called spine-pelvis-hip complex as a coordinated functional unit, that accommodates changes in the position of the acetabulum and femur during postural changes of the body. The coxo-femoral joint represents the fulcrum of the coordinated movement of the spinal-lumbopelvic complex, with its functionality largely depending on the motion of the other anatomically interconnected pelvic components, in order to ensure the compensatory changes during postural changes between the acetabular and femoral components: for example, when performing a given movement, a loss of movement at the pelvic level will determine an equal increase in femoral movement [1].

Terminology

The knowledge of the accurate anatomical and biomechanical environment of the hip joint is essential to plan a proper post-surgical rehabilitation program. To better understand the biomechanical basis of the spinal-lumbopelvic complex, a few parameters should be defined.

- On the sagittal plane, the pelvic incidence is the angle created by the intersection of the line passing through the centre of the femoral head to the midpoint of the sacral plate and the line running perpendicular to the middle of the sacral plate. This parameter represents the physical and functional relationship between the femoral head and the spine and is considered a relatively fixed parameter, characteristics of each individual [2].
- The sacral slope is the orientation of the sacral plate in relation to the horizontal line. It is usually evaluated to define the position of the spine-pelvic junction and the difference in its values between standing and sitting position represents the entity of the pelvic mobility during postural changes [3].
- Pelvic femoral angle is the angle between the femoral axis and the sacrum and can be used to assess the femoral motion during postural changes [4].

Hip muscles

The peri-articular muscle support apparatus plays a fundamental role in maintaining proper joint biomechanics. The hip abductors are the gluteus medius, minimus and tensor fascia lata. Although their action is traditionally the abduction of the femur on the fixed pelvis, this action is not commonly performed during daily life activities, especially against any significant resistance. On the other side, the real function of these muscles in the everyday life is connected to the control of the pelvis' movement on the fixed femur, preventing the adduction of the pelvis on the supporting limb [5].

These muscles, although often considered as a single functional unit, represent two distinct components with their own innervation and function [6]. Moreover, the gluteus medius muscle is composed of three distinct components, that are sequentially activated during gait: the posterior bundles are activated during the initial phase of heel contact with the ground, remaining active until the toe-off phase; the anterior bundles reach maximum activity during upright stance and single stance [7]. Thus, it is thought that the main function of the posterior bundles of the gluteus minimus and gluteus medius, being parallel to the femoral neck, is to stabilize the femoral head within the acetabular cup during different phases of the stride.

The insertion and orientation of the bundles of the gluteus medius support its role as a rotator and abductor stabilizer. The gluteus medius has two distinct insertions on the greater trochanter, on the lateral and postero-superior facet respectively. The direction of the fibres of the anterior and middle portions and the anterior portion of the gluteus minimus suggest that they are the initiators of the abduction movement, which is completed by the tensor fascia lata muscle.

During the gait cycle, the pelvic ring plays a fundamental role by acting as a hinge between the lumbar spine and the hip. Therefore, the knowledge of the interaction between the hip and the spine can improve post-operative rehabilitation outcomes.

A healthy gait pattern requires both hip joint and peri-articular muscle function. Indeed, the simultaneous activation of the hip adductors and abductors muscles of the supporting limb (stance phase) allows the advance of contralateral limb (swing phase). Moreover, gluteus medius, gluteus maximus and tensor fascia lata muscles, also act as shock absorbers of the impact on the limb in the load response phase.

In this context, the different muscle groups of the hip perform different functions:

- the extensor group (gluteus maximus, ischiocruralis, adductor magnus) brakes the anterior rotation of the pelvis in the initial phase of support and decelerates the rotation of the limb in support in the terminal phase of the swing;
- the flexor group intervenes in the initial phase of the swing, with a modest contribution, due to the pendulum mechanism linked to the position of the barycentre;
- the abductor group, in particular the gluteus medius and the anterior bundles of the gluteus maximus, is active from the terminal phase of the swing, has a peak of activation during the first part of the heel contact, and then progressively decreases. The tensor fascia lata muscle has a synergistic action at the hip level. Moreover, it also acts at knee level through the iliotibial band, and remaining active until the end of the intermediate support.

Functional anatomy in pathologic hip

In daily life, the Central Nervous System (CNS) ensures the maintenance of upright statics using two strategies: the alignment of body segments in order to minimize joint loads, muscle intervention and energy consumption and the activation of neuromuscular mechanisms that avoid the static maintenance of posture, potentially harmful to the supporting tissues, and ensure a 'dynamic balance' with the maintenance of the position by the effect of automatic and reflex adaptation mechanisms. In order for these mechanisms to be valid, it is essential that the peri-articular muscular apparatus, as well as motor and sensory control mechanisms, are not compromised.

Based on the previous observations, it is easy

to understand how the muscular damage related to the surgical act, the post-operative pain, together with a delayed or unsuitable rehabilitation program, can lead to a failure in the long-term functional results. Besides the gluteal muscles, it has been demonstrated how the iliotibial tract helps the abductor muscles in preventing Trendelenburg walking, by acting as the primary hip abductor. Therefore, also the release of the fascia lata alone can lead to a positive Trendelenburg sign during walking [8].

Hip degenerative disease leads to a progressive decrease in motion of the anterior hinge of the spine-pelvic complex with a consequent necessity of an increased compensatory movement of the opposite hinge (the lumbo-sacral junction). Therefore, changes in the motility of the anterior hinge of the complex (coxo-femoral joint), may cause an abnormal overload of lumbo-sacral spine. Based on the flexibility of the lumbo-sacral junction and its ability to increase the range of motion for pelvic sagittal rotation, this posterior hinge overload may lead to different degrees of spine degenerative changes [9].

Hip replacement is one of the most successful surgeries in modern orthopaedics, because it allows patients with severe functional deficits to improve their quality of life by restoring joint function and abolishing pain symptoms. However, after the prosthetic replacement, the distribution of loads and tensions is clearly different from the physiological one. Therefore, a correct rehabilitation program should take into count the modified interaction of the different structural components of the functional rachis-pelvis-hip unit. The following paragraphs will show the different tools for instrumental assessment of the anatomy and function of healthy and pathological hip.

Quantitative measures of rehabilitation interest: ultrasound, electrophysiology, gait analysis

In rehabilitation, the use of specific quantitative outcome measures is fundamental for effective patient management [10]. Proficient objective evaluations are desirable in the diagnostic and therapeutic moments for deciding the proper treatment approaches and for constantly evaluating their success [11]. The medical tools useful for these aims are able to provide numerical data, which precisely describe morpho-functional features of the patients. Furthermore, these data can be used to compare the variables in different evaluation times in order to reveal the progression of the condition. Obviously, the association with a precise anamnesis and a specific clinical examination is essential to get a real overview of the patient [12]. Additionally, in rehabilitation, another important issue to keep in mind is the necessity to study the general functionality of the body and not only the integrity of the single organ [13]. For these reasons, other types of outcome measures based on patient perspective are often used. For example, the scales about the patient's independence in daily living or pain perception are fundamental and should be always applied [14]. However, these scales are prone to a variable degree of subjectivity. This limitation may cause misunderstanding for its low precision and, sometimes, scarce reproducibility. Hence, even for the evaluation of general functional performance, the use of quantitative measures should be considered. During the decades some evaluation tools have assumed an increasing importance in the different rehabilitation fields. In particular, ultrasound (US) is able to directly visualize the structures of interest (mainly joints, muscles and nerves), allowing the morphological characterization of the organs [15]. Additionally, the electrophysiological exam (EDX) plays a relevant role to quantify the severity of nerve or muscle dysfunction [16]. The association of US and EDX deserves special attention, because the two exams may together overcome the respective imitations and provide a clear picture of the disease [17]. Finally, for the study of body function and disability the gait analysis (GA) has a special place. It is a computed method to calculate the efficiency of the movement [18]. The aforementioned tools are directly used by specialist in physical medicine and rehabilitation and are especially not invasive. The can be considered as the extension of the clinical evaluation and can contribute in the rehabilitation of mini-invasive prostheses.

Ultrasound

Diagnostic ultrasound (US) is an imaging technique based on the emission and reception of mechanical waves with a frequency higher than 20 MHz. The sound beam goes through the tissues and the ultrasound machine rebuilds the tomographic image of the scanned body segment using the reflected part of the sound waves. The technique is not invasive and is used to study all the tissues between the skin and the bone, which represent an almost absolute obstacle. Hence, many structures can be visualized [19]. Considering the hip, the convex probe of 7-12 MHz is usually employed for the transverse and longitudinal scans. First of all, hip joint components are clearly visible by ultrasound [20]. This allows the identification of bone and inhomogeneity and the eventual presence of bursitis (fig. 1). In cases of arthritis, the bone presents a ridge and thickness and echogenicity alterations may be visible [21].

Additionally, by ultrasound, the physician can find the presence of external compression, like cyst or tumor, or the tendon lesion [22]. Finally, the possibility to perform dynamic evaluation is extremely important. Indeed, ultrasound, differently from the routine magnetic resonance, allows the visualization of the anatomical relationships during the passive or active movement of the joint [23]. However, these just represent a minimal part of the assessable elements. Indeed, ultrasound is able to visualize the muscles. Their normal ultrasound pattern is characterized by a general hypoechoic image interspersed with thin hyperechoic lines (fig. 2).

If the muscle is affected by hypotrophy or direct damage, its ultrasound pattern can reveal different changes. A recent muscular lesion is visualized as a hypoechoic continuity solution inside the muscle, while in the chronic phase, the lesion usually appears hyperechoic. In case of myopathy or muscular damage secondary to neuropathy, the muscle shows a general change with the loss of its normal hypoechogenicity [24]. If these changes about the muscles are based on semiquantitative measures, ultrasound permits the quantification of the muscle dimensions, determining the precise value of diameters and area in the transverse scan. The importance of these evaluations is very high, because they provide fundamental information about muscle atrophy. Considering the necessity of rehabilitation after the intervention of hip prosthesis, the knowledge about muscle wellness supports the development and the application of specific programs aimed at a prompt recovery. Furthermore, nerves and vessels can be studied by ultrasound (fig. 3).

This may be useful before the intervention to exclude the presence of anatomical variants. Albeit the minimally invasive intervention can reduce the risks of operations, ultrasound can be used to assess the nerves in the suspicion of the iatrogenic lesion. In a similar way, the impairment of local arteries and veins is assessable. For these reasons, ultrasound is a significant tool in physicians' hands, giving irreplaceable contributions. Moreover, ultrasound is fundamental in some anesthetic procedures, both for intervention preparation and for the eventual pain treatment in specific patients. Besides the described utilities, additional analysis based on sonographic technology is possible. Power Doppler is a method able to reveal the movement of the particles. Hence, it is proficient in evaluating the vascularization of a district [25]. This is useful to determine if hypervascularization is present and, so, if a process of inflammation is happening. Furthermore, in recent years, elastography has seen constant development. This assesses the stiffness of the tissues, on the basis of the changes of the tissue during compression. Elastography may be useful for adding information about the physical properties of muscles and tendons and for checking their evolution over time [26].

Electrodiagnostic examination

The role of EDX in rehabilitation is well-known. EDX comprises several evaluation techniques that provide information about nerve

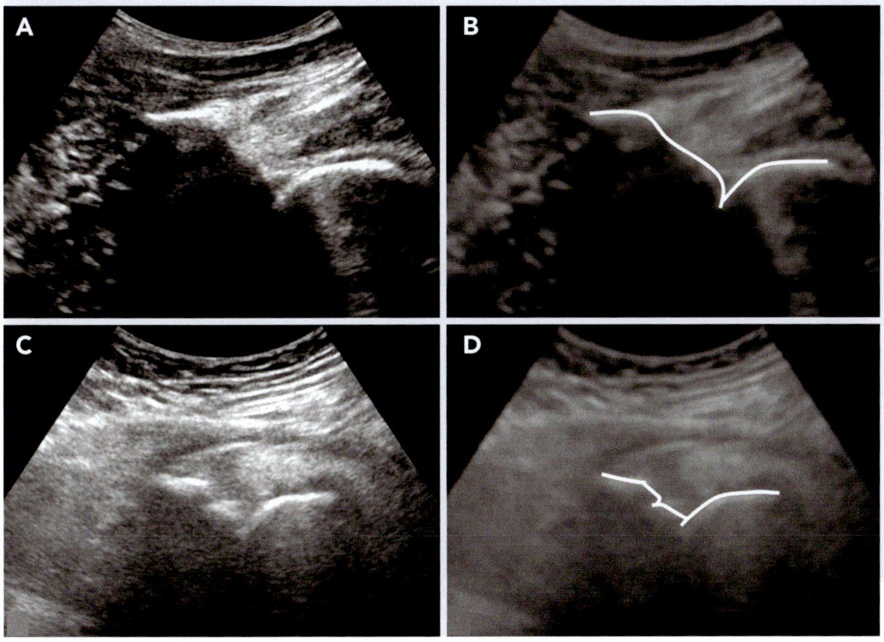

Figure 1 Ultrasound picture of hip. A) Normal subject and its schematic representation (B). C) Patient with hip osteoarthrosis and its representation (D). In B and D, the white lines indicate the osteoarticular elements. In C and D irregular shape is visible

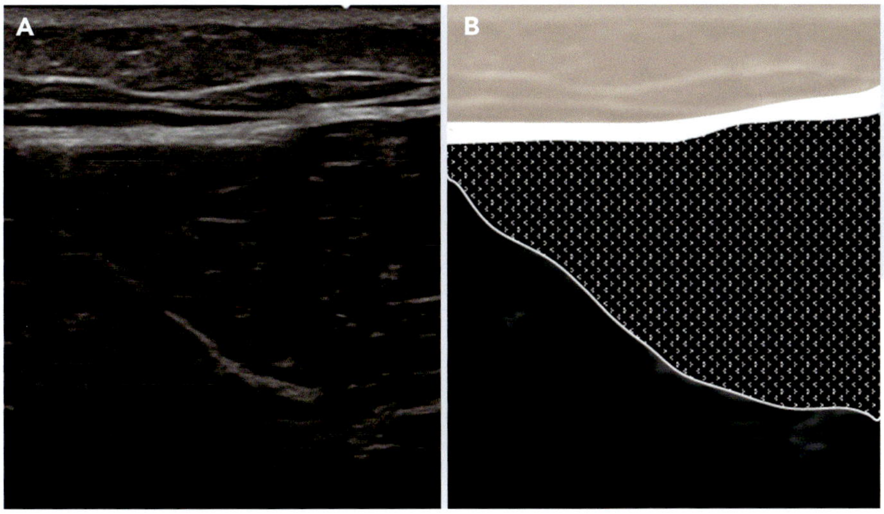

Figure 2 Muscle picture of the normal biceps femori (A) and its schematic view (B)

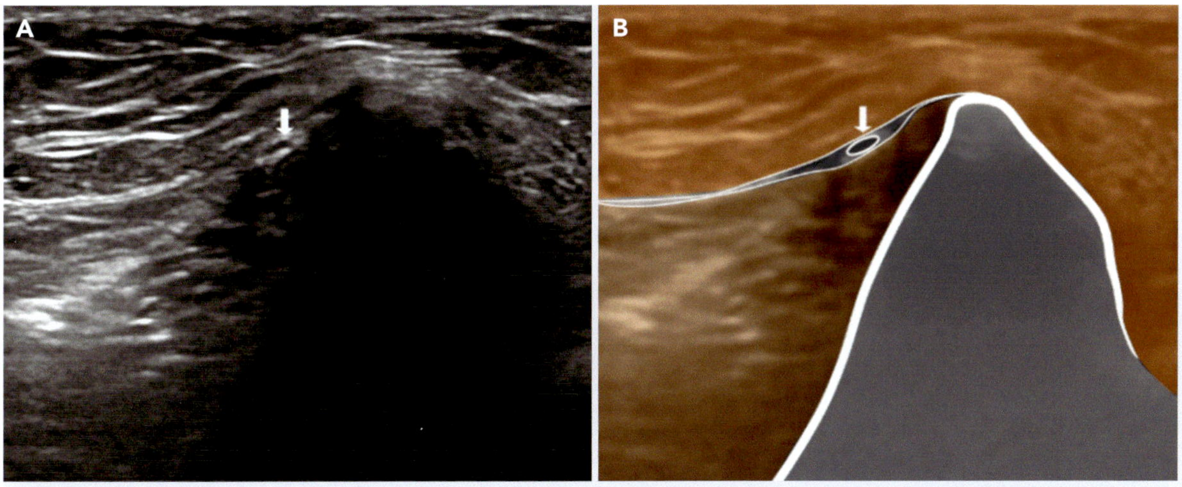

Figure 3 Ultrasound evaluation of the lateral femoral cutaneous nerve (A) and its schematic view (B). The bone shape is relative to the anterior superior iliac spine. The nerve is inside the ligament. In particular, the nerves of the anatomical sites are identifiable to describe the patient's anatomy

and muscle functions. These techniques are based on the registration of electrical potentials at different levels and estimate the type and severity of a dysfunction [27]. Needle electromyography (EMG) exploits the potentials produced by the muscle fibers during rest and voluntary activity. This is a very powerful tool, because it can determine if a clinical muscular involvement is associated with nerve or muscle damage and if it is acute or chronic. In particular, the recording of potentials during the rest is a sign of recent damage. The evaluation of the dimensions and recruitment of motor units during the activity allows the identification of axonal or myopathic damage. EMG is very useful to exclude or confirm the presence of radicular damage that can mimic the symptomatic spectrum of hip arthropathy. In this way, the assessment of the muscular recruitment supports the decision about the best rehabilitation to administer. For example, if a reduction in recruitment is visible (because of underlying disease), the reinforcement of the muscle acquires different importance in comparison with the case of a spared muscle. Besides EMG, the nerve conduction study can be performed in order to evaluate the potentials and the velocity of sensory and motor nerves (fig. 4).
This exam has to be added to the EMG and, in particular, clinical evaluation for the diagnosis of neuropathy [28]. This is an eventuality to keep in mind, because it can help to oversee the patient before and after the surgical intervention. In a few words, the detection of neuropathy or a susceptibility to nerve suffering can help the surgeon to shoot down the rare risks of attribution of medical fault. The integration of information obtainable by EDX, especially when combined with cynical and ultrasound exams, are extremely powerful and can be seen as an aid for the physician. The techniques are inexpensive, a little invasive and relatively fast to perform. Finally, they represent the practical evidence of the proficient collaboration between orthopedics and physiatrists for the diagnosis and the development of the rehabilitation project.

Gait analysis

Gait analysis represents a powerful, complete and precise technique to assess the motor function of walking. It is a computed-based reconstruction of body segments through the use of markers and special cameras. The gait analysis system is able to create a virtual skeleton of the subject and to calculate the variations of the angular movements of the joints during the gait (fig. 5).
The added value of this type of evaluation is determined by its capability to detect the minimal divergences from the normal pattern

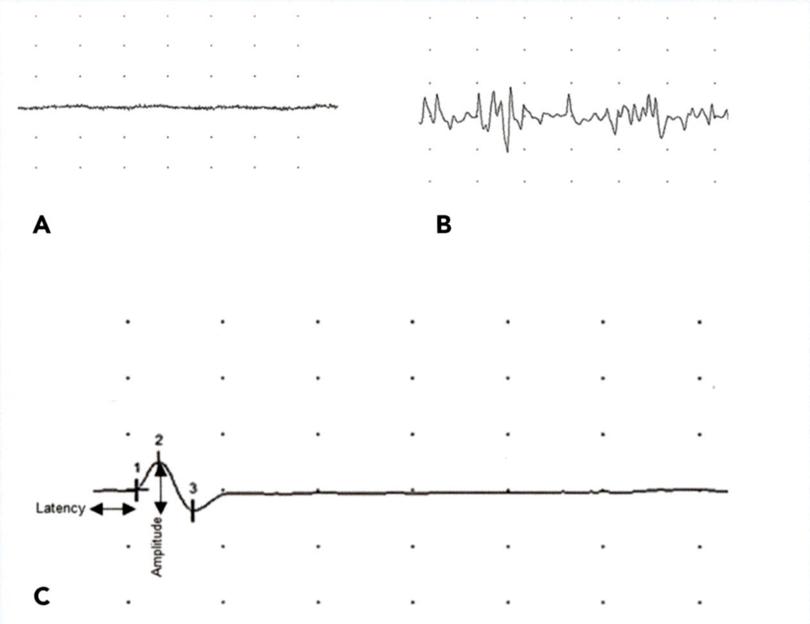

Figure 4
Electromyographic findings in healthy subjects: no rest activity (A) and normal motor units (B). The typical nerve axonal response in nerve conduction study (C)

and the quantification of abnormalities. The clinical importance is determined by the possibility to study complex motor functions and understanding how the different body components interact to produce a task. This is relevant in order to evaluate which mechanical alterations should be treated and to decide the proper rehabilitation programs. In the case of hip dysfunctions, motion analysis can be used to understand how the disease is affecting walking and how we can manage the patients. The reduction of angular movement of the hip, and eventually of the other joints, can be reported and measured. This can be associated with the impairment in force productions. By gait analysis, the physician can prepare the patient to obtain the best results after the surgery, through the administration of personalized motor exercises. Furthermore, gait analysis can be obviously used to quantify the evolution of the disease and the amelioration after the surgical treatment. Finally, in recent years, wearable sensors have been used to study gait, but, usually, just the kinematic data are available [29].

Conclusion

The techniques above described are completions of the clinical evaluation and should be seen as extensions of the physical examination. They can reveal and measure what cannot be seen by the human eye. For this reason, the results of US, EDX and gait analysis should be always compared to the clinical data to reduce the risk of misunderstands and to really add useful information for the patient's management. US may provide data about the morphology of a body segment, EDX about the function, gait analysis about the interaction of more segments. From this point of view, the quantitative evaluation can define the origins and the severity of the disability and can indicate how to treat it. The described diagnostic model should be guided by the ICF approach to extend the potentialities of rehabilitation.

Minimally-invasive hip arthroplasty and rehabilitation: disability and functional outcomes

During the last decades, in the field of hip prosthetic surgery, there has been an evolution, not only in surgical techniques, but also in peri-operative anaesthesia management and in post-operative rehabilitation treatment. These changes have led to a reduction in the average length of stay and a more rapid functional recovery of the patient. Moreover, the introduction of minimally invasive techniques has resulted in a further reduction of

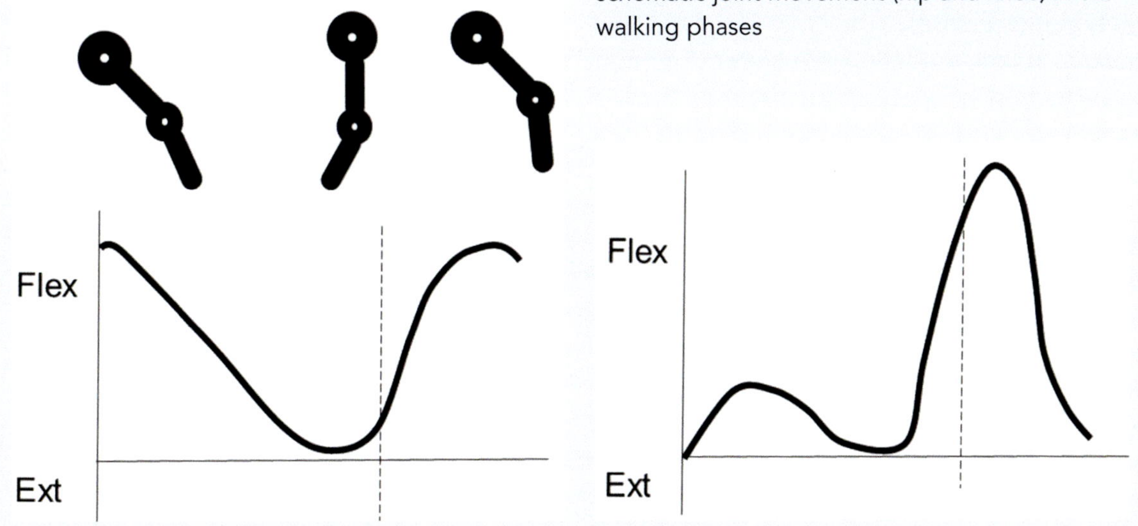

Figure 5 Normal joint angular variation in hip and knee during the walking. The icons represent the schematic joint movement (hip and knee) in the walking phases

these times, also thanks to accelerated rehabilitation protocols.

The primary objective of prosthetic surgery is to allow the patient the recovery of autonomy in the performance of activities of daily living in the absence of pain. As is well known, an individual's activity level varies with gender, age, occupation, schooling, and other factors. The level of physical activity, which in turn depends on the person's activity level, is another key factor in the quality of life. The World Health Organization (WHO) defines the quality of life as a person's perception of his or her place in life in relation to cultural contexts, value system, goals, expectations, and interests. In an orthopaedic patient, correlating quality of life and participation in activities of daily living is fundamental to the rehabilitation process.

The purpose of minimally invasive prosthetic hip surgery is, in fact, to reduce the trauma related to the surgical act, the period of hospitalization, and to improve functional recovery, and therefore, patient satisfaction, goals made possible also by the association with antalgic anaesthesiologic techniques and new rehabilitation protocols. Traditionally, the rehabilitation following prosthetic surgery follows, in fact, very precise and standardized guidelines both in terms of exercise protocols and timing. However, in clinical practice, recovery of mobility and function of the operated hip is frequently observed to be faster than expected. This variability is also related to an intensive post-operative rehabilitation regimen, which allows for better and faster functional outcomes.

There is, in fact, evidence in the literature that the reduction of surgical invasiveness alone cannot explain these benefits, for which adequate anaesthesiologic pain management and an individualized rehabilitation protocol are also fundamental [30]. To confirm this, there are several works showing that there are no substantial differences in length of stay and patient conditions after discharge between those who undergo a standard and minimally invasive procedure and how in the different studies the difference in the post-surgical rehabilitation regimen seems to play a key role in the timing and recovery of patients [31]. It should be noted, however, that the less-invasive nature of the surgical act and the sparing of muscle groups allows an accelerated rehabilitation.

In order to better understand these aspects, it is necessary to premise that following any surgical act at the hip, biomechanical variations occur during walking, which differ depending on the periarticular tissues involved in the surgical incision. Therefore, by preserving anatomical integrity, and consequently muscle function in patients undergoing prosthetic surgery, it is possible to obtain a benefit in terms of improvement of motor performance and reduction of maladaptive compensation mechanisms.

A recent study has shown how the use of the minimally invasive technique in hip prosthetic surgery, determines a better quality of life and a lower incidence of lameness compared to the traditional surgical technique. The latter aspect could be related to the greater muscle damage associated with the classical technique, which shows a higher prevalence of lameness at 8 years after surgery [32].

Lameness is an index of gait disturbance and represents one of the symptoms that most compromises the quality of life of the patient with coxarthrosis. It can be due to several causes and results in altered gait kinematics and reduced stance time on the affected limb and a transfer of the centre of mass to the ipsilateral limb.

Patients treated with the minimally invasive technique showed a reduced prevalence of lameness compared to the traditional technique.

Previous gait analysis studies have reported that after traditional prosthetic surgery, although there is an increase in the range of motion in flexion-extension, the biomechanics of the lower limb is partially compromised with the impossible recovery of physiological values in the joint moments of strength and power of hip, knee and ankle [33]. These observations are confirmed by studies with long-term follow-up (up to 10 years), which have shown suboptimal results in the recovery of hip abductor muscle strength, gait speed, neuromotor control and return to physical activity. The extent of this muscle damage caused by the traditional trans gluteal approach is confirmed by the finding of a significant increase in creatine kinase and markers of inflammation, even months after surgery [34].

A recent work with medium-term follow-up after minimally invasive hip prosthetic surgery showed an improvement in gait parameters and hip kinematics starting from 6 months, compared to the pre-operative period. This was in spite of an increase in joint motion, which, however, did not reach that of a healthy subject of the same age and gender [33]. These data show how, following hip implantation, an improvement in walking performance can be verified, without, however, a restoration of joint motion equal to the values of a healthy subject, further confirming the importance of muscle function in the functional recovery of these patients. The same study also demonstrated an improvement in spatial-temporal parameters (stride length, swing time and double stance, cadence, walking speed) and kinematics 6 months after surgery.

In hip osteoarthrosis, a hyperactivation and a difference in the sequence of spatial-temporal activation of the peri-articular muscles of the hip, in particular of the gluteus maximus, gluteus medius and rectus femoris muscles, has been demonstrated. These abnormalities represent probable maladaptive mechanisms due to the underlying arthritic pathology and pain symptoms. Prosthetic surgery would seem to reduce this phenomenon, through the reduction of the painful stimulus and the improvement of the articular functionality, as suggested by the positive correlation between the improvement of pain, functionality and joint motion of the hip on one hand, and the reduction of the activation of the gluteus maximus muscle on the other hand in subjects undergoing hip prosthesis. However, even after surgery, abnormalities in the sequence of muscle activation during some subphases of gait have been demonstrated, which could be responsible for the failure of optimal recovery of hip joint motion in the medium to long term. Therefore, the rehabilitation program should focus on these aspects and consider specific muscle groups: rectus femoris, gluteus medius and gluteus maximus, as well as work on specific tasks (e.g. balance in single and double stance).

In addition to functional recovery, of fundamental importance is the personal perception of the patient, which, according to the bio-psycho-social model, is a key determinant for the success of the intervention in the long term. Questionnaires on physical and mental well-being, such as the Short Form-36 (SF-36), show a better perception of the patient in functional recovery following minimally invasive surgery. Patients perceive less limitation related to physical impairment resulting in better efficiency in walking and energy use (cardiovascular performance). Activities of daily living are more easily performed.

The minimally invasive approach spares the abductor muscles to a greater extent and, as we know, a pelvis-trochanteric muscle is a fundamental constituent of the functional unit necessary for energetically efficient walking. Damage to the capsular, muscular, and ligamentous components of the joint can result in static and dynamic alteration with N increased risk of falling. There are only a few studies in the literature that have compared the two surgical techniques in terms of rehabilitative outcomes.

The opinions of the scientific community regarding the advantages of the minimally invasive technique are still conflicting, although there is a slight prevalence in favour of the minimally invasive technique.

Moreover, there are concomitant factors that may affect functional outcomes in the long term. Galea et al., in a study on 976 patients undergoing hip replacement with a follow-up of up to 7 years, showed that the mental dimension (emotional issues) and the weight of the patient (reported in terms of BMI) are two factors largely correlated with the incidence of pain, both in the operated and healthy limb and functional limitation.

Similarly, Wiklund et al. showed that patients undergoing minimally invasive hip surgery reported a lower incidence of pain than patients undergoing the classical technique. This aspect would also seem to positively influence other domains, such as general well-being and sociality.

Rehabilitation of minimally invasive hip arthroplasty: literature analysis

In the last ten years, the scientific literature about the rehabilitation of minimally invasive hip arthroplasty has seen, on PubMed, a relative reduction of the number of publications in the middle of the decade and an increase in the last part of the considered period (fig. 6).
This may allow some speculations, mainly the constant interest in the topic and the continued importance of the support of rehabilitation in the management of orthopedic diseases. The papers are from three continent, with a prevalence in Europe. In particular, Germany has the highest number of publications, followed by the United States of America (USA) and China (fig. 7).
The high number of publications from the USA and China is not surprising, because the first is a country historically very productive, while the second is the most populated country in the world, with a large level of scientific production in the last decades in every field. Germany is a less expectable result, but, besides its large population, this result can make underline how the research about this kind of hip arthroplasty is significant. Another interesting result is the absence of some large countries in this research. In particular, India and Brazil do not show any paper in this search. This analysis may indicate the necessity to share more information about the topic to stimulate scientific research.
Concerning the papers obtained by this search, some authors declare the importance of the personalization of rehabilitation programs [35]. Furthermore, an early re-education after surgery is recommended for reducing muscle damage. The exact description of the exercise is missing, but the authors agree on their roles for the recovery [36]. A very important issue to consider is the presence of pain, which can limit the adherence to the rehabilitation protocols [37]. For this reason, even radiofrequency, combined with classical therapeutic exercises, has been proposed to reduce pain [38]. As expected, the improvement of pelvic stabilization has a notable positive impact [39]. The final aim, as rehabilitation always shows, is the improvement of function and patient satisfaction. Obviously, the surgical intervention itself plays its role to reduce the time of rehabilitation, with cost reduction and amelioration of patient's condition. In order to assess the effectiveness of rehabilitation, walking speed should be highly considered. In a few words, rehabilitation programs should improve stability and reduce the risks of falls. Additionally, the length of stay of patients with accelerated rehabilitation is 40% minor than the patients treated with a standard approach [40]. In conclusion, the minimally surgical approach contributes to the rapid gain of function, because it limits the pain, makes faster rehabilitation and recovery.

Bibliography

1. Heckmann N, Tezuka T, Bodner RJ, et al. Functional Anatomy of the Hip Joint. J Arthroplasty. 2021;36(1):374-378.
2. Legaye J, Duval-Beaupère G, Hecquet J, et al. Pelvic incidence: A fundamental pelvic parameter for three-dimensional regulation of spinal sagittal curves. Eur Spine J. 1998;7:99-103.
3. Lazennec JY, Riwan A, Gravez F, et al. Hip spine relationships: Application to total hip arthroplasty. HIP Int. 2007; 17 Suppl 5:S91-104.
4. Philippot R, Wegrzyn J, Farizon F, et al. Pelvic balance in sagittal and Lewinnek reference planes in the standing, supine and sitting positions. Orthop Traumatol Surg Res. 2009;95:70-6.
5. Walker JM. Functional anatomy of the hip. South African J Physiother. 1969;25:8-11.
6. Al-Hayani A. The functional anatomy of hip abductors. Folia Morphol (Warsz). 2009;68:98-103.
7. Soderberg GL, Dostal WF. Electromyographic study of three parts of the gluteus medius

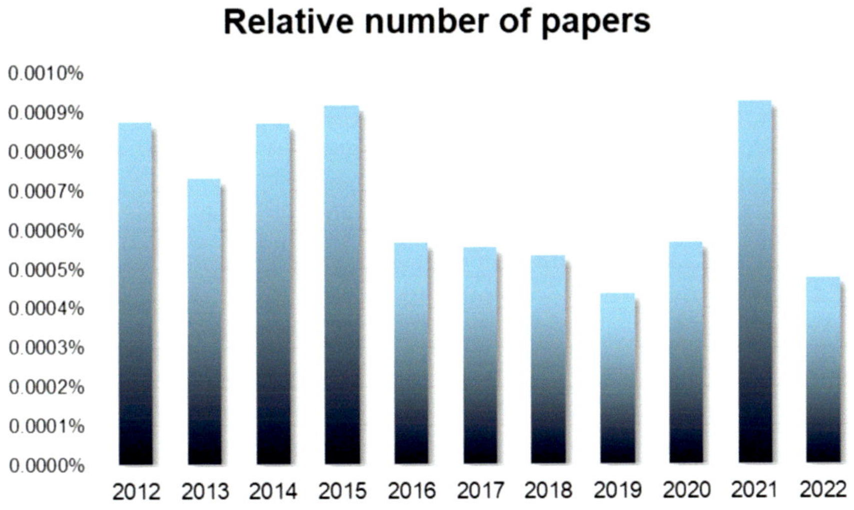

Figure 6 Relative number of papers during the years. The results are normalized for the total number of papers in the world during the years

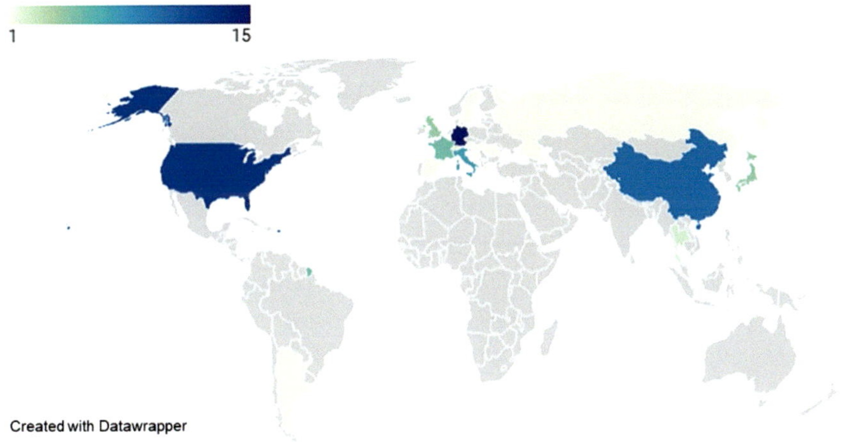

Figure 7 Geographical origins of the selected papers

muscle during functional activities. Phys Ther. 1978;58:691-696.
8. Evans P. The postural function of the iliotibial tract. Ann R Coll Surg Engl. 1979;61:271-80.
9. Pizones J, García-Rey E. Pelvic motion the key to understanding spine-hip interaction. EFORT Open Rev. 2020;5:522-533.
10. Bouwens van der Vlis TAM, Duits A, van de Veerdonk MMGH, et al. Cognitive Outcome After Deep Brain Stimulation for Refractory Obsessive-Compulsive Disorder: A Systematic Review. Neuromodulation. 2022;25(2):185-194.
11. Pardo G, Coates S, Okuda DT. Outcome measures assisting treatment optimization in multiple sclerosis. J Neurol. 2022;269(3):1282-1297.
12. Dubé MO, Langevin P RJ. Measurement properties of the Pain Self-Efficacy Questionnaire in populations with musculoskeletal disorders: a systematic review. Pain Rep. 2021;6:e972.
13. Guiu-Tula FX, Cabanas-Valdés R, Sitjà-Rabert M, et al. The Efficacy of the proprioceptive neuromuscular facilitation (PNF) approach in stroke rehabilitation to improve basic activities of daily living and quality of life: A systematic review and meta-analysis protocol. BMJ Open. 2017;7:e016739.
14. Shah S, Vanclay F, Cooper B. Improving the sensitivity of the Barthel Index for stroke rehabilitation. J Clin Epidemiol. 1989;42:703-9.
15. Wang JC, Wu WT, Chang KV, et al. Ultrasound imaging for the diagnosis and evaluation of sarcopenia: An umbrella review. Life. 2022;12:1-13.
16. Brambilla C, Pirovano I, Mira RM, et al. Combined use of emg and eeg techniques for neuromotor assessment in rehabilitative applications: A systematic review. Sensors. 2021;21:7014.

17. Coraci D, Masiero S, Padua L. Ultrasound advanced techniques for nerve assessment: One of the fires of PrometheUS. Clin Neurophysiol. 2022;135:164-165.
18. Spech C, Paponetti M, Mansfield C, Schmitt L, et al. Biomechanical variations in children who are overweight and obese during high-impact activities: A systematic review and meta-analysis. Obes Rev. 2022;23(6):e13431.
19. Coraci D, Loreti C, Fusco A, et al. Peripheral neuropathies seen by ultrasound: A literature analysis through lexical evaluation, geographical assessment and graph theory. Brain Sci. 2021;11:1-9.
20. Tognolo L, Giordani F, Biz C, et al. Myofascial points treatment with focused extracorporeal shock wave therapy (f-ESWT) for plantar fasciitis: an open label randomized clinical trial. Eur J Phys Rehabil Med. 2022;58(1):85-93.
21. Martinoli C, Garello I, Marchetti A, et al. Hip ultrasound. Eur J Radiol. 2012;81:3824-31.
22. Giard MC, Pineda C. Ganglion cyst versus synovial cyst? Ultrasound characteristics through a review of the literature. Rheumatol Int. 2015;35:597-605.
23. Padua L, Coraci D, Gatto DM, Glorioso D, Lodispoto F. Relationship Between Sensory Symptoms, Mulder's Sign, and Dynamic Ultrasonographic Findings in Morton's Neuroma. Foot Ankle Int. 2020;41:1474-1479.
24. Coraci D, Giovannini S, Hobson-Webb LD, Fusco A, Padua L. Computer-based echotexture comparison of muscles. Exploring innovative analyses of ultrasound images. Clin Neurophysiol. 2020;131(2):583-585.
25. Kara M, Gürçay E, Ekiz T, et al. EURO-MUSCULUS/USPRM global report on musculoskeletal ultrasound publications. Am J Phys Med Rehabil. 2020;99:847-852.
26. Sigrist RMS, Liau J, Kaffas AE, Chammas MC, Willmann JK. Ultrasound elastography: Review of techniques and clinical applications. Theranostics. 2017;7:1303-1329.
27. Gentile L, Coraci D, Pazzaglia C, et al. Ultrasound guidance increases diagnostic yield of needle EMG in plegic muscle. Clin Neurophysiol 2020;131:446-450.
28. Abel NA, De Sousa EA, Govindarajan R, Mayer MP, Simpson DA. Guidelines for ethical behavior relating to clinical practice issues in neuromuscular and electrodiagnostic medicine. Muscle Nerve. 2015;52(6):1122-1129.
29. Ismailidis P, Nüesch C, Kaufmann M, et al. Measuring gait kinematics in patients with severe hip osteoarthritis using wearable sensors. Gait Posture. 2020;81:49-55.
30. Lilikakis AK, Gillespie B, Villar RN. The benefit of modified rehabilitation and minimally invasive techniques in total hip replacement. Ann R Coll Surg Engl. 2008;90:406-11.
31. Woolson ST, Mow CS, Syquia JF, Lannin JV, Schurman DJ. Comparison of primary total hip replacements performed with a standard incision or a mini-incision. Bone Joint Surg Am. 2004;86(7):1353-1358.
32. Vučković M, Ružić L, Tudor A, et al. Difference in patient quality of life after hip arthroplasty with a minimally invasive approach or classic approach. Acta Clin Croat. 202;60:89-95.
33. Ippolito G, Serrao M, Conte C, et al. Direct anterior approach for total hip arthroplasty: Hip biomechanics and muscle activation during three walking tasks. Clin Biomech. 2021;Oct:105454.
34. Xiao C, Gao Z, Zhang S, et al. Comparative prospective randomized study of minimally invasive transpiriformis approach versus conventional posterolateral approach in total hip arthroplasty as measured by biology markers. Int Orthop. 2021;45:1707-1717.
35. Galea VP, Rojanasopondist P, Ingelsrud LH, et al. Longitudinal changes in patient-reported outcome measures following total hip arthroplasty and predictors of deterioration during follow-up: a seven-year prospective international multicentre study. Bone Joint J. 2019;101-B(7):768-778.
36. Dorr LD, Maheshwari AV, Long WT, et al. Early pain relief and function after posterior minimally invasive and conventional total hip arthroplasty. A prospective, randomized, blinded study. J Bone Joint Surg Am. 2007;89(6):1153-1160.
37. Brismar BH, Hallert O, et al. Early gain in pain reduction and hip function, but more complications following the direct anterior minimally invasive approach for total hip arthroplasty: a randomized trial of 100 patients with 5 years of follow up. Acta Orthop. 2018;89:484-489.
38. de Wouters S, Petronilia S, Paulet D, et al. Outpatient total hip arthroplasty: The future? Acta Orthop Belg. 2021;87:313-319.

39. Martinez L, Noé N, Beldame J, et al. Quantitative gait analysis after total hip arthroplasty through a minimally invasive direct anterior approach: A case control study. Orthop Traumatol Surg Res. 2022;108(6):103214.
40. Götz JS, Leiss F, Maderbacher G, et al. Implementing fast-track in total hip arthroplasty: rapid mobilization with low need for pain medication and low pain values: Retrospective analysis of 102 consecutive patients. Z Rheumatol. 2022;81(3):253-262.
41. Urits I, Orhurhu V, et al. Minimally Invasive Therapies for Osteoarthritic Hip Pain: a Comprehensive Review. Curr Pain Headache Rep. 2020;24:37.
42. Benedetti MG, Cavazzuti L, Amabile M, et al. Abductor muscle strengthening in THA patients operated with minimally-invasive anterolateral approach for developmental hip dysplasia. Hip Int. 2021;31:66-74.
43. Petridis G, Nolde M. Sequential Bilateral Total Hip Arthroplasty Through a Minimally Invasive Anterior Approach is Safe to Perform. Open Orthop J. 2017;11:1417-142.